To Dr. Gene Myers with great
appreciation for his warm constant
support and help.

Piero

June 2005

MEDICAL RADIOLOGY
Diagnostic Imaging

Editors:
A. L. Baert, Leuven
K. Sartor, Heidelberg

R. Maroldi · P. Nicolai (Eds.)

Imaging in Treatment Planning for Sinonasal Diseases

With Contributions by

A. R. Antonelli · G. Battaglia · M. Berlucchi · A. Bolzoni · A. Borghesi · D. Farina
D. Lombardi · P. Maculotti · R. Maroldi · I. Moraschi · P. Mortini · F. Mossi · P. Nicolai
L. Palvarini · L. Pianta · C. Piazza · L. Pinelli · V. Portugalli · L.O. Redaelli de Zinis
D. Tomenzoli

Series Editor's Foreword by

A. L. Baert

Foreword by

W. Draf

With 268 Figures in 620 Separate Illustrations, 44 in Color and 14 Tables

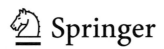 Springer

ROBERTO MAROLDI, MD
Professor, Department of Radiology

PIERO NICOLAI, MD
Professor, Department of Otorhinolaryngology

University of Brescia
Piazzale Spedali Civili 1
25123 Brescia, BS
Italy

MEDICAL RADIOLOGY · Diagnostic Imaging and Radiation Oncology
Series Editors: A. L. Baert · L. W. Brady · H.-P. Heilmann · M. Molls · K. Sartor

Continuation of Handbuch der medizinischen Radiologie
                 Encyclopedia of Medical Radiology

ISBN 3-540-42383-4 Springer Berlin Heidelberg New York

Library of Congress Cataloging-in-Publication Data
Imaging in treatment planning for sinonasal diseases / R. Maroldi, P. Nicolai (eds.) ; with
   contributions by A. R. Antonelli ... [et al.] ; foreword by A. L. Baert.
      p. ; cm. -- (Medical radiology)
   Includes bibliographical references and index.
   ISBN 3-540-42383-4 (alk. paper)
    1. Paranasal sinuses--Imaging. 2. Nose--Imaging. 3. Paranasal
   sinuses--Diseases--Diagnosis. 4. Nose--Diseases--Diagnosis. 5. Paranasal
   sinuses--Diseases--Treatment. 6. Nose--Diseases--Treatment. I. Maroldi, R. (Roberto),
   1954- II. Nicolai, P. (Piero), 1954- III. Antonelli, A. R. IV. Series.
   [DNLM: 1. Paranasal Sinus Diseases--diagnosis. 2. Paranasal Sinus Diseases--therapy.
   3. Diagnostic Imaging--methods. WV 340 I31 2004]
   C8255 2004]
   RF345.I446 2004
   616.2'107²54--dc22   2004045232

Springer is part of Springer Science+Business Media

http//www.springeronline.com
© Springer-Verlag Berlin Heidelberg 2005
Printed in Germany

Medical Editor: Dr. Ute Heilmann, Heidelberg
Desk Editor: Ursula N. Davis, Heidelberg
Production Editor: Kurt Teichmann, Mauer
Cover-Design and Typesetting: Verlagsservice Teichmann, 69256 Mauer

Printed on acid-free paper – 21/3150xq – 5 4 3 2 1 0

To *Elisabetta* and *Daniela*,
for their support and patience

Roberto and Piero

Series Editor's Foreword

This volume not only provides a modern multimodality imaging approach to the pathology of the sinonasal area, based on CT, MR imaging and endoscopy, but also focuses on the treatment strategy and the role of imaging in the decision-making process for each individual patient.

The combined interdisciplinary approach by a radiologist and an ENT surgeon gives this book unique clinical value.

The different chapters comprehensively cover imaging modalities, anatomy, physiology and the complete spectrum of sinonasal diseases. The volume as a whole is eminently readable and superbly illustrated.

The content represents mainly the approach of the editors' institution, based on long clinical experience and innovative research, but also covers other modern views and concepts.

This outstanding volume will serve the needs not only of general radiologists dealing daily with the common sinonasal conditions but also of specialised head and neck radiologists. It can also be recommended highly as an invaluable reference not only to radiologists but also to ENT specialists.

I am confident that this excellent book will meet the same success as previous volumes published in this series.

Leuven   ALBERT L. BAERT

Series Editor's Foreword

Foreword

The time should have passed when the radiologist produced the images he was asked for and the ENT surgeon took them and made his own interpretation as the basis for the decision on conservative or surgical treatment.

The optimal information from images is obtained from interdisciplinary discussion, sitting together as long as time allows. Without a doubt the neuroradiologist or the head and neck radiologist can describe the imaging findings in the most detailed way. On the other hand he or she depends to a high degree on the hopefully precisely formulated questions of the clinical partner. Sometimes the interdisciplinary discussion results in the recommendation of further imaging by the radiologist. This personal contact with the specialty clinician also ensures familiarity with the latest therapeutic options, which eases the interpretation of postoperative images.

This monograph combines in an ideal way the expertise of a superbly skilled head and neck radiologist and a rhinologist who is one of the pioneers of modern endonasal surgery, using endoscope and microscope as indispensable surgical tools. The book gives clear guidance on the necessary imaging and the findings, as well as interpretation of all types of nose and sinus pathology and general guidelines for treatment, particularly surgery, resulting from interdisciplinary discussion. It deals with anatomy, CT and MR techniques of study, inflammatory diseases, tumors, and post-treatment imaging. This is a particularly effective way forward in one of the most fascinating fields of modern otorhinolaryngology.

I wish this book a wide readership among neuroradiologists and head and neck radiologists, as well as ENT, head and neck, and maxillo-facial surgeons.

Fulda   WOLFGANG DRAF

Preface

As there are already many books on imaging of sinonasal tract diseases, one might wonder, "Why bother to compile another one?". In responding to this question, it must be emphasized that cross-sectional imaging (i.e., computed tomography and magnetic resonance) has clearly been one of the backbones which has made possible, in the last decade, the remarkable evolution of treatment strategies for sinonasal tract diseases, in particular microendoscopic sinus surgery.

The purpose of this volume is to provide the knowledge required to properly solve the challenging issues raised by current treatment planning. Accordingly, this book is intended not only for the head and neck expert, or the general radiologist, but for the entire team of physicians (otorhinolaryngologist, maxillo-facial surgeon, radiotherapist, and oncologist) that participate in the decision-making process and who need to be confident with the indications, limitations, and advantages of state-of-the-art imaging techniques.

The book is organized into three main sections. In the first, general aspects such as CT and MR techniques, as well as anatomy and physiology, are thoroughly discussed. In addition, we decided to include a detailed guide to imaging assessment of critical issues, such as bone, orbit, and skull base invasion, in this section. The section is completed by an indispensable overview of a wide spectrum of surgical approaches for the sinonasal tract.

The second part of the book provides step-by-step information on the basic and advanced aspects of clinical presentation, imaging findings, and treatment of sinonasal diseases. For each specific disease, the rationale underlying the treatment strategy is discussed and the imaging findings critical to the decision-making process are identified and discussed. This approach reflects the constant team effort of our two departments, radiology and otorhinolaryngology, over the past 15 years towards integration of clinical and radiological information with the aim of establishing the most appropriate treatment. Special emphasis is placed on the identification of clinical and imaging data that allow selection of a microendoscopic or an external approach in candidates for surgery.

In the third part, the challenging issue of imaging acute or late complications and recurrent lesions is discussed in detail. Moreover, the integration of endoscopic and radiological follow-up in different diseases is thoroughly reviewed. As the book reflects the radiological and clinical experience of a single institution, two topics, namely traumatic lesions and congenital malformations, were not covered as we do not have the required expertise in these fields. We believe that through the correlation of imaging with endoscopic or clinical findings, this book will enable radiologists to familiarize themselves with a more "otorhinolaryngological" point of view and will help clinicians to understand more fully the significance of specific radiological findings. It will also serve as a guide for the selection of imaging techniques.

Finally, we would like to acknowledge Prof. Chiesa (Head of the Department of Radiology) and Prof. Antonelli (Head of the Department of Otorhinolaryngology) who promoted the active cooperation between these two specialties at our university. Without their invaluable support, as well as that of younger colleagues, the writing of this book would have been an impossible challenge.

Brescia

ROBERTO MAROLDI
PIERO NICOLAI

Contents

1 Techniques of Radiological Examination
  D. Farina and A. Borghesi   1

2 CT and MR Anatomy of Paranasal Sinuses: Key Elements
  R. Maroldi, A. Borghesi, and P. Maculotti   9

3 Physiology of the Nose and Paranasal Sinuses
  D. Tomenzoli 29

4 Neoplastic Invasion of Bone, the Orbit and Dural Layers: Basic and Advanced CT
  and MR Findings
  R. Maroldi, D. Farina, and G. Battaglia 35

5 Endonasal and Open Surgery: Key Concepts
  P. Nicolai, A. Bolzoni, C. Piazza, and A. R. Antonelli 47

6 Inflammatory Lesions
  D. Farina, D. Tomenzoli, A. Borghesi, and D. Lombardi 59

7 Cerebrospinal Fluid Leak, Meningocele and Meningoencephalocele
  L. Pianta, L. Pinelli, P. Nicolai, and R. Maroldi 93

8 Benign Neoplasms and Tumor-Like Lesions
  R. Maroldi, M. Berlucchi, D. Farina, D. Tomenzoli, A. Borghesi,
  and L. Pianta 107

9 Malignant Neoplasms
  R. Maroldi, D. Lombardi, D. Farina, P. Nicolai, and I. Moraschi 159

10 Expansile Lesions Arising from Structures and Spaces Adjacent to the Paranasal
   Sinuses
   L. O. Redaelli de Zinis, P. Mortini, D. Farina, and F. Mossi 221

11 Normal and Abnormal Appearance of Nose and Paranasal Sinuses
   After Microendoscopic Surgery, Open Surgery, and Radiation Therapy
   R. Maroldi, P. Nicolai, L. Palvarini, V. Portugalli, and A. Borghesi 255

Legends of Anatomic Structures 295

Subject Index 297

List of Contributors 303

1 Techniques of Radiological Examination

Davide Farina and Andrea Borghesi

CONTENTS

1.1   Incremental and Single-Slice Spiral CT Technique   *1*
1.1.1   CT Protocol Chronic Rhinosinusitis and
        Nasal Polyposis   *1*
1.1.1.1 Patient Preparation   *1*
1.1.1.2 Direct Coronal Plane Acquisition   *1*
1.1.1.3 Axial Plane Acquisition   *2*
1.1.2   CT Protocol in Neoplastic Lesions   *3*
1.1.2.1 Axial Scanning   *3*
1.1.2.2 Coronal Scanning   *3*
1.2   Multislice CT of the Paranasal Sinuses   *3*
1.3   MR Technique   *4*
1.3.1   Designing an MR Protocol: Basic Concepts   *4*
1.3.2.1 MR Protocol   *4*
1.3.2.2 Additional MR Sequences   *5*
1.3.2.3 Signal vs Time Curves in Follow-Up Studies   *6*
        References   *7*

1.1
Incremental and Single-Slice Spiral CT Technique

1.1.1
CT Protocol Chronic Rhinosinusitis and Nasal Polyposis

1.1.1.1
Patient Preparation

Patients affected by chronic rhinosinusitis must receive adequate medical treatment before CT examination of the paranasal sinuses, in order to treat acute infection and solve mucosal edema. Oral antibiotics, nasal steroids and antihistamines – prescribed at least 3 weeks before CT – decrease the risk of overestimating chronic inflammation and polypoid reaction of the mucosa. Additionally, according to the recommendations of several authors, patients should be asked to clear their nose before undergoing the examination (OLIVERIO et al. 1995; PHILLIPS 1997; ZINREICH 1998).

D. FARINA, MD; A. BORGHESI, MD
Department of Radiology, University of Brescia, Piazzale Spedali Civili 1, Brescia, BS, 25123, Italy

Radiation dose is a major concern, especially when CT examination is performed as a screening or presurgical test, in a population that includes a large number of young subjects. In this setting, the rationale of imaging studies is to obtain detailed information on patency/occlusion of mucous drainage pathways, on bone changes (particularly in critical areas such as the skull base and orbit), intrasinusal content (air, fluid, solid, calcifications), and on anatomic variants. As a consequence, conventional radiology should be discarded as an obsolete tool, even though the overall radiation dose delivered to the eye-lens with this technique is rather low (approximately 0.57 mGy) (ZAMMIT-MAEMPEL 1996; PHILLIPS 1997; ZINREICH 1998; SIEVERS et al. 2000).

Computed tomography is a relatively high-dose examination, nevertheless the high natural contrast between air, mucosa and bone enables optimization of low-dose protocols by decreasing tube current down to 30–50 mAs (MACLENNAN 1995; HEIN et al. 2002; HAGTVEDT et al. 2003). This results in a considerable decrease of the eye-lens dose (3.1 mGy when 50 mAs are applied) (SOHAIB et al. 2001) without significant loss of diagnostic information. With MSCT scanners, patient exposure is a primary issue. Recent data demonstrate eye-lens dose higher than single-slice (SS) scanners, even when low-dose protocols (40 mAs) are applied (9.2 mGy). Nevertheless, also with this new tool, exposure is far below the threshold for detectable lens opacities (0.5–2 Gy) (ZAMMIT-MAEMPEL et al. 2003).

1.1.1.2
Direct Coronal Plane Acquisition

Images are electively acquired on coronal plane, as perpendicular to the hard palate as permitted by gantry tilting and patient cooperation. This plane is able to demonstrate patency, width, and morphology of all those airspaces (middle and superior meatus, ethmoid infundibulum) hidden by turbinates and therefore difficult to access at clinical examination. Moreover, coronal imaging clearly depicts both superior and lateral insertion of the middle turbinate, and the cribriform plate. The main weaknesses of this scanning orientation are the poor delineation of the frontal recess (coursing along an oblique-sagittal plane), as well as the impossibility to demonstrate sinusal walls lying in the coronal plane.

Two options are described for patient positioning: supine, with hyperextended head (hanging-head position) (PHILLIPS 1997), or prone. The latter is usually preferred because it is more easily tolerated by the patient and less susceptible to motion artifacts. Additionally, fluid material retained in a maxillary sinus, in the hanging-head position will freely flow towards the ostium, therefore impairing the evaluation of its patency.

The examination area extends from the anterior frontal sinus wall to the posterior border of the sphenoid sinus. Scanning parameters are highly variable according to the clinical issues to be addressed and to the available equipment (ZINREICH 1998). In our experience, optimal demonstration of the ostiomeatal unit and of natural drainage pathways is achieved with:

- Thin slice collimation (1–2 mm), to minimize partial volume artifacts that may mimic mucosal thickenings along small caliber drainage pathways.
- 3- to 4-mm increment/1.5 pitch (sequential or SS spiral equipment, respectively) as a trade-off between dose reduction and the necessity not to miss anatomical structures such as the uncinate process (Table 1.1).

For sinus screening purposes, sufficient information can be obtained with thicker collimation (3–5 mm) and an increment of up to 15 mm.

Table 1.1. Chronic rhinosinusitis, nasal polyposis: scanning parameters, coronal plane

Parameters	Sequential CT	SSCT
Slice thickness	1 mm	2 mm
Increment/ pitch	3 mm	Pitch 1,5
mA/kV	70/133	60/120÷140
Reconstruction algorithm – *kernel**	*Ultrahigh*	A 70÷90

SSCT, single-slice spiral technique. * Siemens equipment

1.1.1.3
Axial Plane Acquisition

This scanning plane enables adequate demonstration of some anatomical structures difficult to assess on coronal plane due to their spatial orientation (such as posterior frontal sinus and sphenoid sinus wall, sphenoethmoid recess). Nonetheless, axial acquisition is recommended only whenever the digital lateral view (topogram) shows excessive dental amalgam or metallic implants, or as a complement after coronal scanning whenever precise information on specific anatomic structures is required.

In the first condition, a data set of thin and contiguous (to avoid aliasing) slices may be acquired with the incremental technique (1–2 mm collimation) or the SS spiral technique (2 mm collimation; pitch 1–1.5; 1–2 mm reconstruction) (Table 1.2). The patient lies in supine position, both his/her sagittal plane and hard palate should be perpendicular to the gantry's scan line, in order to achieve, respectively, optimal symmetry of the anatomical structures on axial plane, and no/minimal gantry tilting. In fact, the quality of MPR is degraded by gantry inclination (stair-step artifacts). Direct scans should be oriented parallel to the hard palate and range from the upper border of frontal sinuses to the alveolar process of maxillary bones; nasal tip and petrous bone should be included in the field of view. Subsequent coronal MPR reformation is obtained for proper assessment of critical anatomical areas either at risk of iatrogenic damage (cribriform plate, fovea ethmoidalis) or playing a key role in mucous drainage (ostiomeatal unit).

When acquired as a complement to the coronal study, axial scans are basically focused on anatomical areas inadequately demonstrated in that orientation (i.e., anterior and posterior walls of maxillary, frontal, and sphenoid sinus, sphenoethmoid recess). Additionally, this scan plane is valuable for the detection of Onodi cells. In this setting, contiguous slices and full coverage of the paranasal area are generally unnecessary, as a consequence, 4- to 5-mm increments can be applied, decreasing both patient exposure and examination time.

Table 1.2. Chronic rhinosinusitis, nasal polyposis: scanning parameters, axial plane

Parameters	Sequential CT	SSCT
Collimation	1÷2 mm	2 mm
Increment/ pitch	1÷5 mm	Pitch 1÷1,5
mA/kV	70/133	60/120÷140
Reconstruction algorithm – *kernel**	*Ultrahigh*	A 70÷90
MPR	COR/SAG	Idem

SSCT, single-slice spiral technique; MPR, multiplanar reconstruction; COR, coronal; SAG, sagittal. * Siemens equipment

1.1.2
CT Protocol in Neoplastic Lesions

The first step in the diagnostic work-up of both benign and malignant sinus neoplasms consists of fiberoptic examination. Endoscopy allows adequate demonstration of the superficial spread of the lesion and may guide a biopsy. The discrimination between benign and malignant tumors and the precise characterization of the lesion are, in most cases, far beyond the capabilities of CT. The main goals of imaging are, therefore, to provide a precise map of deep tumor extension in all those areas blinded at fiberoptic examination, especially anterior cranial fossa, orbit, and pterygopalatine fossa.

In this setting, MR is the technique of choice for several reasons:
- It clearly differentiates tumor from retained secretions
- It allows early detection of perivascular/perineural spread
- It allows higher contrast resolution

On the other hand, the strengths of CT consist of:
- Superior definition of bone structures even in the case of subtle erosions
- Faster and easier performance
- Superior accessibility and lower cost.

As a consequence, in our experience CT indications are restricted to patients who have not undergone a preliminary examination by the otolaryngologist (to rule out non-neoplastic lesions) or to patients bearing contraindications to MR.

1.1.2.1
Axial Scanning

CT protocol consists of native and post-contrast scanning in both axial and coronal planes; it is preferable to start the examination on the axial plane and to complete it with coronal scans, usually limited to the area of the lesion. Both incremental and spiral techniques can be applied, though the latter is faster and requires lower doses of contrast agent.

On the axial plane, the gantry must be parallel to the hard palate. The examination area extends from the superior border of the frontal sinus to the alveolar process of the maxillary bone. Scans are acquired with 2- to 3-mm collimation, 2- to 3-mm increments (sequential CT), pitch 1–1.5 (SS spiral equipment) (Table 1.3). The fastest rotation time should be applied to decrease the risk of motion artifacts. A high

Table 1.3. Neoplasm staging. scanning parameters, axial plane

Parameters	Sequential CT	SSCT
Orientation	Parallel to hard palate	Idem
Collimation	2÷3 mm	2÷3 mm
Increment/ pitch	2÷3 mm	Pitch 1÷1,5
mA/kV	200-240/140	200-240/140
Reconstruction algorithm	*Soft tissue/ bone*	Idem
MPR	COR/SAG	Idem

SSCT single-slice spiral technique; MPR, multiplanar reconstruction; COR, coronal; SAG, sagittal.

contrast resolution is mandatory, therefore a higher radiation dose is required (200–240 mAs, 140 kV) and both soft tissue and bone algorithms are adopted for image reconstruction.

Contrast agent protocol consists of biphasic injection (80–90 ml at a rate of 2.5 ml/s plus 30–40 ml at a rate of 1–1.5 ml/s), and a scanning delay of approximately 80 s. This time interval enables an assessment of the lesion in its window of more intense enhancement, therefore maximizing the detection of lesion boundaries (MAROLDI et al. 1998). Early acquisition in the arterial phase (30s delay) may be indicated when a highly vascular lesion is suspected or to precisely delineate the relationships between the neoplasm and the carotid arteries.

1.1.2.2
Coronal Scanning

Scanning parameters in the coronal plane are comparable to those used for the axial plane. Additional contrast agent administration (40–50 ml at a rate of 2 ml/s) may be suggested. Whenever prone positioning is impossible to obtain, the patient is scanned exclusively in the axial plane (contiguous 2-mm thick slices, no gantry tilting) and multiplanar reconstructions are subsequently obtained.

1.2
Multislice CT of the Paranasal Sinuses

Improvements in CT imaging of the paranasal sinuses provided by multislice technology include fast coverage of the volume of interest, thin collimation (up to 0.75 mm with 16-row MSCT), and acquisition of nearly isotropic (i.e., cubic) voxels. The latter results in high quality multiplanar reformation of the data set, preferably acquired on the axial plane. According to the number of detectors of the equipment employed, the volume of interest is acquired from 4×1 mm up to 16×0.75 mm collimation and no gantry tilting. Data are then reconstructed as 1-mm thick slices with 50% slice overlap, on the axial plane. This set of images is suitable for excellent MPR post-processing (Table 1.4).

Table 1.4. MSCT scanning parameters

Parameters	MSCT (4 rows)	MSCT (16 rows)
Orientation	Axial, no gantry tilting	
Collimation	4×1 mm	16×0.75 mm
Rotation time	0.75 s	0.75 s
mA/kV	70/133	60/120÷140
Reconstruction algorithm – *kernel**	H70h	H70h
Volume reconstruction (**axial plane**)		
Thickness	1.25 mm	1 mm
Interslice gap	0.7 mm	0.5 mm

* Siemens equipment

1.3
MR Technique

MR plays a prominent role in imaging of the paranasal sinuses. Its high contrast resolution combined with multiplanar capability make it a valuable tool in the assessment not only of benign and malignant neoplasms, but also in the evaluation of aggressive inflammatory lesions (invasive mycoses, Wegener granulomatosis, sarcoidosis). In these settings, the high contrast resolution of this technique enables discrimination between the lesion and intrasinusal retained secretions, demonstrating its relationships with adjacent structures, and, in many cases, to providing clues for a differential diagnosis. In contrast, no major indication to MR is found for patients affected by chronic rhino sinusitis or nasal polyposis: scant detail relating to thin bone structures (which are numerous and critical in this area) and high costs are substantial drawbacks (ZINREICH 1998).

1.3.1
Designing an MR Protocol: Basic Concepts

Though modern equipment enables rapid acquisition of nearly all kind of sequences, a basic prin-

ciple guides the design of an MR protocol: the faster the examination time, the lower the risk of motion artifacts. A second key point consists in spatial resolution: nasal cavity and paranasal sinuses are a complex framework of airspaces bordered by thin, bony boundaries. Moreover, a thin osteo-periosteal layer separates the sinonasal region from the anterior cranial fossa (cribriform plate and dura) and the orbit (lamina papyracea and periorbita). An adequate depiction of these structures mandates high field equipment (1.5 T) and a dedicated circular coil (head coil). In addition, a high-resolution matrix (512) should be applied along with the smallest FOV achievable (individually variable, but generally 180–200 mm). Smaller FOV may be obtained but this, of course, requires oversampling in the phase encoding direction to avoid aliasing artifacts, and therefore results in an overall increase of examination time. Acquiring images not exceeding 3–3.5 mm thickness, with an interslice gap ranging from 1.5 mm to 2.4 mm (50%–70%) is also recommended. The parameters listed above, applied to both TSE T2 and SE T1 sequences, are an acceptable compromise between the need to attain small pixel size and the risk of significantly decreasing signal-to-noise ratio.

1.3.2.1
MR Protocol

Symmetric representation of anatomic structures is of the utmost importance, as in many cases the diagnosis may be based on the observation of differences in size and signal intensity of a paired structure when matching the two sides. To achieve this, the internal auditory canals, imaged with a TSE T2 localizer sequence, are taken as a landmark to correctly orientate axial and coronal studies. As for CT protocols, the hard palate is a second point for reference for proper sequence orientation (parallel on axial plane, perpendicular on coronal plane); sagittal studies are aligned to the nasal septum and falx cerebri.

The sequences applied are, basically, TSE T2 and SE T1. The first one provides the best discrimination between solid tissue and fluids (retained secretions, cerebrospinal fluid, colliquated tissues). It is acquired in axial plane and in a second perpendicular plane chosen according to the priority dictated by the lesion site of origin and clinical signs (Table 1.5). SE T1 has the advantage of a superior anatomic resolution, valuable for the definition of the interface between lesion and adjacent structures. Moreover,

Table 1.5. Standard MR protocol

Sequence	TR (ms)	Thickness (mm)	Averages	Matrix	Pixel (mm)	Acquisition time
TSE T2	5680	3–3.5	3	512×256	0.8×0.4×3	2'06"
Gd-DTPA SE T1	400	3–3.5	2	512×256	0.7×0.4×3	2'50"
Total examination time	(2 TSE T2 + 3 SE T1) **12'42"**					
Optional sequences						
FS TSE T2	5960	3–3.5	3	512×256	0.8×0.4×3	2'13"
FS Gd-DTPA SE T1	695	3–3.5	2	512×256	0.7×0.4×3	4'53"

in this sequence fat tissue signal is maximized. This issue enables detection of subtle signal changes in the medullary part of bone, as well as to accurately detect the effacement of fat tissue pads, particularly in critical areas such as the orbit and the pterygopalatine fossa. Plain SE T1 sequence has two major indications:

- Patients examined for lesions of unclear etiology. In this case, additional information is provided regarding signal pattern of the lesion, therefore supporting the differential diagnosis task.
- Patients followed up after treatment. In this scenario a plain SE T1 sequence helps to retrospectively assess the enhancement pattern of a suspect lesion, therefore it offers clues to discriminate a recurrent lesion from scar tissue.

After the administration of paramagnetic contrast agent (Gd-DTPA, 0.2 ml/kg body weight), a SE T1 sequence is acquired in all three planes.

Fat-sat prepulses may be applied to both TSE T2 and enhanced SE T1 sequences to increase lesion conspicuity (particularly in malignant tumors) and to delineate the relationships between a lesion and intraorbital/pterygopalatine fat tissue. The main disadvantage on fat-sat TSE T2 sequences is represented by the loss of a natural contrast agent. Fat tissue (suppressed), bone, and muscular structures all display a hypointense signal, resulting in a difficult delineation of the interface between normal and pathologic tissues. On the other hand, post-contrast fat-sat SE T1 requires a considerable increase of repetition time (TR) that influences both T1 weighting of images and acquisition time. These pitfalls may be solved only by decreasing the number of acquired slices and, therefore, the anatomic coverage. As a result, in our experience, fat-sat technique is preferably applied to SE T1 sequences in collaborative patients, focusing on restricted anatomic areas.

1.3.2.2
Additional MR Sequences

Volumetric interpolated breath-hold imaging (VIBE) is a 3D MR technique aimed at minimizing partial volume effects and maximizing image contrast, and represents a robust alternative to SE T1 sequences. This fat-sat gradient-echo T1 weighted sequence has the potential to provide submillimetric sections, no gaps, and isotropic voxels, thus making it suitable for optimal MPR/MIP reconstructions in all planes.

Due to its high flexibility, it can be optimized for *short acquisition times* (slice thickness 0.7 mm, 144 partitions, matrix size 320, acquisition time 1'26") (Table 1.6). When accurate synchronization of contrast injection and image acquisition is fulfilled, the same sequence may provide high-quality MR angiograms, to correctly demonstrate the relationships between tumor and vessels.

Adequate arrangement of parameters (slice thickness 0.5 mm, 224 partitions, matrix size 448, acquisition time 3'52") converts VIBE into a robust high resolution sequence (Fig. 1.1) that allows full coverage of the paranasal sinuses and skull base, valuable for precise definition of tumor extension and perineural spread (Table 1.6).

Table 1.6. VIBE sequence

	Standard VIBE	High resolution VIBE
TR	6.02 ms	818 ms
TE	2.55 ms	3.47 ms
Scan time	1'26"	3'52"
Voxel size	0.7×0.7×0.7 mm	0.5×0.5×0.5 mm
Partitions	144	244
Coverage	100 mm	0.5 mm
FoV read	320 mm	230 mm
Averages	1	1
Image matrix	320×208	448×208

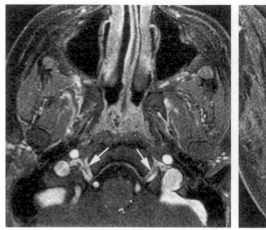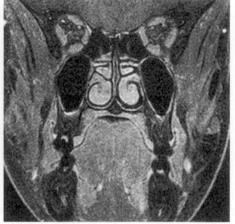

a   b

Fig. 1.1a,b. High resolution VIBE sequence (matrix 448×448, acquisition time 3'48") on axial (**a**) and coronal (**b**) planes. Excellent anatomic definition is demonstrated by the identification of the subtle hypointense hypoglossal nerve, as it courses through the condylar canal, surrounded by enhanced veins (*arrows*)

1.3.2.3
Signal vs Time Curves in Follow-Up Studies

After surgery and/or radiation therapy, precise discrimination between scar tissue and recurrent/persistent tumor is often a hard task. An easy and reliable guide for differential diagnosis may be obtained by comparing signal vs time curves of suspected lesions vs normal mucosa, muscle, or vascular structures. This approach requires a dynamic sequence (GE T1), acquiring the same section with a frame rate of 1/s,

for 1 min. Signal curves are then calculated by placing regions of interest on the suspect lesion and on adjacent normal tissues (vessels, muscles, mucosa) (Fig. 1.2). Helpful information can be obtained by comparing both the average of maximum signal values and the steepness of the curve, in suspect and presumably normal tissues. The main drawback of this application is represented by its limited coverage: the dynamic sequence acquired allows just a single section to be selected after the acquisition of TSE T2 and plain SE T1 sequence.

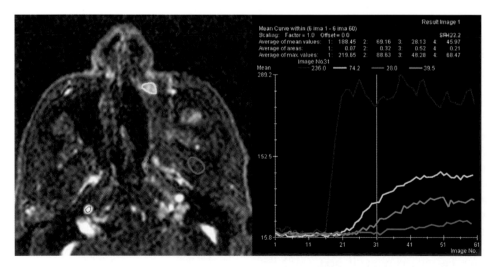

Fig. 1.2. Time versus signal curve. Follow-up MR after radical maxillectomy for adenocarcinoma. Dynamic acquisition (single slice, one scan/s, acquisition time 60 s) after bolus injection of Gd-DTPA. By placing regions of interest on the internal carotid artery (*red*), suspect recurrent tumor (*yellow*), and presumably normal muscle (*green*) and mucosa (*blue*), a time vs signal intensity curve is calculated. Compared to normal tissue, the suspect lesion shows steeper and higher curve. The finding was confirmed at aspiration cytology (true positive)

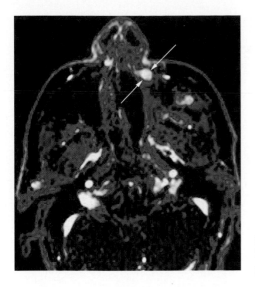

Fig. 1.3. Parametric image obtained from the whole stack of 60 frames. Intensity is related to the slope of the time-enhancement curve. *Arrows* point to the confirmed recurrent tumor

References

Hagtvedt T, Aalokken TM, Notthellen J et al (2003) A new low-dose CT examination compared with standard-dose CT in the diagnosis of acute sinusitis. Eur Radiol 13:976-980

Hein E, Rogalla P, Klingebiel R et al (2002) Low-dose CT of the paranasal sinuses with eye lens protection: effect on image quality and radiation dose. Eur Radiol 12:1693-1696

MacLennan AC (1995) Radiation dose to the lens from coronal CT scanning of the sinuses. Clin Radiol 50:265-267

Maroldi R, Battaglia G, Maculotti P et al (1998) Spiral CT vs subsecond conventional CT in head and neck malignancies. In: Krestin GP, Glazer GM (eds) Advances in CT IV. Springer, Berlin Heidelberg New York, pp 70-75

Oliverio PJ, Benson ML, Zinreich SJ (1995) Update on imaging for functional endoscopic sinus surgery. Otolaryngol Clin North Am 28:585-608

Phillips CD (1997) Current status and new developments in techniques for imaging the nose and sinuses. Otolaryngol Clin North Am 30:371-387

Sievers KW, Greess H, Baum U et al (2000) Paranasal sinuses and nasopharynx CT and MRI. Eur J Radiol 33:185-202

Sohaib SA, Peppercorn PD, Horrocks JA et al (2001) The effect of decreasing mAs on image quality and patient dose in sinus CT. Br J Radiol 74:157-161

Zammit-Maempel I (1996) Radiation dose to the lens from coronal CT scanning of the sinuses. Clin Radiol 51:151

Zammit-Maempel I, Chadwick CL, Willis SP (2003) Radiation dose to the lens of eye and thyroid gland in paranasal sinus multislice CT. Br J Radiol 76:418-420

Zinreich SJ (1998) Functional anatomy and computed tomography imaging of the paranasal sinuses. Am J Med Sci 316:2-12

2   CT and MR Anatomy of Paranasal Sinuses: Key Elements

Roberto Maroldi, Andrea Borghesi, Patrizia Maculotti

CONTENTS

2.1   Introduction   9
2.1.1   Nasal Cavity and Lateral Nasal Wall   9
2.1.2   Ethmoid Bone   10
2.1.3   Frontal Sinus and Frontal Recess   12
2.1.4   Maxillary Sinus, Uncinate Process
        and Ethmoidal Infundibulum   17
2.1.5   Sphenoid Sinus   18
2.2   Development of Nasosinusal Cavities   18
2.3   Surgical Anatomy   18
2.4   Anatomic Variants   19
2.4.1   Nasal Septum and Middle Turbinate   19
2.4.2   Uncinate Process   20
2.4.3   Anterior Ethmoid Cells   20
2.4.4   Onodi Cells and Sphenoid Sinus   21
2.4.5   Asymmetry of Ethmoid Roof   22
2.5   Pterygopalatine Fossa and Pterygoid Process   23
2.6   Nasal Septum   26
        References   26

2.1
Introduction

A conceptual understanding of the anatomic and functional relationships between the nasal cavity and paranasal sinuses is of the utmost importance, particularly when dealing with chronic inflammatory diseases.

According to their drainage pathway, the sinusal cavities may be functionally classified into two subgroups. The first one includes the anterior ethmoid cells, the frontal sinus, and the maxillary sinus; all these cavities drain mucus into the middle meatus. The second group encompasses the posterior ethmoid cells and the sphenoid sinus, both draining into the superior meatus.

R. Maroldi, MD
Professor, Department of Radiology, University of Brescia, Piazzale Spedali Civili 1, Brescia, BS, 25123, Italy
A. Borghesi, MD; P. Maculotti, MD
Department of Radiology, University of Brescia, Piazzale Spedali Civili 1, Brescia, BS, 25123, Italy

2.1.1
Nasal Cavity and Lateral Nasal Wall

Nasal cavities are located in the midface, separated by a median septum; they communicate posteriorly with the nasopharynx through the choanae. The floor of nasal fossae is the hard palate, the cribriform plate and the planum ethmoidalis compose its roof, that separate nasal cavities from the anterior cranial fossa. The nasal septum is made of a "hard" portion (perpendicular lamina of the ethmoid, vomer), and of a "soft" part (septal cartilage).

The lateral nasal wall has a more difficult anatomy, an understanding of it being critical for endonasal surgery planning.

The complex anatomical arrangement of the lateral nasal wall can be more easily understood if related to the embryologic development of turbinates and ethmoid (Wolf et al. 1993).

The ethmoid turbinates originate from ridges in the lateral nasal wall of the fetus. Each of the five ridges (ethmoidoturbinals) has an ascending (more vertical) and descending (more horizontal) portion, being – therefore – similar to the turbinate in the adult. Between the fetal ridges are six grooves. Some ridges and grooves will fuse or disappear – partially or totally – during fetal development to ultimately result in the nasal turbinates of the adult. Key points are:

The first ethmoidoturbinal regresses, i.e. will not develop into a turbinate. The agger nasi is considered a residual of the ascending portion, while the uncinate process is presumably a remnant of the descending portion.

The descending part of the first groove (located between the first and second ethmoidoturbinals) becomes the ethmoidal infundibulum and middle meatus, whereas the ascending part becomes the frontal recess.

The second ethmoidoturbinal gives rise to the bulla lamella, a lamina attached to the lateral nasal wall, a structure that can be observed in few patients because it is usually pneumatized, therefore appearing as the bulla ethmoidalis.

The third and fourth ethmoidoturbinals develop, respectively, into the permanent middle and superior turbinates; and the fifth ethmoidoturbinals become the supreme (uppermost) turbinate.

The superior and uppermost meatus develop from third and fourth fetal grooves.

As a result, ridges fully develop into thin laminae crossing the entire ethmoid to project into the nasal cavity (turbinates) or give rise to incomplete laminae, like the uncinate process. Each bony lamina has a constant portion inserting into the lateral nasal wall (ground lamella) and additional attachments to the lamina cribrosa or to the fovea ethmoidalis (superiorly).

In most subjects, four ground lamellae are usually present, almost each one obliquely oriented, somewhat parallel to one another. The uncinate process – an incompletely developed lamella – is the first one, followed by the bulla lamella. If the latter extends vertically up to the ethmoid roof, the frontal recess becomes separated from the rest of the ethmoid. Pneumatization of this lamella results in the development of the ethmoidal bulla. The third, more constant and complete ground lamella consists of the lateral insertion of the middle turbinate on the lamina papyracea. This lamella separates anterior from posterior ethmoidal cells. A fourth lamella is made by the lateral attachment of the superior turbinate. Occasionally, a fifth lamella may be observed when the supreme turbinate does not regress (KIM et al. 2001).

The spaces among the ground lamellae (interturbinal meatus) are further subdivided by transverse bony septa, resulting in several cells that communicate with the interturbinal meatus only through a small ostium. Rarely these septa are absent. In this latter condition, the original framework of the labyrinth organized into single large cells – corresponding to the interturbinal meatus – can be observed.

Variations or anomalies in the development of ground lamellae and septa will result in a great variability of number, size and morphology of the single ethmoid cells and may additionally reflect on the ratio between the volume of anterior versus posterior cells.

As mentioned above, the *superior meatus* is the drainage pathway of posterior ethmoid cells and sphenoid sinus (the latter through the sphenoethmoid recess).

The middle meatus plays a crucial functional role, as in this area the secretions of several sinuses are collected, namely:

● The ethmoid bulla (roof of the meatus)
● The anterior ethmoid cells and maxillary sinus, both through the hiatus semilunaris, a subtle fissure located in front and below the ethmoid bulla
● The frontal sinus, through the frontal recess

The inferior meatus, although the largest, has a less relevant functional role: in this space only the distal opening of the nasolacrimal duct is found.

2.1.2
Ethmoid Bone

From a practical standpoint, the ethmoid bone can be divided into four structures: two lateral masses, a sagittal midline lamina, and a horizontal plate (Fig. 2.1). The latter (cribriform plate) is the central part of the floor of the anterior cranial fossa. Several microscopic foramina perforate its thin structure, through which course the olfactory nerve filaments with their perineural investment.

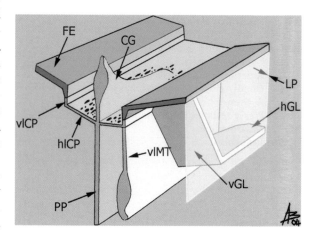

Fig. 2.1. The ethmoid plates and fovea ethmoidalis. A midline (perpendicular plate, *PP*) and two lateral vertical laminae: the medial one made by the vertical lamella of the middle turbinate (*vlMT*) on the top of which is the vertical lamella of the cribriform plate (*vlCP*), the lateral one is the lamina papyracea (*LP*). Horizontal lamella of the cribriform plate (*hlCP*), horizontal (*hGL*) and vertical (*vGL*) – ascending part – of ground lamella of the middle turbinate, crista galli (*CG*), fovea ethmadalis (*FE*)

On the upper part of the sagittal midline lamina (crista galli) – located just above the cribriform plate – inserts the cerebral falx; the inferior part, below the cribriform plate, being referred to as the perpendicular lamina, a component of the nasal septum (Fig. 2.2–2.4).

The lateral masses (ethmoid labyrinth) are made of a variable number (3–18) of pneumatized cells separated by thin bony walls.

Each ethmoid labyrinth is closed by bony margins on its external and internal surfaces only. The external surface is made by the lamina papyracea that separates the cells from the orbit. Dehiscences may be present. As a result, the periosteum of the ethmoid cell comes in contact with the periosteum investing the orbital wall (periorbita). Medially,

the labyrinth is bordered by two constant laminae hanging from the horizontal plate: the middle and superior turbinates. An uppermost small third ethmoid turbinate (supreme turbinate) can seldom be observed.

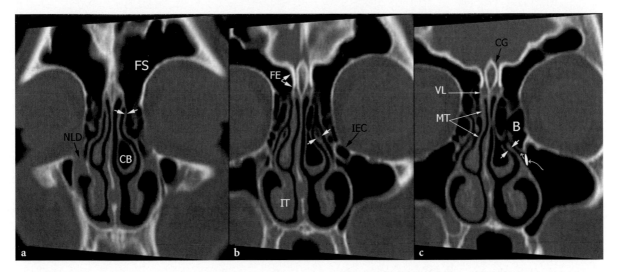

Fig. 2.2a–c. CT coronal reconstructions through the ethmoid labyrinth. **a** Anterior nasal fossa, level of the uppermost insertion of both uncinate processes on the vertical lamellae of the middle turbinates – type 4 according to LANDSBERG and FRIEDMAN (2001) (*white arrows* on *left side*). **b** Bilateral pneumatization of the horizontal (non-attached) free portion of the uncinate processes (*white arrows* on *left side*). **c** The horizontal portion of the uncinate process (*white arrows* on *left side*) and the inferior surface of the ethmoid bulla (*B*) limit the oblique and narrow ethmoid infundibulum. The maxillary sinus ostium is detectable at the bottom of the infundibulum (*white ellipse*). *Curved white arrows* show the path along the ostium and the infundibulum

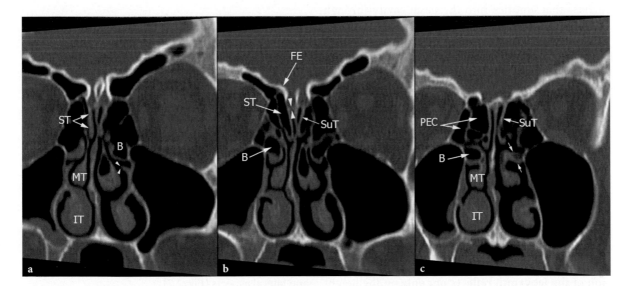

Fig. 2.3a–c. CT coronal reconstructions through the ethmoid labyrinth. **a** Middle nasal fossa at the level of the short horizontal portion of the uncinate process posterior to the ethmoid infundibulum (*white arrowheads* on *left side*). A large ethmoid bulla (*B*) impinges the left middle turbinate on left side. **b** The CT section cuts the posterior part of the bulla (*B*). The horizontal portion of the cribriform plates (*arrowheads*) appears thinner than the bone of the fovea ethmoidalis (*FE*). Bilateral pneumatization of the superior turbinate (*ST*) is present. **c** Lateral attachment of the middle turbinate – the ground lamella (*opposite arrows*) – onto the lateral nasal wall. Posterior ethmoid cells (*PEC*) extend between the lamina papyracea and the supreme turbinate (*SuT*)

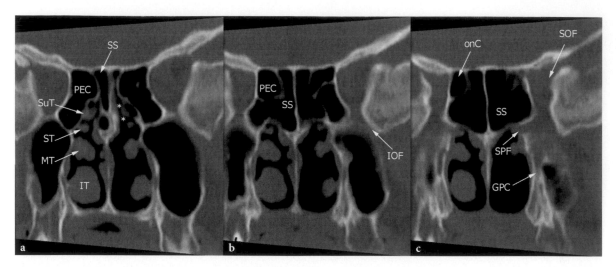

Fig. 2.4a–c. CT coronal reconstructions through the posterior ethmoid labyrinth and the sphenoid sinus. a Level of the sphe-noethmoid recess (*asterisks*). Lateral attachment of all four turbinates (*IT, MT, ST,* and *SuT*) is shown. Anterior aspect of the sphenoid sinus (*SS*) and posterior ethmoid cells (*PEC*) are demonstrated on the same level. A posterior ethmoid cell extends over the right sphenoid sinus – Onodi cell (*onC*) on (**b**) and (**c**). Inferior orbital fissure (*IOF*), superior orbital fissure (*SOF*), sphenopalatine foramen (*SPF*), greater palatine canal (*GPC*)

The middle turbinate – the largest ethmoid lam-ina – separates the labyrinth into anterior and pos-terior cells by means of its middle portion inserting on the lateral nasal wall (ground lamella) (Fig. 2.5).

All the other surfaces of the labyrinth are open, lined only by adjacent structures. Anteriorly, cells open into a narrow cleft – the infundibulum ethmo-idalis – that empties into the nasal cavity through the middle meatus. On the opposite surface, the an-terior aspect of the sphenoid sinus borders the pos-terior ethmoid cells, that empty into another narrow cleft – the sphenoethmoidal recess – draining into the superior meatus and finally into the choanae.

The orbital plate of the frontal bone (fovea eth-moidalis) provides the bony roof of the ethmoid as the cells within the labyrinth extend above the plane of the cribriform plate (LEBOWITZ et al. 2001). The transition between the thicker frontal bone and the thinner, medially located, lateral lamella of the lamina cribrosa can be easily demonstrated on coronal CT planes (Fig. 2.2). The lateral lamella and the lamina cribrosa provide, respectively, the lateral border and the floor of the olfactory fossa. It is im-portant to note that the variability of pneumatiza-tion of the labyrinth reflects not only on the height of the lateral lamella – therefore the relative depth of the olfactory fossa into the nasal cavity – but also on its obliquity and on the transverse size of the lamina cribrosa. Relevant side to side variations are frequently observed.

Moreover, the weakest area of the whole anterior skull base is located where the anterior ethmoidal artery enters the lateral lamella after having crossed the lamina papyracea and the ethmoidal labyrinth. On CT, this area can be detected as a focal, some-times symmetrical, dehiscence on the lateral lamella of the lamina cribrosa.

2.1.3
Frontal Sinus and Frontal Recess

Anterior pneumatization of the frontal recess into the frontal bone gives rise to the frontal sinus (Fig. 2.6). In the sagittal plane its ostium can be identified as the narrowest part of an hourglass space, the upper part widening into the frontal sinus, and the lower empty-ing into the middle meatus through the frontal recess. The latter is not a true tubular structure, as the term "nasofrontal duct" might indicate. In effect, the size and shape of the frontal recess are largely dictated by the adjacent structures: the agger nasi cells anteriorly, the ethmoidal bulla posteriorly, the vertical portion of the uncinate process and the middle turbinate on medial and lateral aspects (Fig. 2.7).

Particularly, the medial and lateral borders of the frontal recess depend on the variable type of the supe-rior attachment of the uncinate process. Six variations have been identified by LANDSBERG and FRIEDMAN (2001) (Fig. 2.8). In type 1, insertion on lamina papy-

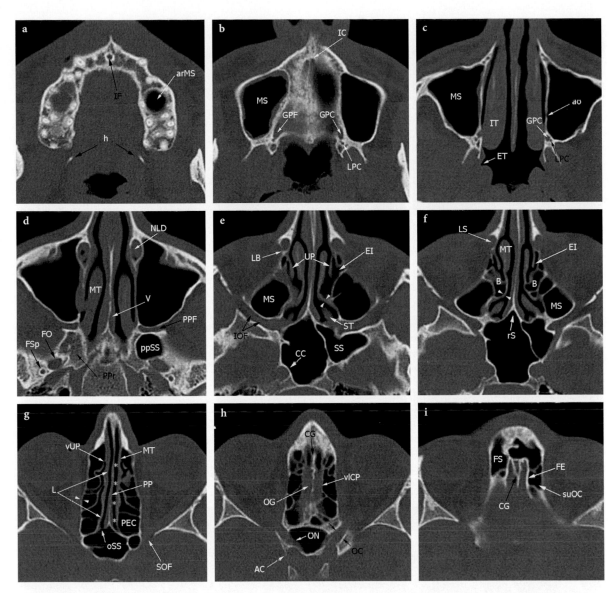

Fig. 2.5a–i. Axial plane. **a** Level of the alveolar process, teeth roots are seen. The inferior portion of medial pterygoid plates – hamulus – is detected (*h*). Alveolar recess of maxillary sinus (*arMS*) **b** Hard palate level. Greater (*GPC*) and lesser (*LPC*) palatine canals result from the articulation of the vertical portion of the perpendicular plate of the palatine bone with the maxillary bone. Opening of the canal – the greater palatine foramen (*GPF*) – appears as an ovoid groove on the *right side*. **c** The inferior concha and the surrounding inferior turbinate (*IT*) are demonstrated. An accessory ostium is located within the posterior third of the medial maxillary sinus wall (*ao*). **d** Level of the inferior aspect of the nasolacrimal ducts (*NLD*). The postero-superior limit of the middle turbinates reaches the choanae (*MT*). **e** Level of the middle meatus. The uncinate processes (*UP*) attach onto the medial aspect of the NLD. The narrow space between the UP and the medial maxillary sinus wall belongs to the ethmoid infundibulum (*EI*). *Arrowheads* indicate the ground lamella of the MT, signing the border between anterior and posterior ethmoid labyrinth (see also **f**), into which the inferior tip of the superior turbinates (*ST*) projects. **f** The ethmoid bullae (*B*) border the posterior limit of the EI. Rostrum of the sphenoid bone (*rs*). **g** The vertical portion of the UP (*vUP*) attaches onto the vertical lamellae of the MT on both sides. A clear separation between anterior and posterior ethmoid cells (*PEC*) cannot be identified on axial planes. The narrow channel-like olfactory fissure (*asterisks*) reach the sphenoethmoidal recess where the ostium of the right sphenoid sinus appears as a small opening close to the midline (*oSS*). Common lamina onto which the middle, superior (and supreme) turbinates attach (*L*). *Arrowheads* indicate the thin lamina papyracea. **h** Olfactory groove (*OG*) level. Because the groove extends down into the labyrinth, it results bordered by ethmoid cells. The thin vertical lamella of the cribriform plate (*vlCP*) separates the groove from the ethmoid cells. **i** At the level of the mid crista galli (*CG*) the olfactory groove is bordered laterally by the thicker frontal bone – fovea ethmoidalis (*FE*). *suOC*, supraorbital ethmoid cell

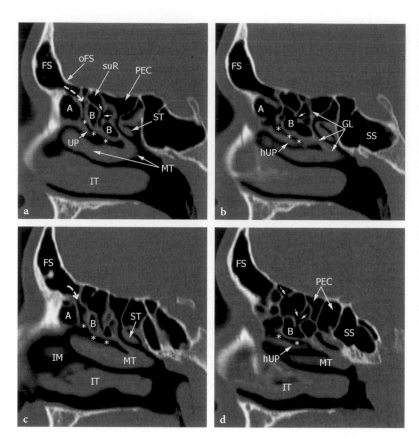

Fig. 2.6a–d. Same patient as in Fig. 2.5. **a,b** Right side. **c,d** Left side. **a** Sagittal plane closer to midline. From the hourglass ostium of the frontal sinus (*oFS*) the mucus follows a curved path (*broken curved arrow*) into the frontal recess between the agger nasi cell (*A*) and the anterior surface of the bulla (*B*). *Asterisks* on (**a**) and (**b**) indicate the course of the hiatus semilunaris bordered by the uncinate process – horizontal (*hUP*) and part of the vertical portion – and the bulla. *suR*, suprabullar recess. **c** Sagittal plane closer to midline. The left frontal sinus ostium is wider than on the opposite side. Because the agger nasi cell (*A*) is smaller, the frontal recess is more vertically oriented (*broken curved arrow*). **d** On a more lateral plane the horizontal portion of the uncinate process is demonstrated (*hUP*). *Asterisks* indicate the hiatus semilunaris. *Small arrows* on (**a**)/(**b**) and (**d**) point to the opening of small anterior ethmoid cells into the bulla ethmoidalis

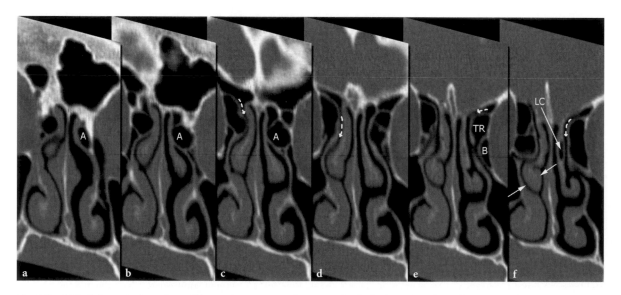

Fig. 2.7a–f. The left vertical portion of the uncinate process inserts on both the lateral surface of a large agger nasi cell (*A*) and the lamina papyracea. As a result, the frontal recess runs medial to the uncinate process (*broken curved white arrows*). Moreover, a terminal recess (*TR*) is created between the superior surface of the bulla and the insertion of the UP onto the lamina papyracea. On coronal scans the agger nasi cell may be differentiated from the bulla ethmoidalis because it is located anterior to the infundibulum ethmoidalis. On the *right side*, a large bulla is associated with a paradoxically curved middle turbinate (*opposite arrows*). Pneumatization of the vertical lamella of left middle turbinate (lamellar concha, *LC*)

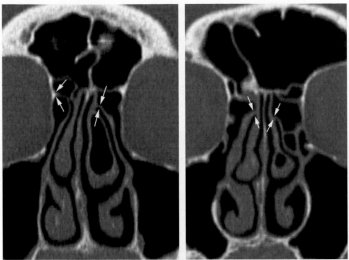

Fig. 2.8a–c. a The vertical portion of the uncinate process inserts onto the lamina papyracea [type 1, according to LANDSBERG and FRIEDMAN (2001)] – right side – and onto the upper aspect of middle turbinate (type 6) – left side. **b** Bilateral insertion of the uncinate process onto the lateral aspect of the middle turbinate. **c** Same patient as in (**b**). The vertical portion of both uncinate processes (*vUP*) reaches the vertical lamella (*vlMT*) of the middle turbinates

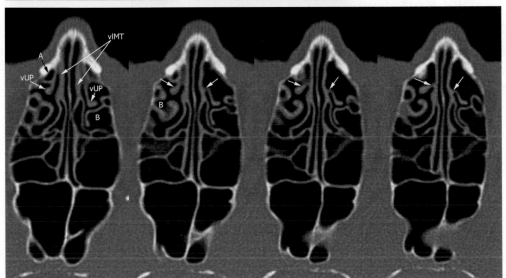

racea, and type 2, insertion on the posteromedial wall of agger nasi cells, the middle turbinate serves as the medial border of the recess and the uppermost uncinate process provides its lateral limit. In type 3, a double insertion – to lamina papyracea (anteriorly) and to the junction of middle turbinate on cribriform plate (posteriorly) – is present. In type 4–6 – insertion to the junction of middle turbinate with the cribriform plate, to the fovea, to the middle turbinate, respectively – the uppermost uncinate process becomes the medial border of the recess, the bulla and lamina papyracea being the lateral limit.

As a result, the frontal recess may empty medial to the uncinate process being separated from the ethmoidal infundibulum (type 1–3), or it may run laterally to the uncinate and join the ethmoidal infundibulum (type 4–6).

Because the frontal recess is bordered, anteriorly, by the agger nasi cells, its width on the sagittal plane depends on the extent of their pneumatization (Fig. 2.6). Furthermore, the posterior border may also vary: it is formed by a single and continuous bony wall when the ground lamella of the bulla ethmoidalis reaches the ethmoid roof. Otherwise, when the ground lamella of the bulla does not insert on the skull base, the frontal recess communicates with a narrow space (sinus lateralis or retrobullar recess) extending above (suprabullar recess cell) and behind the bulla, posteriorly bordered by the ground lamella of the middle turbinate.

Anterior ethmoidal cells developed from the frontal recess may extend into the frontal sinus itself (bulla frontalis), making it rather difficult to distinguish the true frontal sinus from a bulla frontalis cell. Frontal cells have been defined by BENT et al. (1994) to derive from the anterior ethmoid sinus behind the agger nasi and to pneumatize the frontal recess above the agger nasi. Four types have been recognized: a single or several – a tier – frontal cell(s) located over the agger nasi identify type 1, and type 2, respectively. A single large cell extending cephalad into the frontal sinus belongs to type 3. Type 4 identifies a single isolated cell within the frontal sinus (Figs. 2.9–2.11). If not properly identified on a pre-surgical CT examination, the frontal cells type 3 and 4 may be mixed up for the real frontal sinus, potentially resulting in an incorrect procedure.

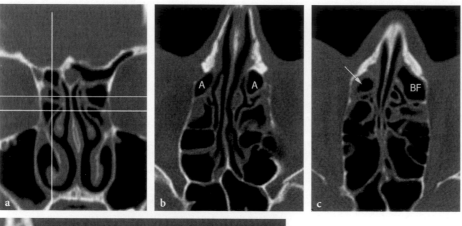

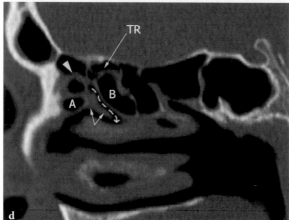

Fig. 2.9a–d. Bulla frontalis type I. a On the coronal image either agger nasi cells and frontal cells type I are shown. The axial plane (b) corresponds to the lower transversal grid on the coronal image. On the postero-medial aspect of the agger nasi cells the attachment of the uncinate processes is visible. The upper transversal grid cuts both frontal cells giving the axial plane in (c). Mucosal thickening on the internal surfaces on the right bulla frontalis (*arrow*). d The plane corresponds to the sagittal grid on (a). The bulla frontalis type I locates on the top of the agger nasi cell, abutting its roof and projecting into the frontal sinus (*arrowhead*). A terminal recess (*TR*) is present. *Small arrows* indicate the uncinate process. The *curved broken arrow* runs along the path of the frontal recess

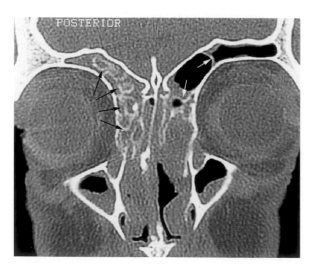

Fig. 2.10. Bilateral bulla frontalis, chronic sinusitis. A tier of several small frontal bullae – type II – is demonstrated on the *right side* (*black arrows*). Air has been replaced by fluid within bullae and frontal sinus (*FS*). A large bulla frontalis on the *left* (type III) is also detected (*white arrows*)

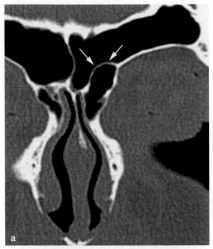

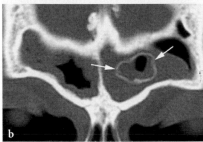

Fig. 2.11. a A large bulla frontalis type III projects into the right frontal sinus (*arrows*). b Demonstration of an isolated frontal cell type IV (*arrows*) with mucosal thickening inside (and within surrounding frontal sinusal walls)

2.1.4
Maxillary Sinus, Uncinate Process and Ethmoidal Infundibulum

Maxillary sinuses are the largest sinonasal cavities, bordered by four bony walls. On the anterior wall the distal opening of the infraorbital canal is found. This canal, through which the terminal branch of maxillary nerve courses (infraorbital nerve), is enclosed within the maxillary sinus roof. The infratemporal wall, which is the thinnest and most fragile, separates the maxillary sinus from the pterygopalatine fossa and masticator space, posteriorly.

The medial wall is more complex, it has a natural ostium (Figs. 2.2, 2.12) towards which mucus is actively transported by cilia, and some accessory ostia, normally bypassed by secretions, located either anteriorly and posteriorly to the maxillary ostium (anterior and posterior fontanellae) (Fig. 2.5). Because the horizontal portion (the fetal descending part) of the uncinate process inserts on the medial wall, the maxillary ostium does not directly communicate with the nasal fossa. Conversely, its ostium opens into the floor of a narrow space – i.e. the inferior aspect of the ethmoidal infundibulum (Fig. 2.12). To arrive into the middle meatus, secretions are transported upward along the ethmoidal infundibulum to reach the hiatus semilunaris, a horizontal 2D plane located between the anterior surface of the bulla ethmoidalis and the free margin of the unci-

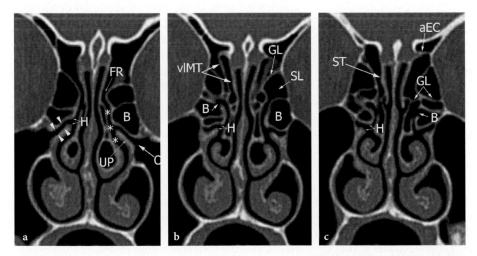

Fig. 2.12a–c. The coronal planes through anterior ethmoid sinus show the different components of the OMU. **a** The maxillary sinus ostium (*O*) communicates with the ethmoid infundibulum (*arrowheads* on *right side*). Ethmoid bulla (*B*) and uncinate process (*UP*) border the infundibulum. The air space between the bulla and the horizontal portion of the uncinate process is part of the hiatus semilunaris (*H*). Frontal recess (*FR*), ethmoid infundibulum and a more posterior opening of the bulla, small arrows on (**b**) and (**c**) open into the middle meatus (*asterisks*). **b** The air space between the attachment of middle turbinate onto the lamina papyracea (ground lamella, *GL*) and the posterior surface of the bulla is the sinus lateralis (*SL*). Pneumatized vertical lamella of the middle turbinate (*vlMT*), superior turbinate (*ST*), anterior canal of the ethmoid (*aEC*)

nate process (Fig. 2.6). The ethmoidal infundibulum is closed anteriorly by the vertical insertion of the uncinate process at the medial maxillary wall, generally forming a sharp angle onto the nasolacrimal duct bony wall (Fig. 2.5). Laterally, the upper portion of the ethmoidal infundibulum is bordered by the lamina papyracea, posteriorly by the ethmoidal bulla. The infundibulum may directly communicate with or be totally separated from the frontal recess depending on the configuration of the uncinate process (see Sect. 2.1.3).

2.1.5
Sphenoid Sinus

Two sinuses, separated by a bony septum that most often lies off the midline, pneumatize the body of sphenoid bone. Septations are frequently demonstrated within the cavities, they are all vertically oriented. Horizontal bony lamellae demonstrated on coronal CT scans belong to posterior ethmoid cells projecting toward or above the sphenoid sinuses. The ostium of sphenoid sinuses is located on the anterior wall, on their superior and medial aspect (Fig. 2.5). It communicates with the sphenoethmoidal recess and the posterior portion of the superior meatus. The sphenoid sinuses are strictly adjacent to relevant anatomic landmarks such as the superior orbital fissure, the optic canal, the cavernous sinus, and the internal carotid artery, laterally; the vault of nasopharynx, below; the hypophysis, above (Fig. 2.1–2.3).

2.2
Development of Nasosinusal Cavities

The size and shape of paranasal sinuses in infants and children differ from those of the adults, resulting in peculiar clinical entities and making surgery more difficult. Their development is linked with the development of the skull and with dentition (ANDERHUBER et al. 1992).

In the newborn only the ethmoid cells – with the uncinate process, ethmoidal bulla, and hiatus semilunaris – are well developed. They are separated by thick connective tissue that progressively reduces as the cells enlarge, resulting in thin bony septa in the adult. The maxillary sinus is just a shallow sac in the lateral nasal wall, the frontal and sphenoid sinuses are blind sacs only, that have not yet reached the frontal and sphenoid cartilage or bone. The turbinates are well developed and bulky. A superior turbinate is demonstrated

in more than 80% of specimens. All nasal meatus are very narrow, causing the newborn to breath through the common nasal meatus.

Between 1–4 years of age, the ethmoid sinus expands in all directions, appearing well developed compared to the other sinuses. The maxillary sinus extends laterally to the infraorbital canal, and caudally to the attachment of the inferior turbinate (WOLF et al. 1993). The frontal and sphenoid sinuses are going to start bone pneumatization, their size being still very small.

Between 4–8 years of age, the ethmoid cells expand more slowly than the frontal and maxillary sinuses. At the age of 7 the frontal sinus extends both medially and laterally into the frontal bone, and the maxillary sinus descends to the middle of the inferior meatus. There are two potentially dangerous situations due to the peculiar anatomy at this age: the uncinate process is close to the medial orbital wall, and the floor of the nose and the floor of the maxillary sinuses are still located at different levels. Uncinate removal is therefore associated with a higher risk of penetrating the lamina papyracea, likewise any attempt to enter the maxillary sinus from the inferior meatus may fail or cause damage of tooth buds.

Between 8–12 years of age, the pneumatization of paranasal sinuses resumes a faster pace. The ethmoid cells are completely developed, and any connective tissue is separating the cells. Due to the eruption of secondary dentition, the maxillary sinus expands causing the choanae to change from circular to rectangular.

Between 12 and 14 years of age, the maxillary sinus reaches the level of the floor of the nasal cavity, and extends to the zygomatic recess, laterally, and to the nasolacrimal duct, medially. The pneumatization of paranasal cavities is almost completed. The sphenoid sinus will reach its permanent size approximately at the age of 22 or 24.

2.3
Surgical Anatomy

Three anatomic areas, corresponding to the narrowest tracts of drainage pathways, are crucial for endoscopic surgery planning: the ostiomeatal (OMU), the frontal recess, and the sphenoethmoid recess.

The OMU is the crossroads of anterior ethmoid, frontal sinus and maxillary sinus mucus transport. This functional unit includes the ethmoidal infundibulum, the maxillary sinus ostium, the ethmoidal bulla, and the uncinate process (Fig. 2.12). The vertical portion of the uncinate process is the real key structure of OMU because its shape and upper attachment determine the morphology of both the ethmoidal infundibulum and the frontal recess.

The ethmoidal infundibulum is the air passage that connects the maxillary sinus ostium to the middle meatus. To simplify, it can be subdivided into two different portions. The anterior part is the air space located between the vertical portion of the uncinate and the anterior surface of the bulla; whereas the posterior part is the air space situated between the horizontal portion (free, unattached portion) of the uncinate process and the inferomedial surface of the bulla or of the orbit, if the sinus lateralis is present. The gap between the ethmoid bulla and the free edge of the uncinate process is the hiatus semilunaris (Fig. 2.6).

The ethmoid bulla is an important surgical landmark: this is actually the most posterior cell in the anterior ethmoid, protruding in the middle meatus. Its size and morphology are highly variable. The middle turbinate is the medial border of the OMU. This subtle, curved bony structure describes a lateral concavity; it has a cranial anchorage on the cribriform plate – through its vertical lamina – and a lateral insertion on the posterior part of lamina papyracea – through its fan-shaped ground lamella.

The width, path, and morphology of the frontal recess are largely determined by the shape and relationships of the upper part of the uncinate process (type 1–6, see Sect. 2.1.3) and by the variable size and pneumatization of adjacent structures, particularly the ethmoid bulla and agger nasi cells.

Moreover, even the configuration of the ethmoidal infundibulum – and its relationship to the frontal recess depend on the anatomy of the uncinate process (LANDSBERG and FRIEDMAN 2001). In most subjects (up to 52%) its lateral insertion on the lamina papyracea (type 1) creates a "roof" that closes the ethmoidal infundibulum in a blind upper pouch (terminal recess) (Fig. 2.7). If the uncinate process attaches anteriorly to the agger nasi cells (type 2, 18%) the ethmoidal infundibulum is closed superiorly by the floor of the agger nasi. In both configurations, the frontal recess and the ethmoidal infundibulum are separated, and the opening of the frontal recess into the middle meatus is medial to the ethmoidal infundibulum, between the uncinate process and the middle turbinate (Fig. 2.7). As in about 17% of subjects (type 3) the upper part of the uncinate process inserts on both the lamina papyracea and the junction of the middle turbinate with the lamina cribrosa, the frontal sinus opens into the middle meatus in approximately 88% of cases (type 1–3). Conversely, if the uncinate process maintains its complete and longest fetal attachment on the ethmoid

roof or medially on the middle turbinate, the frontal recess empties directly into the ethmoid infundibulum, therefore laterally to the uncinate process (Figs. 2.2, 2.8).

From a surgical standpoint, the correct assessment of the frontal recess opening is essential in planning the proper endonasal approach to the frontal recess and the adequate exposure of the frontal sinus. In fact, if the frontal recess opens laterally to the uncinate process, an attempt to find the recess medially to the uncinate would potentially lead toward the olfactory fossa or the frontal lobe.

Because the anterior and uppermost segment of the uncinate process runs obliquely from posterior-inferior to anterior-superior, direct coronal CT scans – obtained perpendicularly to the hard palate – usually do not demonstrate its full course and upper insertion. Multislice CT reconstructions obtained on an oblique plane running along the recess's axis enable a depiction of the actual extent (and insertion) of the unainale process.

The sphenoethmoid recess is outlined by the anterior sphenoid wall and by the posterior wall of posterior ethmoid cells. It conveys sphenoid sinus secretions in the superior meatus (Fig. 2.5).

2.4
Anatomic Variants

Anatomic variants of the OMU structures are relatively frequent; they can be classified as anomalies of size, shape, orientation and entity of pneumatization. In some cases they may impair the physiologic mucous drainage and condition the endoscopic approach. Nevertheless, it must be emphasized that the presence of an anatomic variant does not necessarily imply an increased risk of inflammatory lesion: actually, no direct correlation between anatomic anomalies and nasal obstruction has been clearly demonstrated.

2.4.1
Nasal Septum and Middle Turbinate

Nasal septum deviation is quite a common condition, with its prevalence in asymptomatic subjects reported to range from 20% to 30%; it is usually congenital but may be post-traumatic (WANAMAKER 1996). In most cases it is associated with the presence of a bone spur protruding in the nasal fossa, conflicting with the middle turbinate (less frequently with the inferior), and therefore reducing the diameter of the middle meatus (Fig. 2.13).

Middle turbinate describing a lateral convexity toward the lateral sinusal wall is classified as paradoxical: this variant may hamper an endoscopic approach (Fig. 2.7f). When the bulbous segment is pneumatized, the middle turbinate is referred to as concha bullosa (Figs. 2.2, 2.8). If only the attachment portion of the middle turbinate is pneumatized – with no involvement of the bulbous segment – it is defined lamellar concha (Fig. 2.7f). According to the extent of pneumatization (vertical lamina, bulbous segment, or both) and its entity, this anomaly may narrow or obstruct the ethmoidal infundibulum as well as the middle meatus, and may interfere with nasal airflow, particularly if associated with other anomalies that may obstruct the OMU, such as a large ethmoidal bulla (JOE et al. 2000) (Fig. 2.13). The prevalence of middle turbinate pneumatization on CT studies varies from 14% to 53% (LLOYD 1990; PEREZ et al. 2000). Concha bullosa is often bilateral (Fig. 2.12) and associated with septal deviation.

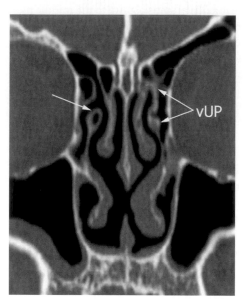

Fig. 2.14. Pneumatization of the vertical portion of the right uncinate process (*arrow*). The left inserts onto the fovea ethmoidalis [type 5 according to LANDSBERG and FRIEDMAN (2001)]. Note the focal nasal septum destruction due to cocaine abuse

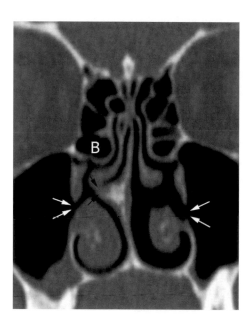

Fig. 2.13. Nasal septum deviation with a bone spur (*black arrows*) protruding into the right nasal fossa. An extensively pneumatized ethmoid bulla is present (*B*). Accessory maxillary sinus ostia (*white arrows*)

2.4.2
Uncinate Process

The most frequent variants are an anomalous curvature with the tip medially and downwardly oriented or the pneumatization of the uncinate process (up to

18% of subjects), the latter generally limited to the apex (uncinate bulla) (BOLGER et al. 1991) (Figs. 2.2, 2.14). Seldom, a hypoplastic uncinate process, tightly

adjacent to the lateral nasal wall or fused to the inferior aspect of the orbital floor or to the lamina papyracea, narrows the ethmoid infundibulum (*atelectatic infundibulum*). As a consequence underdevelopment of the maxillary sinus is observed along with intrasinusal mucous retention. In addition, the hypoplastic maxillary sinus is associated with a lower-than-normal location of the orbital floor. This variant has to be noted because of the higher risk of orbital damage at surgery. More rarely, the uncinate process may be absent.

2.4.3
Anterior Ethmoid Cells

During the development of ethmoid pneumatization, some cells may extend inferiorly and laterally to reach the medial orbital floor and the most inferior portion of the lamina papyracea, below the ethmoid bulla and lateral to the uncinate process (*infraorbital ethmoid cells or Haller cells*) (Fig. 2.15) (STACKPOLE and EDELSTEIN 1997). When large in size, these cells may narrow the ethmoid infundibulum. Size and

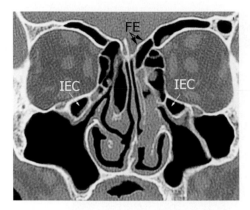

Fig. 2.15. Bilateral infraorbital ethmoid cells (*IEC*; Haller cells). *Black arrows* indicate the asymmetry of the fovea ethmoidalis (*FE*)

morphology of the ethmoid bulla are also highly variable: this cell may dislocate the ethmoid infundibulum and uncinate process (horizontalized). This variant has been considered by some authors to predispose for recurrent maxillary sinusitis. However, the definitive relationship between the presence of this variant and recurrent sinusitis is still debated (STAMMBERGER and WOLF 1988; BOLGER et al. 1991; LAINE and SMOKER 1992).

When extensively pneumatized, the ethmoid bullae may protrude into the middle meatus between the uncinate process and the middle turbinate and may narrow or obstruct the OMU (Figs. 2.3, 2.9, 2.13).

Agger nasi cells are the result of anterior extension of ethmoid cells to pneumatize the lacrimal bones (Figs. 2.6, 2.7, 2.9). Due to their location, agger nasi cells may obstruct the frontal recess.

Bulla frontalis indicates an ethmoid cell extending towards the frontal sinus. It is a rather complex variant and has been described in Sect. 2.1.3

2.4.4
Onodi Cells and Sphenoid Sinus

Onodi cells are the most hazardous variation since, if not reported before surgery, they may be a potential cause of severe complications. There are two definitions of Onodi cells in the literature. In the first they are defined as the most posterior ethmoid cells, superolateral to the sphenoid sinus and associated with a bulging, even if minimal, of the bony wall of the optic nerve (KAINZ and STAMMBERGER 1992) (Fig. 2.16). The second definition describes Onodi cells as posterior ethmoid cells extending into the sphenoid bone, either close to or impressed by the optic nerve bony wall (STAMMBERGER and KENNEDY 1995) (Fig. 2.17). The prevalence has been reported to range between 3.4% to 51%, this differ-

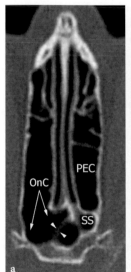

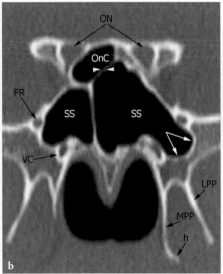

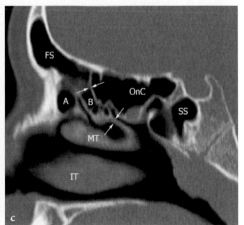

Fig. 2.16a–c. a On the axial plane the Onodi cell (*OnC*) arises on the right side from the posterior ethmoid and extends posteriorly and medially (*arrows*). **b** On the coronal plane the Onodi cell runs over the right and left sphenoid sinus roof (*arrowheads* indicate the thin left sphenoid sinus roof). The left sinus extends laterally into the pterygoid process (*arrows*). **c** On the sagittal plane a single large Onodi cell occupies the whole right posterior ethmoid sinus. *Opposite arrows* point to the ground lamella of the middle turbinate. Left posterior ethmoid cell (*PEC*), sphenoid sinus (*SS*), ethmoid bulla (*B*), frontal sinus (*FR*), agger nasi cell (*A*), middle (*MT*) and inferior (*IT*) turbinates, optic nerve and canals (*ON*), foramen rotundum (*FS*), vidian canal (*VC*), medial (*MPP*) and lateral (*LPP*) pterygoid plates, hamulus of medial pterygoid plate (*h*)

ence probably being related to the criteria used to classify this variant.

The sphenoid sinus itself displays highly variable degrees of pneumatization, including the anterior clinoid and pterygoid processes (Fig. 2.18). These variants may jeopardize endoscopic surgery, particularly when associated with focal areas of dehiscence of the bony walls of the sphenoid sinus. While a complete dehiscence of the bone covering the optic nerve (12%–22%) or the internal carotid artery (8%) has been infrequently found, a paper-thin bony lamina covering these bulgings has been observed more often (KAINZ and STAMMBERGER 1992; DELANO et al. 1996;).

It is important for the radiologist not only to detect thinning or dehiscences of the lateral sphenoid sinus walls but also to precisely assess the relationship of the sphenoid sinus and posterior ethmoid

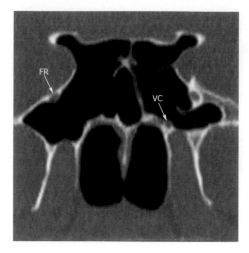

Fig. 2.18. Extensive pneumatization of the anterior clinoid and of the pterygoid processes of both sphenoid sinuses. Foramen rotundum (*FR*), vidian canal (*VC*)

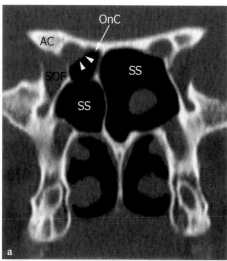

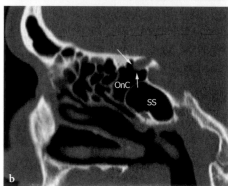

Fig. 2.17a,b. Right Onodi cell (*OnC*) associated with optic nerve canal dehiscence – *arrowheads* on (**a**), *arrows* on (**b**). Sphenoid sinus (*SS*), superior orbital fissure (*SOF*), anterior clinoid (*AC*)

cells with the internal carotid artery and the optic nerve. DELANO et al. (1996) classified the relationship with the optic nerve in four different types. In type 1, the nerve does not contact or impinge either the sphenoid or posterior ethmoid cells. In type 2, the nerve indents the sphenoid sinus, without contacting the posterior ethmoid cells. In type 3, the nerve runs through the sphenoid sinus, and it is surrounded by the pneumatized sinus for at least 50%. In type 4, the nerve courses close to both the sphenoid sinus and posterior ethmoid cells.

2.4.5
Asymmetry of Ethmoid Roof

The morphology of the ethmoid roof is usually inconstant. Asymmetry of the cribriform plate may be seen, directly related to the length of the vertical lamella, that inserts on it (Fig. 2.15). It has been observed in about 10% of patients (DESSI et al. 1994; LEBOWITZ et al. 2001). During surgery, this anomaly entails an increased risk of iatrogenic CSF fistulization or of injury of the anterior ethmoid artery, which courses along the most lateral aspect of the cribriform plate (Fig. 2.12). The depth of the ethmoid roof has been classified by KEROS (1962) in three different types. In type 1 the vertical lamella of the cribriform plate is very short, therefore the olfactory fossa is almost flat; in type 2 the vertical lamella is longer, the olfactory fossa deeper; in type 3 the vertical lamella is particularly long (more than 13 mm) and the roof of the ethmoid is noticeably higher than the cribriform plate. This variation has to be known, because the deeply located olfactory fossa places the thin vertical lamella at risk of penetration during endonasal surgery (KEROS 1962).

Finally, dehiscences and medial deviations can also be found at the level of the lamina papyracea (Fig. 2.19). In most cases they occur close to the insertion of the ground lamella of the middle turbinate into the lamina papyracea. They may be either congenital or due to trauma. Whichever the case excessive medial deviation or dehiscence constitute essential information prior to endonasal surgery. If not known prior to surgery, the risk of intra-orbital penetration is very high.

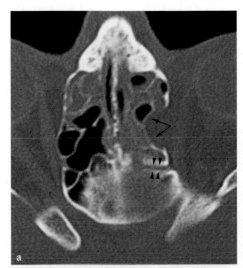

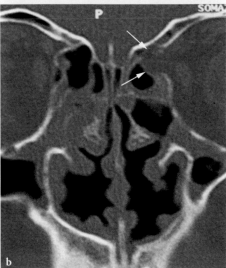

Fig. 2.19a,b. Polyposis and post-traumatic medial deviation of left lamina papyracea (*arrows*) with partial dehiscence of bone. *Arrowheads* point to the posterior ethmoid canal

2.5
Pterygopalatine Fossa and Pterygoid Process

On axial images the pterygopalatine fossa is a thin rectangular fat filled space between the pterygoid process of the sphenoid bone – posteriorly – and the perpendicular plate of the palatine bone – anteriorly, the latter being not separable on CT or MR from the posterior maxillary sinus wall, therefore appearing "fused" into a single bone structure (Fig. 2.20). On sagittal images the space progressively narrows downward where it connects to the pterygopalatine canal (Fig. 2.21).

The pterygopalatine fossa communicates with five different areas: the middle cranial fossa, through the pterygoid (vidian) canal and foramen rotundum/canal; the orbit, through the inferior orbital fissure; the masticator space – or infratemporal fossa – through the pterygomaxillary fissure; the choana, through the sphenopalatine foramen; the oral cavity, through the greater and lesser palatine canals.

Within the pterygopalatine fossa are the pterygopalatine ganglion, part of the maxillary nerve, terminal branches of the internal maxillary artery (the sphenopalatine artery) and fat.

On coronal planes, the pterygoid canal is lower and medial compared to the foramen rotundum, which is higher up, more lateral and larger. Moreover, the foramen rotundum may actually consist of a simple groove – rather than of a complete canal – running on the superior aspect of the pterygoid process (Fig. 2.22). On the axial plane, the pterygoid canal has a more triangular (or "trumpet-like") appearance, being larger at its anterior opening into the pterygopalatine fossa. It communicates, posteriorly, with the foramen lacerum, ending in front of the petrous apex, whereas the foramen rotundum/canal reaches the fluid-content of the Meckel cave. Depending on the degree of sphenoid sinus pneumatization, the pterygoid canal may be almost entirely within the bone, partially or completely surrounded by the sinus.

On coronal MR, the maxillary nerve may be clearly identified using VIBE sequences (Fig. 2.22c). A hypointense rounded structure is shown within the foramen, surrounded by homogeneous enhanced signal, probably due to tiny vessels running along the foramen and the nerve. Due to its smaller size, the pterygoid nerve is not usually demonstrated by this technique, only the enhanced vessels within the canal are detected.

The pterygopalatine fossa transmits the infraorbital nerve and artery to the orbit via the inferior orbital fissure. This fissure separates the orbital

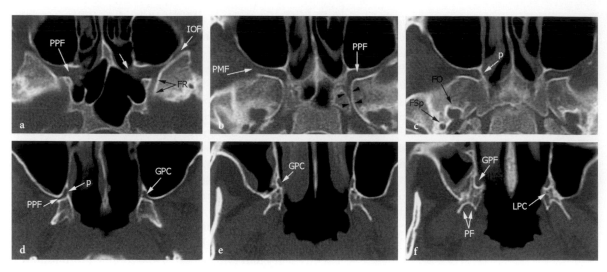

Fig. 2.20a–f. Axial CT through the vertical extent of the pterygopalatine fossa from the upper down to the lower limit. **a** The rectangular pterygopalatine fossa (*PPF*) opens posteriorly into the foramen rotundum (*FR*), superolaterally into the inferior orbital fissure (*IOF*). *Arrow points* to the sphenopalatine foramen. **b** The pterygoid – vidian – canal (*black arrowheads*) has a large anterior opening. Laterally the PPF communicates with the infratemporal fossa via the pterygomaxillary fissure (*PMF*). **c** The foramen ovale (*FO*) and spinosum (*FSp*) are demonstrated on the greater sphenoid wing. Perpendicular plate of the palatine bone (*p*). **d–f** Progressive narrowing of the PPF and onset of greater (*GPC*) and lesser (*LPC*) palatine canals. Greater palatine foramen (*GPF*), pterygoid fossa – scaphoid fossa – (*PF*)

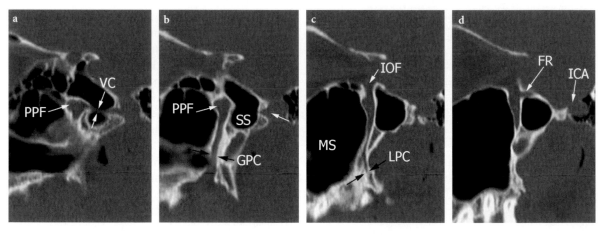

Fig. 2.21a–d. Sagittal CT through the pterygopalatine fossa from medial to lateral. **a** Most medial aspect of the fossa (*PPF*), posteriorly communicating with the pterygoid – vidian –canal (*VC*), completely surrounded by a largely pneumatizing sphenoid sinus (*SS*). **b** The whole vertical extent of the fossa and the greater palatine canal (*GPC*) are located posteriorly to the "fused" perpendicular plate of the palatine bone and posterior maxillary sinus wall. The *white arrow* indicates the posterior opening of the pterygoid canal in front of the petrous apex. **c** The lesser palatine canal (*LPC*) runs laterally and posteriorly to the greater one. The fossa superiorly communicates with the inferior orbital fissure (*IOF*). **d** The most lateral aspect of the fossa, posteriorly it continues into the foramen rotundum (*FR*)

floor from the lateral orbital wall. Because it is angled about 45° to the orientation of the infraorbital canal, the infraorbital nerve has a "bayonet-like" shape as it runs from the infraorbital canal into the pterygopalatine fossa (Fig. 2.23). The infraorbital canal runs parallel to the orbital floor, between the middle and lateral third, except for its anterior por-

tion where it bends downward to the infraorbital foramen (Fig. 2.24).

Laterally, the pterygopalatine fossa communicates with the retromaxillary fat of the masticator space/infratemporal fossa via the pterygomaxillary fissure; medially it transmits the nasopalatine nerve (a branch of the maxillary nerve), posterior supe-

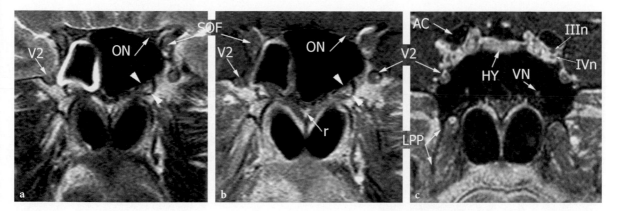

Fig. 2.22a–c. Coronal plane through the pterygoid process. **a,b** TSE T2 and enhanced SE T1 sequences in the same patient. On the *right side* the foramen rotundum is a groove, on the *left* a complete canal. On T2 and Gd-T1, V2 appears as a small hypointense structure within the foramen. *Arrowheads* indicate the anterior (oval) opening of the pterygoid canal. **c** Enhanced VIBE sequence (0.5-mm thickness) shows V2 probably surrounded by enhanced veins, similar to the adjacent cavernous sinus where III and IV nerves are demonstrated. Enhancing vessels surround the pterygoid nerve (*VN*). Bilateral pneumatized anterior clinoids (*AC*). Optic nerve (*ON*), hypophysis (*HY*), superior orbital fissure (*SOF*), rostrum of the splenoid bone (*r*), lateral pterygoid plate (*LPP*)

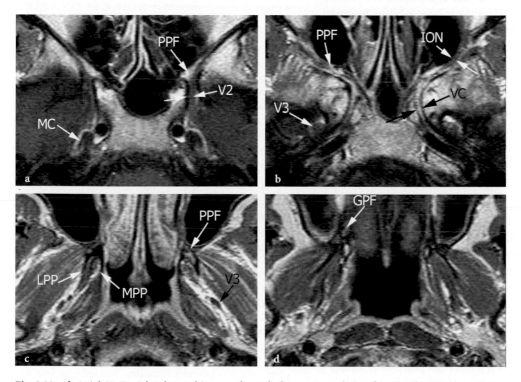

Fig. 2.23a–d. Axial SE T1 Gd-enhanced images through the pterygopalatine fossa. **a** The PPF communicates with the foramen rotundum, posteriorly. The hypointense linear structure running through the foramen rotundum is the maxillary nerve (*V2*). Meckel cave (*MC*). **b** The pterygoid (vidian) canal (*black arrows*, *VC*) has a wider anterior opening into the PPF, it reaches posteriorly the foramen lacerum/petrous apex. *Bayonet-like* course of the infraorbital nerve (*ION*) from PPF into the infraorbital fissure. Mandibular nerve (*V3*). **c** Inferior narrowing of the PPF. Medial (*MPP*) and lateral (*LPP*) pterygoid plates. **d** Opening of the greater palatine canal (*GPF*) at the level of the hard palate

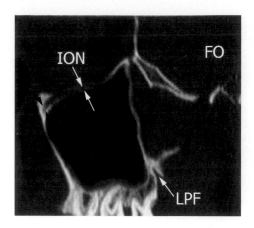

Fig. 2.24. Sagittal plane through the infraorbital canal and infraorbital nerve (*ION*), parallel to the orbital floor until its anterior portion where it turns downward (*arrowheads*) toward the foramen. Foramen ovale (*FO*), lesser palatine foramen (*LPF*)

rior nasal nerves, and the sphenopalatine vessels into the nasal cavity via the sphenopalatine foramen. Inferiorly, the fossa progressively narrows to end in the greater and lesser palatine canals. Along the first are the greater palatine nerve and vessels, the ascending palatine artery and the lesser palatine nerves run within the second canal. The greater palatine foramen opens at the angle formed by the junction of the perpendicular plate with the horizontal plate of the palatine bone (Fig. 2.4).

The anterior two thirds of the hard palate are formed by the palatine processes of the maxillary bones, posteriorly they articulate with the horizontal plates of the palatine bone.

From the pterygoid process arise two plates, the medial more vertically oriented than the lateral one that diverges from the sagittal plane. Posteriorly they enclose a space called the pterygoid – scaphoid – fossa. The lateral – external – pterygoid muscle inserts on the external surface of the lateral plate, the medial – internal – pterygoid muscle arises from the medial surface of the same plate (within the scaphoid fossa). The tensor veli palatini muscle inserts on the medial plate, its tendon runs downward, under a curved process of the medial pterygoid plate (hamulus) to reach the soft palate.

2.6
Nasal Septum

The nasal septum comprises the septal cartilage, anteriorly, the perpendicular plate of the ethmoid bone

supero-posteriorly, and the vomer infero-posteriorly. The rostrum of the sphenoid bone fits into a groove on the superior surface of the vomer (Fig. 2.5). At the base of the nasal septum is the nasal crest formed by the maxillary and palatine bones.

On either side of the upper nasal septum is a narrow space – the olfactory recess – that ends up with the horizontal portion of the cribriform plate. Posteriorly, the olfactory recess widens into the sphenoethmoidal recess (Fig. 2.5).

References

Anderhuber W, Weiglein A, Wolf G (1992) Nasal cavities and paranasal sinuses in newborns and children. Acta Anat (Basel) 144:120-126

Bent J, Cuilty-Siller C, Kuhn FA (1994) The frontal cell as a cause of frontal sinus obstruction. Am J Rhinol 8:185-191

Bolger WE, Butzin CA, Parsons DS (1991) Paranasal sinus bony anatomic variations and mucosal abnormalities: CT analysis for endoscopic sinus surgery. Laryngoscope 101:56-64

DeLano MC, Fun FY, Zinreich SJ (1996) Relationship of the optic nerve to the posterior paranasal sinuses: a CT anatomic study. AJNR Am J Neuroradiol 17:669-675

Dessi P, Moulin G, Triglia JM et al (1994) Difference in the height of the right and left ethmoidal roofs: a possible risk factor for ethmoidal surgery. Prospective study of 150 CT scans. J Laryngol Otol 108:261-262

Joe JK, Ho SY, Yanagisawa E (2000) Documentation of variations in sinonasal anatomy by intraoperative nasal endoscopy. Laryngoscope 110:229-235

Kainz J, Stammberger H (1992) Danger areas of the posterior rhinobasis. An endoscopic and anatomical-surgical study. Acta Otolaryngol 112:852-861

Keros P (1962) On the practical value of differences in the level of the lamina cribrosa of the ethmoid. Z Laryngol Rhinol Otol 41:809-813

Kim SS, Lee JG, Kim KS et al (2001) Computed tomographic and anatomical analysis of the basal lamellas in the ethmoid sinus. Laryngoscope 111:424-429

Laine FJ, Smoker WR (1992) The ostiomeatal unit and endoscopic surgery: anatomy, variations, and imaging findings in inflammatory diseases. AJR Am J Roentgenol 159:849-857

Landsberg R, Friedman M (2001) A computer-assisted anatomical study of the nasofrontal region. Laryngoscope 111:2125-2130

Lebowitz RA, Terk A, Jacobs JB et al (2001) Asymmetry of the ethmoid roof: analysis using coronal computed tomography. Laryngoscope 111:2122-2124

Lloyd GA (1990) CT of the paranasal sinuses: study of a control series in relation to endoscopic sinus surgery. J Laryngol Otol 104:477-481

Perez P, Sabate J, Carmona A et al (2000) Anatomical variations in the human paranasal sinus region studied by CT. J Anat 197(Pt 2):221-227

Stackpole SA, Edelstein DR (1997) The anatomic relevance of the Haller cell in sinusitis. Am J Rhinol 11:219-223

Stammberger H, Kennedy DW (1995) Paranasal sinuses: anatomic terminology and nomenclature. The Anatomic Terminology Group. Ann Otol Rhinol Laryngol Suppl 167:7-16

Stammberger H, Wolf G (1988) Headaches and sinus disease: the endoscopic approach. Ann Otol Rhinol Laryngol Suppl 134:3-23

Wanamaker HH (1996) Role of Haller's cell in headache and sinus disease: a case report. Otolaryngol Head Neck Surg 114:324-327

Wolf G, Anderhuber W, Kuhn F (1993) Development of the paranasal sinuses in children: implications for paranasal sinus surgery. Ann Otol Rhinol Laryngol 102:705-711

3 Physiology of the Nose and Paranasal Sinuses

Davide Tomenzoli

CONTENTS

3.1   Introduction   *29*
3.2   Breathing   *29*
3.3   Mucociliary System   *30*
3.4   Filtration   *30*
3.5   Heating and Humidification   *31*
3.6   Antimicrobial Defense   *31*
3.7   Reflex Action   *31*
3.8   Recovery of Water   *31*
3.9   Resonance   *32*
3.10   Olfactory Function   *32*
3.11   The Role of Paranasal Sinuses   *32*
3.11.1 Lighten the Skull for Equipoise of the Head   *32*
3.11.2 Impart Resonance to the Voice   *32*
3.11.3 Increase the Olfactory Area   *33*
3.11.4 Thermal Insulation of Vital Parts   *33*
3.11.5 Secretion of Mucus to Moisten the Nasal Cavity   *33*
3.11.6 Humidify and Warm the Inspired Air   *33*
3.11.7 Absorption of Stress with Possible Avoidance
        of Concussion   *33*
3.11.8 Influence on Facial Growth and Architecture   *33*
        References   *34*

3.1
Introduction

Many papers and investigations on nasal physiology have been published in the last 40 years; as a consequence, knowledge of nasal functions has now been well established. In contrast, however, the role of the human paranasal sinuses remains as much an enigma today as it was nearly two millennia ago (BLANEY 1990). According to COLE (1998), the conclusive evidence of a functional relevance of the paranasal sinuses has yet to be found. Even though the existence of the paranasal sinuses may be unexplained, their susceptibility to disease is a common

D. TOMENZOLI, MD
Department of Otorhinolaryngology, University of Brescia, Piazzale Spedali Civili 1, Brescia, BS, 25123, Italy

source of suffering for patients and a focus of attention for clinicians.

"Physiologic" breathing occurs through the nose; it may be supplemented by oral respiration under demanding conditions of exercise or of severe nasal obstruction. Nasal fossae may not only be considered the front door of the respiratory system, but are also characterized by peculiar and significant functions other than breathing: conditioning and moistening of the nasal air-flow, filtration of inspired noxious materials, specific and non-specific antibacterial and antiviral activities, reflex action, collection of water from expired airflow, olfactory function.

3.2
Breathing

Every day 10,000 l of ambient air reach lower respiratory airways for pulmonary ventilation. Air enters the nose through the nostrils, as a consequence of a pressure gradient existing between external ambient and pulmonary alveoli, and converges through the so-called nasal valve, positioned in the anterior part of the nasal fossa just behind the nasal vestibulum. The term "nasal valve" refers to an area lying on a perpendicular plane to the anteroposterior axis of the nasal fossa, which is bordered medially by the nasal septum, laterally by the head of the inferior turbinate and superiorly by the posterior margin of the lateral crus of the alar cartilage. This restricted area accounts for about 50% of the total resistance of the respiratory system and gives rise to a laminar airflow. As inspiratory air leaves the narrow valvular area and enters the much larger cross-section of the nasal fossa, its velocity decelerates from 18 m/s to 4 m/s and the laminar airflow becomes turbulent. When airflow reaches nasal fossa it splits into three air streams, the largest of which flows over the superior edge of the inferior turbinate. A second smaller airflow (about 5%–10%) runs along the olfactory mucosa localized on the roof of the nasal fossa, the medial surface of the upper and middle turbinates, and the opposed part of the septum. Finally, a minimal flow runs on the floor of the nasal fossa (Fig. 3.1). The subdivision of the nasal airflow and the presence of a turbulent flow allows the maximal distribution of inspired air throughout the nasal cavity, enabling exchanges of heat, water and contaminants between the inspired air and the respiratory mucosa.

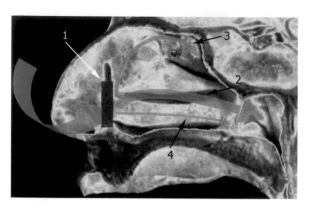

Fig. 3.1. Breathing at rest. Inspired air once it has passed through the nasal valve (*red area*, *1*) divides into three air streams. The main one flows along the middle turbinate (*2*); the second and third flow along the ethmoid roof (*3*) and nasal fossa floor (*4*)

3.3
Mucociliary System

Nasal mucosa presents a ciliated columnar pseudostratified epithelium that lines the nose and the paranasal sinuses and is bounded by squamous epithelium at the level of the nasal vestibulum. The area of the luminal surface of the sinonasal epithelium is greatly expanded by 300–400 microvilli x cell. Also, columnar cells bear about a hundred cilia x cell beating 1000 x/min in sequence with those of neighboring ciliated cells (MYGIND 1978). The cilia beat in a serous periciliary fluid of low viscosity. The beat of a single cilium consists of a rapid forward beat and a slow return beat with a time ratio of 1:3. Within a limited mucosal area all cilia beat in the same direction; the cilia beat synchronously in parallel ranks one after another forming metachronous waves that transport the exogenous particles toward rhinopharynx. Cilia are plunged in a mucus blanket that is made up of a double liquid layer: a superficial viscous sheet

of mucus and an underlying layer of serous fluid. This fluid is deep enough to avoid entanglement of the cilia with the viscoelastic mucus that floats on its surface enabling the mucus (which contains entrapped contaminants, microorganisms and debris) to be propelled along well-established routes to the pharynx, where it is swallowed (Fig. 3.2). Serous and seromucinous glands localized in the intermediate layer of the lamina propria, and the intraepithelial goblet cells are the producers of the periciliary fluid and the thick viscoelastic mucus (COLE 1998; NISHIHIRA and McCAFFREY 1987).

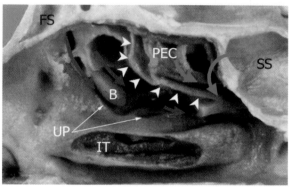

Fig. 3.2. Prechambers and paths of normal mucous drainage. Structures are demonstrated after subtotal removal of middle turbinate. Frontal sinus, anterior ethmoid cells, and maxillary sinus drain into the middle meatus (*red arrows*). The sphenoid sinus and posterior ethmoid cells drain into the superior meatus (*blue arrows*). *Arrowheads* indicate the insertion of the middle turbinate's ground lamella on the lateral nasal wall. *FS*, frontal sinus; *B*, bulla ethmoidalis; *PEC*, posterior ethmoid cells; *SS*, sphenoid sinus; *UP*, uncinate process; *IT*, inferior turbinate

3.4
Filtration

The inspired air contains a great amount of suspended exogenous particulate material. The upper respiratory tract, especially the nose, must act as the first line of defense and plays a significant role as a protective filter for particles as well as for irritant gases. Turbulence and impingement cause deposition of particles just behind the constricted area of the nasal valve. Thus, the nose is normally the principal site of particle deposition, but the efficacy of this nasal filter depends on the diameter of the particles inhaled (MUIR 1972). Few particles greater than 10 µm are able to penetrate the nose during breathing at rest, while particles smaller than 1 µm are not filtered out, reaching the delicate structures of the alveoli. Deposited particles, between 10 and 1 µm in diameter, are removed from the nasal mucosa within 6–15 min depending on the efficacy of the mucociliary system.

3.5
Heating and Humidification

The blood vessels of the nasal mucosa are of paramount importance for the functions of heating and humidification. As reported by detailed studies (CAUNA 1970) the arterioles of the nasal mucosa are characterized by the total absence of the internal elastic membrane so that the endothelial basement membrane is continuous with the basement membrane of the smooth muscle cells. In addition, nasal blood vessels are also characterized by porosity of endothelial basement membrane so that the subendothelial musculature of these vessels may be rapidly influenced by agents and drugs carried in the blood. Between the capillaries and the venules are interposed the cavernous sinusoids; these are localized in the lower layer of the lamina propria especially on the inferior turbinates. Cavernous sinusoids are regarded as specialized capillaries adapted to some of the functional demands of the airway, i.e. moistening and heating of the inspired air. Nasal blood vessels can be classified according to their principal function into capacitance, resistance and exchange vessels. The amount of sinonasal blood volume depends on the tone of the capacitance vessels (mainly venous vessels and cavernous sinusoids), while the blood flow on the tone of resistance vessels (mainly small arteries, arterioles and arteriovenous anastomoses). Finally, transport through the walls of vessels takes place in the exchange vessels (mainly capillaries).

Nasal air condition also depends on a number of factors other than nasal blood vessels such as seromucous glands, goblet cells, plasmatic transudate and lacrimal secretion. Furthermore, the nose has additional properties that contribute to heating and humidifying inspired air such as: maximum wall contact for the mixed flow of air (laminar and turbulent, according to the different areas of the nasal cavities); the ability to change the turbinates cross-section depending on the variation in temperature and humidity of the ambient air; the large amount of blood flowing rapidly through the arteriovenous anastomoses of the turbinates; the contribution to the inhaled air of atomized watery secretion from serous glands.

3.6
Antimicrobial Defense

In addition to physical removal of microorganisms and other noxious materials by mucociliary transport, an important line of defense is provided by the surface fluids that contain macrophages, basophils and mast cells, leucocytes, eosinophils, and antibacterial/antiviral substances that include immunoglobulins, lactoferrin, lysozymes and interferon. These cells and substances discourage microbial colonization and enhance the protective properties of the sinonasal mucosa against infections.

3.7
Reflex Action

Nasal mucosa is supplied by nerves from the somatic and autonomic systems. The sensory fibers travel with the trigeminal nerve, while the parasympathetic fibers are derived from the facial nerve and the sympathetic fibers from the superior cervical ganglion.

Afferent impulses are transported via the sensory fibers to the central nervous system giving rise to tickling or pain. Efferent impulses are propagated through autonomic, vasomotor and secretory-motor nerve fibers. The stimulation of nasal mucosa results in sneezing, watery rhinorrhea and changes in blood flow (ALLISON and POWIS 1971).

Other than nasal effects, the stimulation of the nasal mucosa can produce systemic reflexes as the inhibition of respiration due to an increase in airway resistance or laryngospasm. Furthermore, an increase in resistance in vessels of the skin, muscle, splanchnic and kidney circulation can be observed. Finally, cardiac output is reduced during nasal stimulation as a result of bradycardia (ANGELL and DALY 1972).

3.8
Recovery of Water

During expiration warm air coming from the lower airway condenses in the anterior part of the nose, which has a temperature 4°C lower than that of the lung. With this mechanism, called the "piggy bank" function, the nose is able to recover about 100 ml of water everyday. Nevertheless, during nasal breath-

ing at room temperature the daily total loss is about
500 ml of water and 300 kcal (INGELSTEDT and
TOREMALM 1961).

3.9
Resonance

Even though it can not be considered a vital function,
the nose acts as a resonance box which gives its contribution, together with paranasal sinuses and pharynx,
to the characterization of the tone of the voice.

3.10
Olfactory Function

The superior turbinate, the cribriform plate, the
upper surface of the middle turbinate and the opposed part of the nasal septum are covered by a
specialized epithelium containing receptors cells.
The sense of smell is mediated via stimulation
of these olfactory receptors by volatile chemicals.
Five different types of cells form the olfactory epithelium: the bipolar olfactory neuron, which is a
primary sensory neuron with an olfactory knob
from which several olfactory cilia extend; the basal
cell, which replaces the bipolar neuron cells every
7 weeks; sustentacular cell, which acts as a support
cell supplying nutrients for bipolar neuron cells;
microvillar cell, which have no clearly defined role
except to perhaps assist olfaction; Bowman's glands,
which provide a serous component to the mucous
layer covering the olfactory epithelium (RICE and
GLUCKMAN 1995).

The exact mechanism of olfaction is somewhat
vague. Multiple theories have been proposed but
none have really been supported scientifically. There
is some suggestion that different odors produce different patterns of activity across the olfactory mucosa. Whatever the explanation at the molecular
level, depolarization of the bipolar neurons occurs,
resulting in an action potential that is transmitted
along the olfactory nerve, and the information is
processed centrally in the olfactory tubercle, pyriform cortex, amygdaloid nucleus, and hypothalamus. Interestingly enough, olfactory receptor cells
are the only nerve cells capable of regeneration,
allowing for (at least theoretically) the possibility
of regeneration after severe injury (LAFFORT et al.
1974).

3.11
The Role of Paranasal Sinuses

No conclusive theory on the role of paranasal sinuses
has been accepted yet. Some authors have suggested
a functional role, while others have argued that the
paranasal sinuses in higher primates are merely non-
functional remnants of a common mammalian an-
cestor. The following sections review the different
theories.

3.11.1
Lighten the Skull for Equipoise of the Head

This is the oldest of all theories. The first objection
came from BRAUNE and CLASEN (1877), who claimed
that if the sinuses were filled with spongy bone the
total weight of the head would be increased by only
1%. Despite statements that man's musculature is adequate to maintain head poise regardless of the state
of paranasal sinuses (FLOTTES et al. 1960), it was not
until 1969 that an electromyographic investigation
was made of the activity of human neck muscles in
response to loading the anterior aspect of the head.
It was concluded that the human paranasal sinuses
are not significant as weight reducers of the skull for
maintenance of equipoise of the head (BIGGS and
BLANTON 1970).

3.11.2
Impart Resonance to the Voice

In the seventeenth century, Bartholinus asserted that
paranasal sinuses are important phonatory adjuncts
in that they aid resonance. This theory received support from HOWELL (1917), when he stated that the
peculiar quality or timbre of the individual voice
arises from the accessory sinuses and the bony framework of the face. This conclusion was related to the
observation that Maori – who have a small frontal
sinus – possess a peculiarly dead voice. BLANTON
and BIGGS (1969) also supported this theory on the
basis that the howling monkeys possess particularly
large paranasal sinuses. Nevertheless, a few authors
discounted the resonance theory by observing that
animals with loud voices such as the lion can have
small sinuses (PROETZ 1953), or that other animals,
such as the giraffe and rabbit, have small or shrill,
non-resonant voices despite having large sinus cavities (NEGUS 1958). Finally, FLOTTES et al. (1960)
reported that the physical properties of paranasal

sinuses make them poor resonators and added that sinus surgery does not modify the voice.

3.11.3
Increase the Olfactory Area

This theory arose when Cloquet (1830) incorrectly stated that the human maxillary sinus was lined with olfactory epithelium such as in some mammals. On the contrary, the mucous membrane of the human paranasal sinuses is made up of non-olfactory epithelium, but is lined by a thinner, less vascular mucosa which is more loosely fixed to the bony wall than that of the respiratory region of the nasal cavity.

3.11.4
Thermal Insulation of Vital Parts

This theory was originally proposed by Proetz (1953) who compared the paranasal sinuses to an air-jacket enveloping the nasal fossae. Nevertheless, Eskimos often possess no frontal sinus, while African Negroes possess large frontal sinuses (Blaney 1990).

3.11.5
Secretion of Mucus to Moisten the Nasal Cavity

This theory is also discounted on the basis of histology. First advocated by Haller (1763, reported by Wright 1914) it proposes that the sinuses are important for moistening the nasal olfactory mucosa. However, Skillen (1920) and Negus (1958) observed that an adequate amount of mucus for this purpose cannot be secreted by the human paranasal sinuses lining. In contrast to the nose with its 100,000 submucosal glands, the sinuses have only 50–100 glands (Dahl and Mygind 1998).

3.11.6
Humidify and Warm the Inspired Air

It has long been known that air exchange takes place in the sinuses during respiration. However, a debate existed as to whether this exchange occurs to enable humidification and warming of inspired air. Aerated sinuses develop in large swiftly moving mammals with an active respiration, while slow moving mammals, especially those living in a humid medium like the hippopotamus, have small sinuses (Flottes et

al. 1960). However, some authors demonstrated that exchange of gases between the nose and paranasal sinuses is negligible and thus also the contribution of the sinuses to the conditioning of the inspired air proves to be insignificant (Paulsson et al. 2001).

3.11.7
Absorption of Stress with Possible Avoidance of Concussion

This theory originated from Negus' work on horned ungulates (Negus 1958). He noted that the air spaces which extend over the cranial vault and into the horns, such as the ox and goat, are sometimes explained as stress distributors. However, in other horned ungulates such as the moose, the horns are attached directly to the cranium without air spaces. Rui (1960) observed that the sinus complex could be considered as a pyramidal buffer with the base situated anteriorly and the apex at the sphenoid thus forming an architectural structure suited to a protective function of endocranial structures.

3.11.8
Influence on Facial Growth and Architecture

According to Proetz (1953) the paranasal sinuses are the result of a plastic rearrangement of the skull as a consequence of a disproportionate growth of the face and cranium and associated structures after they are fully or partly ossified. However, Negus (1958) documented that individuals with a single frontal sinus do not show a defective facial growth. Eckel (1963) attributed the presence of sinus cavities to strains and stress of the skull created solely by the pressure exerted by the chewing apparatus. However, Takahashi (1984) emphasized that the shape of the neurocranium and cranial base must also be considered important elements. He stated that in the evolution of mammals from primates to humans, sinuses originally acted as an aid to olfaction, but were influenced by the retraction of the maxillofacial box and by the process of cerebral enlargement. The development of human paranasal sinuses is thus the result of an increase in the angle between the forehead and frontal cranial base, and decrease in the angle of the cranial base at the sella turcica.

In conclusion, according to Blaney (1990), it is becoming apparent that an architectural theory is far more likely in that it is known that craniofacial form has an important bearing on paranasal sinus morphology. Further research into craniofacial form and development needs to be done before the exact role of the paranasal sinuses in humans can be definitively clarified or established. It is encouraging that the more recent studies have emphasized the importance of differential sinuses (TAKAHASHI 1984; BLANEY 1986). With the advent of new imaging techniques much accurate data about paranasal sinus size and morphology can be collected and further differential growth studies performed.

References

Allison DJ, Powis DA (1971) Adrenal catecholamine secretion during stimulation of the nasal mucous membrane in the rabbit. J Physiol (Lond) 217:327-339

Angell JJ, Daly MB (1972) Reflex respiratory and cardiovascular effects of stimulation of receptors in the nose of the dog. J Physiol (Lond) 220:673-696

Biggs NL, Blanton PL (1970) The role of paranasal sinuses as weight reducers of the head determined by electromyography of postural neck muscles. J Biomech 3:255-262

Blaney SPA (1986) An allometric study of the frontal sinus in gorilla, pan and pongo. Folia Primatol 47:81-96

Blaney SPA (1990) Why paranasal sinuses? J Laryngol Otol 104:690-693.

Blanton PL, Biggs NL (1969) Eighteen hundred years of controversy: the paranasal sinuses. Am J Anat 124:135-147

Braune W, Clasen FE (1877) Die Nebenhöhlen der Menschlichen Nase in ihre Bedeutung für den Mechanismus des Riechens. Z Anat Entwicklungsgesch 2:1-15

Cauna N (1970) Electron microscopy of the nasal vascular bed and its nerve supply. Ann Otol 79:443-450

Cloquet H (1830) A system of human anatomy. Machlachlan and Steward, Edinburgh

Cole P (1998) Physyology of the nose and paranasal sinuses. Clin Rev Allergy Immunol 16:25-54

Dahl R, Migynd N (1998) Anatomy, physiology and function of the nasal cavities in health and disease. Adv Drug Deliv Rev 5:3-12

Eckel W (1963) Untersuchungen zur Grössenentwicklung der Kieferhöhlen. Arch Ohren Nasen Kehlkopfheilkd 182:479-484

Flottes L, Clerc P, Rui R et al (1960) La physiologie des sinus. Libraire Arnette, Paris

Howell HP (1917) Voice production from the standpoint of the laryngologist. Ann Otol Rhinol Laryngol 26:643-655

Ingelstedt S, Toremalm NG (1961) Air flow pattern and heat transfer within the respiratory tract. Acta Physiol Scand 51:1-4

Laffort P, Patte F, Etcheto M (1974) Olfactory coding on the basis of physiochemical properties. Ann NY Acad Sci 237:193-208

Muir DCF (1972) Clinical aspects of inhaled particles. Heinemann, London

Mygind N (1978) Nasal allergy. Blackwell Scientific, Oxford

Negus V (1958) The comparative anatomy and physiology of the nose and paranasal sinuses. Livingstone, London

Nishihira S, McCaffrey TV (1987) Reflex control of nasal blood vessels. Otolaryngol Head Neck Surg 96:273-277

Paulsson B, Dolata J, Larsson I, Ohlin P, Lindberg S (2001) Paranasal sinus ventilation in healthy subjects and in patients with sinus disease evaluated with the 133-xenon washout technique. Ann Otol Rhinol Laryngol 110:667-674

Proetz AW (1953) Applied physiology of the nose, 2nd edn. Annals Publishing, St Louis

Rice DH, Gluckman JL (1995) Physyology. In: Donald PJ, Gluckman JL, Rice DH (eds) The sinuses. Raven Press, New York, pp 49-56

Rui L (1960) Contribution a l'étude du role des sinus paranasaux. Rev Laryngol Otol Rhinol (Bordeaux) 81:796-839

Skillen RH (1920) Accessory sinuses of the nose, 2nd edn. Lippincott Company, Philadelphia

Takahashi R (1984) The formation of paranasal sinuses. Acta Otolaryngol Suppl (Stockh) 408:1-28

Wright J (1914) A history of laryngology and rhinology, 2nd edn. Lea and Febiger, New York

4 Neoplastic Invasion of Bone, the Orbit and Dural Layers: Basic and Advanced CT and MR Findings

Roberto Maroldi, Davide Farina, Giuseppe Battaglia

CONTENTS

4.1   Introduction   35
4.2   Patterns of Bone Invasion on CT and MR   36
4.2.1 Bone Remodeling   36
4.2.2 Cortical Destruction   37
4.2.3 Intra-diploic/Medullary Growth   37
4.2.4 Permeative Invasion   37
4.2.5 Sclerosis   38
4.3   CT and MR Findings of Orbital Invasion   39
4.4   CT and MR Findings of Skull Base and
       Dura Mater Invasion   42
       References   46

4.1 Introduction

In the sinonasal area several thick or thinner bony laminae divide the nasal cavity and paranasal sinuses from the orbit and the brain. These bone structures act as a barrier against tumor spread.

Conventional radiology and CT obtained findings suggesting bone invasion upon changes of the normal appearance of these interfaces (Som and Shugar 1980; Som et al. 1991; Lloyd et al. 2000). However, the single absence (lysis) of the mineral content of the lamina papyracea *per se* does not correctly predict, for example, orbital invasion at CT.

In fact, it is well known that the most effective barrier to the spread of neoplastic or inflammatory aggressive lesions beyond sinusal walls is the periosteum rather than the mineralized bony wall (Kimmelman and Korovin 1988). Therefore, neoplastic extent be-

yond the periosteum of the sinusal walls is critical for therapeutic planning.

Nevertheless, the limitation of CT in assessing the presence of a residual demineralized barrier (the periosteum) does not necessarily apply to MR.

In fact, though the mineral content does not give up signal on MR, the cortical bone – its periosteal covering included – can be adequately demonstrated using high resolution matrix and thin voxels, because it appears as a homogeneous hypointense structure (Som et al. 1987) (Fig. 4.1).

This signal actually results from the sum of both cortical bone and its investing thin fibrous periosteal layers. It can be recognized on MR independently of the degree of bone mineralization (Maroldi et al. 1996).

For all these reasons, the information provided by imaging should not simply regard the state of the mineralized wall, but it should be refocused on assessing the normality of the periosteum lining the bony "box."

In addition, the bony interfaces between the sinonasal cavities and brain have a more complex structure, because the intracranial surface of these bones is covered by a specialized connective layer: the dura mater. Like the periosteum, this layer prevents intra-cranial invasion by neoplasms or aggressive inflammatory lesions. The dura mater differs from the periosteum because in most cases it reacts in front of the advancing lesion by significantly increasing its thickness and vascularization (Eisen et al. 1996).

As a result, the assessment of the relationships between tumor and the adjacent bony walls – lined by periosteum or by the dura – will include basic (regular vs. irregular demineralization) and more advanced findings (demonstration of the periosteum, changes of the dura mater layer).

As both focal invasion and the simple contact between tumor and the periosteum/dura mater layer significantly influence the treatment planning, the meticulous assessment of these findings is a relevant part of the imaging work up.

R. Maroldi, MD
Professor, Department of Radiology, University of Brescia, Piazzale Spedali Civili 1, Brescia, BS, 25123, Italy
D. Farina, MD; G. Battaglia, MD
Department of Radiology, University of Brescia, Piazzale Spedali Civili 1, Brescia, BS, 25123, Italy

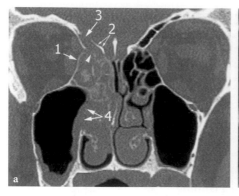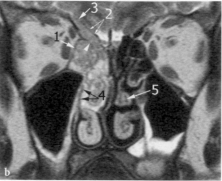

Fig. 4.1a,b. Coronal CT and TSE T2 MR of right ethmoid inverted papilloma. Moderate lateral displacement and reabsorption of the lamina papyracea (*1*) well detectable on MR image because of replacement of the air content within the ethmoid cells by thickened mucosa and tumor. Thinning of the fovea ethmoidalis (*2*) is correctly shown by the two techniques. Laterally, the orbital plate of the frontal bone (*3*) appears completely demineralized, its border undetectable. On MR, a thin hypointense line suggests that the lesion is still confined by the periosteal/dural interface. Similarly, the thin lamella reaching the anterior ethmoid canal (*arrowhead*) and part of the medial maxillary sinus wall (*4*) are better shown by MR. Middle left concha (*5*)

4.2
Patterns of Bone Invasion on CT and MR

In the sinonasal area, the bone framework is composed not only of thin laminae (as the lamina papyracea or the lamina cribrosa) but also of thick osseous structures as the zygomatic bone or the pterygoid process and the great wing of the sphenoid.

The interaction between thin laminae or thick medullary bones and lesions with variable degrees of aggressiveness results in four patterns of bone changes.

4.2.1
Bone Remodeling

Bone remodeling consists of displacement and – usually – thinning of bony walls. In most cases, it is observed in tumors contacting very thin walls as cribriform plate, lamina papyracea, turbinates, and medial maxillary sinus wall. Bone remodeling is a continuously occurring adaptive dynamic process involving both osteoblasts and osteoclasts (GIACCHI et al. 2001). Activation of this process is triggered by mechanical stress – exerted by expansile lesions – as well as by chemical mediators – released in both infectious and non-infectious inflammatory conditions. Bone remodeling is a sort of balance between the activity of osteoblasts and osteoclasts. As a result, thinning and displacement of subtle bone structures may be observed mixed with sclerosis of thicker sinusal walls.

The high spatial and contrast resolution of CT enables the detection of even subtle abnormalities in the mineral content of the remodeled bone (SOM and SHUGAR 1980) (Fig. 4.2). Whereas demineralization of thin cortical interfaces cannot be detected by MR, wall displacement and integrity of the periosteum may be demonstrated on condition that the wall does not contact air on one of its surfaces (MAROLDI et al. 1996) (Fig. 4.1).

Basically, in normal sinuses there are two different physiological and anatomic conditions: air on one side, fat/fluid on the opposite one (lamina papyracea and orbital fat, cribriform plate and CSF); air on both sides (medial maxillary sinus wall).

In the first condition, the displaced and demineralized medial orbital wall or cribriform plate – with

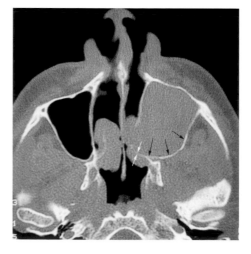

Fig. 4.2. Bone remodeling of the posterolateral (*black arrows*), anterior, and medial maxillary sinus wall in an inverted papilloma. *White arrows* point to demineralization of the inferior concha.

their periosteal layers – can be detected by MR as hypointense (absent) linear signals enclosed in a sort of sandwich between the lesion (on one side) and the orbital fat and CSF (or dura and subarachnoid spaces), respectively, on the other side (ISHIDA et al. 2002) (Fig. 4.3). Of course, the proper frequency encoding direction has to be selected in order to avoid asymmetric appearance of cortical bone due to chemical shift artifact (DICK et al. 1988).

In the second condition, remodeling of the medial maxillary sinus wall or of the sphenoid sinus floor may be shown by MR if a sufficiently thick mucosal layer invests the opposite surface or retained secretions fill the sinus (MAROLDI et al. 1996).

The bone remodeling pattern can be observed in benign neoplasms and in some chronic inflammatory lesions as the mucocele and polyposis, less frequently in malignant neoplasms.

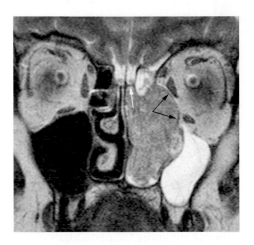

Fig. 4.3. Adenocarcinoma of the ethmoid, TSE T2 sequence. Even if the lamina papyracea is laterally displaced, a continuous sharp hypointense interface separates the orbital fat from the mass (*black arrows*), indicating absence of periorbital penetration. The horizontal (*white arrow*) and lateral (vertical) cribriform plate are demonstrated because tumor and mucous filling the frontal sinus contact the bone from below

4.2.2
Cortical Destruction

Cortical destruction is detected at CT as a break of the mineralized bone through its whole thickness, whereas on MR a defect of the continuous hypointense thickness of the cortex, replaced by solid tissue, implies invasion also of the periosteum (MAROLDI et al. 1996). It can be observed in aggressive inflammatory lesions (both non-invasive and invasive fungal rhinosinusitis), some benign, but aggressive, neo-

plasms as inverted papilloma and juvenile angiofibroma and in malignant tumors (SOM et al. 1991) (Fig. 4.4).

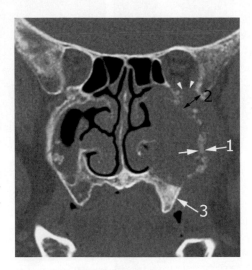

Fig. 4.4. Squamous cell carcinoma of the left maxillary sinus. Irregular destruction of the posterolateral wall (*1*). Tumor spreads into the fat content of the infratemporal fossa and inferior orbital fissure (*2*). *Arrowheads* indicate the extent into the inferior limit of the superior orbital fissure. Sclerotic changes of the alveolar process (*3*)

4.2.3
Intra-diploic/Medullary Growth

Intra-diploic/medullary growth relates to the characteristic path of intra-osseous spread demonstrated by malignant tumors and the juvenile angiofibroma (Fig. 4.5). The density and signal of the spongiosa is replaced by solid tissue characterized by trabecular destruction on plain CT and fat replacement on MR (LLOYD et al. 1999). This intra-osseous tissue usually enhances like the primitive tumor mass. For instance, the typical high enhancement of juvenile angiofibroma can be detected within the diploe (Fig. 4.6).

4.2.4
Permeative Invasion

Permeative invasion with or without sclerosis is a peculiar pattern observed mostly in lymphomas and in adenoid cystic carcinoma (SUEI et al. 1994; YASUMOTO et al. 2000). In this pattern, the most relevant finding is the extensive replacement of the medullary bone even in the absence of evident cortical erosion.

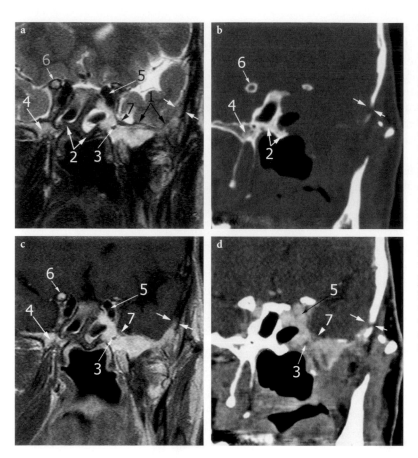

Fig. 4.5a–d. Recurrent myxosarcoma. TSE T2 (**a**), plain CT (**b**), enhanced T1 (**c**), and enhanced CT (**d**). Intraspongiotic spread within the greater wing, pterygoid process, lateral sinus wall and floor of the left sphenoid bone. Whereas plain CT shows lysis of cortical and diploic mineral content of the bone, TSE T2 demonstrates a hypointense interface (*1*) still separating the tumor from the subarachnoid spaces, indicating that the lesion is confined to the dura. Neoplastic erosion extends into the lateral portion of the greater wing (*opposite arrows*). Because of sclerotic changes, the medullary bone within the intersinusal sphenoid septum and the residual sphenoid sinus floor is more hypointense on TSE T2 and enhanced T1 (*2*) than the adjacent pterygoid process (*4*). Residual pterygoid canal content (*3*), internal carotid artery (*5*), anterior clinoid with cortical rim and medullary content (target-like appearance) (*6*), maxillary nerve (*7*)

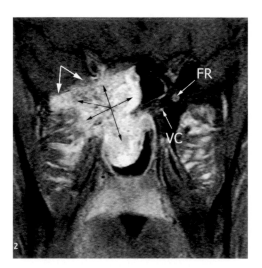

Fig. 4.6. Persistent juvenile angiofibroma. In the GE Gd-enhanced coronal image, the persistent lesion replaces the medullary bone of the greater wing of the right sphenoid (*white arrows*), and projects into the sphenoid sinus, the superior orbital fissure, and into the choana (*black arrows*). Foramen rotundum (*FR*), pterygoid (vidian) canal (*VC*)

In this setting, a very subtle moth-eaten appearance of the hypointense cortical/periosteal lining can be detected only if proper CT and MR techniques are used. This model of sub-periosteal spread can be missed on plain and enhanced CT, particularly in adenoid cystic carcinomas, because only faint areas of denser spongious bone may be present. Conversely, MR is more sensitive because it combines the information provided by different sequences: on both T2 and plain T1, the fat tissue is replaced by hypointense signal; moreover, non homogeneous areas of enhancement can be demonstrated after contrast application, more evident when the fat-sat technique is applied (Fig. 4.7).

4.2.5
Sclerosis

Sclerosis is characterized on MR by the above-mentioned changes on T2 and plain T1 sequences, usually without any contrast enhancement. Extensive sclerosis can be, of course, obvious on CT (Fig. 4.5). This is a chronic inflammatory reaction of the spongiosa

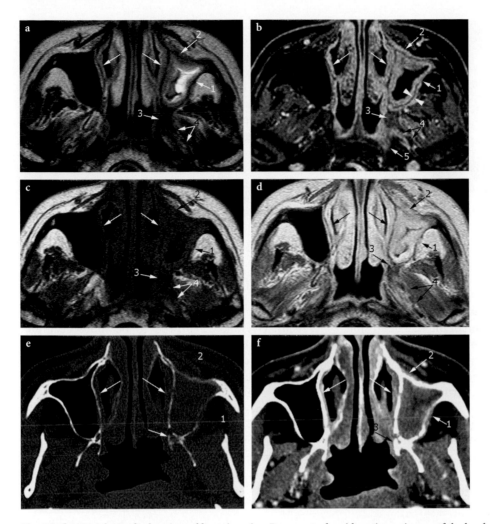

Fig. 4.7a-f. MR and CT of subperiosteal bone invasion. Recurrent adenoid cystic carcinoma of the hard palate. MR sequences: TSE T2 (**a**), Gd-enhanced VIBE (**b**), plain (**c**) and Gd-enhanced T1 (**d**). Bone window CT, plain study (**e**), enhanced CT (**f**). The anterior, medial, and posterolateral walls of left maxillary sinus are invaded through subperiosteal spread. Apart from areas of focal erosion (*1*), subperiosteal spread results in rather subtle CT changes: diffuse demineralization of maxillary sinus walls, and minimal soft tissue thickening along the external surfaces of the walls (*2*). Conversely, MR clearly shows tumor spread on both the inner and outer surfaces of the sinus, leaving the residual walls (hypointense on all sequences) between two layers of neoplastic signal (*arrowheads* in **b**). On TSE T2, subperiosteal spread presents as a plaque-like lesion with a multilayer appearance with a double hypointense layer (neoplastic) investing both sides of the bony walls, the inner being covered by the mucosa (intermediate-to-hyperintense signal layer). This pattern is clearly shown at the medial maxillary sinus wall (*arrows*), where the the diffuse bulging of the mucosa on left side is due to subperiosteal/submucosal invasion. The plaque-like neoplastic layer, which is hypointense on plain T1, enhances after Gd admministration on T1 and VIBE, similarly to the mucosa. Erosion and intramedullary invasion of the left petrygoid process is also shown (*3*). Mandibular nerve (*4*). Extent into the left nasopharyngeal wall is shown (*5*)

present in a wide range of inflammatory and neoplastic conditions (CHANG et al. 1992).

4.3
CT and MR Findings of Orbital Invasion

Most nasosinusal neoplasms invade the orbit through the floor (maxillary sinus squamous cell carcinomas) or the medial wall (ethmoid adenocarcinomas). The other walls are less frequently involved by primitive tumors. In fact, it is more likely to observe this path of orbital invasion by recurrent neoplasms or metastases. Apart from the infrequent event of perineural spread along the infraorbital nerve, rarely tumors extend into the orbit through the fissures or canals.

As both the medial wall and the orbital floor are very thin, they are often displaced by tumors arising

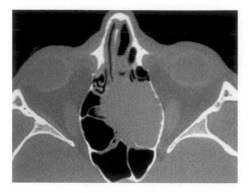

Fig. 4.8. Adenocarcinoma of left ethmoid abutting the lamina papyracea. Mild sclerotic changes combined with focal areas of erosion are shown

in the adjacent sinuses (Fig. 4.8). Chronic pressure exerted by the mass is usually associated with thinning and demineralization of the wall or erosion.

Surgical strategy is controversial in the presence of erosion of the lamina papyracea. According to some authors this condition indicates orbital exenteration (Ketcham et al. 1973). Nevertheless, criteria defining the indications for orbital preservation or exenteration have changed throughout the last three decades. Recent evidence in the surgical literature supports a conservative approach even in the presence of bone erosion on condition that the periorbita is not invaded (Lund et al. 1998; Cantu et al. 2000). More re-

cently, data provided by other investigators (Tiwari et al. 2000 Imola and Schramm 2002;) advocate more advanced criteria for orbital preservation. An additional distinct fascial layer surrounding the periocular fat and separating it from the periorbita has been reported by Tiwari et al. (1998). Invasion of the fascia prevents orbital preservation. In the series by Imola and Schramm (2002), full thickness periorbital invasion was treated by microscopically assisted dissection, enabling even limited removal of the orbital fat.

Thus, imaging the periorbita is crucial for CT and MR. Prediction of orbital invasion has been based on the detection of positive findings graded through progressive steps: tumor contacting the periorbita (sensitivity of CT and MR 90%); fat obliteration (positive predictive value: CT 86%, MR 80%); extraocular muscle involvement (positive predictive value of MR 100%) (Eisen et al. 2000). Overall, CT proved to be more accurate than MR. By comparison, in our series of 49 sinonasal malignancies the absence of orbital invasion has been correctly predicted in 40 orbits with tumor contacting the wall more than 10 mm of length (negative predictive value of CT 75%, MR 100%) (Maroldi et al. 1996, 1997). Detection of a hypointense/absent linear signal indicating the periorbita was the more specific predictor with overall accuracy of MR significantly better than CT (95.4% vs 81%) (Fig. 4.9–4.13).

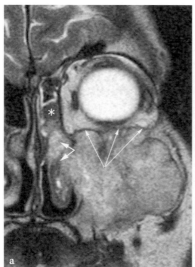
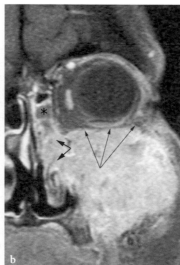
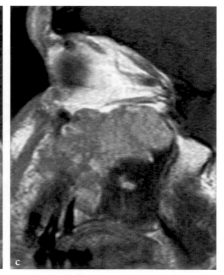

Fig. 4.9a-c. Squamous cell carcinoma of left maxillary sinus. On coronal TSE T2 (a) and VIBE (b), upward displacement of the orbital floor by the tumor is observed. A hypointense interface between the mass and the orbital fat can be recognized (*long arrows*). Tumor invades the middle meatus (*short arrows*) blocking the anterior ethmoid. Hypointense fluid (high protein concentration) within the ethmoid bulla (*asterisk*). On sagittal GD-enhanced T1 (c) a hypointense interface cannot be demonstrated, only the sharp limits suggest that the lesion is limited by the periorbita

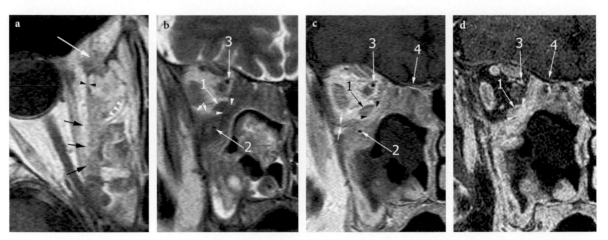

Fig. 4.10a-d. Spindle cell naso-ethmoid carcinoma. The hypointensity of the lamina papyracea/periorbita can be appreciated only in its anterior third (*black arrowheads*). In the posterior two thirds of the medial orbital wall, neoplastic spread through the lamina papyracea/periorbita (*black arrows*) appears as several short solid finger-like projections into the orbital fat. An ethmoid cell wall – same thickness of the papyracea – can be adequately detected by MR (*white arrowheads*). Invasion of the right nasal bone (*white long arrow*). In the same patient as (**a**), TSE T2 (**b**), Gd-enhanced T1 (**c**) and VIBE (**c**) coronal planes show invasion of the medial orbital wall with solid - and enhancing - tissue (*arrowheads*) replacing the orbital fat medially to the rectus inferior muscle (*1*). Invasion of the lateral orbital floor (*small white arrows* on **b** and *opposite arrows* on **c**) is also present. The signal void of the infraorbital artery is surrounded by tumor (*2*). Ophthalmic artery (*3*), minimal dural thickening at the fovea ethmoidalis (*4*)

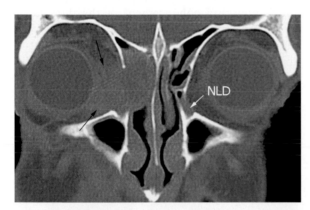

Fig. 4.11. Adenocarcinoma of right ethmoid sinus invading the orbit (*arrows*) through the erosion of the lamina papyracea and lacrimal bone. *NLD*, nasolacrimal duct

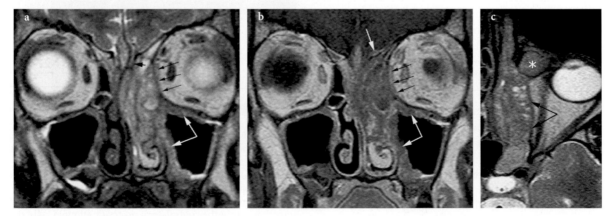

Fig. 4.12a–c. Sinonasal non-Hodgkin lymphoma. Permeative pattern of invasion through the lamina papyracea (*black arrows*) and extent into the maxillary sinus along the bony walls (*white arrows*). The horizontal and lateral (vertical) lamella of the cribriform plate are well demonstrated on TSE T2 [*short black arrow* on (**a**)]. Focal dural enhancement is appreciated on (**b**) at the level of the orbital plate of the frontal bone (white arrow). Lacrimal sac dilatation (*asterisk*)

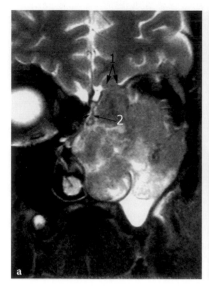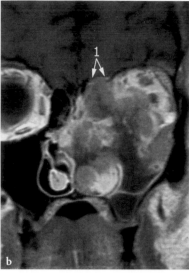

Fig. 4.13a,b. Squamous cell carcinoma of left nasal cavity with extensive orbital infiltration. Invasion through the bony/periosteal hypointense interface of the fovea ethmoidalis (*1*) with minimal enhancement of the dural layer. Residual vertical lamella of the middle torbinate (*2*)

Although preoperative imaging may aid in surgical planning, in ambiguous cases of orbital invasion the intra-operative mapping of the orbital wall, with gross examination or frozen sections, is necessary.

Orbital invasion is considered a negative prognostic factor, even though some authors specify that decrease in survival may reflect the wider extension of lesions invading the orbit (SHAH et al. 1997).

MR has been reported to be more precise than CT. Early observations emphasized the usefulness of T2 (and T1 sequences) in separating the low signal of bone from the high signal of CSF (Fig. 4.14). Thickening and enhancement of the dura mater invaded by tumor were mentioned by WEISSMAN and CURTIN (1994). Other investigators reported that enhanced MR sequences could demonstrate leptomeningeal invasion (VOLLE et al. 1989; KRAUS et al. 1992a). Moreover, in the series by ISHIDA et

4.4
CT and MR Findings of Skull Base and Dura Mater Invasion

Assessment of the deep extent of sinonasal tumors toward the dural layer is one of the issues that significantly influence the treatment planning.

Like in the invasion of orbital walls, bone destruction of the skull base is better demonstrated by CT. However, here the imaging findings differ from those observed in the other bone interfaces of the sinonasal area because when the skull base is invaded, the dura mater usually shows abnormal thickening and enhancement that can be due either to neoplastic invasion or to inflammatory, non-neoplastic reaction.

Since dural invasion implies both a worse prognosis and a surgical resection not limited to the eroded bone, the goals of imaging focus on establishing the depth of skull base invasion (KRAUS et al. 1992b; SHAH et al. 1997).

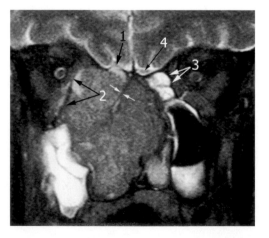

Fig. 4.14. Naso-ethmoidal adenocarcinoma, intestinal-type, TSE T2. Upward displacement of the right fovea ethmoidalis (*1*) due to a small mucocele underneath (showing hyperintense signal) secondary to tumor (that shows homogeneous intermediate intensity). The tumor abuts the right medial orbital wall, remodeled, but not invaded (*2*). Because of fluid retention within the contralateral posterior ethmoid cells, the papyracea/periorbita is well demonstrated (*3*). *Opposite arrows* point to the right residual vertical lamella of the middle concha. Olfactory tract (*4*)

al. (2002), as well as in our own, specific changes in the appearance of the hypointense/absent signal of bone and the overlying dura proved to correctly predict dural invasion.

A key diagnostic observation concerns the signal intensity of the three structures located at the interface between the ethmoid roof and brain at the anterior cranial fossa: cribriform plate and its double periosteal covering, dura mater, subarachnoid space.

On enhanced sagittal and coronal MR spin echo T1 or 3D GE fat sat T1 sequences the three layers give rise to a "sandwich" of different signals (bone-periosteum complex, dura, CSF) (ISHIDA et al. 2002).

If a malignant sinonasal neoplasm approaches the ACF floor, three different conditions may occur: (a) the neoplasm appears in close contact with an uninterrupted, hypointense cribriform plate or fovea ethmoidalis (Fig. 4.15); (b) the neoplasm erases the hypointensity of the cribriform plate, extends into the ACF and displaces an uninterrupted, hyperintense and thickened dura (Fig. 4.16); (c)

the neoplasm encroaches the dural hyperintensity without erasing the hypointense signal of CSF (Fig. 4.17, 4.18); (d) the neoplasm extends beyond the dura encroaching the hypointense CSF and invades brain tissue (Fig. 4.19).

This last sign is easier to detect if the signal intensity of the neoplasm is lower than the enhanced dura surrounding the invaded segment (MAROLDI et al. 1997).

Resectability of tumors invading the brain does not stand only upon the assessment by imaging of the depth of tumor extent into the brain or on the detection of bilateral brain invasion. It requires a thorough evaluation of several other issues, the most important being the histotype and patient's performance status. Patients with limited brain invasion treated by craniofacial resection are reported to have non-significant decrease in survival compared to those with dural invasion only.

Contraindications to surgery other than brain invasion are considered to be the involvement of the internal carotid artery or of the cavernous sinus (SHAH et al. 1997) (Fig. 4.20)

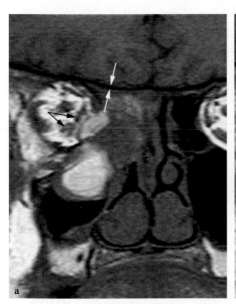
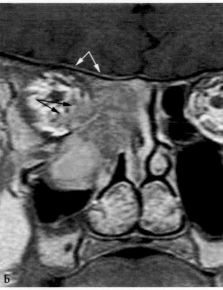

Fig. 4.15a,b. Ethmoidal adenocarcinoma, intestinal-type, plain (**a**) and Gd-enhanced T1 (**b**). The black signal of the planum ethmoidalis/fovea is continuous and regular [*opposite white arrows* on (**a**)]. Mild and uniform enhancement of the dura is detected after Gd administration [*white arrows* on (**b**)]. Invasion of medial wall and part of the floor of the orbit (*black arrows*)

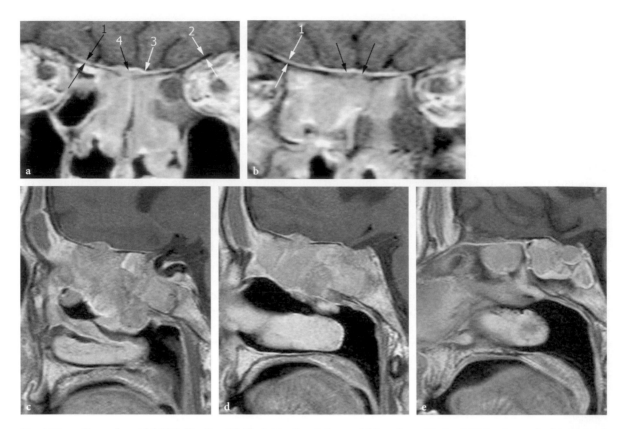

Fig. 4.16a–e. Naso-ethmoidal SCC, T1 after Gd administration. Intracranial invasion with dural thickening and subtotal dural infiltration. **a** Minimal dural thickening at the periphery of the lesion (*1*), normal frontal bone appearance at the orbital roof (*2*). Focal thickening of the dura (*3*) more hyperintense than the tumor's signal (*4*). **b** No sign of dural layer trespassing at this level, bone has been eroded (*black arrows*). Mild dural thickening (*1*). **c–e** On the sagittal planes, bone erosion and subtotal replacement of the hyperintense signal of the focally thickened dura suggest intracranial extradural invasion. Posterior sphenoid sinus wall destruction with hypophysis invasion is present. Blockage of frontal sinus drainage is associated with mucous retention and mucosal thickening

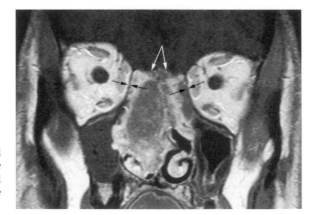

Fig. 4.17. Sinonasal undifferentiated carcinoma, Gd-enhanced T1. Midline invasion of the anterior cranial fossa floor (*white arrows*) without dural thickening (intracranial intradural spread). No sign of brain edema. Lamino papyraces (*opposite arrrows*)

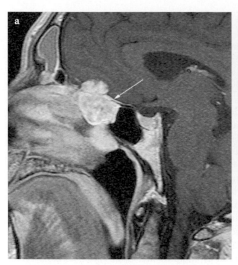
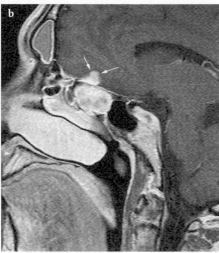

Fig. 4.18a,b. Adenocarcinoma of the ethmoid sinus, Gd-enhanced T1. **a** Tumor and the enhanced dura have similar signal intensity. The thickened dura is seen investing the planum ethmoidalis posteriorly to neoplastic invasion (*arrow*). **b** Intracranial intradural spread without brain invasion (*arrows*)

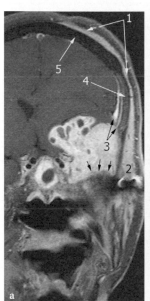
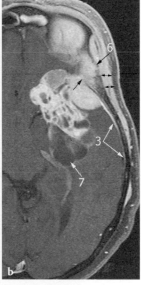

Fig. 4.19a,b. Recurrent adenoid cystic carcinoma, left maxillary sinus was the primary site, Gd-enhanced GE-T1 sequences. Galea capitis (*1*) and temporal muscle (*2*) invasion. The intracranial mass arises from spread through the greater wing of the left sphenoid [*black arrows* in (**a**)]. Intracranial intradural spread exhibits a mushroom-like appearance. Double layer enhancement along the inner surface of the temporal and parietal bones (*3*) may be correlated to dural spread (it does not extend into the sulci), the more hyperintense layer abutting brain tissue, and to sub-periosteal spread, the less hyperintense layer closer to the bone. Intra-diploic enhancement is present: compare abnormal (*4*) to normal (*5*) diploic signal. Bone is clearly invaded at the temporal fossa (*6*). A cyst-like mass is demonstrated on the posterior aspect of the intracranial tumor (*7*)

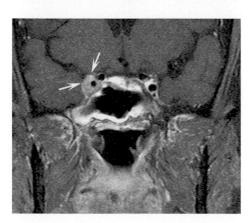

Fig. 4.20. Recurrent SCC of the posterior ethmoid, Gd-enhanced GE coronal plane. Encasement of right internal carotid artery (*arrows*) with cavernous sinus invasion

References

Cantu G, Solero C, Mattavelli F et al (2000) Resezione cranio-facciale anteriore per tumori maligni: esperienza di 200 casi. Acta Otorhinolaryngol Ital 20:91-99

Chang T, Teng MM, Wang SF et al (1992) Aspergillosis of the paranasal sinuses. Neuroradiology 34:520-523

Dick BW, Mitchell DG, Burk DL et al (1988) The effect of chemical shift misrepresentation on cortical bone thickness on MR imaging. AJR Am J Roentgenol 151:537-538

Eisen MD, Yousem DM, Montone KT et al (1996) Use of preoperative MR to predict dural, perineural, and venous sinus invasion of skull base tumors. AJNR Am J Neuroradiol 17:1937-1945

Eisen MD, Yousem DM, Loevner LA et al (2000) Preoperative imaging to predict orbital invasion by tumor. Head Neck 22:456-462

Giacchi RJ, Lebowitz RA, Yee HT et al (2001) Histopathologic evaluation of the ethmoid bone in chronic sinusitis. Am J Rhinol 15:193-197

Imola MJ, Schramm VL Jr (2002) Orbital preservation in surgical management of sinonasal malignancy. Laryngoscope 112:1357-1365

Ishida H, Mohri M, Amatsu M (2002) Invasion of the skull base by carcinomas: histopathologically evidenced findings with CT and MRI. Eur Arch Otorhinolaryngol 259:535-539

Ketcham AS, Chretien PB, van Buren JM et al (1973) The ethmoid sinuses: a re-evaluation of surgical resection. Am J Surg 126:469-476

Kimmelman CP, Korovin GS (1988) Management of paranasal sinus neoplasms invading the orbit. Otolaryngol Clin North Am 21:77-92

Kraus DH, Lanzieri CF, Wanamaker JR et al (1992a) Complementary use of computed tomography and magnetic resonance imaging in assessing skull base lesions. Laryngoscope 102:623-629

Kraus DH, Sterman BM, Levine HL et al (1992b) Factors influencing survival in ethmoid sinus cancer. Arch Otolaryngol Head Neck Surg 118:367-372

Lloyd G, Howard D, Phelps P et al (1999) Juvenile angiofibroma: the lessons of 20 years of modern imaging. J Laryngol Otol 113:127-134

Lloyd G, Lund VJ, Howard D et al (2000) Optimum imaging for sinonasal malignancy. J Laryngol Otol 114:557-562

Lund VJ, Howard DJ, Wei WI et al (1998) Craniofacial resection for tumors of the nasal cavity and paranasal sinuses – a 17-year experience. Head Neck 20:97-105

Maroldi R, Farina D, Battaglia G et al (1996) Risonanza Magnetica e Tomografia Computerizzata a confronto nello staging delle neoplasie rino-sinusali. Valutazione di costo-efficienza. Radiol Med (Torino) 91:211-218

Maroldi R, Farina D, Battaglia G et al (1997) MR of malignant nasosinusal neoplasms. Frequently asked questions. Eur J Radiol 24:181-190

Shah JP, Kraus DH, Bilsky MH et al (1997) Craniofacial resection for malignant tumors involving the anterior skull base. Arch Otolaryngol Head Neck Surg 123:1312-1317

Som PM, Shugar JM (1980) The significance of bone expansion associated with the diagnosis of malignant tumors of the paranasal sinuses. Radiology 136:97-100

Som PM, Braun IF, Shapiro MD et al (1987) Tumors of the parapharyngeal space and upper neck: MR imaging characteristics. Radiology 164:823-829

Som PM, Lawson W, Lidov MW (1991) Simulated aggressive skull base erosion in response to benign sinonasal disease. Radiology 180:755-759

Suei Y, Tanimoto K, Taguchi A et al (1994) Radiographic evaluation of bone invasion of adenoid cystic carcinoma in the oral and maxillofacial region. J Oral Maxillofac Surg 52:821-826

Tiwari R, van der Wal J, van der Waal I et al (1998) Studies of the anatomy and pathology of the orbit in carcinoma of the maxillary sinus and their impact on preservation of the eye in maxillectomy. Head Neck 20:193-196

Tiwari R, Hardillo JA, Mehta D et al (2000) Squamous cell carcinoma of maxillary sinus. Head Neck 22:164-169

Volle E, Treisch J, Claussen C et al (1989) Lesions of skull base observed on high resolution computed tomography. A comparison with magnetic resonance imaging. Acta Radiol 30:129-134

Weissman JL, Curtin HD (1994) Advances in treatment of tumors of the cranial base. Advances in imaging. J Neurooncol 20:193-211

Yasumoto M, Taura S, Shibuya H et al (2000) Primary malignant lymphoma of the maxillary sinus: CT and MRI. Neuroradiology 42:285-289

5 Endonasal and Open Surgery: Key Concepts

Piero Nicolai, Andrea Bolzoni, Cesare Piazza, and Antonino R. Antonelli

CONTENTS

5.1   Introduction   47
5.2   Microendoscopic Surgery: Knowledge of
        the Basic Principles   47
5.2.1   Inflammatory Diseases   48
5.2.1.1 Uncinectomy   49
5.2.1.2 Middle Antrostomy   49
5.2.1.3 Ethmoidotomy   50
5.2.1.4 Sphenoidotomy   51
5.2.1.5 Clearance of the Frontal Recess   51
5.2.2   Neoplastic Lesions   53
5.3   Open Surgery: Basic Knowledge of
        the Most Frequently Used Approaches   53
5.3.1   Maxillectomies   53
5.3.2   Osteoplastic Flap Sinusotomy   56
5.3.3   Anterior Craniofacial Resection   57
        References   58

5.1
Introduction

Surgery plays a role of paramount importance in the management of both inflammatory and neoplastic lesions of the sinonasal tract. During the last two decades a clear tendency to limit the indications of external approaches in favor of endonasal procedures with the help of endoscopes and/or the microscope has been observed. However, external approaches have still a role in the management of some selected cases of inflammatory diseases and benign tumors and they must be considered the gold standard for malignant tumors. The aim of this chapter will not be to review all the numerous surgical techniques which have been reported along the years in the literature, but instead to focus on those which are nowadays more commonly used and which should be necessarily included in the armamentarium of any otorhinolaryngologist or maxillo-facial surgeon with special interest in sinonasal diseases.

P. Nicolai, MD, Professor
A. Bolzoni, MD; C. Piazza, MD
A. R. Antonelli, Professor and Chairman
Department of Otorhinolaryngology, University of Brescia, Piazzale Spedali Civili 1, Brescia, BS, 25123, Italy

5.2
Microendoscopic Surgery: Knowledge of the Basic Principles

Microscopic and endoscopic surgery of the nose and paranasal sinuses were separately developed in Europe at the end of the 1950s and in the early 1970s thanks to Heermann (1958) and Messerklinger (1972, 1978), respectively. Among others, Draf (1991; Draf and Weber 1993) for microscopic surgery, and Stammberger (1986a,b) and Wigand (1981) for endoscopic surgery have contributed tremendously to spreading the use of these techniques all around the world. The microscope has the advantage of a binocular view, which gives a tridimensional perspective and a better sense of depth; furthermore, the surgeon can use both hands for surgical maneuvers, a peculiarity which can be extremely helpful in situations of massive bleeding. Endoscopes are available with lenses of different angulation (Fig. 5.1); this enables a good view of the most remote recesses of the sinonasal compartment (i.e., frontal recess and sinus, maxillary sinus), something which is not feasible with a microscope. Furthermore, endoscopes, which are presently used coupled with a camera connected with a high-resolution video, are excellent for photodocumentation. After a period of disputes opposing supporters

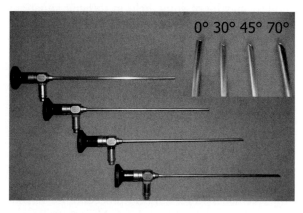

Fig. 5.1. Endoscopes available for endoscopic surgery with lenses of various angulation (0°, 30°, 45°, 70°)

of the two techniques, a reasonable compromise, recognizing advantages and limitations inherent to each technique and suggesting that both techniques could be used in a combined fashion, has been found. This has led to the coining of the term "microendoscopic surgery" (STAMM and DRAF 2000), which will be used in the present book.

The technique for systematic endoscopic evaluation of the lateral nasal wall developed by MESSERKLINGER (1972) confirmed that most inflammatory diseases of the paranasal sinuses secondarily arise from an inflammatory process taking origin in one or more of the narrow spaces (called "pre-chambers") which collect the mucus drainage from the different sinuses. The ostiomeatal unit has a key role in the ventilation and drainage of the maxillary and frontal sinuses and of the anterior ethmoid cells, much like the spheno-ethmoid recess has for posterior ethmoid cells and sphenoid sinus. Any anatomic variant narrowing those spaces may impair the mucociliary clearance efficacy, predisposing to obstruction and contributing to the pathogenesis of sinusitis.

As a logical consequence of physiopathologic observations, a new concept of a selective, more conservative surgery has resulted. MESSERKLINGER (1972) observed that surgical removal of the primary disease at the level of the lateral nasal wall by means of a limited procedure ("pre-chamber" surgery) resulted in the recovery of sinus diseased mucosa without resorting to any surgical aggressive procedure on the sinus itself. Endoscopic surgery was first described as a one-handed technique in which one of the surgeon's hands handles the endoscope, while the other manages different instruments using the shaft of the endoscope as a safe guide to advance in the nasal fossa, positioning it as far as possible behind the instrument. Having an experienced assistant who helps the surgeon with suction (so-called two-handed techniques) may be of some help in difficult situations such as massive bleeding.

The aim of this section is to briefly analyze the standard surgical steps of a microendoscopic dissection taking into account the differences in the management philosophy between inflammatory and neoplastic lesions.

5.2.1
Inflammatory Diseases

Any microendoscopic surgical procedure for inflammatory diseases should be planned by taking into account the nature and extent of the disease together with

the specific anatomy of the single patient. For example, whenever a patient presents with a disease limited to a specific sinus (maxillary, frontal, or sphenoid), the aim of surgery should be opening, clearance, and reventilation of the affected sinus through the more conservative approach. In contrast, most patients with sinonasal polyposis require a complete marsupialization of all the cavities (Fig. 5.2), which is achieved by combining different surgical steps: uncinectomy, middle antrostomy, ethmoidotomy, sphenoidotomy, and clearance of the frontal recess. These steps will be described in detail to give a better understanding of the path that the surgeon has to follow during the dissection along the lateral nasal wall (Fig. 5.3) and, consequently, of the

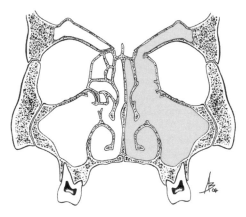

Fig. 5.2. On the right, complete marsupialization of all ethmoidal cells, maxillary and frontal sinuses, with preservation of the inferior and middle turbinates can be observed

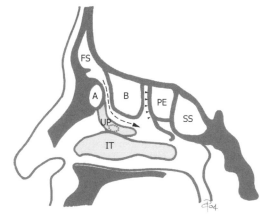

Fig. 5.3. The structures of the lateral wall of the nasal cavity, after removal of the middle and superior turbinates, are visible. The ground lamella (*arrowheads*) divides the anterior (*B*, bulla ethmoidalis; *A*, agger nasi) from the posterior ethmoid (*PE*). The natural ostium of the maxillary sinus (*black arrow*) is hidden behind the uncinate process. *Dashed line* indicates the path of drainage of the frontal sinus into the middle meatus. *FS*, frontal sinus; *UP*, uncinate process; *IT*, inferior turbinate; *SS*, sphenoid sinus

information coming from CT analysis he should clearly have in mind.

5.2.1.1
Uncinectomy

Uncinectomy is the first surgical step to gain access to the ostiomeatal complex. In the case of isolated disease of the maxillary sinus, resection can be limited to the inferior part of the uncinate process just to expose the natural ostium of the maxillary sinus and the area of the posterior fontanelle (Fig. 5.4a). On the other hand, when the patient presents inflammatory changes only in the frontal sinus, superior uncinectomy may enable an adequate exposure of the frontal recess (Fig. 5.4b). Whenever the surgeon is dealing with extensive disease, the uncinate process must be entirely resected (Fig. 5.4c). CT scan, other than supplying information regarding possible anatomic variations of the uncinate process (i.e., pneumatization, paradoxical curvature) and the configuration of its upper part in relation to adjacent structures, clearly shows the relationship between the uncinate process and the lamina papyracea. This allows the surgeon to minimize the risk to penetrate the orbit during surgical maneuvers.

5.2.1.2
Middle Antrostomy

In some patients with recurrent maxillary sinusitis, inflammatory changes at the level of the inferior part of the ethmoid infundibulum interfere with the patency of the natural ostium, but only minimal mucosal alterations are present within the sinus. Whenever, after performing an inferior uncinectomy and removing with atraumatic technique the polyps possibly present in the inferior part of the ethmoid infundibulum, the natural ostium is well evident and patent, harvesting a middle antrostomy is unnecessary. Conversely, this is required when the maxillary sinus presents extensive disease. Widening its natural ostium in an anterior direction is limited by the presence of the nasolacrimal duct; therefore, one should be very careful not to injure it, to avoid a lacrimal pathway stenosis. Therefore, we prefer to create the antrostomy by enlarging the ostium posteriorly at the expense of the posterior fontanellae, where the maxillary and nasal mucosa stick together without bony interposition (Fig. 5.5). Whenever a dehiscence at this level (accessory ostium) is present, both ostia must be included in the antrostomy to guarantee an

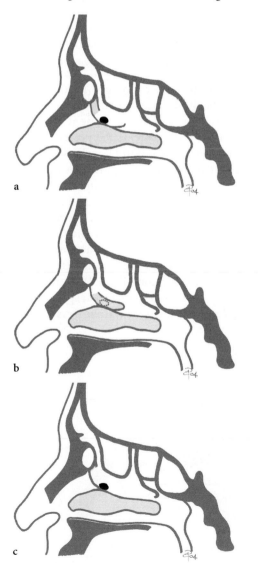

Fig. 5.4a-c. Three different types of uncinectomy are displayed: partial inferior (**a**); partial superior (**b**); total (**c**)

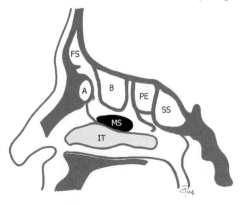

Fig. 5.5. After performing a total uncinectomy, middle antrostomy is harvested by posteriorly enlarging the natural ostium. *MS*, maxillary sinus; *B*, bulla ethmoidalis; *A*, agger nasi; *PE*, posterior ethmoid; *FS*, frontal sinus; *IT*, inferior turbinate; *SS*, sphenoid sinus

effective drainage, to avoid the phenomenon of mucus recirculation, and to prevent a persistent mucus discharge from the maxillary sinus.

Using angled endoscopes and curved instruments it is possible to easily work through a middle antrostomy inside the maxillary sinus. However, some areas of the medial maxillary wall or of the alveolar recess which are hidden to a transnasal view, may be easily reached through a canine fossa approach, a transoral small opening in the anterior wall obtained with a trocar. Surgical instruments may be used through the canine fossa into the maxillary sinus under the control of an angled endoscope inserted transnasally or vice versa (Fig. 5.6).

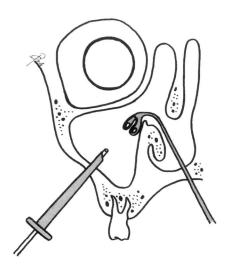

Fig. 5.6. Canine fossa approach: the endoscope is introduced into the trocar through the anterior wall of the maxillary sinus; different surgical instruments may be used through the nasal cavity

5.2.1.3
Ethmoidotomy

The term "ethmoidotomy" will be used instead of "ethmoidectomy" since the aim of endonasal surgery for inflammatory diseases is generally to remove all the bony septa which made up the ethmoid labyrinth apart from the peripheral walls of the box, which are left intact. Any effort should also be paid to preserve as much as possible the peripheral mucosa, thus avoiding denudation of the bone and slowing of the healing process. The use of cutting instruments and of a microdebrider, which has been designed for precise removal of only soft tissues, helps tremendously in obtaining a very conservative dissection.

The bulla ethmoidalis is usually the largest and more constant cell of the anterior ethmoid: its opening is recommended at the level of the inferomedial corner, a safe area far away from the lamina papyracea and the skull base. After the bulla has been removed (Fig. 5.7), the course of the ground lamella can

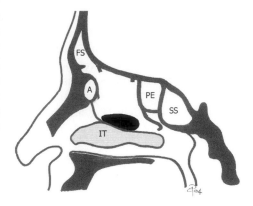

Fig. 5.7. The bulla ethmoidalis has been removed. *A*, agger nasi; *PE*, posterior ethmoid; *FS*, frontal sinus; *IT*, inferior turbinate; *SS*, sphenoid sinus

usually be followed with the endoscope. Its identification may be difficult because of pathologic changes or anatomic variations and also because it is not always a smooth flat bony plate. If the posterior ethmoid must be opened, the ground lamella should be perforated on its inferomedial corner. It is of paramount importance not to remove the inferior part of the lamella, which would result in destabilization of the middle turbinate with a high risk of lateralization and secondary closure of frontal recess and maxillary ostium. The posterior ethmoid is now accessible and the surgeon proceeds to open all the cells to obtain an adequate marsupialization (Fig. 5.8). During the dissection along the lamina papyracea, special care should be taken not to injure and transgress it, with

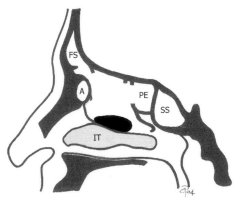

Fig. 5.8. The ground lamella has been perforated to approach the posterior ethmoidal cells. *A*, agger nasi; *PE*, posterior ethmoid; *FS*, frontal sinus; *IT*, inferior turbinate; *SS*, sphenoid sinus

the potential risk of determining a lesion of the medial rectus muscle or of the optic nerve. The presence of an Onodi cell, which by definition contains in its lateral wall the optic nerve, should be identified on CT scan and kept well in mind by the surgeon during this phase of the operation.

One of the major sources of debate among rhinosurgeons is how to manage the middle turbinate during ethmoid surgery. In our opinion, every effort should be made to spare this anatomic structure, which plays an important role in modulating the air flow through the nasal fossa and also contributes to olfactory function, but there are indeed situations, when it becomes unstable or it is covered by a mucosa with massive polypoid changes, which make its sacrifice necessary. Whenever the surgeon is faced with a pneumatized middle turbinate which is itself diseased or causes obstruction of the ostiomeatal complex, a partial sagittal turbinectomy, leaving intact the medial part, is indicated (Fig. 5.9).

and, on the other, by the anatomical configuration of each single patient. A transnasal approach to the sphenoid sinus is generally elected when an isolated disease of the sinus is present and there is enough space between the septum and the middle-superior turbinates to have direct access to the sphenoethmoid recess and the sphenoid ostium. Whenever the surgeon is faced with an unfavorable anatomic situation or the disease involves both the ethmoid and the sphenoid, the transethmoid approach is preferable. However, one should keep in mind that a transethmoid approach does not lead to the anterior wall of the sphenoid in the region of its natural ostium, but superiorly and laterally to it. Access to the sinus has therefore to be gained inferiorly and medially by down-fracturing the anterolateral wall; sphenoidotomy is then progressively enlarged to include the sphenoid ostium. An alternative technique (BOLGER et al. 1999; ORLANDI et al. 1999), which we personally prefer for its safety, consists first in the identification of the sphenoid ostium by resecting the inferior part of the superior turbinate, and subsequently in its progressive enlargement in an inferolateral direction.

Whatever technique has been chosen, the size of a sphenoidotomy should be large enough to prevent any possible scar closure (Fig. 5.10).

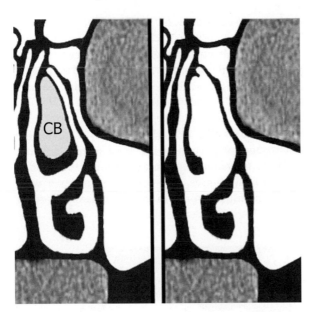

Fig. 5.9. On the left, a concha bullosa (*CB*) is represented. On the right, a partial sagittal turbinectomy, leaving intact the medial part, has been performed

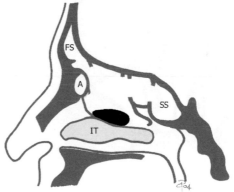

Fig. 5.10. A wide sphenoidotomy has been performed. *A*, agger nasi; *FS*, frontal sinus; *IT*, inferior turbinate; *SS*, sphenoid sinus

5.2.1.4
Sphenoidotomy

There are two main routes to approach the sphenoid sinus with microendoscopic surgery: through the ethmoid or through the nasal fossa, by passing in between the septum and the middle-superior turbinates. The choice between the two options is dictated, on one hand, by the type and extent of disease

5.2.1.5
Clearance of the Frontal Recess

The approach to the frontal recess and to the frontal sinus is by far the most difficult step in the learning curve of microendoscopic surgery. This is mainly due to the extremely complex and variable anatomy of a very narrow area, where mucosal and bony alterations related to the disease make the identification of the surgical landmarks even more challenging. Understanding the anatomy of the single patient through a careful analysis of imaging studies and, in general, the use of a very gentle and atraumatic dissection technique are key elements for being successful in managing frontal sinus inflammatory diseases without significant complications.

The less invasive approach to the frontal sinus, which, in most patients with inflammatory diseases, makes obtaining good re-ventilation and a satisfactory control of specific symptoms such as frontal headache possible, simply includes a careful clearance of the frontal recess. This is achieved by removing the upper part of the uncinate process, the posterosuperior wall of the agger nasi cell and the ethmoid bulla, whenever hypertrophic (Fig. 5.11). It is worth mentioning that in selected patients with favorable anatomy, the ethmoid bulla can be preserved. Removal of the entire floor of the frontal sinus by alternatively using a burr and cutting instruments, a technique known as Draf's type IIB

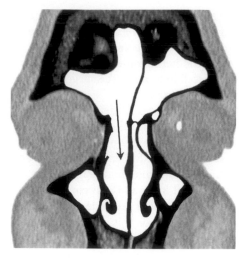

Fig. 5.12. Type IIB approach to the frontal sinus according to WEBER et al. (2001). The entire floor of the frontal sinus between the lamina papyracea and the nasal septum has been removed

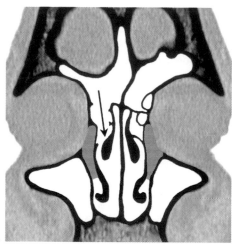

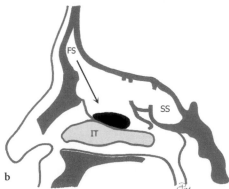

Fig. 5.11. a Clearance of the frontal recess: the posterosuperior wall of the agger nasi cell has been removed (*orange* indicates lacrimal pathways). **b** Resection of the ethmoid bulla is also visible. *FS*, frontal sinus; *IT*, inferior turbinate; *SS*, sphenoid sinus

drainage (WEBER et al. 2001) (Fig. 5.12), guarantees a wider access to the sinus in case of extensive inflammatory changes or small benign lesions, such as osteoma or inverted papilloma. The more advanced endonasal microendoscopic technique for frontal sinus diseases is Draf's type III median drainage (DRAF 1991), also known in the US literature as modified Lothrop procedure (GROSS et al. 1995) (Fig. 5.13). By removing the anterosuperior portion of the nasal septum together with the intersinus septum and drilling the floor of both frontal sinuses, this operation creates a wide common drainage for both frontal sinuses. According

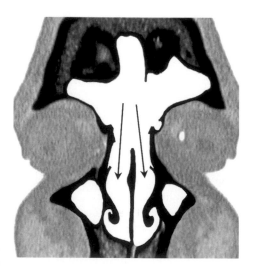

Fig. 5.13. Type III approach to the frontal sinus (median drainage) according to DRAF (1991)

to DRAF et al. (2000), when the size of the frontal sinus is such that the anteroposterior diameter measured on axial CT is less than 0.8 cm, it is very difficult to end up with a patent frontal sinusotomy. Another limitation of the technique is exposure of the far lateral part of extensively pneumatized frontal sinuses.

5.2.2
Neoplastic Lesions

In the last two decades the indications for micro-endoscopic surgery have been greatly expanded to include most benign lesions of the sinonasal tract (SCHICK et al. 2001; TOMENZOLI et al. 2004) and na-sopharynx (ROGER et al. 2002; NICOLAI et al. 2003) and even selected cases of early malignant tumors (STAMMBERGER et al. 1999; GOFFART et al. 2000, ROH et al. 2004).

Since the usual principle of achieving a radical excision, which is the main goal of oncologic surgery, must be fulfilled as in any external procedure, the microendoscopic technique must be adapted to the different nature of the lesions. Therefore, dissection has to be carried out along the subperiosteal plane whenever the surgeon is dealing with benign lesions without any sign of bony resorption. Resection of the underlying bone is routinely required instead for malignant lesions and also for benign lesions when cross sectional imaging suggests the presence of bony thinning or resorption.

En-bloc resection is feasible when the lesion is limited in size and involves the nasal fossa and/or the ethmoid, but it is difficult to achieve when the lesion entirely fills the nasal fossa or extends into the maxillary sinus. In such situations, one must resort to removing that portion of the lesion which is freely growing into the nasal cavity and does not invade the adjacent structures to create enough space for surgical maneuvers. Another important surgical trick is to transect the tumor in two or more pieces, possibly with the help of a laser which makes it possible to work in a bloodless field, so that it becomes easier to have a good view over the limits of the lesion and to perform the dissection along the proper planes.

Much data on the management of benign lesions with microendoscopic approaches has been accumulated in the literature so that general consensus on indications and limitations is well established. These will be discussed for the specific lesions in the pertinent chapters. On the contrary, the experience on malignant lesions is still very limited in terms of sample size and follow-up to allow any meaningful conclu-

sion. A microendoscopic approach seems presently justified for early low-grade lesions and should be performed only in highly specialized centers, where the members of the surgical team have adequate experience also in external procedures and proper co-operation with other specialists (i.e., neurosurgeons) is easily available, should the intraoperative findings dictate the need for an external more invasive approach (STAMMBERGER et al. 1999).

5.3
Open Surgery: Basic Knowledge of the Most Frequently Used Approaches

5.3.1
Maxillectomies

This term includes a wide spectrum of surgical procedures, varying from partial resections of different types in relation to the site of origin of the lesion (inferior maxillectomy, medial maxillectomy, subtotal maxillectomy), to the standard radical maxillectomy, to the extended radical maxillectomies, in which the operation includes clearance or resection of one or more adjacent anatomic structures (orbit, premaxillary soft tissues and skin, zygomatic bone, pterygoid process, pterygomaxillary fossa, infratemporal fossa).

Access to the lesion may be obtained through a transoral approach, as for tumors involving the inferior half of the maxillary sinus, which are amenable to partial inferior maxillectomy (Fig. 5.14).

Medial maxillectomy, which is usually associated to an ethmoidectomy (Fig. 5.15), is indicated for benign (i.e., inverted papilloma) and malignant lesions limited to the lower part of the ethmoid, the nasal cavity,

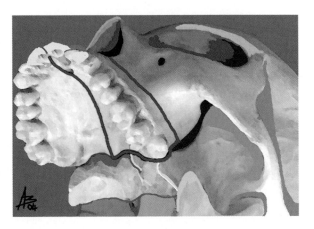

Fig. 5.14. Partial inferior maxillectomy

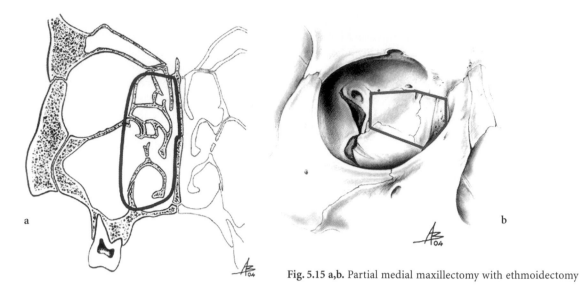

Fig. 5.15 a,b. Partial medial maxillectomy with ethmoidectomy

and/or the medial wall of the maxillary sinus. In many benign lesions, the operation can also be performed transnasally with a microendoscopic approach, but for most malignant lesions an external approach is still the option of choice. Medial maxillectomy has been traditionally performed through a lateral rhinotomy approach (Fig. 5.16), but in recent years a common tendency to resort to midfacial degloving (CASSON et al. 1974) has been observed. This surgical technique is characterized by the association of sublabial and rhinoplastic incisions, with or without osteotomies at the level of nasal bones and the frontal process of the maxilla (Fig. 5.17).

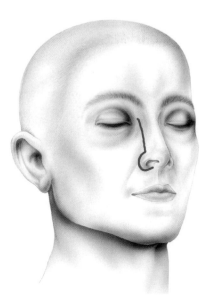

Fig. 5.16. Lateral rhinotomy incision

The first step is a bilateral intercartilaginous incision at the level of the nasal vestibulum; the procedure then proceeds with nasal soft tissue dissection from lateral cartilages and nasal septum by means of an incision that divides it from the columella. The intercartilaginous incisions go on bilaterally until the floor of the vestibulum, joining together with the septal incision. The second step is another incision at the level of mucosa of the superior buccal vestibulum extended to the third molar bilaterally, followed by a subperiosteal dissection which exposes the anterior wall of both maxilla, the inferolateral margins of the pyriform fossa, and the infraorbital nerves up to the inferior frame of the orbits. At this point, the nasal-maxillary cavity is entered by entirely resecting the anterior wall of the maxillary sinus. In the case of benign lesions or of malignant lesions not involving the anterior wall, it can be temporarily removed and fixed back at the end of the operation with microplates in titanium or in reabsorbable material.

Midfacial degloving, which currently represents the gold standard for the surgical treatment also of neoplasms of the nasopharynx (i.e., juvenile angiofibroma) not amenable to microendoscopic surgery, has the advantage of avoiding evident scars and of maintaining good vascularization of the facial flap. Major limitations are, however, an anterior extension of the neoplasm with involvement of the nasal bones, lacrimal pathways, and/or pre-maxillary soft tissues, a superior growth into the frontal sinus, and all the situations in which the inferior and/or the medial walls of the orbit are eroded by the lesion and a careful dissection from the periorbit is therefore required. In all these situations a lateral rhinotomy approach, with or without

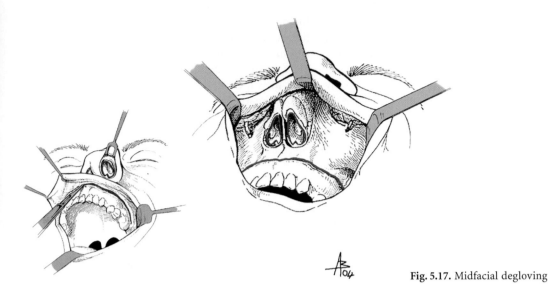

Fig. 5.17. Midfacial degloving

superior lip splitting (Fig. 5.16), which gives an excellent exposure of the surgical field and ensures a good control of the dissection along the inferior and medial orbital walls, is still indicated.

The same access is recommended for radical maxillectomy (Fig. 5.18) and extended radical maxillectomies, which may require the association of an infratemporal approach or a frontal craniotomy whenever the lesion extends far posteriorly or superiorly to invade the skull base, respectively.

The goal of modern oncologic surgery of the sinonasal tract is not only to provide a radical extirpation of the lesion, but also to preserve to the best possible extent functions such chewing, eating, and speaking, as well as aesthetic appearance. Different techniques can be employed principally in relation to the entity of the ablative procedure.

A prosthetic obturator is a simple solution for a small defect after inferior maxillectomy. A clasp-retained obturator can later be substituted by a more stable one based on bone-anchored implants. Problems of prosthetic stability derive from excision of more than half the palate. In such cases, a tripod-like stabilization of the obturator can be obtained by means of bone graft or, even better, with one of the more reliable revascularized free osseous flaps (from scapula, iliac crest, fibula, or radium) (FUNK et al. 1998). In toothless patients, soft tissue flaps can be sufficient to separate the sinonasal tract from the oral cavity. For less than half-palate defects, a pedicled temporalis muscle flap can still be considered an option, particularly when in combination with total or extended maxillectomy; it is easy to harvest and the risk of failure is very low (COLMENERO et al. 1991). On the other hand, larger palatal excision

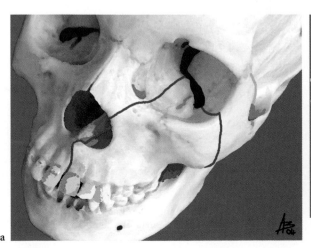

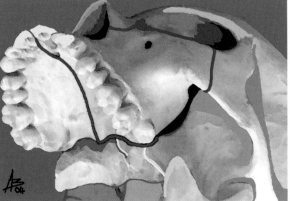

Fig. 5.18 a,b. Radical maxillectomy

without need of dental rehabilitation should be closed by a radial free flap or with the muscular portion of other composite flaps (scapular, fibular, or iliac crest).

Iliac crest, scapula, and fibula, if appropriately harvested and oriented, can be even used to adequately restore the anterior maxillary contour and three-dimensional projection of the face when the anterior wall of the maxillary and zygomatic bones have been removed.

When more than half of the orbital floor needs to be resected, reconstruction with split calvarial bone is mandatory to prevent sequelae such as diplopia or enophthalmos. Moreover, the membranous portion of cranial bones like the parietal one, seems to be reabsorbed less frequently than the endochondral bones previously used (rib and iliac crest), even during radiotherapy (Zins and Whitaker 1993). However, meticulous coverage of the graft by soft tissues should be always obtained.

In the case of extended maxillectomies, a number of different situations can be encountered depending on the specific structures removed. Large cheek or scalp defects can be closed by free flaps (radial, rectus abdominis or parascapular) with the appropriate bulk. External nose and auricular defects are usually restored by prostheses; pedicled or free flaps simply play the role of cover for the surgical wound to prepare tissues for prosthesis retention. Orbital exenteration usually poses more challenging problems. A pure soft lining of the orbital cavity can be achieved by the temporalis muscle, over which a prosthesis will be later positioned (Turner et al. 1999). The orbit can be alternatively filled by soft tissue transfer if an adjacent skull base defect demands it or when ocular prosthesis is not desired.

5.3.2
Osteoplastic Flap Sinusotomy

This operation is currently considered the gold standard whenever an external approach to the frontal sinus is required after failure of previous endonasal procedures or when the disease cannot be adequately reached transnasally. The anterior wall of the frontal sinus may be exposed through a coronal incision, which is carried out far posteriorly to be hidden by the hair line, or a "butterfly" or "seagull" incision, which is performed along the superior border of the eyebrows (Fig. 5.19). Our preference is for coronal incision, since the latter may leave the patient with a visible scar and some numbness of the forehead. Soft tissue dissection is then carried along the plane between the galea and

the pericranium to leave the pericranium adherent to the underlying bone, so as to maintain an adequate vascularization to the bone. With the help of a template of the frontal sinus, obtained from a Caldwell view the superior margin of the sinus is identified and a cut is made in the bone along this margin with an oscillating saw (Fig. 5.20). Using a chisel, the bony flap is gently down-fractured attached to the pericranium

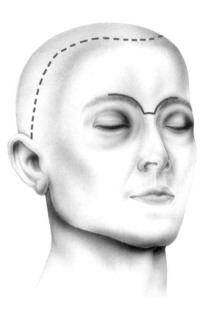

Fig. 5.19. Different incisions for osteoplastic frontal sinusotomy: coronal incision (*broken red line*) and "butterfly" or "seagull" incision (*solid red line*)

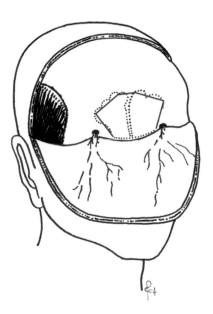

Fig. 5.20. A skin-galeal frontal flap has been dissected and downward reflected. With the help of a template, a bony flap is created and down-fractured

and the frontal sinus is entirely exposed. The original technique includes careful removal of the disease (i.e., mucocele, osteoma) together with all the mucosa lining the sinus, plugging of both frontal infundibula with cartilage and/or muscle, and obliteration of the sinus with fat obtained through a small incision made in the abdominal wall. In our experience, in selected patients who have an extremely localized disease not involving the infundibulum area in an otherwise well ventilated sinus, obliteration of the sinus may be avoided.

A coronal approach is routinely indicated for osteomyelitis of the frontal bone, which usually complicates an acute frontal rhinosinusitis. The entity of bony resection must be tailored to the extent of the osteomyelitic process. If the anterior wall is involved, obliteration of the sinus with fat is obtained and reconstruction of the bony wall is secondarily performed, when there will be clear clinical and radiological signs that the inflammatory process has been controlled. When osteomyelitis affects the posterior wall of the frontal sinus, this needs to be resected; cranialization of the sinus is performed after sealing both frontal infundibula with cartilage or muscle to prevent any contamination from the nasal cavities.

5.3.3
Anterior Craniofacial Resection

Even though anecdotal examples of operative techniques anticipating the concept of anterior craniofacial resection were published in the 1940s (DANDY 1941) and 1950s (MALECKI 1959), KETCHAM et al. (1963) must be credited with the first results on a group of 19 patients with malignant tumors, most originating from the sinonasal tract, who had received anterior craniofacial resection. This surgical technique can be considered the major innovative procedure among the external approaches of the last four decades, since it has markedly contributed to improving the prognosis of malignant tumors encroaching the anterior skull base. The basic concept of the operation is to obtain additional exposure of the tumor from above and to ensure even superiorly a free margin of resection. This is usually achieved through a coronal incision and a frontal craniotomy, which, accoording to RAVEH et al. (1993), is harvested as low as possible to obtain a good view on the anterior skull base without undue retraction of the frontal lobes (Fig. 5.21). A midfacial degloving, a lateral rhinotomy approach, or even in selected cases a transnasal microendoscopic approach (THALER et al. 1999) is associated to perform the dissection of the inferior part of the surgical specimen.

Whenever the lesion is in close contact with the skull base, but there are no radiologic and intraoperative signs of bony involvement, the procedure can be carried out extradurally and the dissection superiorly includes the cribriform plate and the fovea ethmoidalis. Those lesions eroding the skull base and possibly infiltrating the dura dictate instead a wide resection of the dura. The ablative part of the operation must be further extended to include a variable amount of brain parenchyma when the lesion is clearly in contact or even infiltrates the frontal lobe(s). Dura defects require multiple-layer duraplasty which can be performed with different autologous and/or homologous materials. An anteriorly-pedicled pericranium flap down-folded and fixed posteriorly to the planum sphenoidale is commonly used to reinforce the duraplasty and to offer a nicely vascularized barrier, which divides the sinonasal tract from the cranium.

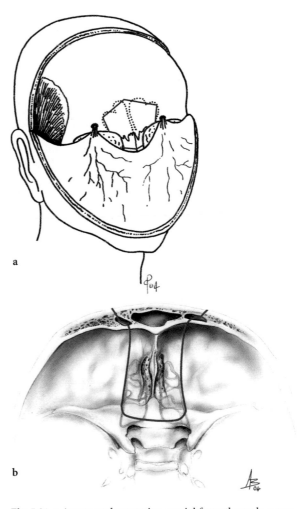

Fig. 5.21. a Access to the anterior cranial fossa through a coronal incision (*red line*, frontal craniotomy). **b** Posteriorly the resection reaches the planum sphenoidale

References

Bolger WE, Keyes AS, Lanza DC (1999) Use of the superior meatus and superior turbinate in the endoscopic approach to the sphenoid sinus. Otolaryngol Head Neck Surg 120:308-313

Casson PR, Bonanno PC, Converse JM (1974) The midfacial degloving procedure. Plast Reconstr Surg 53:102-113

Colmenero C, Martorell V, Colmenero B et al (1991) Temporalis myofascial flap for maxillofacial reconstruction. J Oral Maxillofac Surg 49:1067-1073

Dandy WE (1941) Orbital tumors. Oskar Priest Publications, New York

Draf W (1991) Endonasal micro-endoscopic frontal sinus surgery, the Fulda concept. Op Tech Otolaryngol Head Neck Surg 2:234-240

Draf W, Weber R, Keerl R et al (2000) Endonasal and external micro-endoscopic surgery of the frontal sinus. In: Stamm A, Draf W (eds) Microendoscopic surgery of the paranasal sinuses and the skull base. Springer-Verlag, Berlin Heidelberg New York, pp 257–278

Draf W, Weber R (1993) Endonasal pansinus operation in chronic sinusitis. I: Indication and operation technique. Am J Otolaryngol 14:394-398

Funk GF, Arcuri MR, Frodel JL (1998) Functional dental rehabilitation of massive palatomaxillary defects: cases requiring free tissue transfer and osseointegrated implants. Head Neck 20:38-51

Goffart Y, Jorissen M, Daele J et al (2000) Minimally invasive endoscopic management of malignant sinonasal tumors. Acta Otorhinolaryngol Belg 54:221-232

Gross CW, Gross WE, Becker DG (1995) Modified transnasal endoscopic Lothrop procedure: frontal drillout. Op Tech Otolaryngol Head Neck Surg 6:193-200.

Heermann H (1958) Endonasal surgery with the use of the binocular Zeiss operating microscope. Arch Klin Exp Ohren Nasen Kehlkopfheilkd 171:295-297

Ketcham AS, Wilkins RH, van Buren JM et al (1963) A combined intracranial facial approach to the paranasal sinuses. Am J Surg 106:698-703

Malecki J (1959) New trends in frontal sinus surgery. Acta Otolaryngol (Stockh) 50:137-140

Messerklinger W (1972) Technik und Möglichkeiten der Nasenendoskopie. HNO 20:133-135

Messerklinger W (1978) Endoscopy of the nose. Urban and Schwarzenberg, Munich

Nicolai P, Berlucchi M, Tomenzoli D et al (2003) Endoscopic surgery for juvenile angiofibroma: when and how. Laryngoscope 113:775-782

Orlandi RR, Lanza DC, Bolger WE et al (1999) The forgotten turbinate: the role of the superior turbinate in endoscopic sinus surgery. Am J Rhinol 13:251-259

Raveh J, Leadrach K, Speiter M et al (1993). The subcranial approach for fronto-orbital and anteroposterior skull-base tumors. Arch Otolaryngol Head Neck Surg 119: 385-393

Roger G, Tran Ba Huy P, Froehlich P et al (2002) Exclusively endoscopic removal of juvenile nasopharyngeal angiofibroma: trends and limits. Arch Otolaryngol Head Neck Surg 128:928-935

Roh HJ, Batza PS, Citazdi, MJ et al (2004) Endoscopic resection of sinonasal malignancies: a preliminary report. Am J Rhinol 18:239-248

Schick B, Steigerwald C, el Tahan R et al (2001) The role of endonasal surgery in the management of frontoethmoidal osteomas. Rhinology 39:667-670

Stamm AC, Draf W (2000) Micro-endoscopic surgery of the paranasal sinuses and the skull base. Springer, Berlin Heidelberg New York

Stammberger H (1986a) Endoscopic endonasal surgery-concepts in treatment of recurring rhinosinusitis, part I. Anatomic and pathophysiologic considerations. Otolaryngol Head Neck Surg 94:143-147

Stammberger H (1986b) Endoscopic endonasal surgery-concepts in treatment of recurring rhinosinusitis, part II. Surgical technique. Otolaryngol Head Neck Surg 94:147-156

Stammberger H, Anderhuber W, Walch C et al (1999) Possibilities and limitations of endoscopic management of nasal and paranasal sinus malignancies. Acta Otorhinolaryngol Belg 53:199-205

Thaler ER, Kotapka M, Lanza DC et al (1999) Endoscopically assisted anterior cranial skull base resection of sinonasal tumors. Am J Rhinol 13:303-310

Tomenzoli D, Castelnuovo P, Pagella F et al (2004) Different endoscopic surgical strategies in the management of inverted papilloma of the sinonasal tract: experience on 47 cases. Laryngoscope 114:193–200

Turner GE, Cassisi NJ (1999) Maxillofacial prosthetics. In: Maniglia AJ, Stucker FJ, Stepnick DW (eds) Surgical reconstruction of the face and anterior skull base. Saunders, Philadelphia, pp 245-258

Weber R, Draf W, Kratzsch B et al (2001) Modern concepts of frontal sinus surgery. Laryngoscope 111:137-146

Wigand ME (1981) Transnasal ethmoidectomy under endoscopic control. Rhinology 19:7-15

Zins JE, Whitaker LA (1983) Membranous versus endochondral bone: implications for craniofacial reconstruction. Plast Reconstr Surg 72:778-784

6 Inflammatory Lesions

Davide Farina, Davide Tomenzoli, Andrea Borghesi, and Davide Lombardi

CONTENTS

6.2 Acute Rhinosinusitis and Its Complications 59
6.2.1 Definition, Epidemiology, Pathophysiology, and Etiology 59
6.2.2 Clinical and Endoscopic Findings 60
6.2.3 Treatment Guidelines 61
6.2.4 Key Information to Be Provided by Imaging 62
6.2.5 Imaging Findings 62
6.3 Chronic Rhinosinusitis and Polyposis 65
6.3.1 Definition, Epidemiology, Pattern of Growth 65
6.3.2 Clinical and Endoscopic Findings 66
6.3.3 Treatment Guidelines 67
6.3.4 Key Information to Be Provided by Imaging 68
6.3.5 Imaging Findings 68
6.3.5.1 Infundibular Pattern 68
6.3.5.2 Ostiomeatal Unit Pattern 68
6.3.5.3 Sphenoethmoid Recess Pattern 69
6.3.5.4 Pattern of Nasal Polyposis 69
6.3.5.5 Sporadic Pattern 71
6.3.5.6 Chronic Rhinosinusitis: Staging Systems 72
6.4 Fungal Rhinosinusitis 72
6.4.1 Definition, Epidemiology, and Pathophysiology 72
6.4.2 Clinical and Endoscopic Findings 73
6.4.3 Treatment Guidelines 74
6.4.4 Key Information to Be Provided by Imaging 75
6.4.5 Imaging Findings 75
6.5 Aggressive Granulomatous Lesions 77
6.5.1 Wegener Granulomatosis 77
6.5.1.1 Definition and Epidemiology 77
6.5.1.2 Clinical and Endoscopic Findings 78
6.5.1.3 Treatment Guidelines 79
6.5.1.4 Key Information to Be Provided by Imaging 80
6.5.2 Cocaine Induced Destructive Lesions 80
6.5.2.1 Definition and Epidemiology 80
6.5.2.2 Clinical and Endoscopic Findings 80
6.5.2.3 Treatment Guidelines 81
6.5.2.4 Key Information to Be Provided by Imaging 81
6.5.3 Sarcoidosis 81
6.5.3.1 Definition and Epidemiology 81
6.5.3.2 Clinical and Endoscopic Findings 82
6.5.3.3 Treatment Guidelines 82
6.5.3.4 Key Information to Be Provided by Imaging 83
6.5.4 Imaging Findings 83
References 88

D. Farina, MD
Department of Radiology, University of Brescia, Piazzale Spedali Civili 1, Brescia, BS, 25123, Italy
D. Tomenzoli, MD
Department of Otorhinolaryngology, University of Brescia, Piazzale Spedali Civili 1, Brescia, BS, 25123, Italy
A. Borghesi, MD
Department of Radiology, University of Brescia, Piazzale Spedali Civili 1, Brescia, BS, 25123, Italy
D. Lombardi, MD
Department of Otorhinolaryngology, University of Brescia, Piazzale Spedali Civili 1, Brescia, BS, 25123, Italy

6.2
Acute Rhinosinusitis and Its Complications

6.2.1
Definition, Epidemiology, Pathophysiology, and Etiology

Rhinosinusitis is defined as an inflammation of the mucosa of the nose and paranasal sinuses. It is classified as acute, subacute, and chronic according to whether the duration of symptoms persists as long as 4 weeks, between 4 and 12 weeks, and more than 12 weeks, respectively (Brook et al. 2000). More than \$2 billion is spent annually in the United States for over-the-counter medications for rhinosinusitis (National Center for Health Statistics 1994).

Even though data regarding the incidence of rhinosinusitis in the world population are scarce in the literature, every year approximately 16% of adults in the United States receive a diagnosis of rhinosinusitis (National Center for Health Statistics 1994).

If the forms of rhinosinusitis exclusively arising in a single paranasal sinus, such as the maxillary sinus, in relation to tooth disease, facial trauma, or paranasal sinus neoplasms are excluded, the first step in the pathophysiology of most rhinosinusitis is almost invariably an inflammation with edema of the mucosa which involves one or both "pre-chambers" (ostiomeatal complex, sphenoethmoidal recess). This causes an obstruction of the dependent sinus outflow and creates an ideal environment for pathogen and saprophytic bacteria. In acute rhinosinusitis, the most frequently isolated bacteria are *Streptococcus pneumoniae*, *Haemophilus influenzae*, and *Moraxella catharralis* in 41%, 35%, and 7% of cultures, respectively (Wald 1998).

Apart from the duration of symptoms, acute and subacute rhinosinusitis may be regarded as the same disease, since they share the same etiology (infectious), pathogenesis (obstruction of the sinus drainage), medical therapy, and complications. For this reason, they will be discussed together under the term *acute rhinosinusitis*.

Despite the widespread use of broad-spectrum antibiotics, complications of acute rhinosinusitis may still be a fatal event in a percentage ranging from 1% to 3.7% (PATT and MANNING 1991; YOUNIS et al. 2002a). BRADLEY et al. (1984) and YOUNIS et al. (2002b) reported the occurrence of complications in 0.5% and 11% of patients admitted to their institutions for rhinosinusitis, respectively. Intraorbital and intracranial complications are more frequently reported, while osteomyelitis and toxic shock syndrome are rarely encountered (LUSK 1992; YOUNIS et al. 2002a,b).

Orbital complications may be subdivided into five groups (CHANDLER et al. 1970):
- *Group 1.* Preseptal cellulitis. Edema of the eyelids without tenderness and with no associated visual loss or limitation of extraocular motility
- *Group 2.* Orbital cellulitis without abscess. Diffuse edema of the adipose tissue in the orbit with no abscess formation
- *Group 3.* Orbital cellulitis with subperiosteal abscess. Abscess formation between the orbital periosteum and orbital bone; the abscess displaces the globe, usually down and laterally; if the proptosis is severe, it will be associated with limitation of ocular motility and perhaps decreased visual acuity
- *Group 4.* Orbital cellulitis with abscess within the orbital fat. Proptosis may be purely frontally directed and not laterally or inferiorly displaced as in subperiosteal abscess; severe limitation of extraocular motility results and visual loss due to optic neuropathy may ensue
- *Group 5.* Cavernous sinus thrombosis. Orbital phlebitis extends into the cavernous sinus and across the basilar venous plexus to the opposite side, resulting in bilateral disease

In decreasing order of frequency, *intracranial complications* are: subdural empyema, intracerebral abscess, extradural abscess, meningitis, and, more rarely, cavernous and superior sagittal sinus thrombosis (JONES et al. 2002).

According to some authors (LANG et al. 2001; NOORDZIJ et al. 2002; YOUNIS et al. 2002a,b) complicated rhinosinusitis more frequently affects children and adolescents, with a male/female ratio of 3:1 (KRAUS and TOVI 1992).

Sinonasal infections reach the orbit and the intracranial cavity spreading through the neurovascular foramina, congenital or acquired bony dehiscences, or via a retrograde flow through the diploic valveless veins secondary to a thrombophlebitis. Since in children the cranium has more diploic veins than in adults, infections spread more deeply and more rapidly. This accounts for a higher incidence of severe complications in children (LUSK 1992; LANG et al. 2001; YOUNIS et al. 2002b).

6.2.2
Clinical and Endoscopic Findings

Patients with acute rhinosinusitis commonly complain of nasal obstruction, rhinorrhea, headache, facial pain, and dysosmia.

The occurrence of an orbital complication may be suspected when fever, exacerbation of headache, and ocular symptoms appear (YOUNIS et al. 2002a). In the presence of preseptal cellulitis, erythema and edema of the eyelid without ophthalmoplegia or visual loss are observed. When proptosis, chemosis, and impairment of extraocular movement occur, a subperiosteal or intraorbital abscess must be suspected. When the patient complains of a unilateral impairment or loss of visual acuity, a compression of the optic nerve or the ophthalmic artery or the small retinoic vessels must be excluded. Acute headache, fever, and painful paresthesia in the distribution of the trigeminal nerve are the early symptoms of cavernous sinus thrombosis; they can be followed by afferent pupillary defect, extraocular motility palsy, and hyperesthesia of the cornea as a consequence of trigeminal nerve inflammation (LUSK 1992). An ominous sign is the appearance of bilateral orbital involvement, which indicates a propagation of the infection to the opposite side through the cavernous sinus plexus (SHAHIN et al. 1987).

Whenever an orbital complication is observed, ophthalmologic consultation is mandatory to disclose any possible sign (optic disc pallor, papilledema, decreased venous pulsation) suggesting an impairment of blood flow.

In a patient with acute rhinosinusitis, the onset of an acute or gradually worsening headache is the most important symptom indicating an intracranial complication. Nausea, vomiting, alteration of mental status, affective changes, seizures, lethargy, and coma may also be observed. If the frontal lobe is involved,

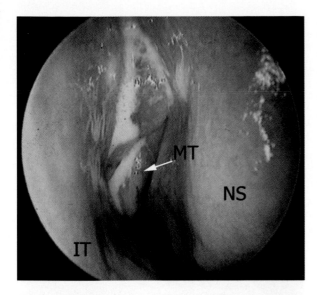

Fig. 6.1. Acute bacterial rhinosinusitis. At nasal endoscopy (0° rigid endoscope), whitish, purulent secretion covers the right middle turbinate (*MT*). Nasal septum, *NS*; inferior turbinate, *IT*

signs and symptoms may be absent, with only mild personality changes until the infection spreads.

Nasal endoscopy shows an inflamed, congested mucosa covered by purulent secretions, flowing from the ostiomeatal complex and the sphenoethmoidal recess when the entire ethmoid is affected by the infection (Fig. 6.1). Isolated involvement of the anterior or posterior compartment of the ethmoid is suggested by the presence of purulent discharge into the middle or superior meatus, respectively. Sometimes, a micropolyposis secondary to the infection can be appreciated. There are no peculiar endoscopic findings which differentiate an uncomplicated from a complicated acute rhinosinusitis; therefore, only an accurate clinical evaluation may alert the physician.

6.2.3
Treatment Guidelines

The treatment of choice of acute rhinosinusitis is antibiotic therapy. The most frequently used antibiotics for non-complicated rhinosinusitis are amoxicillin-clavulanate and second generation cephalosporins for at least 10 days. If the patient does not improve within 72 h, an alternative antibiotic should be used. In the very rare event medical therapy fails, microendoscopic surgery, based on a preoperative CT, is indicated. This may encompass a very limited dissection aimed at restoring the ventilation of the involved paranasal sinus(es), by removing only those bony structures (i.e., uncinate process, ethmoid bulla, pneumatized middle turbinate) which impair the outflow of secretions. There is no need to perform any stripping of mucosa, which will revert to a normal status within a short period.

Most orbital complications respond to intravenous broad-spectrum antibiotics within 48–72 h. According to YOUNIS et al. (2002a), surgery is required when at least one of the following five circumstances is present:
- CT evidence of abscess formation
- 20/60 (or worse) visual acuity on initial evaluation
- Severe orbital complications (i.e., blindness or an afferent pupillary reflex on initial evaluation)
- Progression of orbital signs and symptoms despite therapy
- Lack of improvement within 48 h despite maximum medical therapy

While in the past orbital complications have been routinely treated through external procedures, in the last decades microendoscopic surgery has emerged as the surgical modality of choice for acute rhinosinusitis with an orbital complication, particularly in case of subperiosteal or intraorbital abscesses with a medial location (LUSK 1992; NOORDZIJ et al. 2002; SOBOL et al. 2002). Surgical steps include uncinectomy, anterior and posterior ethmoidotomy, followed by subtotal removal of the lamina papyracea to drain the abscess. Conversely, abscesses located laterally in the orbit require an external approach. For cavernous sinus thrombophlebitis, other than intravenous broad-spectrum antibiotics, steroids, and drainage of the sinonasal area infected (generally the sphenoid or the ethmoid sinus), anticoagulants may be indicated (AMRAN et al. 2002).

Treatment of intracranial complications consists of broad-spectrum intravenous antibiotics crossing the blood–brain barrier. Surgical treatment is indicated if no improvement is noted within 48 h, provided the patient's neurologic condition is stable. Microendoscopic surgery may be employed, apart from the patients who have obvious CT signs of osteomyelitis of the frontal bone. In this circumstance, a coronal approach with wide resection of diseased bone is mandatory. When the posterior wall of the frontal sinus is also involved and needs to be removed, cranialization is required.

6.2.4
Key Information to Be Provided by Imaging

- Extent of the disease
- Presence of anatomic variants altering the physiologic drainage of paranasal sinuses and favoring the occurrence of an acute infection
- Presence of anatomic variants which may increase the risk of intraoperative complications
- Presence of resorption of sinusal walls, particularly the lamina papyracea and the anterior skull base floor
- Presence of abundant scar tissue due to previous sinus surgery
- Identification of complications and assessment of their extent

6.2.5
Imaging Findings

Acute rhinosinusitis does not require a radiologic study of the paranasal sinuses because the symptoms reported by the patient in association with the endoscopic examination are the only diagnostic steps required for making a correct diagnosis (PHILLIPS 1997).

When an *orbital complication* is suspected, generally secondary to acute ethmoiditis, CT permits differentiation between edema, phlegmon, and abscess, and precise identification of the site of the lesion, which is necessary for proper treatment planning (HÄHNEL et al. 1999). CT may discriminate between preseptal cellulitis, subperiosteal inflammation, and intraorbital (extra- or intraconal) spread. Involvement of orbital muscles and posterior extension of the inflammatory collection towards orbital fissures are additional critical issues, the latter entailing an obvious risk of intracranial spread.

Preseptal cellulitis (Group 1 according to CHANDLER et al. 1970) is confined to the anterior compartment of the orbit (eyelid, periorbital soft tissues). CT shows thickening of the orbital septum, increased density of orbital septum and periorbital soft tissues without involvement of the orbital cavity or exophthalmos (OLIVERIO et al. 1995).

Increased density of intraorbital fat tissue is the hallmark of orbital cellulitis (Group 2 according to CHANDLER et al. 1970). It is often observed at the level of the retrobulbar space amid muscles and optic nerve.

Subperiosteal abscess is located between the inner surface of the orbital walls and the periorbita (Group 3 according to CHANDLER et al. 1970) (Fig. 6.2). Both CT and MR may demonstrate a fluid collection with

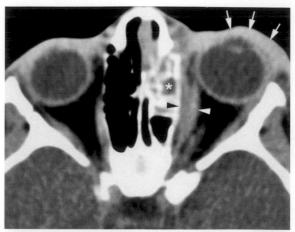
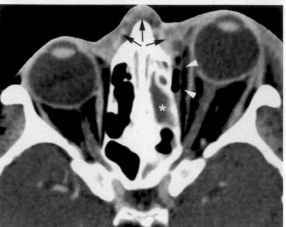

Fig. 6.2 a,b. Complicated acute rhinosinusitis: subperiosteal abscess. Axial CT after contrast administration. **a** Fluid inflammatory material occupies the left ethmoid labyrinth (*asterisk*). Thickening and increased density of periorbital soft tissues at the level of medial orbital angle, eyelid, and nasal pyramid: preseptal edema (*arrows*). An inflammatory collection is detected between the lamina papyracea and the medial rectus muscle (*arrowheads*). **b** The small gas bubbles in the upper section contained in the collection is bordered by a thin hypodense line, probably the periorbita (*arrowheads*): subperiosteal abscess. Thickening of the prenasal tissue (*black arrows*)

a peripheral enhancing rim. CT better depicts subtle defects of the bony walls adjacent to the abscess (YOUSEM 1993). Gas bubbles within the collection herald the presence of anaerobic agents or indicate fistulization from contiguous paranasal cavities.

Abscesses (Group 4 according to CHANDLER et al. 1970) secondary to ethmoid sinusitis are generally observed along the lamina papyracea, displacing the orbit anteriorly and laterally, whereas fluid collections complicating frontal sinusitis are located along the superior orbital wall and dislocate the ocular bulb anteriorly and inferiorly. A key point to be ruled out at CT is intraconal extension of the abscess through a breach of the periorbita. In this case, a precise assessment of the relationships between the lesion, extrinsic muscles, ocular bulb, and optic nerve is necessary (Fig. 6.3).

MR better demonstrates further vascular complications, such as superior ophthalmic vein or cavernous sinus thrombosis (Group 5 according to CHANDLER et al. 1970) (YOUSEM 1993; OLIVERIO et al. 1995).

The entity of bone changes – perfectly depicted at CT – is widely variable: intraorbital spread of inflammation in the absence of detectable defects of the lamina papyracea can often be observed in pediatric patients. More aggressive inflammatory processes may induce osteitis or osteomyelitis. Both CT and MR may demonstrate irregular areas of sclerosis – indicating chronic osteitis – as well as bone destruction with sequestration, typical of active osteomyelitis (Fig. 6.4).

Overall, CT may provide a correct diagnosis of orbital complication in up to 91% of cases, being significantly more accurate than clinical examination alone (81%) (YOUNIS et al. 2002c).

Intracranial complications are generally secondary to frontal sinusitis. They are observed even in the absence of sinus wall defects, as they may be secondary to thrombophlebitis of valveless diploic veins (LERNER et al. 1995). Imaging is mandatory, in order to correctly assess the degree of involvement of in-

tracranial structures. In this setting, MR should be considered the technique of choice, its accuracy being superior to CT, in particular in differentiating dural reaction from epidural/subdural or intracerebral abscess, and in demonstrating thrombosis of sagittal or cavernous sinus (HÄHNEL et al. 1999; RAO et al. 2001; YOUNIS et al. 2002c).

CT findings of meningitis may be unremarkable. Early signs are represented by mild enlargement of ventricles and subarachnoid spaces. Large amounts of inflammatory exudate may efface subarachnoid spaces, inducing marked enhancement of the meninges. This is probably related to extravasation of contrast agent from small vessels or to the presence of granulation tissue. Dural enhancement is also demonstrated at MR, on Gd-enhanced SE T1 images, especially at the level of the falx, tentorium, and convexity (YOUNIS et al. 2002c).

At CT, subdural/epidural abscess is detected as an extracerebral hypodense fluid collection with a convex shape, separated from the parenchyma by a thick and enhancing rim (Fig. 6.5).

The CT appearance of brain abscesses is widely variable in the different phases of evolution. During the cerebritic phase, a focal hypodense area may be observed, characterized by a superficially gyriform and deeply granular pattern of enhancement.

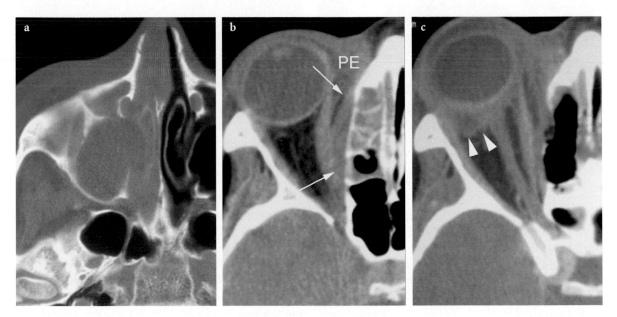

Fig. 6.3a–c. Complicated acute rhinosinusitis: from subperiosteal to intraconal abscess. Plain CT scan on the axial plane (**a,b**); contrast enhanced CT scan obtained 24 h after surgery (**c**). Acute rhinosinusitis: maxillary sinus and ethmoid labyrinth are occupied by inflammatory secretions. Preseptal edema (*PE*) and a subperiosteal abscess – bordered by medial rectus muscle – (*arrows*) are demonstrated in (**b**). CT scan performed 24 h after surgery (**c**) shows a large residual cavity after partial ethmoidotomy and a breach in the medial orbital wall. Though subperiosteal abscess has been drained, an intraconal inflammatory collection has developed behind the eyeball (*arrowheads*)

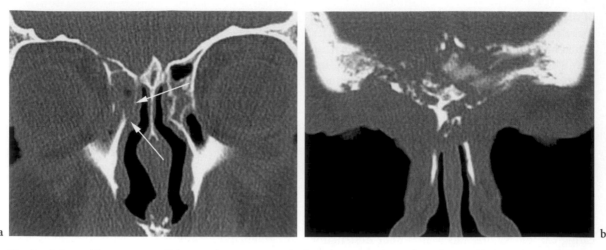

Fig. 6.4a,b. Frontal bone osteomyelitis secondary to acute right frontal sinusitis due to frontal recess blockage (*arrows*)

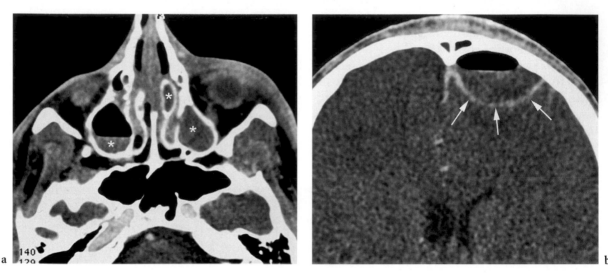

Fig. 6.5a,b. Complicated acute rhinosinusitis. Axial CT after contrast administration. (**a**) Fluid material occupies both maxillary sinuses (a level is observed on the *right*) and a left concha bullosa (*asterisks*). The more cranial scan (**b**) shows an air–fluid collection within the anterior cranial fossa, bordered by thick and enhancing dura (*arrows*): epidural abscess. The absence of macroscopic defects of posterior frontal sinus wall suggests intracranial spread of infection through small veins perforating the diploe of frontal bone

Subsequently, an overall increase in volume occurs as the result of an increase of central necrosis and peripheral edema. These components are undifferentiated at plain CT, whereas contrast administration demonstrates an irregular and enhancing rim separating them (Fig. 6.6). The abscess phase is characterized by the presence of a spontaneously hyperdense thin rim showing strong and homogeneous enhancement, and smooth inner surface. This peripheral ring may be pluriloculated or it may show small satellite rings, generally along its thinner medial border. Perilesional edema is a common finding, absent only in immunocompromised patients or in subjects under steroid therapy.

MR findings of cerebral abscesses are more sensitive. This technique actually better depicts subtle changes observed in the early cerebritic phase, such as sulcus effacement, mass effect, patchy enhancement along sulci and gray matter. Pus collections generally display the typical MR signal pattern of fluids (hyper T2, hypo T1, no enhancement), whereas the capsule bordering the abscess shows hypo T2 and hyper T1 signal with vivid contrast enhancement.

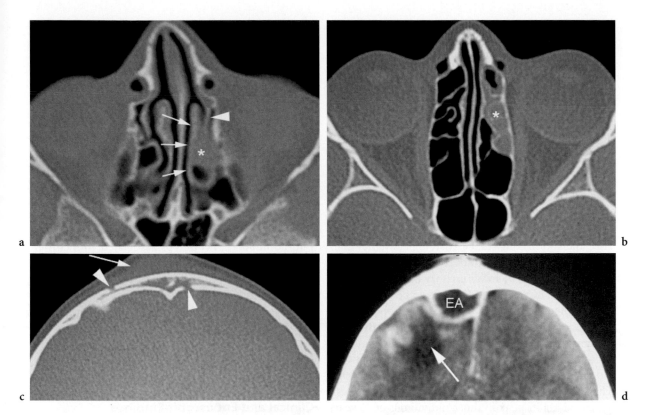

Fig. 6.6a–d. Complicated acute rhinosinusitis. CT scan before (**a–c**) and after (**d**) contrast administration, on the axial plane. **a,b** Acute rhinosinusitis with ostiomeatal unit pattern: inflammatory material (*asterisk*) is detected in the middle meatus – between the middle turbinate (*arrows*) and the uncinate process (*arrowhead*) – and in the anterior ethmoid. **c** A more cranial scan also shows thickening of subcutaneous soft tissue in the frontal region (*arrow*). Focal discontinuities of cortical bone are detected on both inner and outer cortical surfaces of frontal bone (*arrowheads*). **d** After contrast injection, both epidural (*EA*) and intraparenchymal abscess (*arrow*) are demonstrated

6.3
Chronic Rhinosinusitis and Polyposis

6.3.1
Definition, Epidemiology, Pattern of Growth

Chronic rhinosinusitis is defined as an inflammation of the mucosa of the nose and paranasal sinuses lasting more than 12 weeks (BROOK et al. 2000). In the last decade, this disease has ranked first among the most frequently reported chronic medical conditions in the United States (WAGNER 1996). Chronic rhinosinusitis is a multifactorial disease and the most important predisposing factors are: nasal allergy, recurrent upper respiratory tract infections, environmental pollutants, ASA syndrome, dental infections, sinonasal anatomic variants, immunodeficiencies, mucociliary anomalies (such as primary ciliary dyskinesia, Young's syndrome and cystic fibrosis), and iatrogenic factors (mechanical ventilation, nasogas-

tric tubes, nasal packing, scar tissue in the ostiomeatal complex as a consequence of sinonasal surgical procedures). Finally, in recent years many studies have been published suggesting that fungi may have a role in the pathophysiology of chronic rhinosinusitis (PONIKAU et al. 1999; BRAUN et al. 2003).

Even though little is known in detail about the etiology of chronic rhinosinusitis, all the aforementioned conditions may cause the onset of the disease by inducing damage of the sinonasal mucosa. Recent data suggest that enzymes stored in the eosinophil granules and released in the presence of fungi may play a role in the damage occurring to the cilia and to the epithelial cells of sinonasal mucosa (PONIKAU et al. 1999). As a consequence, thickening of the mucosa and polyps formation may be observed. These mucosal changes lead to stagnation and inspissation of secretions inside the sinus, resulting in a pH decrease. These modifications maintain sinus inflammation and create an ideal milieu for saprophytic bacteria or pathogens coming from nasal fossa (GWALTNEY et al. 1995).

All the bacteria implicated in acute rhinosinusitis may be cultured in chronic rhinosinusitis, but there is a shift in their relative prevalence. By several accounts, the role of *Staphylococcus aureus* and respiratory anaerobes is higher while classic pathogens of acute rhinosinusitis are less frequently isolated (WALD 1998).

Sinonasal polyposis is a quite common finding in chronic rhinosinusitis, ranging from 2% to 16% of cases (SETTIPANE 1996; HOLMSTRÖM et al. 2002).

Macroscopically, nasal polyps appear as edematous formations, very often yellow-white in appearance and soft in consistency. Histologically, they consist of respiratory epithelium covering an edematous stroma infiltrated by inflammatory cells. Eosinophils are found in 80% of cases (KRAMER and RASP 1999), whereas neutrophils predominate when polyps are associated with cystic fibrosis, primary ciliary dyskinesia syndrome, or Young's syndrome. Sinonasal polyps occur in all races and social classes and are equally divided between males and females (SETTIPANE 1996). The frequency of sinonasal polyposis increases with age, reaching its peak in those individuals of 50 years and older (LARSEN and TOS 2002). Several predisposing factors have been reported, such as fungal rhinosinusitis, ASA syndrome, Kartagener's syndrome, cystic fibrosis, and adult asthma, all of which present an incidence of associated polyposis in 80%, 36%, 27%, 20% and 9%, respectively.

Neither etiology nor pathogenesis of sinonasal polyposis are fully clarified. Recently, BACHERT et al. (2001), by detecting high levels of specific IgE antibodies to staphylococcal enterotoxins in nasal polyps samples, pointed to a possible role of bacterial superantigens in the onset of eosinophilic inflammation and then in the pathophysiology of nasal polyposis. In regards to pathogenesis, LARSEN et al. (1992) proposed a hypothesis on polyps formation called the "epithelial rupture theory," which includes five stages that may schematically be summarized as follows: (1) epithelial damage leading to a prolapse of the lamina propria; (2) epithelialization of the prolapsed lamina propria; (3) new gland formation; (4) enlargement and elongation of the glands of the polyp; (5) changes of the epithelium and stroma of the well-developed polyp, changes of density in goblet cells, cell infiltration, and vascularity of the stroma.

STAMMBERGER (1991, 1997) has greatly contributed to clarifying the site of origin of sinonasal polyps, as well as to providing a classification, which is very helpful for clinical work-up, and for planning surgical and medical therapy. According to his data, polyps arising into the sinonasal tract show the following distribution in relation to the site of origin: 80% from the uncinate-turbinate-infundibulum space, 65% from the face of the bulla-hiatus semilunaris-infundibulum, 48% from the frontal recess, 42% from the "turbinate sinus," 30% inside the bulla, 28% from the "lateral sinus," 27% from the posterior ethmoid (superior meatus), and 15% from the middle turbinate. The classification identifies five different groups of nasal polyps: (1) antrochoanal polyp; (2) large isolated choanal polyps; (3) polyps associated with chronic rhinosinusitis (non eosinophil-dominated); (4) polyps associated with chronic rhinosinusitis (eosinophil-dominated as diffuse nasal polyposis in aspirin intolerance, allergic fungal chronic rhinosinusitis, and asthma patients); (5) polyps associated with specific diseases (cystic fibrosis, malignancies, etc.).

6.3.2
Clinical and Endoscopic Findings

Many patients with chronic rhinosinusitis present nasal obstruction as the primary complaint. Other symptoms include nasal discharge, postnasal drip, facial pain, dysosmia, chronic cough, and headache. Headache is usually dull and radiating to the top of the calvarium or bitemporal for sphenoid or posterior ethmoid disease. Pain at the glabella, inner canthus, or between the eyes suggests anterior ethmoid or frontal rhinosinusitis. Pain over the cheeks most frequently suggests maxillary rhinosinusitis.

Patients with sinonasal polyposis complain of symptoms similar to those reported by patients with chronic rhinosinusitis, as the two diseases frequently coexist. Conversely, when an isolated polyp arises in a nasal fossa, unilateral signs and symptoms are generally reported. Among sinonasal inflammatory diseases, sinonasal polyposis is the one most frequently associated with bronchial hyperresponsiveness, with a percentage of up to 50% (HOLMSTRÖM et al. 2002). This association is more evident in patients with diffuse eosinophilic sinonasal polyposis.

In chronic rhinosinusitis, endoscopy shows an edematous and inflamed mucosa with a thick mucous or mucopurulent secretion outflowing from the ostiomeatal complex and/or the sphenoethmoid recess. Anatomical anomalies or small polyps obstructing the middle meatus may also be observed (Fig. 6.7).

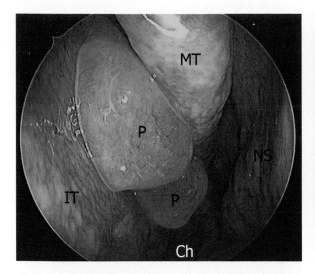

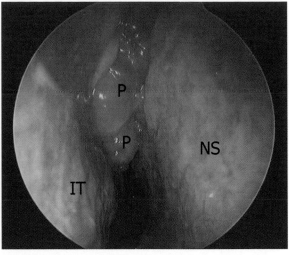

Fig. 6.7. Isolated polyps within the middle meatus. At endoscopy (30° rigid endoscope) of the right nasal fossa, two inflammatory polyps (*P*), coming out from the middle meatus, are evident. Choana (*Ch*), inferior turbinate (*IT*), middle turbinate (*MT*), nasal septum (*NS*)

Fig. 6.8. Massive polyposis (*P*) of right nasal fossa (0° rigid endoscope). Middle turbinate and uncinate process are not visible, since they are completely hidden by the polyps. Inferior turbinate *IT*; nasal septum, *NS*

In the presence of a diffuse sinonasal polyposis, endoscopy displays multiple soft, lobular and mobile formations, variable in size, with a smooth and shiny surface, bluish-gray or pink in color, more frequently arising in the middle meatus (Fig. 6.8). As a consequence of sinonasal ostia obstruction, also in sinonasal polyposis endoscopic signs of acute rhinosinusitis can be observed. Antrochoanal polyp, which is considered a separated entity, is a lonely neoformation originating from the mucosa of the maxillary sinus which bulges, due to its considerable size, into the nasopharynx through the choana.

6.3.3
Treatment Guidelines

The goals of medical therapy for chronic rhinosinusitis are control of infection, reduction of tissue edema, and improvement of ostia patency and sinus drainage. Reduction or elimination of irritating environmental factors is also important. Medical therapy is mainly based on: (1) antibiotics, which help to control infection in the closed sinus cavities. A 3-week antibiotic course has been suggested as minimum treatment for chronic rhinosinusitis (WAGNER 1996). Bacterial growth probably does not take so long to be suppressed, but a high risk of relapse does exist if damaged mucosa is not allowed to heal; (2) decongestants, which may help to maintain ostial patency; (3) secretolytics, which facilitate drainage by decreasing secretion density; (4) topical or oral steroids, which produce a strong antiedematous and antiinflammatory effect by decreasing the synthesis and release of a series of cytokines (i.e., IL-3 and IL-8) and adhesion molecules which are up-regulated in chronic rhinosinusitis, concomitantly with the reduction of the release of leukotrienes and prostaglandins (BACHERT et al. 2001).

Surgery is indicated in recurrent rhinosinusitis and chronic rhinosinusitis with persistent symptoms after 6 months of adequate medical therapy, in patients with systemic diseases, such as bronchial asthma, ASA syndrome, cystic fibrosis, ciliary dyskinesia, and in the presence of complications (YOUNIS and LAZAR 1996). In the last decades, functional microendoscopic surgery has gained much popularity for the treatment of chronic rhinosinusitis, so that external approaches are becoming obsolete in the management of this specific disease. The operation should be planned after a 5- to 10-day course of antibiotic and steroid therapy aimed at minimizing the inflammatory status of the mucosa and at eradicating possible bacterial infections. The extent of the dissection must be graduated according to the extent of the disease. After surgery, a meticulous follow-up including periodic endoscopic evaluations is mandatory to modulate the possible need for medical therapy, particularly in patients with bronchial hyperresponsiveness who have a high risk of persistent symptoms.

The same philosophy applies to sinonasal polyposis, which in the diffuse form requires a balanced combination of medical and surgical therapy, specifically tailored to each patient to improve his/her quality of life. Steroids are the only drug which have largely been proven to be effective in diffuse sinonasal polyposis, while antibiotics and antihistamines are used when infection or allergy are present, respectively (MYGIND 1999). In approximately 80% of patients, steroid therapy delays surgery for several months, even though most cases revert to the initial endoscopic findings at the end of medical therapy (VAN CAMP and CLEMENT 1994). Antrochoanal and other choanal polyps are the only forms which benefit exclusively from a surgical approach.

The likelihood of recurrence after surgery in patients with sinonasal polyposis is very high in patients with the diffuse eosinophilic form associated with bronchial hyperresponsiveness, is lower in patients without risk factors, and minimal in any form of choanal polyp.

6.3.4
Key Information to Be Provided by Imaging

- Extent of the disease
- Presence of anatomic variants altering the physiologic drainage of paranasal sinuses, supporting the vicious circle which leads to chronic inflammation
- Presence of anatomic variants which may increase the risk of intraoperative complications
- Presence of resorption of sinusal walls, particularly the lamina papyracea and the anterior skull base floor
- Presence of abundant scar tissue due to previous sinus surgery

6.3.5
Imaging Findings

CT evaluation of patients complaining of *chronic rhinosinusitis* is essentially focused on an accurate delineation of those elements – inflammatory mucosal changes and/or predisposing anatomic factors – that may impair mucociliary drainage.

According to SONKENS et al. (1991), at CT five different patterns of chronic rhinosinusitis may be described based on obstruction of different drainage pathways.

6.3.5.1
Infundibular Pattern

Infundibular pattern is the most limited model, occurring in the ostiomeatal area. Ethmoid infundibulum and maxillary sinus alone are involved, whereas ethmoid and frontal sinus are preserved.

This pattern is mainly due to the presence of mucosal thickenings or isolated polyps along the infundibulum. Anatomic predisposing factors are infraorbital cells, uncinate process variants, and hypoplasia of the maxillary sinus. At CT, infundibular obstruction and inflammatory changes of maxillary sinus mucosa are promptly detected (Fig. 6.9).

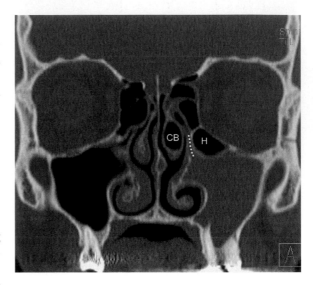

Fig. 6.9. Infundibular model. The ethmoid infundibulum (*dotted line*) is obstructed by thickened mucosa and markedly narrowed by a large infraorbital ethmoid cell, Haller cell (*H*), and a concha bullosa (*CB*)

6.3.5.2
Ostiomeatal Unit Pattern

Ostiomeatal unit pattern reflects the obstruction of all drainage systems in the middle meatus. As a consequence, it is heralded by maxillary, frontal, and anterior ethmoid sinusitis. Nonspecific mucosal thickenings as well as nasal polyps most commonly induce ostiomeatal unit pattern, whereas marked septal deviation and concha bullosa are anatomic predisposing factors (Fig. 6.10). Additionally, this model can also be observed in the presence of neoplastic lesions arising from the lateral nasal wall, such as inverted papilloma.

6.3.5.3
Sphenoethmoid Recess Pattern

Sphenoethmoid recess pattern is rather rare, consisting of sphenoid sinusitis and (not infrequently) posterior ethmoiditis, secondary to sphenoethmoid recess obstruction. Obliteration of the recess and inflammatory mucosal thickenings within sphenoid and posterior ethmoid are better depicted with axial CT (Fig. 6.11).

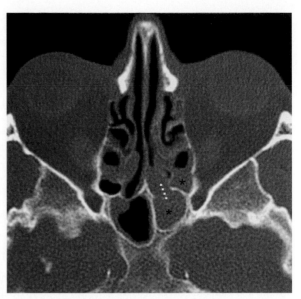

Fig. 6.11. Sphenoethmoid recess pattern. Mucosal thickening along the path of sphenoethmoid recess (*dotted line*), thickened mucosa, and retained secretions within posterior ethmoid cells and sphenoid sinus (*asterisks*)

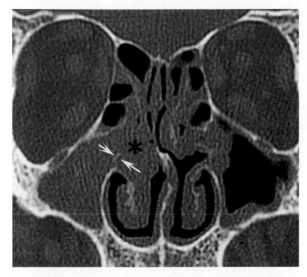

Fig. 6.10. Ostiomeatal unit pattern. Polypoid thickening of the mucosa in the middle meatus (*asterisk*). Retained secretions fill the maxillary sinus; mucosal thickenings in the anterior ethmoid. Incomplete resorption of the uncinate process, only partially visible (*arrows*)

6.3.5.4
Pattern of Nasal Polyposis

The pattern of *nasal polyposis* is characterized in most cases by bilateral involvement of middle meati, ethmoid infundibula (often widened), and paranasal cavities. Inflammatory polyps most frequently arise in the middle meatus from the mucosa investing the middle turbinate, the ethmoid infundibulum, and the uncinate process. They also originate from the anterior part of ethmoid bulla or frontal recess. At CT, they appear as solid lobulated lesions filling the ethmoid, nasal fossae and sinusal cavities, in most cases with bilateral extension. Bone remodeling is associated, triggered by mechanical pressure exerted by the polyps but also by the local release of inflammatory mediators and by bacterial invasion of bone and periosteum (GIACCHI et al. 2001). This

process is a complex balance between the activity of osteoblasts and osteoclasts. As a result, thinning and displacement of subtle bone structures such as ethmoid labyrinth and lamina papyracea (often exhibiting inversion of its normal medial convexity) may be observed along with sclerosis of thicker sinusal walls, such as posterolateral maxillary sinus wall (Fig. 6.12a).

Two additional signs are described as common features of sinonasal polyposis. (1) Widening of ethmoid infundibulum can be observed in several different conditions, including antrochoanal polyp and inverted papilloma. The specificity of this finding, however, is increased by bilateral presentation. (2) Truncation of middle turbinate (bilateral in up to 80% of cases) is easily recognized on CT scans as an amputation of the more distal, bulbous part, the vertical lamella usually being spared. In a series of 100 patients (LIANG et al. 1996) affected by chronic rhinosinusitis, this sign was observed exclusively in the subgroup with sinonasal polyposis, in 58% of cases.

MR signal pattern of inflammatory polyps does not differ from that of mucosal cysts, it is composed of hyper T2 signal and a combination of hyperintensity (mucosa) and hypointensity (edematous stroma) on contrast-enhanced T1 (Fig. 6.12b).

Even though bone changes and bilateral pattern of growth are quite typical, it must be emphasized

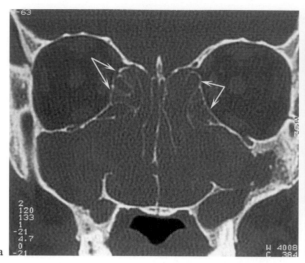
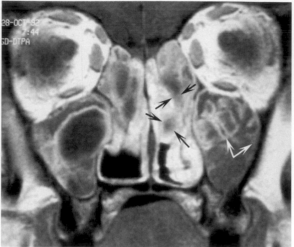

a   b

Fig. 6.12a,b. Nasal polyposis. Coronal CT (**a**) and Gd-DTPA SE T1 (**b**) scans through the anterior ethmoid. Nasal fossae, maxillary sinuses and ethmoid cells are completely filled by polyps. Dehiscence and remodeling of bone structures of the lateral nasal walls; pressure exerted by polyps remodels and laterally displaces both laminae papyraceae [*arrows* in (**a**)]. MR better delineates the hypointense stromal component of polyps [*black arrows* in (**b**)], deep to the mucosal surface. Within the maxillary sinus the folds of hypertrophic mucosa are detected [*white arrows* in (**b**)]

that density/signal pattern of nasal polyps is not completely specific; therefore several authors recommend thorough evaluation of surgical specimens.

A peculiar variant of sinonasal polyp is represented by *antrochoanal polyp*. This lesion arises in the maxillary sinus and protrudes in the middle meatus (through its natural drainage pathway or through an accessory ostium), where it extends between the middle turbinate and the lateral nasal wall. In its further posterior growth, the lesion typically reaches the choana. CT density of antrochoanal polyp is low (fluid-like), MR appearance resembles that of inflammatory polyps (Figs. 6.13, 6.14). *Sphenochoanal* and *ethmoidochoanal polyps* are described as extremely rare variants.

As a consequence of their natural history (growth through ostia), all sinochoanal polyps are subject to vascular compromise, because the waist of the polyp may be strangled as it passes through constrictive ostia. When this occurs, the intranasal portion of the sinochoanal polyp shows dilation and stasis of feeding vessels combined with edema. This vascularly compromised part of the lesion exhibits bright enhancement, possibly due to stasis in dilated vessels and is referred to as an *angiomatous polyp* (BATSAKIS and SNEIGE 1992; DE VUYSERE et al. 2001) (Fig. 6.14). Prolonged vascular damage may induce complete necrosis of the polyp, finally resulting in autopolypectomy (PRUNA 2003).

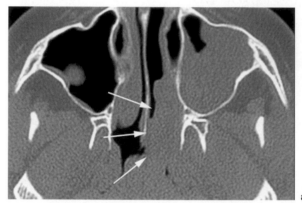

a

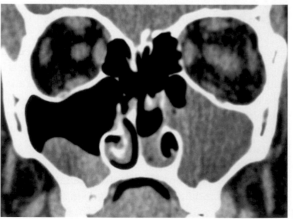

b

Fig. 6.13a,b. Antrochoanal polyp. Axial (**a**) and coronal (**b**) CT scan. Polypoid lesion occupies the left maxillary sinus, protruding into the nasal fossa and, through the choana, in the nasopharynx (*arrows*). Note in (**b**) the low density of the lesion

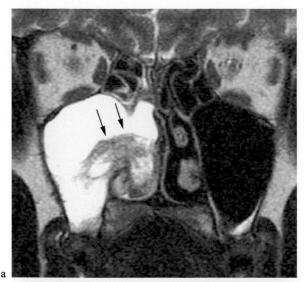

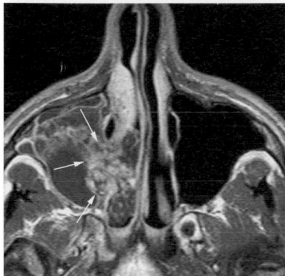

Fig. 6.14a,b. Antrochoanal polyp. Coronal SE T2 (**a**), axial Gd-DTPA SE T1 (**b**). The maxillary sinus is occupied by a lesion protruding through an accessory ostium into the middle meatus and then posteriorly reaching the choana. The signal pattern of the lesion resembles that of a common nasal polyp. The part of the lesion passing through the ostium (*arrows*) shows hypointense T2 signal and vivid enhancement, possibly due to stasis of contrast agent within dilated vessels. This vascularly compromised component of the lesion is referred to as an angiomatous polyp

6.3.5.5
Sporadic Pattern

Sporadic pattern includes a wide list of different conditions (such as isolated sinusitis, retention cyst, mucocele, post-surgical changes) unrelated to impairment of any of mucociliary drainage patterns.

Mucosal thickenings are an extremely common finding in maxillary and sphenoid sinus whereas, within ethmoid cells, it is often impossible to differentiate them from inflammatory polyps or retained secretions.

CT findings consist of partial or complete obliteration of a sinusal cavity by means of thickened mucosa with smooth – occasionally lobulated – surface and homogeneously low density. This appearance is, actually, a radiographic counterpart of chronic inflammatory edema of the mucosal/submucosal layer. No relevant bone changes are generally associated.

At MR, thickened mucosa shows a uniformly bright signal on SE T2 sequences, whereas SE T1 after contrast administration demonstrates hyperintensity of the enhancing mucosa combined with hypointense signal of the edematous submucosal layer.

CT and MR appearance of retained secretions is strictly related to the composition of the entrapped fluid. Protein content and viscosity of chronically retained secretions progressively increase, resulting in higher CT density. Raised HU values are also observed within pus or blood collections. At MR, an inverse correlation is observed between protein concentration and T2 signal. On plain T1 sequence, signal rises to a peak (at about 40% protein concentration) and then progressively decreases to hypointensity (SOM et al. 1989).

Retention cysts are more frequently observed in the maxillary sinus (in the alveolar recess or at the level of the roof close to the infraorbital canal). They are secondary to obstruction of a mucosal or minor salivary gland. At CT, retention cysts appear as hypodense lesions (fluid-like HU levels) with smooth and convex borders, and variable size (ranging from a few millimeters to centimeters). They are attached to a sinus wall (generally without remarkable bone changes); their location is unchanged varying patient's decubitus (Fig. 6.15). MR signal pattern is similar to the one described for retained secretions.

Nonetheless, it must be emphasized that all abnormalities included in the sporadic pattern can be observed as incidental findings in up to 38% of patients submitted to imaging studies of the head for nonsinusal pathologies (WANI et al. 2001). In the majority of cases no significant correlation exists with clinical symptoms, outlining the basic role of clinical history and physical examination (including nasal endoscopy) in the diagnosis of acute and chronic rhinosinusitis (COOKE and HADLEY 1991; WANI et al. 2001).

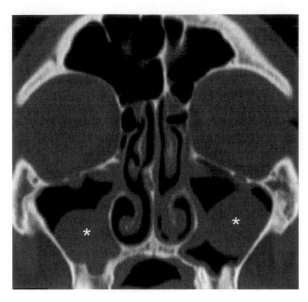

Fig. 6.15. Retention cysts. In both maxillary sinuses smooth sharply marginated lesions (*asterisks*) are observed, unrelated to drainage pathway impairment. No relevant bone changes are observed, particularly at the site of attachment of both lesions

6.3.5.6
Chronic Rhinosinusitis: Staging Systems

Besides the above-mentioned more traditional classification in five patterns reflecting the pathophysiology of chronic rhinosinusitis, several efforts were made to measure the severity of this disease entity based on both clinical manifestations and on CT findings. Among the latter, the Lund-Mackay system (LUND and MACKAY 1993) is the most popular because of its high inter- and intra-observer agreement rate, as well as its simplicity and reproducibility.

The Lund-Mackay classification applies a three point scale (0, no opacification; 1, partial opacification; 2, total opacification) to each major paranasal cavity (maxillary, frontal and sphenoid sinus, anterior and posterior ethmoid). A score is similarly assigned to the ostiomeatal complex, graded as patent (0) or obstructed (2). The total sum of CT alterations may therefore range from 0 to 24.

The impact of CT-based staging systems is still controversial. Several reports failed to demonstrate a direct correlation between patient complaints at presentation and imaging findings (STEWART et al. 1999; BHATTACHARYYA and FRIED 2003). This seems to decrease the possible role of CT in the assessment of disease severity. In contrast, some correlation was demonstrated between CT scan severity and endoscopic appearance (KENNEDY 1992). In addition, af-

ter surgery a more significant improvement of symptoms was observed in the subgroup of patients with high pretreatment CT scores (STEWART et al. 1999). Thus, CT should essentially be considered an invaluable tool for proper surgical planning and for anatomic landmark delineation.

6.4
Fungal Rhinosinusitis

6.4.1
Definition, Epidemiology, and Pathophysiology

Fungal rhinosinusitis can be defined as an infection of paranasal sinuses in which fungi play a role of primary pathogens or an inflammation due to the presence of fungi in the sinonasal tract.

The first publication of a patient with fungal rhinosinusitis dates back to 1791 (PLAIGNAUD 1791) and until the 1980s fungal infections of paranasal sinuses were considered a rare entity. However, during the last two decades, the observation of fungal rhinosinusitis has increased in relation to the growing occurrence of situations impairing immunologic system activity: diabetes mellitus with ketoacidosis, congenital or acquired (secondary to HIV infection, organ transplantation, chemotherapy for solid neoplasms, or lymphoproliferative diseases) immunodeficiencies, and long-term broad-spectrum antibiotic or steroid therapy. A concomitant improvement in histologic, microbiologic and radiologic techniques and a higher awareness of the disease has made it easier to establish a proper diagnosis (DE CARPENTIER et al. 1994).

DESHAZO et al. (1997) were the first authors to propose a classification of fungal rhinosinusitis based on the presence or absence of invasion of sinonasal mucosa and to separate noninvasive from invasive forms. The former included mycetoma and allergic fungal rhinosinusitis, and the latter comprised acute fulminant rhinosinusitis, chronic invasive fungal rhinosinusitis and granulomatous invasive fungal rhinosinusitis. Refinement in the knowledge of the pathophysiology of noninvasive forms has recently led some authors to update the terminology by recommending the use of the term "fungus ball" instead of "mycetoma" and the use of the adjective "eosinophilic" instead of "allergic" (PONIKAU et al. 1999) as more indicative of the real nature of the disease.

Fungus ball, which generally affects immunocompetent and nonatopic subjects, is localized in the maxillary sinus in about 80% of patients. It is characterized by a mass of inspissated fungal debris and mucus progressively growing in the sinus lumen, without invasion of the underlying mucosa.

Eosinophilic fungal rhinosinusitis is a diffuse process, histologically characterized by the presence of eosinophils and eosinophil degranulation byproducts, called Charcot-Leyden crystals. Abundant quantity of mucins may completely fill one or more sinuses. The disease is associated with polyposis or rhinosinusitis recalcitrant to common medical therapies apart from high-dose steroids, and affects more commonly asthmatic patients. Until 1999, it was thought that eosinophils detected in the diseased mucosa were recruited by a type I allergic reaction to fungal colonization of paranasal sinuses (MANNING and HOLMAN 1998). However, PONIKAU et al. (1999) have recently observed that eosinophils are present in a high concentration not only in the tissue of patients with chronic rhinosinusitis, but also in the mucus where they cluster and degranulate around fungi hyphae, which are subsequently destroyed by a massive release of eosinophilic cytokines (PONIKAU et al. 2002). Furthermore, allergy skin tests were positive only in 25% of patients. The conclusion that the authors draw from their observations was that eosinophils migrate intact through the epithelium in response to the presence in the lumen of fungi, which therefore do not act as pathogens but simply elicit a series of biochemical events which mainly involves eosinophils. For this reason, PONIKAU et al. (2002) proposed the use of the term "eosinophilic."

Acute fulminant rhinosinusitis is an aggressive, angioinvasive process. It is characterized by a rapidly progressive and often fatal course, with early invasion of orbital content or extension to the anterior and middle cranial fossa. The infection generally occurs in immunocompromised patients (GILLESPIE et al. 1998).

Chronic invasive fungal rhinosinusitis is a slowly progressive disease characterized by fungal tissue invasion without angioinvasion. Patients may be or may not be immunocompromised (BUSABA et al. 2002).

Finally, *granulomatous invasive fungal rhinosinusitis*, which occurs in immunocompetent patients with a geographic predominance in Sudan, is a slowly progressive chronic infection that extends beyond the boundaries of the sinus involved. Histologically, it differs from chronic invasive fungal rhinosinusitis for the presence of pseudotubercles consisting of a granulomatous reaction with giant cells, histiocytes, lymphocytes, plasma cells, and newly formed capillaries (YAGI et al. 1999).

Aspergillus species are the fungi most frequently cultured in fungus ball, while a spectrum of about 40 different species have been observed in the other forms of fungal rhinosinusitis. In particular, paranasal sinus mucormycosis is an opportunistic infection which affects diabetic patients with ketoacidosis (RUOPPI et al. 2001).

6.4.2
Clinical and Endoscopic Findings

Patients with maxillary sinus fungus ball generally complain of symptoms similar to those of a chronic maxillary sinusitis (unilateral nasal obstruction, purulent rhinorrhea, cacosmia, and facial pain), even though the disease may silently progress for a long time. When the fungus ball is located in the sphenoid sinus, vertex headache is the main complaint reported by the patient, while nasal symptoms may be less evident.

Nasal endoscopy often shows nonspecific changes as medialization of the uncinate process, edema of the mucosa of the ostiomeatal complex or of the sphenoethmoid recess, with thick mucous or mucopurulent secretion outflowing from the middle or superior meatus, respectively. Sometimes, the fungus ball may become evident in the middle or superior meatus or in the nasal fossa. Its appearance varies from a friable material of greenish, brownish, or grayish color to a thick material with a "pudding-like" consistency (Fig. 6.16).

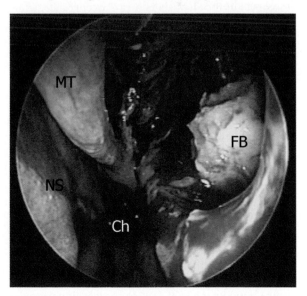

Fig. 6.16. Intraoperative view of left nasal fossa (0° rigid endoscope). After uncinectomy, a fungus ball (*FB*) filling the maxillary sinus is detected. Choana (*Ch*); middle turbinate (*MT*); nasal septum (*NS*)

Eosinophilic fungal rhinosinusitis generally causes bilateral nasal obstruction, watery or mucopurulent rhinorrhea, anosmia, facial pain, and headache. Proptosis and diplopia may seldom be observed as a consequence of lamina papyracea resorption and compression of orbital content by ethmoid disease, while neurologic symptoms due to skull base erosion are a less frequent complaint.

Patients with eosinophilic fungal rhinosinusitis generally had several nasal polypectomies, and bronchial asthma has been reported in more than 50% of cases. Nasal endoscopy displays an edematous and inflamed mucosa, multiple polyps and a thick, viscous secretion, described as "peanut butter" in one or both nasal fossae.

According to YAGI et al. (1999), who reported their experience on 43 Sudanese patients affected by granulomatous fungal rhinosinusitis, symptoms and signs more frequently observed were nasal obstruction with purulent rhinorrhea, headache, swelling of the medial canthus, of the forehead, or of the cheek, proptosis and visual disturbances. The ethmoid was more frequently affected, followed by maxillary and frontal sinuses. Nasal polyposis may be the only visible sign at nasal endoscopy in about 40% of cases. Other endoscopic findings are gelatinous gray-green oil rhinorrhea and firm rubbery tissue, brownish in color, occupying the nasal fossa.

Signs and symptoms of chronic invasive fungal rhinosinusitis are quite similar to those reported by patients with the granulomatous form. At nasal endoscopy, nasal polyposis is a rare occurrence, while a pale and edematous mucosa, not bleeding during debridement, with concomitant mucosal and bony necrosis, may be observed.

Finally, acute fulminant fungal rhinosinusitis usually presents in an immunocompromised patient with nonspecific signs and symptoms mimicking an acute rhinosinusitis. However, pathognomonic symptoms may rapidly arise, such as black nasomucosal spots, severe facial pain and cheek swelling, epistaxis, headache, ophthalmoplegia, proptosis, and signs of endocranial invasion.

At endoscopy, nasal mucosal changes may be observed, reflecting ischemia induced by fungal vasculitis (Fig. 6.17). Early, erythematous or edematous mucosa becomes dusky or necrotic, before progressing to ulceration beneath an eschar. Crusting may overlay a gangrenous, insensitive inferior turbinate. According to DE CARPENTIER et al. (1994), the last sign precedes the rapid onset of facial swelling, orbital symptoms, and systemic dissemination, with involvement of the lungs, liver, and spleen.

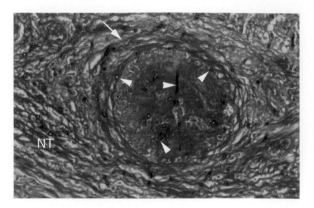

Fig. 6.17. Acute fulminant fungal rhinosinusitis. Fungal hyphae (*arrowheads*) are present within the lumen and the wall (*arrow*) of a vessel. Necrotic tissue (*NT*) is also visible. (Grocott specific histochemical staining). Original magnification 40×

6.4.3
Treatment Guidelines

Endonasal removal under microendoscopic guidance is unanimously considered the treatment of choice for fungus ball (KLOSSEK et al. 1997). When the lesion is localized in the maxillary sinus, an inferior partial uncinectomy and a wide middle antrostomy with conservation of middle turbinate are the only surgical steps required to allow the extirpation of the fungal disease. Maxillary mucosa must always be spared even though it appears inflamed and edematous. In fact, the restoration of physiologic ventilation and drainage of the affected sinus allows quick healing of the maxillary mucosa. When the fungus ball grows inside the sphenoid sinus, a transnasal microendoscopic sphenoidotomy may generally be performed when no septal deviation or middle turbinate hyperpneumatization are present. Otherwise, a trans-ethmoidal approach is preferable. Finally, if the fungus ball occupies the frontal sinus, a superior partial uncinectomy with clearance of the frontal recess is usually indicated. Sinus lavages under pressure may be very useful for completely removing fungal debris from the frontal sinus. Medical therapy (i.e., antibiotics and topical steroids) is generally not indicated.

At present, no general consensus exists on the treatment of eosinophilic fungal rhinosinusitis. Therapy should be tailored to each patient, based on the extent of the disease, the severity of symptoms, and the response to steroid therapy (local and/or systemic), which is usually the more effective. When medical therapy fails to control symptoms, microendoscopic surgery is indicated to reestablish a good ventilation of the sinuses, to remove eosinophilic mucins which entrap fungi, and to make sinonasal mucosa more accessible to topical treatments. Recently, high-dose itraconazole, an oral antifungal agent, has been proposed (RAINS and MINECK 2003) in an attempt to break the vicious circle elicited by the presence of fungi and to reduce the need for frequent surgery and long-term oral steroids. Even irrigations of the sinonasal cavities with antifungal agents such as Amphotericin B (PONIKAU et al. 2002; RICCHETTI et al. 2002) seem to provide good control of the disease. However, no prospective randomized studies on the efficacy of antifungal agents have been published yet.

Finally, the treatment recommended for invasive fungal rhinosinusitis consists of systemic, intravenous, Amphotericin B, and aggressive surgical debridement, which can require microendoscopic surgery for chronic indolent and granulomatous forms and even total maxillectomy and orbital exenteratio for the fulminant form. Moreover, for the latter some authors advocate prolonged postoperative treatment with oral antifungal drugs for up to 1 year. Even with the combination of surgery and antifungal drugs, fulminant invasive fungal rhinosinusitis carries a mortality rate ranging from 50% to 80% (GILLESPIE et al. 1998).

6.4.4
Key Information to Be Provided by Imaging

- Site and extent of the mycotic process
- Presence of bone erosion
- Presence of invasion of the orbital content and of the cavernous sinus
- Presence of skull base erosion

6.4.5
Imaging Findings

Both CT and MR findings of *fungus ball* are conditioned by the high content of heavy metals (iron and manganese) and calcium within fungal hyphae. As a result, CT density of the fungus ball is spontaneously hyperdense; microcalcifications can be observed, scattered within the lesion (Fig. 6.18). Though extremely specific, these signs lack sensitivity (DHONG et al. 2000). The MR pattern may often be misleading: actually, the paramagnetic properties of iron and manganese combined with the low number of freely moving protons provoke both T1 and T2 shortening. Consequently, on both sequences, MR demonstrates

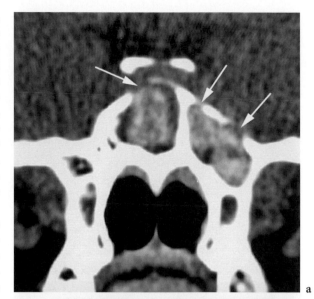

a

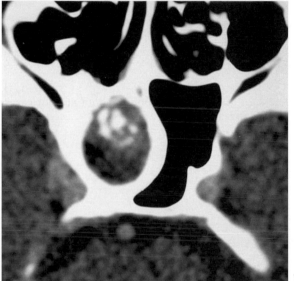

b

Fig. 6.18a,b. Fungus ball. Plain CT, coronal (**a**) and axial (**b**) plane. In (**a**) both sphenoid sinuses are completely filled by spontaneously hyperdense material. Focal areas of pressure demineralization are depicted at the roof of sinuses (*arrows*). In (**b**) some scattered calcifications are demonstrated within the fungus ball

a hypointense lesion bordered by hyperintense (T2) and enhancing (T1, after contrast administration) mucosa (RAO et al. 2001). In some cases, T1 and T2 shortening may be so marked to result in a signal void, making discrimination between fungus ball and intrasinusal air nearly impossible (Fig. 6.19).

In *eosinophilic fungal rhinosinusitis*, the CT density and MR paramagnetic characteristics of fungal material, as well as progressive dehydration of eo-

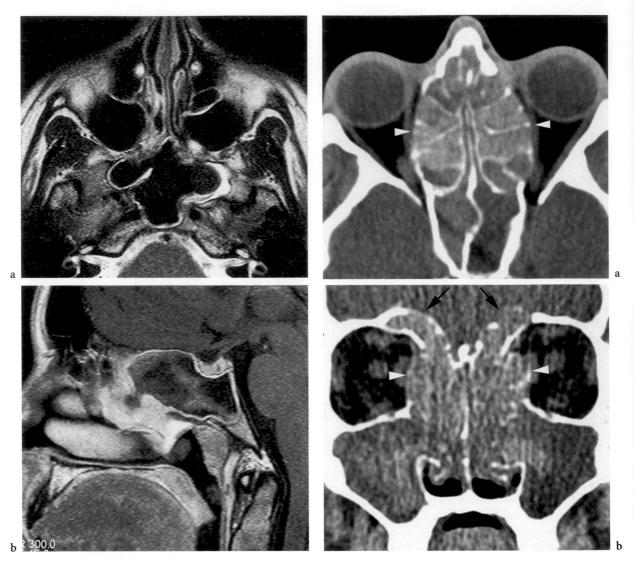

Fig. 6.19a,b. Fungus ball. Axial SE T2 (**a**), sagittal Gd-DTPA SE T1 (**b**). Retained fungal hyphae exhibit on both pulse sequences marked hypointensity, resembling an empty sinus. The non-invasive nature of this form of fungal infection is heralded by the complete preservation of the mucosa, detectable as a thin and continuous hyperintense and enhancing layer

Fig. 6.20a,b. Nasal polyposis, eosinophilic fungal rhinosinusitis. Ethmoid, nasal fossae, and maxillary sinuses are completely filled by polypoid material exhibiting scattered areas of spontaneous hyperdensity. Extensive bone remodeling and dehiscence at the level of the medial orbital walls, both pushed laterally (*arrowheads*). Focal areas of demineralization are also observed at the roof of the frontal sinuses (*arrows*)

sinophilic mucin, produce signal patterns similar to fungus ball (Fig. 6.20). The differentiation is based on localization of the disease – isolated and unilateral in 94% of fungus balls, diffuse and scattered in 95% of eosinophilic fungal rhinosinusitis – and association with nasal polyposis, which is more common in eosinophilic fungal rhinosinusitis (DHONG et al. 2000).

Bone changes in both fungus balls and eosinophilic fungal rhinosinusitis follow the same model exhibited by chronic rhinosinusitis and nasal polyposis. Mechanical pressure and osteoclastic activ-

ity result in bone demineralization, whereas sclerotic thickening is observed in the case of prevalent osteoblastic activity. Sinus expansion and bone thinning are more commonly observed in eosinophilic fungal rhinosinusitis (93% vs 3.6%) (MUKHERJI et al. 1998; FERGUSON 2000), whereas sclerosis of sinusal walls is more typical in fungus balls.

Invasive mycoses may manifest in two main forms, namely acute fulminant and chronic, the discrimination between the two being based on the clinical course. A rare invasive form involving immunocompetent patients has been reported in Southeast Asia and Africa, referred to as *granulomatous or "indolent" fungal rhinosinusitis*. Its CT and MR appearance is not yet clearly defined. Imaging findings of *acute fulminant fungal rhinosinusitis* basically consist of aggressive destruction of bony sinusal walls and invasion of adjacent soft tissues. At MR, abnormal changes of the sinusal investing mucosa (effacement of the hyperintense – T2 – and of the enhancing mucosal layer) are the direct demonstration of the invasive nature of the infection (Fig. 6.21). Intrasinusal hyperdensities are far less common than in noninvasive forms. Spread to the pterygopalatine fossa, orbit, anterior and/or middle cranial fossa is a particularly severe complication (SALEH and BRIDGER 1997). CT and MR appearance of *chronic invasive fungal rhinosinusitis* does not significantly differ from the acute fulminant form: intracranial and intraorbital infiltration is almost always observed, usually with inhomo-

geneous enhancing tissue invading the orbital apex or the cavernous sinus (CHAN et al. 2000; RUMBOLDT and CASTILLO 2002) (Fig. 6.22). The differential diagnosis between these two entities is mainly based on the celerity and severity of the clinical course.

6.5
Aggressive Granulomatous Lesions

6.5.1
Wegener Granulomatosis

6.5.1.1
Definition and Epidemiology

Wegener granulomatosis is a chronic, granulomatous vasculitis mainly affecting the respiratory tract and

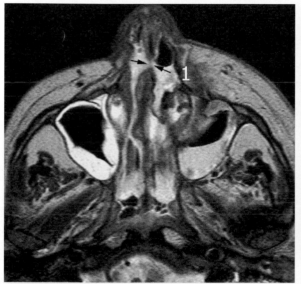

a

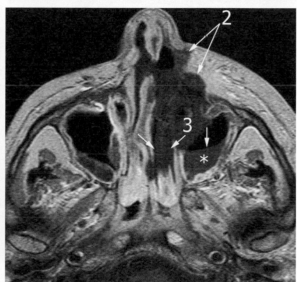

b

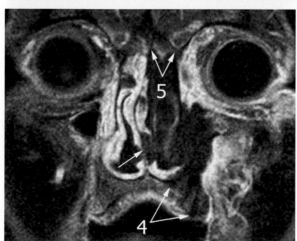

c

Fig. 6.21a–c. Acute fulminant fungal rhinosinusitis. TSE T2 axial plane (**a**), Gd-DTPA SE T1 axial plane (**b**), VIBE coronal plane (**c**). Inhomogenous inflammatory material centered at the level of vertical process of maxillary bone and along medial wall of maxillary sinus. Note the absence of contrast uptake, related to ischemic necrosis (invasion and obliteration of vessels). Extensive bone destruction is detected, involving nasal septum (*1*), infiltration of premaxillary subcutaneous fat tissue (*2*), middle turbinate (*3*), hard palate and alveolar process of maxillary bone (*4*). The lesion contacts the ethmoid roof (*5*) with no signs on intracranial extension

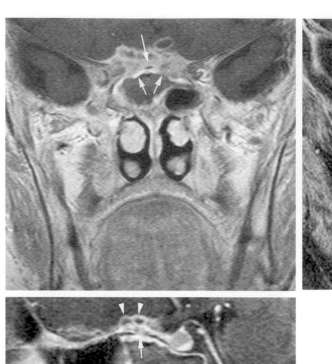

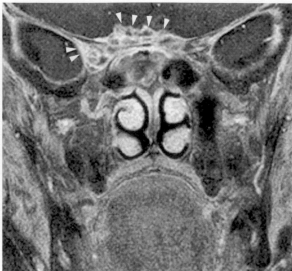

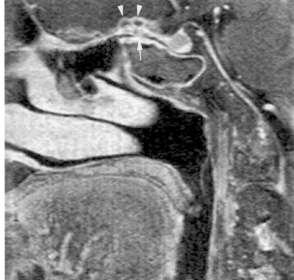

Fig. 6.22a–c. Chronic invasive fungal rhinosinusitis. Coronal Gd-DTPA SE T1 (**a**), coronal Gd-DTPA VIBE (**b**), reformatted sagittal Gd-DTPA VIBE (**c**). A hypointense fungus ball is retained within the sphenoid sinus. At the level of the sinus roof both the hyperintense mucosa and the hypointense cortical bone are focally interrupted (*arrows*). A plaque-like inhomogeneous lesion is demonstrated along the intracranial surface of the planum sphenoidale invading the right superior orbital fissure (*arrowheads*)

the kidneys. More rarely, other organs and systems may be involved. A sinonasal tract localization is present in up to 91% of patients with systemic Wegener granulomatosis (YUCEL et al. 2002). An isolated form of involvement, without other localizations, has also been described (LLOYD et al. 2002).

The etiology of the disease is still unknown; however, the hypothesis of an autoimmune process is at present the most favored.

The incidence ranges between 0.5 and 8 new cases per 1,000,000 inhabitants per year (TAKWOINGI and DEMPSTER 2003). The age at presentation is extremely variable, varying from 9 to 78 years (HOFFMAN et al. 1992; TAKWOINGI and DEMPSTER 2003), thus confirming that the observation in the pediatric age is not exceptional. Moreover, there is a moderate predominance in male patients.

6.5.1.2
Clinical and Endoscopic Findings

Wegener granulomatosis is characterized by a great variety of presentations, including systemic and local manifestations. General symptoms may be weakness, arthralgia, neurologic deficits, unexplained fever, malaise, and weight loss. Otitis media and hearing loss, subglottic stenosis, and oropharyngeal lesions, such as ulcers, are common presentations in the otolaryngologic district. However, the sinonasal tract is by far the most frequently involved area, with

85% and 68% of patients suffering from sinusitis and rhinitis, respectively. The most common complaints are epistaxis, crusting, and nasal obstruction. Nasal mucosa appears covered by crusts, with superficial hemorrhages. Especially in advanced stages and/or in the presence of an aggressive form of the disease, it is possible to identify necrosis and resorption of the septal cartilage, turbinates, and lateral bony walls of the nasal cavities; mucosa is even more friable and inclined to hemorrhage (Fig. 6.23). Patients with an extensive septal perforation may present a typical deformity of the nasal pyramid called "saddle nose". When the granulomatous process directly involves the lacrimal pathway or the presence of abundant scar tissue obstructs the nasolacrimal duct, chronic dacryocystitis with epiphora may be observed.

Orbital involvement may occur in different forms. Exophthalmos and diplopia may be related to intraorbital pseudotumor, cranial nerve palsy, or lacrimal gland enlargement; visual impairment due to compression of the optic nerve is also possible. Direct ocular globe involvement may present with uveitis, episcleritis, conjunctivitis, or retinitis (PROVENZALE et al. 1996).

Diagnosis is based on clinical, serological, histological, and imaging data. The clinical picture may sometimes be slightly nonspecific; however, nasal crusting and otitis media resistant to common antibiotic therapy must arouse the suspicion of Wegener granulomatosis. Among laboratory tests, "antineutrophil cytoplasmic antibodies" with a cytoplasmic pattern (c-ANCA) positivity is the most accurate indicator for Wegener granulomatosis. In the systemic form, serologic titer of this antibody is sensitive and specific, with values reaching 92% and 100%, respectively (YANG et al. 2001). In localized Wegener granulomatosis, however, this test lacks sensitivity (LLOYD et al. 2002). The erythrocyte sedimentation rate is elevated in most patients with active disease; it may be used as a predictor of treatment outcome and therefore as a prognostic index (TAKWOINGI and DEMPSTER 2003). In patients without c-ANCA positivity, it is otherwise crucial to obtain a biopsy at the level of involved areas. At histology, characteristic elements for Wegener granulomatosis are necrotizing vasculitis, with fibrinoid necrosis of small and medium vessels wall (LLOYD et al. 2002).

Differential diagnosis includes all the conditions that can present with a midline destructive lesion: lymphoproliferative disorders (T-cell lymphoma and angiocentric natural killer T-cell lymphoma), sarcoidosis, tuberculosis, and cocaine induced lesions.

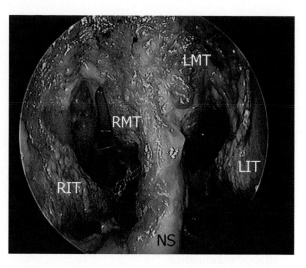

Fig. 6.23. Extensive destruction of the nasal septum (*NS*), with partial resorption of right (*RMT*) and left middle turbinate (*LMT*) (0° rigid endoscope). The mucosa is covered by crusts suggestive of an active phase of the disease. Left inferior turbinate (*LIT*), right inferior turbinate (*RIT*)

6.5.1.3
Treatment Guidelines

In the pre-immunosuppressant era, the prognosis for patients affected by Wegener granulomatosis was dismal, with a mortality rate of 82% and 90% within 1 and 2 years, respectively (KERR et al. 1993; TAKWOINGI and DEMPSTER 2003). Introduction of steroids and cytotoxic drugs (cyclophosphamide, prednisolone, azathioprine) has dramatically changed the clinical course, with a 5-year survival rate of up to 75% (HOFFMAN et al. 1992; YANG et al. 2001; TAKWOINGI and DEMPSTER 2003) and a mortality rate ranging from 5% to 20% in the adult population (TAKWOINGI and DEMPSTER 2003). Antimetabolites, antibiotics, saline washings, and emollients are also important in order to improve nasal airflow and to avoid bacterial superinfections.

The role played by surgery is quite limited. Under endoscopic control it is possible to perform debridement of crusting, cautery of bleeding points, and biopsy of lesions in case of possible relapse of the disease. Endoscopic surgery can be a valid tool for removing inflammatory polyps and for treating acute and/or complicated sinusitis, not responsive to medical therapy. However, long-term outcome is not satisfactory, unless the disease is in a remission phase. In fact, abundant scar tissue and crusting cause an obstruction of the surgical cavities and a relapse of symptoms. The same negative effects are observed when an endoscopic dacryocystorhinostomy is performed; a silicon stent left in place for up to 6 months does not prevent late re-obstruction of the lacrimal pathway.

6.5.1.4
Key Information to Be Provided by Imaging

- Presence and entity of mucosal thickening
- Bony and cartilaginous alterations, with regard to the entity of resorption and/or to the presence of neo-osteogenesis
- Cranial nerve involvement
- Middle ear involvement
- Extension into deep spaces, such as pterygopalatine fossa and masticator space, not appreciable at clinical examination
- Detection of acute and/or complicated sinusitis, requiring surgical treatment
- In the presence of exophthalmos, identification of lacrimal gland involvement or of intraorbital pseudotumor

6.5.2
Cocaine Induced Destructive Lesions

6.5.2.1
Definition and Epidemiology

Cocaine is an alkaloid, derived from *Erythroxilon coca* leaves, which has been used for centuries for its euphoric and analgesic properties. Even though debated for its side effects, the use of cocaine as a vasoconstrictor agent in local anesthesia procedures is still licit in common medical practice (KASEMSUWAN and GRIFFITHS 1996; DE et al. 2003). Cocaine abuse is a social problem of increasing importance. For instance, in the United States up to 6 million inhabitants can be considered habitual or occasional users, and 30 million have used it at least once in their life (SEYER et al. 2002).

Addiction to such a drug may have local or systemic effects, which depend on abuse duration, the form of administration, and the amount of the doses. The frequent observation of sinonasal lesions is due to the fact that inhalation (or "snorting") of cocaine powder is the most common form of administration. Nevertheless, addiction may exert also systemic negative effects, such as an increase in blood pressure and in the risk of arrhythmias and heart ischemia, due to vasoconstriction. Local damage may be attributed to several factors, including decreased mucocili-

ary beat frequency (HOFER et al. 2003), vasoconstriction, traumatic effect of crystals insufflated at high velocity, local superinfection, and irritant action of adulterants (LANCASTER et al. 2000; TRIMARCHI et al. 2001; VILELA et al. 2002).

6.5.2.2
Clinical and Endoscopic Findings

Cocaine abuse through nasal insufflation may remain clinically silent, but may also cause signs and symptoms which are related to different degrees of involvement of sinonasal structures. The nasal mucosa is the first to suffer from cocaine addiction: the most frequent presenting complaints are epistaxis, nasal crusting, obstruction, hyposmia, and headache. At endoscopy, it is possible to detect crusts that may be localized on the nasal septum, in the case of short-term use, or may be widely present in the nasal cavities when faced with long-standing and high-dose abuse. Superficial hemorrhages and ischemic areas are also visible, especially in the case of recent abuse. It is worth mentioning that a direct proportional relationship between number of doses, entity, and length of drug addiction and damage on nasal and paranasal structures is not always observed. In the presence of more severe involvement, mucosal ulcers and septal perforation may be detected. Less frequently, massive necrosis involving bone and cartilage, which can lead to hard and soft palate perforation (MARÌ et al. 2002; SMITH et al. 2002; TRIMARCHI et al. 2003), complete ethmoid, turbinates, and nasal septum resorption (SEYER et al. 2002) (Fig. 6.24), collapse of the nasal pyramid due to columella and alar cartilage destruction (CARTER and GROSSMAN 2000; VILELA et al. 2002; TRIMARCHI et al. 2003), can be detected. In patients presenting with these lesions, differential diagnosis with other pathologic conditions, such as Wegener granulomatosis, lymphoproliferative disorders, sarcoidosis, and tuberculosis, may be intriguing. Clinical history is the key element in order to reach a correct diagnosis. Based upon our experience, it is not possible to rely upon identification of urine catabolites, since patients, especially if addicted, often refuse their consensus for the examination. In regards to serology, some of the cocaine abusers show a c-ANCA positivity pattern (SMITH et al. 2002), which is not distinguishable from the typical profile of Wegener granulomatosis (TRIMARCHI et al. 2001, 2003). A more detailed analysis demonstrated that there is a difference in the antigens recognized in cocaine abusers and in vasculitis patients (TRIMARCHI et al. 2001, 2003). Moreover, cocaine abusers do not

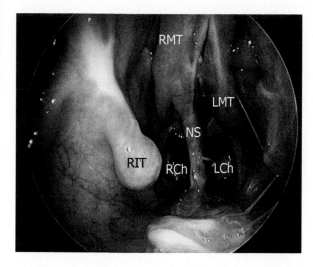

Fig. 6.24. Endoscopic appearance (0° rigid endoscope) of nasal fossae in a long-term cocaine abuser. Almost complete destruction of the right inferior turbinate (*RIT*) and cartilaginous nasal septum (*NS*) is well evident. Mucosa, without crusts and superficial hemorrhages, suggests cessation of drug addiction. Left choana (*LCh*); left middle turbinate (*LMT*); right choana (*RCh*); right middle turbinate (*RMT*)

show alterations in inflammatory parameters, which are by contrast elevated in Wegener granulomatosis patients.

At histology, cocaine addiction induces vascular alterations, such as perivenulitis, microabscesses of the vessel wall, leukocytoclastic vasculitis, and fibrinoid necrosis; these features are frequently found also in vasculitic patients. However, Cocaine does not cause extravascular changes which, by contrast, are frequent in diseases like Wegener granulomatosis.

6.5.2.3
Treatment Guidelines

The most effective treatment for cocaine abusers is obviously cessation of addiction. In the presence of minimal lesions, conservative treatment aimed at removing crusts and necrotic tissue and moistening mucosa, includes the use of saline solution irrigations and emollients. Bacterial infection, which is mostly due to *Staphylococcus aureus*, is treated by topical or systemic antibiotics, according to cultures. Whenever major destruction is present, no reconstructive surgery should be planned until cocaine abuse has been ceased and the lesion has remained stable for at least 1 year (LANCASTER et al. 2000). Pedicled or revascularized free flaps could warrant a good functional and aesthetic outcome. Hard palate perforation could benefit from the ap-

plication of an obturator prosthesis, that may reduce negative effects of oronasal reflux (MARÌ et al. 2002; TRIMARCHI et al. 2003).

6.5.2.4
Key Information to Be Provided by Imaging

- Extent of cartilaginous and bony destruction
- Status of structures such as turbinates, hard and soft palate, nasal pyramid, skull base, the involvement of which is more suggestive of drug addiction

6.5.3
Sarcoidosis

6.5.3.1
Definition and Epidemiology

Sarcoidosis is a systemic non-caseating granulomatous disease that mainly involves lungs (80-90% of all patients) (FERGIE et al. 1999) and the upper respiratory tract, including the nasal fossae and paranasal sinuses (KRESPI et al. 1995; DESHAZO et al. 1999). Other extra-respiratory localizations are lymph nodes, liver, spleen, eye, skin, bones, brain, salivary and lacrimal glands (DESHAZO et al. 1999; MAZZIOTTI et al. 2001).

The etiology of sarcoidosis is still unknown. Some immunological alterations (i.e., depression of T-lymphocyte function, elevated B-lymphocyte activity and serum levels) are frequently found in affected subjects and are hypothesized to play a relevant role in the onset of the disease. Also infective agents, such as *atypical Mycobacteria*, are listed among the potential etiologic factors (FERGIE et al. 1999).

Incidence can vary from 1.2 to 19 cases per 1000,00 per year in Caucasians and from 36.5 to 81.8 in African Americans (ZEITLIN et al. 2000). Female are estimated to have a slight preponderance in incidence, with a sex ratio ranging from 1:1 to 2.4:1 (ZEITLIN et al. 2000). The mean peak of occurrence is between 20 and 40 years.

Head and neck manifestations are detected in up to 15% of patients (SHAH et al. 1997; DAMROSE et al. 2000; ZEITLIN et al. 2000). Sinonasal involvement is a rare event, which was observed in less than 1% of patients by McCAFFREY and McDONALD (1983), in their study on Mayo Clinic experience. This rate, obtained through a retrospective analysis, seems to underscore the problem, since nasal symptoms may not have been evident at presentation. More recent reports, however, confirmed sinonasal tract involvement in no more than 6% of all cases of sarcoidosis (MARKS and GOODMAN et al. 1998; DAMROSE et al. 2000; ZEITLIN et al. 2000).

6.5.3.2
Clinical and Endoscopic Findings

The pattern of sinonasal involvement is variable and different symptoms and signs are detected in relation to the duration of the active phase of the disease. In fact, sarcoidosis is characterized by periods of spontaneous remission and exacerbation, with a very variable clinical course. At presentation, nasal obstruction is the most common complaint; other frequent signs and symptoms are epistaxis, rhinorrhea, crusting, hypo-anosmia, epiphora. The clinical presentation reflects the alterations of the mucosa. In the early stages, nasal mucosa may appear dry and friable, with occasional congestion possibly anticipating the formation of polyps. In the presence of chronic disease, however, the most frequent lesions are ulcers, crusting and also perforations affecting specific sites such as the nasal septum. Prolonged disease with relevant involvement of paranasal sinus mucosa may lead to bacterial rhinosinusitis and, therefore, to the onset of nasal discharge, headache, and/or facial pain.

Diagnosis must take into account clinical history and examination, serological tests, imaging evaluation, and histology.

Clinical examination has to evaluate the presence of the aforementioned nasal mucosal and osteocartilaginous alterations, along with other complaints which may suggest the possible systemic nature of the disease.

Laboratory tests include a complete blood count, ANCA titers, erythrocyte sedimentation rate, and levels of angiotensin converting enzyme, which are elevated in sarcoidosis and may be an index of an active phase of the disease (DAMROSE et al. 2000).

At imaging, besides CT and/or MR evaluation of the sinonasal tract, chest X-ray and/or CT are indicated to identify lung lesions, present in up to 90% of patients.

Histologic evaluation should look for non-caseating granulomas and rule out the presence of vasculitis, an element that could point diagnosis towards other conditions, the most frequent and serious being Wegener granulomatosis.

DESHAZO et al. (1999) identified different diagnostic criteria which can help in establishing the diagnosis of sarcoidosis of the sinonasal tract:

- Mucoperiosteal thickening or opacification of a sinus as detected by plain film, CT, or MR imaging
- Histopathologic demonstration of non-caseating granulomas in material taken from sinus. Special stains for fungus and mycobacteria must be negative, and no evidence of vasculitis should be present
- Negative serologic response for syphilis and negative ANCA response
- No evidence on chest X-ray or clinical history of other diseases associated with granulomatous nasal or sinus inflammation (tuberculosis, syphilis, Wegener granulomatosis, fungal infection, or berylliosis)

It becomes clear that the diagnosis of sarcoidosis is basically made by exclusion, since many of the elements indicated are nonspecific and in common with other diseases.

Differential diagnosis includes all the granulomatous diseases, such as Wegener granulomatosis, tuberculosis, rhinoscleroma, syphilis, berylliosis, leprosy, fungal infection, and also cocaine addiction. Diagnosis is made easier by the presence, in up to 50% of patients, of lupus pernio (i.e., a violaceous skin lesion mostly located at the level of the nose, ear, and cheeks). Of course, the presence of pulmonary involvement leads to the correct diagnosis.

6.5.3.3
Treatment Guidelines

The mainstay of treatment is medical therapy based upon steroid agents, which are effective in controlling the disease, either localized or systemic. Medical therapy has to be tailored to the length and severity of the disease and to the response of patients to the treatment itself. In the presence of complications, such as acute rhinosinusitis, antibiotics and decongestants must be administered.

According to KRESPI et al. (1995), three different stages of sinonasal sarcoidosis (mild, moderate, severe) may be recognized, according to the entity of the disease. Mild sinonasal tract involvement (Stage I) may be treated by topical steroids. Nasal irrigations and emollients play a role in removing crusts and necrotic tissue, thus avoiding bacterial superinfections and restoring more "physiologic" conditions for the mucosa. Stage II disease (moderate but reversible disease or mild disease not responsive to treatment) could benefit also from intra-lesional injections of steroids. Stage III sarcoidosis (severe, irreversible disease) must be treated also with systemic steroids.

Surgery should be reserved to symptomatic patients whose sinonasal involvement can not be treated with medical therapy. Events such as a complicated rhinosinusitis, mucocele, inflammatory adhesions, and obstructive polyposis are elective conditions for surgical treatment. As in other chronic inflammatory diseases, surgery in patients with sarcoidosis appears to be effective in the short term, but shows no satisfactory long-term outcomes (MARKS and GOODMAN 1998). In selected cases, persistent frontal sinusitis and headache may be effectively treated by osteoplastic sinusotomy with fat obliteration (MARKS and GOODMAN 1998).

6.5.3.4
Key Information to Be Provided by Imaging

- Presence of thickened nasal and paranasal sinus mucosa
- Entity of bony and cartilaginous alterations
- Presence of sinusitis, with particular attention to complications requiring surgical treatment
- Entity of intraorbital involvement in those patients with ocular symptoms (diplopia, exophthalmos, reduced visual acuity)
- Atypical pattern of diffusion, like perineural spread (MAZZIOTTI et al. 2001)

6.5.4
Imaging Findings

Among all the small vessel vasculitides listed in the Chapel Hill classification, *Wegener granulomatosis* is by far the most common in the ENT area (up to 90% of patients) (JENNETTE and FALK 1997), basically involving three anatomic subsites, namely, sinonasal cavities and orbit, middle ear and mastoid, and larynx.

Wegener granulomatosis manifestations in the nose and paranasal sinuses are extremely polymorphic; they may consist of mucosal and/or bone changes. Mass-like pseudotumor lesions are reported more commonly in the orbit.

In Wegener granulomatosis, optimal imaging techniques should provide high contrast resolution to accurately depict subtle soft tissue changes observed in the sinonasal area as well in the adjacent deep spaces of the face. For these reasons, though CT enables excellent demonstration of bone changes, MR should be considered as the first line imaging technique whenever Wegener granulomatosis is suspected at clinical examination and laboratory tests.

According to a recent classification (MUHLE et al. 1997), mucosal changes in the early stage of the disease result in rather nonspecific MR findings. Thickening combined with TSE T2 hyperintensity of the epithelial and submucosal layer of the nose and sinus cavities can be observed, reflecting edema and inflammatory cell infiltration in the areas of vasculitis. Though sensitive, this MR signal pattern can be nonspecific in up to 37% of patients.

In the late stage of the disease, signal intensity of mucosa and submucosa switches to hypointensity on both TSE T2 and SE T1 sequences, with variable degrees of contrast enhancement (Fig. 6.25). This is mostly due to submucosal accumulation of dense collagen fibers with granuloma formation. In this stage, the specificity of MR significantly increases (up to 100%) (MUHLE et al. 1997).

Evidently, CT discrimination between early and late stage of Wegener granulomatosis is almost impossible as both conditions are displayed as nonspecific mucosal thickenings at times associated with intrasinusal fluid levels (LLOYD et al. 2002).

In advanced stages of the disease, inflammatory infiltrate and granulomatous lesions within small vessel walls lead to obliteration of the lumen and, as a consequence, to avascular necrobiosis. This is the pathologic basis of bone destruction, a hallmark of this disease, reported with different rates of prevalence (8%–75%) (MUHLE et al. 1997; TRIMARCHI et al. 2001; LLOYD et al. 2002;). The width of this process is also somewhat controversial. Whenever an early diagnosis of Wegener granulomatosis is obtained and proper treatment promptly instituted, this finding is rare (12% of patients) and limited to the nasal septum (TRIMARCHI et al. 2001). Conversely, in late stages of the disease, a bilateral symmetric destructive pattern, also involving the middle and inferior turbinate, medial maxillary sinus wall, lamina papyracea, and cribriform plate, is described (LLOYD et al. 2002).

Alternatively, new bone apposition may prevail resulting in sclerotic thickening of bony structures such as sinus walls. Within sclerotic bone, hypodense areas have been described (LLOYD et al. 2002) with fat tissue signal on MR, probably reflecting bone marrow accumulation.

Mass-like pseudotumoral lesions are more commonly described in the orbit (Fig. 6.26), either as a primary involvement or as a secondary spread from contiguous deep spaces of the face, such as the pterygopalatine fossa or masticator space (Fig. 6.27)

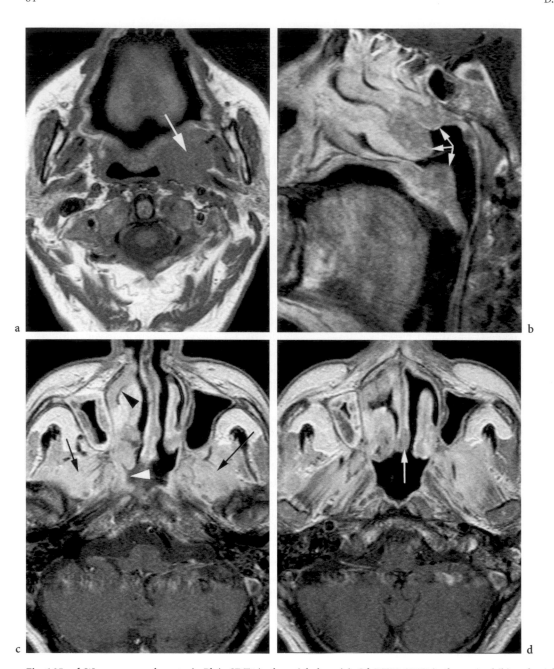

Fig. 6.25a–d. Wegener granulomatosis. Plain SE T1 in the axial plane (**a**), Gd-DTPA SE T1 in the sagittal (**b**) and axial plane (**c–d**). Hypointense mildly enhancing submucosal localizations of the disease are identified as pseudomasses (at the level of the soft palate, tonsillar fossa, nasal septum, and posterior tip of the middle and inferior turbinates) (*white arrows*). Plaque-like submucosal thickening is seen along the right lateral nasal (*black arrowhead*) and nasopharyngeal wall (*white arrowhead*). Extensive involvement of masticator spaces is demonstrated by vivid enhancement of pterygoid muscles (*black arrows*)

(NISHINO et al. 1993; PROVENZALE and ALLEN 1996; MARSOT-DUPUCH et al. 2002). CT detection is mainly based on effacement of adjacent fat tissue planes; however, the limited contrast resolution of this technique makes discrimination between lesions and adjacent muscular structures very difficult to achieve. This information can be obtained with MR, whereby a granulomatous lesion exhibits hypointense signal on TSE T2 and plain SE T1 sequences. Contrast enhancement ranges between mild inhomogeneous (MUHLE et al. 1997) to bright (PROVENZALE and ALLEN 1996). Differential diagnosis of orbital pseudotumoral lesions encompasses a long list of disease entities, including fungal in-

Fig. 6.26. Wegener granulomatosis. TSE T2 in the coronal plane. Bilateral orbital pseudomasses (*arrows*), extraconal on the *left*, intraconal on the *right,* where the lesion contacts the optic nerve

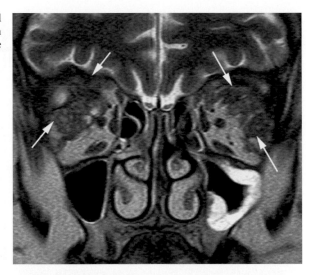

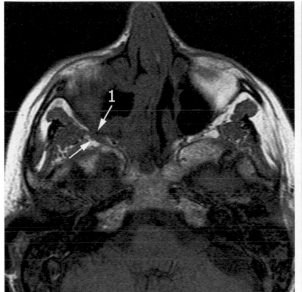
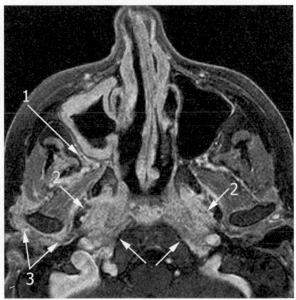

a   b

Fig. 6.27a,b. Wegener granulomatosis. Plain SE T1 (**a**) and enhanced VIBE (**b**) in the axial plane. On plain SE T1, relevant thickening of the mucosa lining the right maxillary sinus is seen, combined with soft tissue signal within the pterygopalatine fossa (*1*). **b** Marked enhancement of both the tissue in the pterygopalatine fossa and along the maxillary sinus walls is demonstrated. The fat suppressed sequence clearly shows the relevant enhancement of parapharyngeal spaces and nasopharyngeal walls (*2*). Soft tissue thickening and enhancement at the right temporomandibular joint (*3*) is also observed

fection, sarcoidosis, connective tissue diseases, and neoplastic lesions (basically lymphomas, metastases, and fibrous tumors) (DALLEY 1999; WEBER et al. 1999). In all these conditions, imaging findings should be carefully matched with clinical information and laboratory tests, as even sophisticated information provided by MR are, in itself, often insufficient to provide the diagnosis.

Neurologic manifestations of Wegener granulomatosis may be related to central/peripheral nerve involvement as well as to central nervous system localization of the disease. Cranial nerve involvement, a process triggered by small vessel vasculitides of the vasa nervorum (DRACHMAN 1963), is rather uncommon (6.5% of cases) (NISHINO et al. 1993); very rarely it has been described as the unique manifestation of the disease. MR findings include asymmetric nerve thickening, enlargement and destruction of the related foramina and fissures, and abnormal signal pattern resembling that described

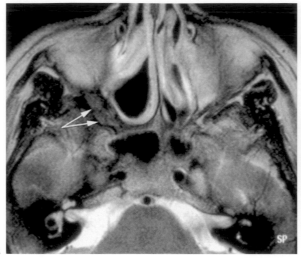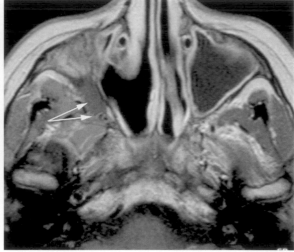

a   b

Fig. 6.28a,b. Wegener granulomatosis. SE T2 (**a**) and Gd-DTPA SE T1 (**b**) in the axial plane. Thickening of the maxillary nerve (*arrows*) as it courses through the pterygopalatine fossa. Note hypointense signal and mild enhancement, indicating granulomatous tissue surrounding the nerve

in mucosal lesions and in pseudotumors (Fig. 6.28). CT is less sensitive to nerve abnormalities: actually, this technique enables the detection of late indirect signs such as pressure erosion and/or enlargement of skull base foramina and fissures.

Otologic manifestations of Wegener granulomatosis are related to the involvement of the Eustachian tube or of the middle ear. Active granulomatous tissue within the middle ear may exhibit enhancement differently from retained fluid observed in serous otitis media (MAROLDI et al. 2001) (Fig. 6.29).

Cerebral vasculiti is rather uncommon: it may result in an intraparenchymal or subarachnoid hemorrhage, or in a stroke. The latter may also be secondary to vessel compression from mass-like pseudotumoral lesions. Remote granulomatous lesions may affect the brain parenchyma (rarely) (PROVENZALE and ALLEN 1996) or dura. Plaque thickening and marked contrast enhancement of the dura (without pial involvement) are reported, promptly responding to immunosuppressive treatment. Similar findings are detected in a list of different conditions including neurosarcoidosis, primary and secondary dural tumors, infectious diseases, hypertrophic pachymeningitis.

Destruction of central facial bone structures is the hallmark of *cocaine induced midline destructive lesions*. This process shows a centrifugal pattern of progression, starting from the nasal septum (eroded in 100% of patients) to involve turbinates

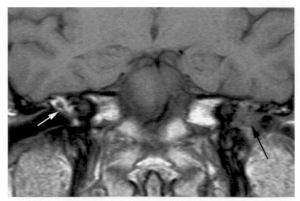

a

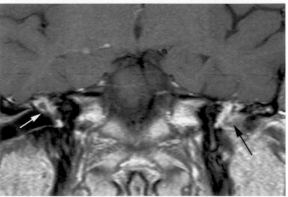

b

Fig. 6.29a,b. Wegener granulomatosis. SE T1 before (**a**) and after (**b**) Gd-DTPA administration. On the *right side* an hyperintense signal fills the middle ear, suggesting dehydrated fluid collection (*white arrows*). **b** On the *left side*, there is relevant enhancement of the retained material in the middle ear, consistent with granulation tissue (*black arrows*). Part of the ossicular chain is demonstrated on both sides

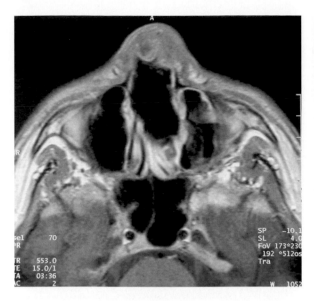

Fig. 6.30. Cocaine induced midline destructive lesions. Gd-DTPA enhanced SE T1, axial plane. Extensive destruction of midline nasal structures with involvement of the nasal septum and both inferior turbinates. Distortion of the inferior portion of the nose is also seen

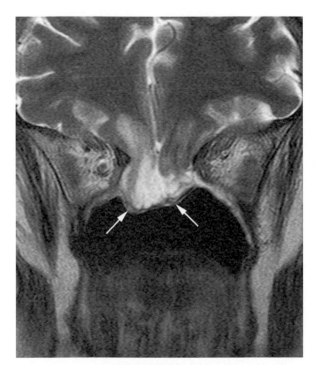

Fig. 6.31. Cocaine induced midline destructive lesions. TSE T2, coronal plane. Bilateral meningoencephalocele (*arrows*) secondary to extensive destruction of all centrofacial structures

(inferior 75%, middle 62.5%), lateral nasal wall (medial maxillary sinus wall, lamina papyracea), both roof and floor of nasal cavities (hard and soft palate) (Fig. 6.30, 6.31). The concept of centrifugal progression is strengthened by the correlation demonstrated between the area of septal erosion and the degree of midfacial structure destruction (TRIMARCHI et al. 2001).

Mucosal inflammation may also be detected on MR: signal characteristics are quite similar to those described for Wegener granulomatosis, namely T2 hypointensity combined with nonhomogeneous and decreased enhancement.

The differential diagnosis between cocaine induced midline destructive lesions and Wegener granulomatosis is rather difficult as these two entities exhibit overlapping histopathologic features and because ANCA testing may give positive results also in cocaine induced midline destructive lesions. Moreover, cocaine abusers are obviously inclined to deny drug addiction. Two elements may help to solve the diagnosis: hard and soft palate are generally spared by Wegener granulomatosis (LLOYD et al. 2002); in addition, mucosal areas with abnormal MR signal in cocaine abusers are generally confined to the septum or turbinates, where deposition of insufflated crystals occurs (TRIMARCHI et al. 2001).

A very limited number of studies in the literature focus on imaging findings of sinonasal sarcoidosis – reflecting the low incidence of this condition. CT and MR findings may consist, in moderate stages, of isolated mucosal thickenings, intrasinusal air–fluid levels, and hypertrophy of turbinates, impossible to differentiate from a mere chronic sinusitis (KRESPI et al. 1995). In advanced stages, submucosal granulomas and bone erosions may be observed, shifting the differential diagnosis towards Wegener granulomatosis and cocaine induced midline destructive lesions. MR signal pattern of sarcoid granulomas resembles that of Wegener granulomatosis lesions (T2/T1 hypointensity, variable enhancement) (Fig. 6.32). Bone destruction may be rather extensive, both the hard and soft palate may be affected.

Actually, these three non-infectious destructive inflammatory diseases may have highly overlapping manifestations, making a CT/MR based differential diagnosis nearly impossible. The main task of imaging, therefore, is to precisely assess the extent of the lesions, particularly in deep spaces of the face.

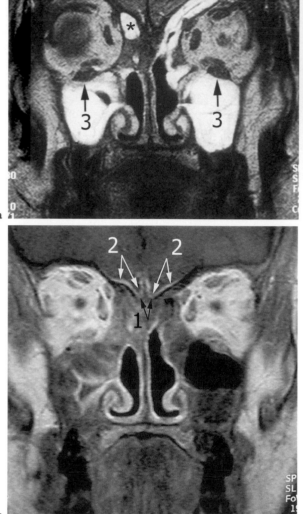

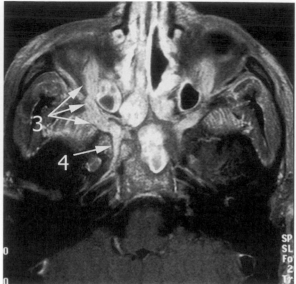

Fig. 6.32a–c. Sarcoidosis. TSE T2 in the coronal plane (**a**), fat suppressed Gd-DTPA SE T1 (**b**) in the axial plane, Gd-DTPA SE T1 (**c**) in the coronal plane; examination obtained 8 months after microendoscopic sinus surgery. A hypointense, mildly enhancing pseudomass occupies the roof of the residual ethmoid, obstructing the frontal sinus (*asterisk*) and encroaching the floor of anterior cranial fossa (*1*). Reactive changes of the adjacent dura are present (*2*). Bilateral thickening of infraorbital and vidian nerves (*3–4*); hypointense signal on T2 and vivid enhancement indicate granulomatous involvement

References

Amran MA, Sidek DS, Hamzah M et al (2002) Cavernous sinus thrombosis secondary to sinusitis. J Otolaryngol 31:165-169

Bachert C, Hörmann K, Mösges R et al (2003) An update on the diagnosis and treatment of sinusitis and nasal polyposis. Allergy 58:176-191

Bachert C, Gevaert P, Holtappels G et al (2001) Total and specific IgE in nasal polyps is related to local eosinophilic inflammation. J Allergy Clin Immunol 107:607-614

Batsakis JG, Sneige N (1992) Choanal and angiomatous polyps of the sinonasal tract. Ann Otol Rhinol Laryngol 101:623-625

Bhattacharyya N, Fried MP (2003) The accuracy of computed tomography in the diagnosis of chronic rhinosinusitis. Laryngoscope 113:125-129

Brandley PJ, Manning KP, Shaw MD (1984) Brain abscess secondary to paranasal sinusitis. J Laryngol Otol 98:719-725

Braun H, Buzina W, Freudenschuss K et al (2003) Eosinophilic fungal rhinosinusitis: a common disorder in Europe? Laryngoscope 113:264-269

Brook I, Gooch WM III, Jenkins SG (2000) Medical management of acute bacterial sinusitis. Recommendations of a clinical advisory committee on pediatric and adult sinusitis. Ann Otol Rhinol Laryngol 109:2-20

Busaba NY, Colden DG, Faquin WC et al (2002) Chronic invasive fungal sinusitis: a report of two atypical cases. Ear Nose Throat J 81:462-466

Carter EL, Grossman ME (2000) Cocaine-induced centrofacial ulceration. Cutis 65:73-76

Chan LL, Singh S, Jones D et al (2000) Imaging of mucormycosis skull base osteomyelitis. AJNR Am J Neuroradiol 21:828-831

Chandler JR, Langenbrunner DJ, Stevens ER (1970) The pathogenesis of orbital complications in acute sinusitis. Laryngoscope 80:1414-1428

Cooke LD, Hadley DM (1991) MRI of the paranasal sinuses: incidental abnormalities and their relationship to symptoms. J Laryngol Otol 105:278-281

Dalley RW (1999) Fibrous histiocytoma and fibrous tissue tumors of the orbit. Radiol Clin North Am 37:185-194

Damrose EJ, Huang RY, Abemayor E (2000) Endoscopic diagnosis of sarcoidosis in a patient presenting with bilateral exophthalmos and pansinusitis. Am J Rhinol 14:241-244

De Carpentier JP, Ramamurthy L, Denning DW et al (1994) An algorithmic approach to aspergillus sinusitis. J Laryngol Otol 108:314-318

De R, Uppal HS, Shehab ZP et al (2003) Current practices of cocaine administration by UK otorhinolaryngologists. J Laryngol Otol 117:109-112

De Vuysere S, Hermans R, Marchal G (2001) Sinochoanal polyp and its variant, the angiomatous polyp: MRI findings. Eur Radiol 11:55-58

DeShazo RD, O'Brien M, Chapin K et al (1997) A new classification and diagnostic criteria for invasive fungal sinusitis. Arch Otolaryngol Head Neck Surg 123:1181-1188

DeShazo RD, O'Brien MM, Justice WK et al (1999) Diagnostic criteria for sarcoidosis of the sinuses. J Allergy Clin Immunol 103:789-795

Dhong HJ, Jung JY, Park JH (2000) Diagnostic accuracy in sinus fungus balls: CT scan and operative findings. Am J Rhinol 14:227-231

Drachman DA (1963) Neurological complications of Wegener's granulomatosis. Arch Neurol 8:145-155

Fergie N, Jones NS, Havlat MF (1999) The nasal manifestations of sarcoidosis: a review and report of eight cases. J Laryngol Otol 113:893-898

Ferguson BJ (2000) Fungus balls of the paranasal sinuses. Otolaryngol Clin North Am 33:389-398

Giacchi RJ, Lebowitz RA, Yee HT et al (2001) Histopathologic evaluation of the ethmoid bone in chronic sinusitis. Am J Rhinol 15:193-197

Gillespie MB, O'Malley BW Jr, Francis HW (1998) An approach to fulminant invasive fungal rhinosinusitis in the immunocompromised host. Arch Otolaryngol Head Neck Surg 124:520-526

Gwaltney JM Jr, Jones JG, Kennedy DW (1995) Medical management of sinusitis: educational goals and management guidelines. The International Conference on sinus Disease. Ann Otol Rhinol Laryngol [Suppl] 167:22-30

Hähnel S, Ertl-Wagner B, Tasman AJ et al (1999) Relative value of MR imaging as compared with CT in the diagnosis of inflammatory paranasal sinus disease. Radiology 210:171-176

Hofer E, Neher A, Gunkel AAR et al (2003) In vitro study on the influence of N-chlorotaurine on the ciliary beat frequency of nasal mucosa. Am J Rhinol 17:149-152

Hoffman GS, Kerr GS, Leavitt RY et al (1992) Wegener granulomatosis: an analysis of 158 patients. Ann Inter Med 116:488-498

Holmstöm M, Hlmberg K, Lundblad L et al (2002) Current perspectives on the treatment of nasal polyps: a Swedish opinion report. Acta Otolaryngol (Stockh) 122:736-744

Jennette JC, Falk RJ (1997) Small-vessel vasculitis. N Engl J Med 337:1512-1523

Jones NS, Walker JL, Bassi S et al (2002) The intracranial complications of rhinosinusitis: can they be prevented? Laryngoscope 112:59-63

Kasemsuwan L, Griffiths MW (1996) Lignocaine with adrenaline: is it as effective as cocaine in rhinologic practice? Clin Otolaryngol 21:127-129

Kennedy DW (1992) Prognostic factors, outcomes and staging in ethmoid sinus surgery. Laryngoscope 102:1-18

Kerr GS, Fleisher TA, Hallahan CW et al (1993) Limited prognostic value of changes in antineutrophil cytoplasmic antibody titer in patients with Wegener's granulomatosis. Arthritis Rheum 36:365-371

Klossek JM, Serrano E, Peloquin L et al (1997) Functional endoscopic sinus surgery and 109 mycetomas of paranasal sinuses. Laryngoscope 107:112-117

Kramer MF, Rasp G (1999) Nasal Polyposis: eosinophils and interleukin-5 Allergy 54:669-680

Kraus M, Tovi F (1992) Central nervous system complications secondary to oto-rhinologic infections. An analysis of 39 pediatric cases. Int J Ped Otolaryngol 24:217-226

Krespi YP, Kuriloff DB, Aner M (1995) Sarcoidosis of the sinonasal tract: a new staging system. Otolaryngol Head Neck Surg 112:221-227

Lancaster J, Belloso A, Wilson CA et al (2000) Rare case of naso-oral fistula with extensive osteocartilaginous necrosis secondary to cocaine abuse: review of otorhinolaryngological presentation in cocaine addicts. J Laryngol Otol 114:630-633

Lang EE, Curran AJ, Patil N et al (2001) Intracranial complications of acute frontal sinusitis. Clin Otolaryngol 26:452-457

Larsen K, Tos M (2002) The estimated incidence of symptomatic nasal polyps. Acta otolaryngol (Stockh) 122:179-182

Larsen PL, Tos M, Kuijpers W et al (1992) The early stages of polyp formation. Laryngoscope 102:670-677

Lerner DN, Choi SS, Zalzal GH et al (1995) Intracranial complications of sinusitis in childhood. Ann Otol Rhinol Laryngol 104:288-293

Liang EY, Lam WW, Woo JK et al (1996) Another CT sign of sinonasal polyposis: truncation of the bony middle turbinate. Eur Radiol 6:553-556

Lloyd G, Lund VJ, Beale T et al (2002) Rhinologic changes in Wegener's granulomatosis. J Laryngol Otol 116:565-569

Lund VJ, Mackay IS (1993) Staging in rhinosinusitis. Rhinology 31:183-184

Lusk PR (1992) Pediatric sinusitis. Raven, New York

Manning SC, Holman M (1998) Further evidence for allergic pathophysiology in allergic fungal sinusitis. Laryngoscope 108:1485-1496

Marì A, Arraz C, Gimeno X et al (2002) Nasal cocaine abuse and centrofacial destructive process: report of three cases including treatment. Oral Surg Oral Med Oral Pathol Oral Radiol Endod 93:435-439

Marks SC, Goodman RS (1998) Surgical management of nasal and sinus sarcoidosis. Otolaryngol Head Neck Surg 118:856-858

Maroldi R, Farina D, Palvarini L et al (2001) Computed tomography and magnetic resonance imaging of pathologic conditions of the middle ear. Eur J Radiol 40:78-93

Marsot-Dupuch K, de Givry SC, Ouayoun M (2002) Wegener granulomatosis involving the pterygopalatine fossa: an unusual case of trigeminal neuropathy. AJNR Am J Neuroradiol 23:312-315

Mazziotti S, Gaeta M, Blandino A et al (2001) Perineural spread in a case of sinonasal sarcoidosis: a case report. AJNR Am J Neuroradiol 22:1207-1208

McCaffrey TV, McDonald TJ (1983) Sarcoidosis of the nose and paranasal sinus. Laryngoscope 93:1281-1284

Muhle C, Reinhold-Keller E, Richter C et al (1997) MRI of the nasal cavity, the paranasal sinuses and orbits in Wegener's granulomatosis. Eur Radiol 7:566-570

Mukherji SK, Figueroa RE, Ginsberg LE et al (1998) Allergic fungal sinusitis: CT findings. Radiology 207:417-422

Mygind N (1999) Advances in the medical treatment of nasal polyps. Allergy 54:12-16

National Center for Health Statistics (1994) Vital and health statistic: current estimates from National Health Interview Survey no 190. US Department of Health and Human Service, Washington DC

Nishino H, Rubino FA, DeRemee RA et al (1993) Neurological involvement in Wegener's granulomatosis: an analysis of 324 consecutive patients at the Mayo Clinic. Ann Neurol 33:4-9

Noordzij JP, Harrison SE, Mason JC et al (2002) Pitfalls in the endoscopic drainage of subperiosteal orbital abscesses secondary to sinusitis. Am J Rhinol 16:97-101

Oliverio PJ, Benson ML, Zinreich SJ (1995) Update on imaging for functional endoscopic sinus surgery. Otolaryngol Clin North Am 28:585-608

Patt BS, Manning SC (1991) Blindness resulting from orbital complications of sinusitis. Otolaryngol Head Neck Surg 104:789-795

Phillips CD (1997) Current status and new developments in techniques for imaging the nose and sinuses. Otolaryngol Clin North Am 30:371-387

Plaignaud M (1791) Observations sur un fongus du sinus maxillaire. J Chir 1:111-116

Ponikau JU, Sherris DA, Kern EB et al (1999) The diagnosis and incidence of allergic fungal sinusitis. Mayo Clin Proc 74:877-884

Ponikau JU, Sherris DA, Kita H et al (2002) Intranasal antifungal treatment in 51 patients with chronic rhinosinusitis. J Allergy Clin Immunol 110:862-866

Provenzale JM, Allen NB (1996) Wegener granulomatosis: CT and MR findings. AJNR Am J Neuroradiol 17:785-792

Provenzale JM, Mukherji S, Allen NB (1996) Orbital management by Wegener's granulomatosis: image findings. AJR Am J Roentgenol 166:929-934

Pruna X (2003) Morpho-functional evaluation of osteomeatal complex in chronic sinusitis by coronal CT. Eur Radiol 13:1461-1468

Rains BM 3rd, Mineck CW (2003) Treatment of allergic fungal sinusitis with high-dose itraconazole. Am J Rhinol 17:1-8

Rao VM, Sharma D, Madan A (2001) Imaging of frontal sinus disease: concepts, interpretation, and technology. Otolaryngol Clin North Am 34:23-39

Ricchetti A, Landis BN, Maffioli A et al (2002) Effect of antifungal nasal lavage with amphtericin B on nasal polyposis. J Laryngol Otol 116:261-263

Rumboldt Z, Castillo M (2002) Indolent intracranial mucormycosis: case report. AJNR Am J Neuroradiol 23:932-934

Ruoppi P, Dietz A, Nikanne E et al (2001) Paranasal sinus mucormycosis: a report of two cases. Acta Otolaryngol 121:948-952

Saleh HA, Bridger MW (1997) Invasive aspergillosis of the paranasal sinuses: a medical emergency. J Laryngol Otol 111:1168-1170

Settipane GA (1996) Epidemiology of nasal polyps. Allergy Asthma Proc 17:231-236

Seyer BA, Grist W, Muller S (2002) Aggressive destructive midfacial lesion from cocaine abuse. Oral Surg Oral Med Oral Pathol Oral Radiol Endod 94:465-470

Shah UK, White JA, Gooey JE et al (1997) Otolaryngologic manifestations of sarcoidosis: presentation and diagnosis. Laryngoscope 107:67-75

Shahin J, Gullane PJ, Dajal VS (1987) Orbital complications of acute sinusitis. J Otolaryngol 16:23-27

Smith JC, Kacker A, Anand VK (2002) Midline nasal and palate destruction in cocaine abusers and cocaine's role in rhinologic practice. Ear Nose Throat J 81:172-177

Sobol SE, Marchand J, Tewfik TL et al (2002) Orbital complication of sinusitis in children. J Otolaryngol 31:131-136

Som PM, Dillon WP, Fullerton GD et al (1989) Chronically obstructed sinonasal secretions: observations on T1 and T2 shortening. Radiology 172:515-520

Sonkens JW, Harnsberger HR, Blanch GM et al (1991) The impact of screening sinus CT on the planning of functional endoscopic sinus surgery. Otolaryngol Head Neck Surg 105:802-813

Stammberger H (1991) Functional endoscopic sinus surgery. Decker, Philadelphia

Stammberger H (1997) Rhinoscopic surgery. In: Settipane GA, Lund VJ, Bernsein JM, Tos M (eds) Nasal polyps: epidemiology, pathogenesis and treatment. OceanSide, Providence

Stewart MG, Sicard MW, Piccirillo JF et al (1999) Severity staging in chronic sinusitis: are CT scan findings related to patient symptoms? Am J Rhinol 13:161-167

Takwoingi Y, Dempster JH (2003) Wegener's granulomatosis: an analysis of 32 patients seen over a 10-year period. Clin Otolaryngol 28:187-194

Trimarchi M, Gregorini G, Facchetti F et al (2001) Cocaine-induced midline destructive lesions: clinical, radiographic, histopathologic, and serologic features and their differentiation from Wegener granulomatosis. Medicine 80:391-404

Trimarchi M, Nicolai P, Lombardi D et al (2003) Sinonasal osteocartilaginous necrosis in cocaine abusers: experience in 25 patients. Am J Rhinol 17:33-43

Van Camp C, Clement PA (1994) Results of oral steroid treatment in nasal polyposis. Rhinology 32:5-9

Vilela RJ, Langford C, McCullagh L et al (2002) Cocaine-induced oronasal fistulas with external nasal erosion but without palate involvement. Ear Nose Throat J 81:562-563

Wagner W (1996) Changing diagnostic and treatment strategies for chronic sinusitis. Cleve Clin J Med 63:396-405

Wald ER (1998) Microbiology of acute and chronic sinusitis in children and adults Am J Med Sci 316:13-20

Wani MK, Ruckenstein MJ, Parikh S (2001) Magnetic resonance imaging of the paranasal sinuses: incidental abnormalities and their relationship to patient symptoms. J Otolaryngol 30:257-262

Weber AL, Romo LV, Sabates NR (1999) Pseudotumor of the orbit. Clinical, pathologic, and radiologic evaluation. Radiol Clin North Am 37:151-168

Yagi HI, Gumaa SA, Shumo AI et al (1999) Nasosinus aspergillosis in Sudanese patients: clinical features, pathology, diagnosis, and treatment. J Otolaryngol 28:90--94

Yang C, Talbot JM, Hwang PH (2001) Bony abnormalities of the paranasal sinuses in patients with Wegener's granulomatosis. Am J Rhinol 15:121-125

Younis RT, Lazar R (1996) Criteria for success in pediatric

functional endonasal sinus surgery. Laryngoscope 106:869-873

Younis RT, Lazar RH, Bustillo A et al (2002a) Orbital infection as a complication of sinusitis: are diagnostic and treatment trends changing? Ear Nose Throat J 81:771-775

Younis RT, Lazar RH, Anand VK (2002b) Intracranial complications of sinusitis: a 15-year review of 39 cases. Ear Nose Throat J 81:636-644

Younis RT, Anand VK, Davidson B (2002c) The role of computed tomography and magnetic resonance imaging in patients with sinusitis with complications. Laryngoscope 112:224-229

Yousem DM (1993) Imaging of sinonasal inflammatory disease. Radiology 188:303-314

Yucel EA, Keles N, Ozturk AS et al (2002) Wegener's granulomatosis presenting in the sinus and orbit. Otolaryngol Head Neck Surg 127:349-351

Zeitlin JF, Tami TA, Baughman R et al (2000) Nasal and sinus manifestations of sarcoidosis. Am J Rhinol 14:157-161

7 Cerebrospinal Fluid Leak, Meningocele and Meningoencephalocele

Luca Pianta, Lorenzo Pinelli, Piero Nicolai, and Roberto Maroldi

CONTENTS

7.1   Definition, Epidemiology, Classification   93
7.2   Clinical and Endoscopic Findings   94
7.3   Diagnosis   95
7.4   Treatment Guidelines   96
7.4.1   Follow-Up   98
7.5   Key Information to Be Provided by Imaging   98
7.6   Imaging Findings   98
7.6.1   Integration of Imaging into the
         Diagnostic Work-Up   98
7.6.1.1 CSF Leak Associated with Persistent
         or Intermittent Rhinorrhea   98
7.6.1.2 CSF Leak Presenting with Recurrent Meningitis   102
7.6.2   Invasive Imaging Techniques   104
         References   105

7.1
Definition, Epidemiology, Classification

The term "cephalocele" encompasses the extracranial extension of any intracranial structure through a congenital or acquired defect in the cranium and dura, that is an external brain hernia. Apart from atretic cephaloceles (*formes frustes* of cephaloceles occurring only in the parietal and occipital regions), cephaloceles can be essentially subdivided into two types: *meningoceles*, in which the structures protruding consist solely of leptomeninges and CSF; *meningoencephaloceles*, in which the structures protruding consist of leptomeninges, CSF and brain (Naidich et al. 1992). When an abnormal communication develops between the subarachnoid space and the sinonasal tract and/or the middle ear/mastoid system CSF rhinorrhea occurs.

According to Ommaya's classification (Ommaya 1983), *CSF leaks* can be divided into *traumatic* (accidental or iatrogenic) and *spontaneous* (associated with high or normal CSF pressure).

Approximately 80% of CSF leaks are caused by head trauma with skull base fractures and 16% are the result of sinus or skull base surgery (Beckhardt et al. 1991). The prevalence of CSF leak in head traumas is approximately 2%, whereas CSF leak complicates about 25% of facial fractures (Zlab et al. 1992; Eljamel 1994). Microendoscopic sinus surgery is associated with a 0%–3% prevalence of CSF leak (Gjuric et al. 1996).

Spontaneous fistulas, which are estimated to be responsible for only 3%–4% of CSF leaks (Beckhardt et al. 1991; Nachtigal et al. 1999), are more frequently observed in females (males/females ratio 1:2) in the fourth decade of life.

While the pathogenesis of traumatic fistulas is intuitive, spontaneous leaks recognize a multifactorial origin: intracranial pressure, brain pulsation, cranial base pneumatization, and arachnoid pits (the so-called four P's of fistula formation) are thought to play a major role. The presence of elevated intracranial pressure may cause a gradual distension of the meningeal sac and the formation of a cephalocele through congenital defects of the skull base or a natural avenue of least resistance such as the sellar diaphragm. Eventually, the meninges break down and CSF leak occurs. The fistula can be considered as a pressure relief valve, and the leakage is very difficult to be controlled until intracranial pressure is restored to normal values. Brain pulsation may be responsible for thinning and erosion of the bone of the skull base and the development of a cephalocele through a congenital or traumatic defect. In hyperpneumatized paranasal sinuses and temporal bones the skull base is very thin and may have different paths of least resistance for the development of a fistula. The presence of arachnoid villi in communication with basal meningeal veins along the skull base cause the "pitting"

L. Pianta, MD
Department of Otorhinolaryngology, University of Brescia, Piazzale Spedali Civili 1, Brescia, 25123, Italy
L. Pinelli, MD,
Department of Radiology, Neuroradiology Section, University of Brescia, Piazzale Spedali Civili 1, Brescia, 25123, Italy
P. Nicolai, MD
Professor, Department of Otorhinolaryngology, University of Brescia, Piazzale Spedali Civili 1, Brescia, 25123, Italy
R. Maroldi, MD
Professor, Department of Radiology, University of Brescia, Piazzale Spedali Civili 1, Brescia, 25123, Italy

of the cranial floor. If pits occur over a hyperpneumatized area they may transmit brain pulsations that eventually erode the bone of the skull base (NUSS and COSTANTINO 1995).

The association between CSF leak and primary empty sella is well known: SHETTY et al. (2000) reported 90% of patients with sphenoid spontaneous CSF leak having complete (63%) or partially (27%) empty sella. Very recently, SCHLOSSER and BOLGER (2003) found similar percentages of patients with complete or partially empty sella (63% and 33%, respectively) having spontaneous encephaloceles and associated CSF leak. Before stabilizing on high pressure values, benign intracranial hypertension is thought to start with intermittent mild episodes frequently leading to the development of an empty sella (SCHLOSSER and BOLGER 2003). This would explain why up to 15% of patients with empty sella will develop benign intracranial hypertension, but up to 94% of patients with benign intracranial hypertension already have an empty sella (ZAGARDO et al. 1996). Other causes of CSF leak with increased intracranial pressure are intracranial tumors and hydrocephalus (ZLAB et al. 1992; CLARK et al. 1994).

CSF leak with normal intracranial pressure may be observed in connective tissue disorders like Marfan's syndrome and osteogenesis imperfecta (MOKRI et al. 2002), as well as in tumors arising in the sinonasal tract, chronic sinus diseases, skull base osteomyelitis, syphilis, and leprosy (TOLLEY 1991).

The presence of bony defects in the skull base is responsible for the development of congenital cephaloceles. This condition shows a peculiar distribution: while the reported incidence varies from 1:35,000 to 1:40,000 live births in the West, higher values have been observed in Southeast Asian countries (1:5,000 live births in Thailand) (MAHAPATRA and SURI 2002).

Congenital cephaloceles involving the skull base are classified into: temporal, fronto-ethmoidal, spheno-orbital, spheno-maxillary, and nasopharyngeal (NAIDICH et al. 1992). Nasopharyngeal cephaloceles, in which the defect lies within the ethmoid, sphenoid or basioccipital bones, are possible causes of CSF leak. They are subcategorized into transethmoidal, spheno-ethmoidal, transsphenoidal and transbasioccipital types according to the specific site of the ostium.

While other forms of cephaloceles are typically detected prenatally (by obstetric ultrasound) or at birth (by clinical presentation of a subcutaneous "mass"), nasopharyngeal cephaloceles may escape detection for years, and first present in childhood or even adulthood, sometimes being the unexpected cause of an "idiopathic" CSF rhinorrhea.

In general, the herniated brain contents of meningoencephaloceles have been considered dysplastic and non-functioning; this is true in most cases, but the concept has been recently questioned, as long as in some occipital and transsphenoidal cephaloceles functioning brain may be found within the sac (OI et al. 1994)

7.2
Clinical and Endoscopic Findings

Unilateral/bilateral watery persistent or intermittent rhinorrhea, a previous history of head trauma or surgery on the sinonasal tract, middle ear/mastoid or skull base, and recurrent meningitis are the clinical findings which should alert the physician to the diagnosis of CSF leak.

Nasal discharge usually increases or may be elicited by maneuvers elevating CSF pressure (i.e., compression of the internal jugular veins, Valsalva maneuver). In case of a leak through the temporal bone, CSF reaches the nasopharynx via the Eustachian tube and becomes evident in most cases as bilateral clear rhinorrhea. The onset of CSF rhinorrhea after trauma occurs within the first 48 h in 80% of patients, whereas 95% will present within 3 months of the accident. The so-called "reservoir sign" is a peculiar finding which is particularly suggestive for the presence of a CSF fistula: CSF tends to accumulate in the sphenoid sinus while the patient is recumbent, and remains in the sinus until the patient resumes the erect position and the head is leaned forward. At that moment, the fluid exits the sphenoid ostium and sudden profuse rhinorrhea becomes evident (NUSS and COSTANTINO 1995).

Patients with intermittent CSF leak frequently complain of headache, which appears whenever rhinorrhea stops and CSF pressure increases (BECKHARDT et al. 1991). Symptoms and signs such as headache, vomit, or edema of the papilla are suggestive for intracranial hypertension. If CSF leak is secondary to a neoplasm of the sinonasal tract invading the skull base, nasal obstruction, mucous rhinorrhea, epistaxis, visual impairment, and alterations of eye motility may be present. Both intracranial neoplasms and lesions involving the skull base from adjacent sites may cause neurologic signs and symptoms.

In case of a cephalocele, signs and symptoms depend on its location. Transethmoidal cephaloceles herniate into the nasal cavity and may be characterized by unilateral nasal obstruction; less frequently, this is the heralding symptom of transsphenoidal encephaloceles. Endoscopic evaluation may reveal a smooth isolated polypoid mass coming from the olfactory fossa (Fig. 7.1) or sphenoid sinus. In this setting, removal or biopsy of the lesion is contraindicated unless appropriate radiologic evaluation has been obtained. Fronto-ethmoidal and spheno-orbital cephaloceles herniate into the soft tissues of the nose region and of the orbit(s), respectively, and are characterized by swelling, proptosis, and hypertelorism. In these cases, an association with facial deformities and cleft palate is frequently observed (MAHAPATRA and SURI 2002).

In a patient with persistent CSF leak, rarely nasal endoscopy identifies the site of CSF leakage. Watery rhinorrhea and mucosal bulging at the olfactory fossa is the most favorable situation suggesting a CSF leak coming from a cephalocele. An unexpected sinonasal neoplasm can also be detected by endoscopy.

Recurrent meningitis, even in the absence of rhinorrhea, should raise a suspicion of CSF leak. The prevalence of meningitis and brain abscess is reported to be up to 40% in traumatic non-intermittent fistulae, whereas their incidence greatly varies in spontaneous leaks (BECKHARDT et al. 1991; ELJAMEL 1994; WAX et al. 1997).

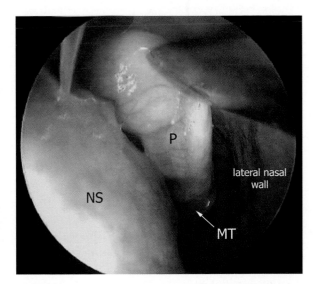

Fig. 7.1. Meningocele of the left nasal fossa. Endoscopic evaluation with a 0°-angled rigid endoscope: an isolated bluish polypoid mass (*P*) projecting from the left olfactory fossa is visible. Nasal septum, *NS*; middle turbinate, *MT*

7.3
Diagnosis

Physicians can be faced with two main different scenarios: patients with persistent or intermittent watery rhinorrhea highly suggestive for CSF leak and patients who had one or more bouts of meningitis apparently without any specific cause. In the first situation, which is the most frequent, diagnosis should include first chemical methods to analyze the nasal discharge in order to obtain confirmation of its nature, while in the second an immediate imaging examination and fluorescein test are indicated (Fig. 7.2).

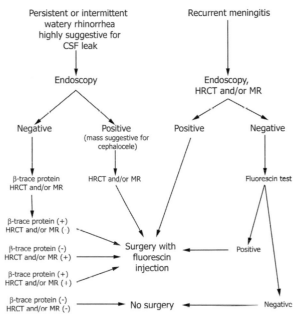

Fig. 7.2. Work-up in the case of suspected spontaneous or traumatic CSF leak. High resolution CT (HRCT)

Chemical methods for glucose, protein, or chloride have been used for many years to confirm CSF leak. However, they are nowadays considered highly nonspecific (OBERASCHER and ARRER 1986) and beta-2 transferrin (B2T) assay has taken their place in the confirmation of CSF rhinorrhea diagnosis. B2T is a polypeptide involved in ferrous ion transport: while beta-1 transferrin is present in serum, nasal secretions, tears, and saliva, B2T has been demonstrated in CSF, perilymph, and aqueous humor only. The reported sensitivity and specificity for B2T test in the diagnosis of CSF rhinorrhea is 100% and 95%, respectively (NANDAPALAN et al. 1996; SKEDROS et al. 1993). Furthermore, the procedure is absolutely noninvasive, the amount of fluid necessary for analysis is very small (0.5 ml), detection of B2T can be achieved within 3 h, and contamination by other body fluids does not invalidate the method. Beta-trace protein (BTP) is another brain specific protein that is produced mainly in the leptomeninges and the choroid plexus; it is the second most abundant protein in CSF after albumin. This protein has also been detected in other body fluids such as serum and perilymph at much lower concentrations than in CSF. Recently, a BTP nephelometric assay for the quantification and detection of CSF in nasal fluid has shown sensitivity of 91.17% and specificity of 100% (BACHMANN et al. 2000). Compared with B2T assay, BTP assay is less time-consuming . Therefore, B2T and BTP assays are nowadays considered the first line test in confirming the diagnosis of CSF rhinorrhea.

The recommended fluorescein test protocol is based on the employment of 1 ml of 5% sodium fluorescein solution diluted with 10 ml of patient's CSF. The patient is put in Trendelenburg position and the solution is slowly injected intrathecally through a lumbar puncture (STAMMBERGER 1991). Rare adverse effects of intrathecal injection of fluorescein have been reported (temporary paresthesias of the lower limbs, weakness of the extremities, dizziness, dysphasia, hemiparesis and status epilepticus) (MOSELEY et al. 1978); however, the occurrence of these symptoms seems to be related to the use of higher concentrated solutions of the dye (SENIOR et al. 2001).

7.4
Treatment Guidelines

Although most traumatic CSF fistulas can spontaneously heal with conservative measures such as bed rest, head supraelevation, administration of laxatives and antiemetics, and positioning of a lumbar drainage, a surgical corrective procedure is recommended in case these measures fail within 10–15 days (HEGAZY et al. 2000).

Immediate surgical correction is instead indicated in the case of traumatic fistulas associated with intracranial lesions requiring craniotomy and in all cases of iatrogenic leaks occurring during skull base surgery and sinus surgery (HEGAZY et al. 2000).

WIGAND (1981) first reported the endoscopic endonasal approach for CSF leaks occurring during microendoscopic sinus surgery for inflammatory conditions. From this first experience, microendoscopic repair gained popularity and is now considered the treatment of choice.

External approaches are still the mainstay in the treatment of frontoethmoidal, spheno-orbital and spheno-maxillary cephaloceles, while nasopharyngeal lesions may be amenable with a microendoscopic approach.

A large spectrum of materials can be used for duraplasty: abdominal fat, septal mucoperichondrium, turbinate bone, temporalis muscle and fascia, cadaver pericardium, lyophilized dura, fascia lata, and hydroxyapatite (ZWEIG et al. 2000).

Transnasal surgical repair involves mainly three techniques: underlay, overlay and tobacco pouch (SCHICK et al. 2001). The *underlay technique* is ideal for defects located in the fovea ethmoidalis (Fig. 7.3). Graft material (bone from the middle turbinate or cartilage from the septum) is positioned between the dura and the skull base or intracranially over the dura. A free mucoperichondral graft, harvested from the septum, is subsequently placed, as a second layer, on the endonasal surface of the skull base to reinforce the plasty.

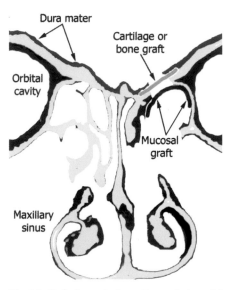

Fig. 7.3. Underlay technique. Coronal view of the anterior skull base showing the repair of a defect in the fovea ethmoidalis with "underlay technique." Grafting material (autologous cartilage from nasal septum or bone from middle turbinate) is positioned between the skull base and the dura. A mucosal graft from nasal septum or middle turbinate is placed as a second layer to reinforce the plasty

The *overlay technique* is generally employed for defects located in the lamina cribra, where the presence of olfactory phyla makes it difficult to dissect dura from the adjacent skull base (Fig. 7.4). A free cartilaginous or bony graft is first placed on the extracranial surface of the skull base to close the bony gap; similarly to underlay technique, duraplasty is then completed with a second layer of free mucoperichondrium. This technique can be also used in the lateral wall of extensively pneumatized sphenoid sinuses, where the leak is usually coming from a defect in the floor of the middle cranial fossa. In this setting, extensive drilling of the pterygoid process is required to ensure an adequate exposure (CASIANO and JASSIR 1999).

The *tobacco pouch technique* is an alternative procedure for sphenoid sinus defects: after careful removal of the entire mucosa investing the sinus, fascia lata plus Gel foam or abdominal fat is positioned into the sinus and then sealed by a mucoperichondral graft (WEBER et al. 1996; SCHICK et al. 2001) (Fig. 7.5).

A review of the literature indicates high success rates for microendoscopic procedures, varying from 75.9% to 97% after primary repair, up to 100% after revision surgery. These results are independent

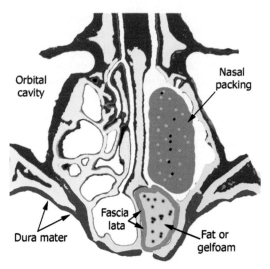

Fig. 7.5. Tobacco pouch technique. Axial view of the skull base showing the repair of a defect in the posterior wall of a sphenoid sinus with "tobacco pouch technique." A double layer packing with fascia lata and abdominal fat or Gelfoam is positioned into the sinus

from the surgical technique and grafting materials (DODSON et al. 1994; BURNS et al. 1996; LANZA et al. 1996; CASTILLO et al. 1999; MARSHALL et al. 1999; NACHTIGAL et al. 1999; MAO et al. 2000; ZWEIG et al. 2000; SCHICK et al. 2001).

Important clues for a successful repair are represented by: precise location and exposure of the defect with adequate removal of the surrounding mucosa, removal of unstable bony fragments around the breech, and use of an oversized graft (GASSNER et al. 1999; CASTELNUOVO et al. 2001; SCHICK et al. 2001).

An elevated body mass index, a finding frequently associated with spontaneous CSF leak (SCHLOSSER and BOLGER 2003), has also been recently shown to be related with failure of repair (LINDSTROM et al. 2004).

Although some authors consider perioperative antibiotic therapy unnecessary, or even contraindicated, for potential positive selection of resistant bacteria, it is generally recommended for at least 48 h after surgery to decrease the incidence of postoperative meningitis (CHOI and SPANN 1996; NACHTIGAL et al. 1999; HEGAZY et al. 2000; ZWEIG et al. 2000).

Some authors recommend the use of a lumbar drainage and its maintenance for at least 72 h after surgery (MCCORMACK et al. 1990; PERSKY et al. 1991; MAO et al. 2000). According to more recent and numerous series, its use should be limited to those patients who have an associated hydrocephalus and/ or intracranial hypertension (DODSON et al. 1994; CASIANO and JASSIR 1999; HEGAZY et al. 2000).

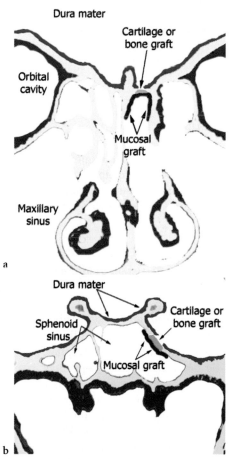

Fig. 7.4a,b. Overlay technique. **a** Coronal view of the anterior skull base showing the repair of a defect in the olfactory fossa with "overlay technique." Autologous cartilage or bone and mucosal graft are positioned endonasally under the dural defect. **b** Coronal view of the middle skull base showing the repair of a defect in the lateral wall of a hyperpneumatized sphenoid sinus with "overlay technique." After drilling of the pterygoid process a double layer plasty is positioned

The success rate of the microendoscopic approach (superior to external techniques) and the low incidence of postoperative complications make it the treatment of choice. External approaches are nowadays justified in the case of repeated failures of microendoscopic techniques, multifocal fronto-basal fractures, association with brain lesions requiring craniotomy, and fistulae not endoscopically treatable (posterior wall of the frontal sinus).

7.4.1
Follow-Up

Although most CSF leak recurrences generally occur within days or months after surgical repair, late recurrences have been described even after years. Periodic endoscopic evaluations are therefore mandatory, while BTP or fluorescein tests and imaging techniques are indicated in the case of suspicious symptoms such as persistent rhinorrhea and meningitis. Patients with intracranial hypertension should be considered at risk for a recurrent lesion or a second meningocele at a different site; periodic MR may therefore be indicated for early detection of this occurrence.

7.5
Key Information to Be Provided by Imaging

- Presence of intra- and extracranial pathology possibly related to the CSF fistula (empty sella, paranasal sinuses diseases, skull or head and neck tumors or infections) and/or contraindicating lumbar puncture possibly necessary for fluorescein or contrast-medium injection (acute posttraumatic lesions, hydrocephalus, brain tumors)
- Radiological confirmation of the CSF leak
- Side, site, size and possible number of the fistula(e)
- "Nature" of the lesion primarily causing CSF rhinorrhea (bony dehiscence, meningocele, meningoencephalocele)

7.6
Imaging Findings

The development of highly accurate chemical methods to confirm CSF leak has recently shifted the use of imaging from its *traditional* primary purpose of directly demonstrating the leakage, as evidence of its existence, to different – though not less challenging – tasks.

As a direct consequence, there is less need to use *invasive* "cisternographic" imaging techniques, which have the purpose of tracking the fistulous tract by means of radiopaque or radioactive "markers" previously injected into the CSF. Therefore, nowadays, the identification of intra- and extracranial lesions possibly causing CSF leak and the detailed demonstration of the anatomic/topographic features of the fistula(e) are the main objectives of imaging.

This information may be achieved by "plain" *noninvasive* imaging techniques, aimed at identifying lesions involving the skull base or to detect osseous/dural defects. Interestingly, MR – the more recently introduced imaging technique – enables the identification of the fistula by means of special sequences that enhance the CSF signal (MR cisternography), therefore providing findings similar to those obtained by *invasive* "cisternographic" techniques.

7.6.1
Integration of Imaging into the Diagnostic Work-Up

The use of imaging – as for the employment of either fluorescein test or BTP test – is dictated by the clinical presentation of CSF leak that can be separated into persistent or intermittent rhinorrhea vs. recurrent meningitis (Fig. 7.2)

7.6.1.1
CSF Leak Associated with Persistent or Intermittent Rhinorrhea

When persistent or intermittent watery rhinorrhea suggests CSF leak, endoscopy is the first line examination. An endonasal expansile lesion (cephalocele? glioma?) may be detected or endoscopy may give a negative result. In the first case, BTP test is unnecessary, as CSF leak is assumed to be related to the endonasal lesion. Additionally, having detected a nasal mass, the main clinical issue is to defining its relationship with intracranial structures. In this setting, MR is preferable to high resolution CT. In fact, T2 and MR cisternographic sequences are superior in demonstrating the uninterrupted CSF signal extending from the subarachnoid space into the mass, or into paranasal sinuses/nasal cavity or into middle ear, with or without brain tissue (STAFFORD et al. 1996) (Fig. 7.6).

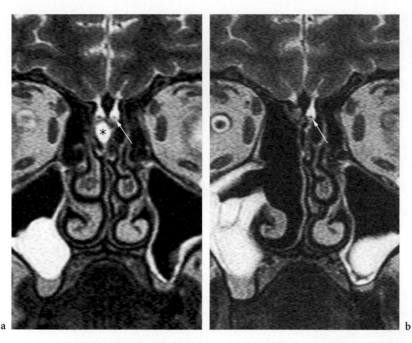

Fig. 7.6a,b. Small spontaneous meningocele through the right cribriform plate. Coronal TSE T2 before (**a**) and after (**b**) surgical repair. **a** A small rounded fluid collection (proved to be a meningocele at surgery) is seen under the right cribriform plate (*asterisk*); both olfactory bulbs are clearly visible over the cribriform plate in this patient with a "deep" olfactory fossa (the *left one* indicated by *arrows*). Subtle mucosal thickening in both maxillary sinuses, with retention cyst on the right side. **b** After successful endoscopic repair with overlay technique, the CSF collection in the right olfactory cleft is no longer visible. Note the post-surgical changes on the right side due to middle turbinectomy, uncinectomy, middle antrostomy, and ethmoidotomy

CT has a complementary role, related to its superior depiction of bony detail. At MR, the cephalocele appears as a round "mass" with sharp margins, isointense to CSF in all sequences (meningocele) or containing some tissue isointense to brain parenchyma (meningoencephalocele), protruding from the intracranial cavity into the nasal cavity or paranasal sinuses. The lumen of the lesion is continuous with the subarachnoid space and often has a constriction in the portion passing through the bone defect (the "neck" of the cephalocele) (Fig. 7.7). CT clearly shows the sclerotic margins of the bone defect. Cerebral MR may show the associated brain anatomy "distortion", presumably due to the effect of the brain pulsation in utero, which "pushed" the pliable unmyelinated brain outward through the defect (TRUWIT et al. 1996). The result is a general tendency of the ventricles and subarachnoid spaces, which subtend the cephalocele, to be stretched and elongated, "pointing" toward the calvarial defect. This finding is usually observed in patients with large occipital or parietal cephaloceles.

Cephaloceles may be isolated anomalies, but may also be seen in conjunction with other congenital brain malformations or as a part of a syndrome. The radiologist must therefore also look for associated anomalies, such as agenesis or hypogenesis of the corpus callosum, Dandy-Walker malformation, or malformations of cortical development (NAIDICH et al. 1992).

Among lesions to be differentiated from cephaloceles is the so-called nasal glioma (heterotopic brain tissue). It consists of a variable amount of dysplastic brain tissue (especially glia cells, whereas neurons are present in only about 10% of cases), located within the nasal cavity or in the nasal subcutaneous tissue. It is thought to result from the herniation of brain tissue into a dural projection that normally extends through the foramen cecum during the embryologic development. Regression of the more superior portion of this dura projection leads to complete separation of the nasal glioma from the intracranial contents. If inferiorly the dural projection remains adherent to the skin of the nose and fails to involute, but no brain tissue herniates through it; a dermal sinus tract is present. It is usually suggested by a small dimple on the surface of the nose. Along the path of the dermal sinus tract (epi)dermoids may develop.

MR is clearly superior to CT in the evaluation of nasal gliomas, because it directly shows the lack of communication with the subarachnoid space, which is the hallmark of cephaloceles. Furthermore, the dysplastic brain tissue of nasal glioma appears hyper-

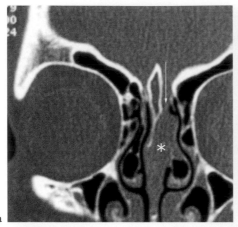
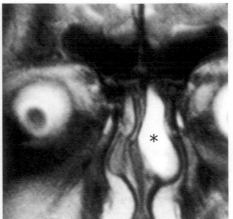

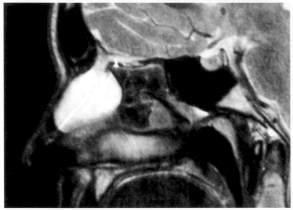

Fig. 7.7a–c. Fronto-ethmoidal spontaneous meningocele in an 8-year-old girl. Coronal high resolution CT (**a**), TSE T2 in the coronal (**b**) and sagittal (**c**) planes. **a** Bone defect in the left cribriform plate (*arrow*), associated with soft-tissue density in the left nasal cavity (*asterisk*). **b** The outpouching of CSF in the left nasal cavity is clearly identified as fluid signal (hyperintense) on TSE T2 images (*asterisk*). Even if the signal intensity of CSF is slightly brighter than that of nasal mucosa, an inflammatory polyp could be a differential diagnosis. **c** On sagittal image, the direct communication between the fluid collection in the nasal cavity and the frontal subarachnoid space is clearly depicted (*arrow*). There is no brain parenchyma extending into the endonasal CSF collection

intense to gray matter in both T1- and T2-weighted images (Fig. 7.8).

When no endonasal mass is detected by endoscopy, BTP test is indicated, its sensitivity for CSF leak being more than 90% (Bachmann et al. 2000).

If post-traumatic rhinorrhea is investigated, positivity of BTP will confirm the diagnosis. In this setting, high resolution CT is the first line imaging technique, having a reported sensitivity ranging from 50% up to 100% (Dietrich et al. 1993; Lloyd et al. 1994, Zapalac 2002). It is obtained without intrathecal or intravenous contrast agent administration, using thin (1- or 2-mm) contiguous axial and coronal planes. Scans or multiplanar reconstructions are orientated parallel and perpendicular to the anterior cranial fossa floor, respectively. The whole skull base needs to be examined, including the mastoid cells.

Because CSF leak is not directly detectable on high-resolution CT, the identification of a bony defect is indirectly taken as the possible site of the CSF leak, even if the bone defect itself does not necessarily correspond to the site of dural tear (Tolley et al. 1992). However, bony dehiscences are not infrequent in the skull base (Tolley et al. 1991), having

been demonstrated in about 14% of ethmoid bones (Ohnishi 1981). Similar dehiscences have been described in the sphenoid and, less commonly, in the frontal sinus. As a consequence, a simple bony defect cannot be considered a reliable sign of CSF fistula. Conversely, when a bony defect, located at the edge between skull base and paranasal sinus/nasal cavity, is associated with fluid collection and/or mucosal thickening within the adjacent sinus/nasal cavity, it can be assumed to be located close to the dural breach site (Fig. 7.9). By combining these findings, the specificity of high-resolution CT raised to 86% in a series of 15 patients with traumatic (accident or iatrogenic) fistulae (Lloyd et al. 1994).

However, precise location of the fistula(e) may be rather difficult, if not impossible, in the presence of comminuted fractures, particularly when scar tissue partially replaces the skull base or invests its endonasal interrupted surface. In this case, CT findings may indicate more than a single potential site of CSF leak, therefore not enabling a sufficiently tailored surgical approach. MR may provide additional findings, like showing signal intensity consistent with CSF within the scar tissue or across the interrupted skull base.

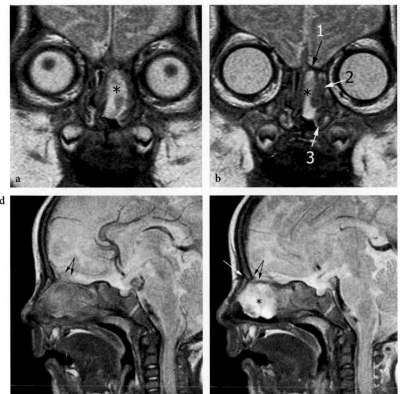

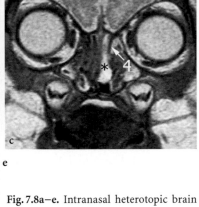

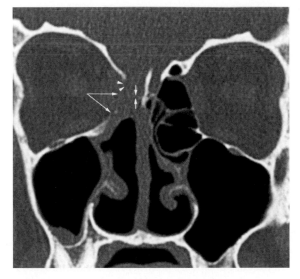

Fig. 7.8a–e. Intranasal heterotopic brain tissue (nasal glioma). Coronal (a–c) and sagittal (d–e) TSE T2. a The mass (*asterisk*) arises from left olfactory fissure, the left nasal cavity is completely occupied. b The nasal glioma abuts the inferior surface of the cribriform plate (*1*) without any connection with subarachnoid space. Middle (*2*) and inferior (*3*) turbinates are compressed. c The vertical lamina of the middle turbinate limits the lateral aspect of the nasal glioma. d On midline sagittal plane, the crista galli (*black arrows*) shows intermediate signal. e On off-midline sagittal plane, the nasal glioma (*asterisk*) appears bordered superiorly by the lateral aspect of the crista galli (*black arrows*). A normal nasofrontal suture is present (*white arrow*)

Figure 7.9. Traumatic iatrogenic CSF fistula, post-microendoscopic sinus surgery. Coronal high resolution CT at the level of the olfactory fossa. A large bone defect is demonstrated to involve the horizontal (*short arrows*) and the lateral lamella (*arrowhead*) of the right cribriform plate. The right lamina papyracea is not recognizable (*long arrows*). Note the absence of the middle turbinate and ethmoid labyrinth on the right side, due to previous endonasal surgery

In particular, MR cisternography has been proposed as a non-invasive cisternographic technique. It consists of turbo spin echo sequences with fat-suppression (to null signal from bone marrow) that greatly increase CSF signal intensity and suppress the background, providing heavily T2 images with detailed anatomic information of the subarachnoid cisterns. If necessary, a small number of images (usually between two and eight) may be compressed into composite images using maximum intensity projection algorithms. Composite images may be useful to detect fistulae with irregular and tortuous tracks (EL GAMMAL and BROOKS. 1994). In detecting CSF fistulae, MR cisternography yielded sensitivity of 87%, specificity ranging from 57% up to 100%, and accuracy of 78%–89% (EL GAMMAL et al. 1998, SHETTY et al. 1998). Although MR cisternography may be added to the diagnostic work-up, at present precise identification of the fistula(e) is made possible at surgery by fluorescein leakage detection, which is more accurate than imaging techniques.

In fact, even fistulae due to incomplete damage of the meninges causing permeation rather than a complete breech are shown with this technique. The fluoroscein tracer is administered via lumbar puncture, and a special light filter is necessary to endoscopically detect small fistulae. In case of spontaneous fistula, a positive BTP test requires the patient to be investigated either by CT, adding the high resolution CT technique to the standard examination of the head, and by MR. Detection of paranasal sinuses or temporal bone hyperpneumatization will prompt the accurate assessment of the whole skull base to rule out bone dehiscences. The presence of an empty sella with or without a fluid-like broad-based lesion on sphenoid walls may arouse the suspicion of benign intracranial hypertension. In this setting, intermittent CSF leak may be associated with other imaging findings suggesting idiopathic intracranial hypertension, as increased CSF amount surrounding the optic nerves along their intraorbital course (Suzuki et al. 2001). Furthermore, any fluid-like broad-based lesion hanging on the extracranial surface of the skull base may indicate a cephalocele located beyond the limit of diagnostic endoscopy (Stone et al. 1999).

However, the presence of a high signal on T2 images within paranasal sinuses or mastoid cells or adjacent to the skull base may be due to thickened mucosa, mastoiditis or rhinosinusitis, and not necessarily to CSF accumulation. Therefore, a CSF fistula may be suspected whenever the high signal of the fistulous tract appears to be in *direct* continuity with the intracranial subarachnoid space. This point is relevant, as high signal intensities on T2 sequences are shown in up to 25% of patients examined by MR for non-sinonasal diseases (Moser et al. 1991).

Indirect evidence of CSF fistula is provided by a low-lying gyrus rectus when the leak is located at the cribriform plate area ("gyrus rectus sign"), probably related to the negative pressure created by the fistula (Shetty et al. 1998).

Finally, unexpected intracranial or extracranial tumors, hydrocephalus, or skull base inflammatory lesions may be demonstrated by CT or MR.

When BTP test, high resolution CT, and MR are all negative, the diagnosis of CSF has to be considered unlikely or spontaneous healing of the dural defect(s) might have occurred during the diagnostic work-up.

In a series of 42 spontaneous and post-traumatic CSF leaks examined by high-resolution CT, radionuclide cisternography, and CT cisternography, spontaneous resolution of CSF leakage within 1 month from imaging studies was observed in all patients negative at high resolution CT (29%) (Stone et al. 1999).

7.6.1.2
CSF Leak Presenting with Recurrent Meningitis

In this second group of patients, CSF leak is suspected because of recurrent meningitis in the absence of rhinorrhea. In this setting, the first line approach entails both endoscopy and imaging. BTP is, of course, unhelpful.

Endoscopy, CT and/or MR may succeed in demonstrating lesions both in post-traumatic and spontaneous fistulae. Compared to patients with CSF leak and rhinorrhea, the main difference consists in the absence of imaging findings of active leak (i.e., fluid collection within sinonasal cavities or focal mucosal thickening adjacent to bone dehiscences or to skull-base fractures).

Being based on indirect findings, high-resolution CT may be positive in inactive and active leaks with similar rates because it does not depend on the amount of CSF leakage at the time of investigation (Fig. 7.10).

Recently, a three-dimensional (3D), heavily T2-weighted sequence (3D CISS, constructive interference in steady state), has been proposed for CSF fistula detection (Jayakumar et al. 2001). 3D-CISS, being heavily T2-weighted with better CSF-brain-bone-air contrast, and allowing thinner (sub-millimeter) sections and multiplanar reconstructions, seems to be ideally suited for the demonstration of CSF leak (Fig. 7.11). Its very short TE enables a minimization of signal loss from magnetic susceptibility effects at the air–bone interface. The main advantage of this sequence is its ability to reduce artifacts from CSF pulsations. Unfortunately, in CISS sequence fat tissue appears moderately bright, so that anatomical details at the skull base/CSF interface may be obscured. Jayakumar et al. (2001) reported a sensitivity of 100% in a series of six patients: larger series have to be provided to establish the role of this promising technique.

If both endoscopy and non-invasive imaging are negative, the fluorescein test is considered more useful than *invasive* cisternographic techniques, because their sensitivity is insufficient in patients with inactive leak.

In the case of a positive fluorescein test, endoscopy may or may not precisely identify the fistula, as the defect can be located beyond diagnostic endoscopy limits. Microendoscopic surgery with fluorescein injection is indicated.

A negative fluorescein test makes the diagnosis of CSF leak unlikely.

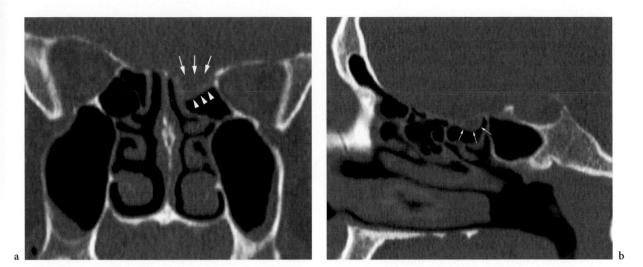

a   b

Fig. 7.10a,b. Traumatic (due to car accident) CSF fistula. Coronal high resolution CT (**a**), with reformatted sagittal section (**b**). On the left side, the posterior aspect of the fovea ethmoidalis is not visible (*arrows*): a soft tissue density is clearly demonstrated (*arrowhead*) strictly adjacent to the large bone defect

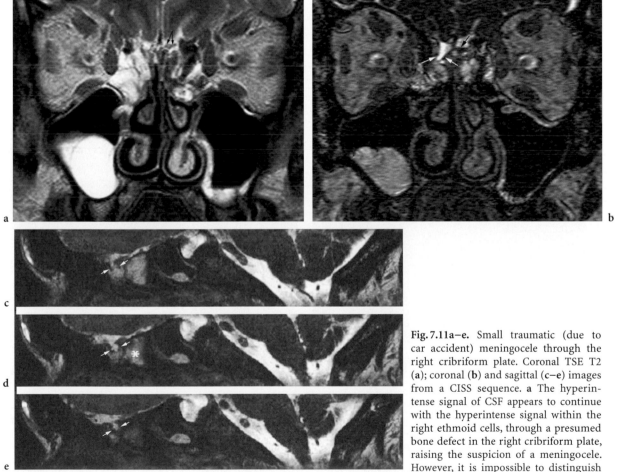

Fig. 7.11a–e. Small traumatic (due to car accident) meningocele through the right cribriform plate. Coronal TSE T2 (**a**); coronal (**b**) and sagittal (**c–e**) images from a CISS sequence. **a** The hyperintense signal of CSF appears to continue with the hyperintense signal within the right ethmoid cells, through a presumed bone defect in the right cribriform plate, raising the suspicion of a meningocele. However, it is impossible to distinguish the CSF possibly present in the ethmoidal cells from the thickened mucosa and/or sinus secretions. Only the left olfactory bulb is seen (*arrow*). **b** On coronal CISS sequence – 0.7 mm of thickness, obtained at the same level as (**a**) – the small meningocele (*white arrows*) shows the same signal as intracranial CSF, brighter than mucosal thickening. The contralateral olfactory bulb is demonstrated (*black arrow*). **c–e** The CISS sagittal reformatted sections show the small meningocele "neck" (*arrows*)

7.6.2
Invasive Imaging Techniques

In the past, several invasive "cisternographic" nuclear medicine and radiologic techniques have been developed to confirm and locate the site of CSF leaks. Since "cisternographic techniques" rely on demonstrating the passage of some "marked" CSF through the bone/dural defect, their sensitivity strictly depends on the amount of CSF crossing the defect at the time of the examination. Nowadays they are indicated in very few cases.

Among invasive techniques, *radionuclide cisternography* has been the first to successfully detect the site of CSF rhinorrhea (CROW et al. 1956). Unfortunately, most CSF leaks are intermittent, causing its accuracy to reduce from approximately 70% in patients with active leaks to 28% in patients with inactive leaks (ELJAMEL et al. 1994).

CT cisternography has been considered one of the most reliable techniques in CSF fistula detection, although the rate of positive studies has been quite variable in large reported series, ranging from 36%–40% in inactive leaks, and up to 81%–92% in active leaks (MANELFE et al. 1982; COLQUHOUN 1993; ELJAMEL et al. 1994). It requires intrathe-

cal injection of contrast agent (usually via lumbar puncture). A few minutes after contrast agent injection, thin CT slices (1–3 mm) are obtained, with both soft tissue and bone algorithms, preferably in the coronal plane (DRAYER et al. 1977). Not to miss any potential CSF leakage site, scans should extend from the anterior frontal sinus wall to the posterior surface of the petrous bone. In fact, CSF rhinorrhea due to leakage through the petrous bone into the middle ear and then, via Eustachian tube, into the nasopharynx – where the CSF may emerge via the nasal cavity – has been reported (SHETTY et al. 1997). CT cisternography may directly demonstrate the contrast agent passage through bony and dural defects and/or the pooling of the contrast agent within nasal cavity or paranasal sinuses (Fig. 7.12).

Positive findings consist of direct demonstration of contrast agent passage through the bone/dural defect or of bone defect(s) associated with contrast agent pooling within ipsilateral sinus. Equivocal findings entail detection of bone defect(s) and/or the presence of contrast agent within the ipsilateral nasal pledget. *Negative* findings require no extracranial contrast agent or bone defect demonstrated (MANELFE et al. 1982).

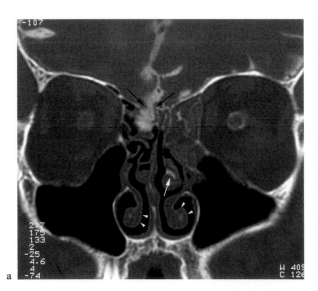 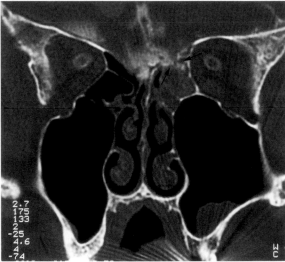

Fig. 7.12a,b. Multiple traumatic CSF fistulae due to fractures of the anterior skull base floor. CT cisternography, coronal sections (**a,b**). **a** Contrast agent flows from the right frontobasal subarachnoid space into the ethmoid cells through the right fovea ethmoidalis fracture (*black arrows*). The superficial lining of the mucosa investing nasal structures is hyperdense (*arrowheads*) due to layering and absorption of contrast agent leaking from the fistula. On the *left side*, a thicker collection of contrast agent fills a cleft in the middle turbinate (*white arrow*). These findings prompt a careful examination of the CT scan set, looking for other CSF fistulae. **b** A more posterior coronal section discloses a fovea ethmoidalis fracture on the *left side* (*arrows*), with leak of a small amount of contrast agent into the ethmoidal cells

Failures to demonstrate "marked CSF" *along* the fistula path may also be due to excessive tortuosity of the track or, conversely, to a very large defect, that does not retain enough "marked CSF". The presence of fresh blood or small bony septa within paranasal sinuses may be misinterpreted as contrast agent pooling or tracks. Conversely, the hyperdense subarachnoid CSF may obscure small bone defects of the skull base.

Recently, *invasive* MR cisternography has been obtained by intrathecal administration of Gd-based contrast agent in a small series of patients without relevant collateral effects.

References

Bachmann G, Nekic M, Michel O (2000) Clinical experience with beta-trace protein as a marker for cerebrospinal fluid. Ann Otol Rhinol Laryngol 109:1099–1102

Beckhardt RN, Setzen M, Carras R (1991) Primary spontaneous cerebrospinal fluid rhinorrhea. Otolaryngol Head Neck Surg 104:425:432

Burns JA, Dodson EE, Gross CW (1996) Transnasal Endoscopic Repair of Cranionasal Fistulae: A Refined Technique With Long-term Folllow-up. Laryngoscope 106:1080–1083

Casiano RR, Jassir D (1999) Endoscopic cerebrospinal fluid rhinorrhea repair: is a lumbar drain necessary? Otolaryngol Head Neck Surg 121:745–750

Castelnuovo P, Mauri S, Locatelli D, et al (2001) Endoscopic Repair of Cerebrospinal Fluid Rhinorrhea: Learning from Our Failures. Am J Rhinol 15:333–342

Castillo L, Jaklis A, Paquis P, et al (1999) Nasal endoscopic repair of cerebrospinal fluid rhinorrhea. Rhinology 37:33–36

Choi D, Spann R (1996) Traumatic cerebrospinal fluid leakage: risk factors and the use of prophylactic antibiotics. Br J Neurosurg 10:571–575

Clark D, Bullock P, Hui T, et al (1994) Benign intracranial hypertension: a cause of CSF rhinorrhea. J Neurol Neurosurg Psychiatry 57:847–849

Colquhoun IR (1993) CT cisternography in the investigation of cerebrospinal fluid rhinorrhoea. Clin Radiol 47:403–408

Crow HJ, Keogh C, Northfield DWC (1956) The localization of cerebrospinal-fluid fistulae. Lancet 271:325–327

Dietrich U, Felges A, Sievers K, et al (1993) Localisation of fronto-basal traumatic cerebrospinal fluid fistulas. Comparison of radiologic and surgical findings. Zentrab Neurochirurgie 54:24–31

Dodson EE, Gross CW, Swerdloff JL, et al (1994) Transnasal endoscopic repair of cerebrospinal fluid rhinorrhea and skull base defects: A review of twenty-nine cases. Otolaryngol Head Neck Surg 111:600–605

Drayer BP, Wilkins RH, Boehnke M et al (1977) Cerebrospinal fluid rhinorrhoea demonstrated by metrizamide CT cisternography. AJR Am J Roentgenol 129:s149–151

El Gammal T, Brooks BS (1994) MR cisternography: initial experience in 41 cases. AJNR Am J Neuroradiol 15:1647–1656

El Gammal T, Sobol W, Wadlington VR, et al (1998) Cerebrospinal fluid fistula: detection with MR cisternography. AJNR Am J Neuroradiol 19:627–631

Eljamel M, Pidgeon C, Toland J, et al (1994) MRI cisternography, and the localization of CSF fistula. Br J Neurosurg 8:433–437

Eljamel MS (1994) Fractures of the middle third of the face and cerebrospinal fluid rhinorrhea. Br J Neurosurg; 8:289–293

Gassner HG, Ponikau JU, Sherris DA, et al (1999) CSF Rhinorrhea: 95 Consecutive Surgical Cases with Long Term Follow-Up at the Mayo Clinic. Am J Rhinol 13:439–447

Gjuric M, Goede U, Keimer H, et al (1996) Endonasal endoscopic closure of cerebrospinal fluid fistulas at the anterior cranial base. Ann Otol Rhinol Laryngol 105:620–623

Hegazy HM, Currau RL, Snyderman CH, et al (2000) Transnasal Endoscopic Repair of Cerebrospinal Fluid Rhinorrhea: A Meta-Analysis. Laryngoscope 110:1166–1172

Jayakumar PN, Kovoor JME, Srikanth SG, et al (2001) 3D steady-state MR cisternography in CSF rhinorrhoea. Acta Radiol 42:582–584

Johnson DB, Brennan P, Toland J, et al (1996) Magnetic resonance imaging in the evaluation of cerebrospinal fluid fistulae. Clin Radiol 51:837–841

Lanza DC, O'Brien DA, Kennedy DW (1996) Endoscopic Repair of Cerebrospinal Fluid Fistulae and Encephaloceles. Laryngoscope 106:1119–1125

Lindstrom DR, Toohill RJ, Loehrl TA, et al (2004) Management of cerebrospinal fluid rhinorrhea: the Medical College of Wisconsin experience. Laryngoscope 114:969–974

Lloyd MN, Kimber PM, Burrows EH (1994) Post-traumatic cerebrospinal fluid rhinorrhoea: modern high-definition computed tomography is all that is required for the effective demonstration of the site of leakage. Clin Radiol 49:100–103

Lund VJ, Savy L, Lloyd G, Howard D (2000) Optimum imaging and diagnosis of cerebrospinal fluid rhinorrhoea. J Laryngol Otol 114:988–992

Mahapatra AK, Suri A (2002) Anterior Encephaloceles: A study of 92 Cases. Pediatr Neurosurgery 36:113–118

Manelfe C, Cellerier P, Sobel D, et al (1982) Cerebrospinal fluid rhinorrhoea: evaluation with metrizamide cisternography. AJR Am J Roentgenol 138:471–476

Mao VH, Keane WM, Atkins JP, et al (2000) Endoscopic repair of cerebrospinal fluid rhinorrhea. Otolaryngol Head Neck Surg 122:56–60

Marshall AH, Jones NS, Robertson IJA (1999) An algorhithm for the management of CSF rhinorrhea illustrated by 36 cases. Rhinology 37:182–185

McCormack B, Cooper PR, Persky M (1990) Extracranial repair of cerebrospinal fluid fistulas: technique and results in 37 patients. Neurosurgery 27:412–417

Mokri B, Maher CO, Sencakova D (2002) Spontaneous CSF leaks: Underlying disorders of connective tissue. Neurology 58:814–816

Moseley JH, Carton CA, Stern WE (1978) Spectrum of complications in the use of intratechal fluorescin. J Neurosurg 48:765–767

Moser FG, Panush D, Rubin JS, et al (1991) Incidental paranasal sinus abnormalities on MRI of the brain. Clin Radiol 43:252–254

Nachtigal D, Frenkiel S, Yoskovitch A, et al (1999) Endoscopic Repair of Cerebrospinal Fluid Rhinorrhea: Is It the Treatment of Choice? J Otolaryngol 28: 129–133

Naidich TP, Altman NR, Braffman BH et al (1992) Cephaloceles and related malformations. AJNR Am J Neuroradiol 13:655–690

Nandapalan V, Watson ID, Swift AC (1996) Beta-2-transferrin and cerebrospinal fluid rhinorrhea. Clin Otolaryngol 21:259–264

Nuss DW, Costantino PD (1995) Diagnosis and Management of Cerebrospinal Fluid Leaks. Highlights of the Instructional Courses of the American Academy of Otolaryngology- Head and Neck Surgery. Edited by: Frank E Lucente, Volume 8, 1995, Mosby-Yearbook Publishers.

Oberascher G, Arrer E (1986) Efficency of various methods of identyfying cerebrospinal fluid in oto- and rhinorrhea. O.R.L. 48:320–325

Ohnishi T (1981) Bony defects and dehiscences of the roof of the ethmoid cells. Rhinology 19:195–202

Oi S, Saito M, Tamaki N, et al (1994) Ventricular volume reduction technique – a new surgical concept for the intracranial transposition of encephalocele. Neurosurgery 34: 443–448

Ommaya AK (1983) Spinal fluid fistulae. Clin Otolaryngol 8:317–327

Persky MS, Rothstein SG, Breda SD, et al (1991) Extracranial repair of cerebrospinal fluid otorhinorrhea. Laryngoscope 101:134–136

Schick B, Rainer I, Brors D, et al (2001) Long-Term Study of Endonasal Duraplasty and Review of the Literature. Ann Otol Rhinol Laryngol 110:142–147

Schlosser RJ, Bolger WE (2003) Significance of empty sella in cerebrospinal fluid leaks. Otolaryngol Head Neck Surg 128:32–38

Senior BA, Jafri K, Benninger M (2001). Safety and Efficacy of Endoscopic Repair of CSF Leaks and Encephaloceles: A Survey of the Memebers of the American Rhinologic Society. Am J Rhinol 15:21–25

Shetty PG, Shroff MM, Fatterpekar GM, et al (2000) A retrospective analysis of sphenoid sinus fistula: MR and CT findings. AJNR Am J Neuroradiol 21:337–342

Shetty PG, Shroff MM, Kirtane MV, et al (1997) Cerebrospinal fluid otorhinorrhea in patients with defects through the lamina cribrosa of the internal auditory canal. AJNR Am J Neuroradiol 18:478–481

Shetty PG, Shroff MM, Sahani DV, et al (1998) Evaluation of high-resolution CT and MR cisternography in the diagno-sis of cerebrospinal fluid fistula. AJNR Am J Neuroradiol 19:633–639

Stammberger H (1991) Detection and Treatment of Cerebrospinal Fluid leaks. In: Functional Endoscopic Sinus Surgery. BC Decker, Philadelphia, pp 437–438

Stone JA, Castillo M, Neelon B, et al (1999) Evaluation of CSF leaks: High-resolution CT compared with contrast-enhanced CT and radionuclide cisternography. AJNR Am J Neuroradiol 20:706–712

Suzuki H, Takanashi J, Kobayashi K, et al (2001) MR imaging of idiopathic intracranial hypertension. AJNR Am J Neuroradiol 22:196–199

Tolley NS (1991) A clinical study of spontaneous CSF rhinorrhea. Rhinology 29:223–230

Tolley NS, Brookes BG (1992) Surgical management of cerebrospinal fluid rhinorrhea. J R Coll Surg Edimb 37:12-15

Tolley NS, Lloyd G, Williams H (1991) Radiological study of primary spontaneous CSF rhinorrhoea. The Journal of Laryngology and Otolology 105:274–277

Truwit CL, Barkovich AJ (1996) Disorders of brain development. In: Scott WA (ed) Magnetic Resonance Imaging of the Brain and Spine, 2nd edition. Lippincott-Raven Publishers, Philadelphia, pp179–264

Wax MK, Ramadan HH, Ortiz O, et al (1997) Contemporary management of cerebrospinal fluid rhinorrhea. Otolaryngol Head Neck Surg 116:442–449

Weber R, Keerl R, Draf W, et al (1996) Management of dural lesions occurring during endonasal sinus surgery. Arch Otolaryngol Head Neck Surg 122:732–736

Wigand ME (1981) Transnasal ethmoidectomy under endoscopic control. Rhinology 19:7–15

Zagardo MT, Cail WS, Kelman SE, et al (1996) Reversible empty sella in idiopathic intracranial hypertension: an indicator of successful therapy? AJNR Am J Neuroradiol 17:1953–1956

Zapalac JS, Marple BF, Schwade ND (2002) Skull base cerebrospinal fluid fistulas: A comprehensive diagnostic algorithm. Otolaryngol Head Neck Surg 126:669–676

Zlab MK, Moore GF, Daly DT, et al (1992) Cerebrospinal Fluid Rhinorrhea: A Review of the Literature. Ear Nose Throat J 71:314–317

Zweig JL, Carrau RL, Celin SE, et al (2000) Endoscopic repair of cerebrospinal fluid leaks to the sinonasal tract: Predictors of success. Otolaryngol Head Neck Surg 123:195–201

8 Benign Neoplasms and Tumor-Like Lesions

Roberto Maroldi, Marco Berlucchi, Davide Farina, Davide Tomenzoli, Andrea Borghesi, and Luca Pianta

CONTENTS

8.1   Osteoma   107
8.1.1   Definition, Epidemiology, Pattern of Growth   107
8.1.2   Clinical and Endoscopic Findings   108
8.1.3   Treatment Guidelines   108
8.1.4   Key Information to Be Provided by Imaging   109
8.1.5   Imaging Findings   109
8.1.6   Follow-Up   110
8.2   Fibrous Dysplasia and Ossifying Fibroma   110
8.2.1   Definition, Epidemiology, Pattern of Growth   110
8.2.2   Clinical and Endoscopic Findings   111
8.2.3   Treatment Guidelines   112
8.2.4   Key Information to Be Provided by Imaging   112
8.2.5   Imaging Findings   112
8.2.6   Follow-Up   114
8.3   Aneurysmal Bone Cyst   114
8.3.1   Definition, Epidemiology, Pattern of Growth   114
8.3.2   Clinical and Endoscopic Findings   115
8.3.3   Treatment Guidelines   115
8.3.4   Key Information to Be Provided by Imaging   115
8.3.5   Imaging Findings   115
8.3.6   Follow-Up   116
8.4   Sinonasal Mucocele   117
8.4.1   Definition, Epidemiology, Pattern of Growth   117
8.4.2   Clinical and Endoscopic Findings   117
8.4.3   Treatment Guidelines   117
8.4.4   Key Information to Be Provided by Imaging   118
8.4.5   Imaging Findings   118
8.4.6   Follow-Up   121
8.5   Abnormal Sinus Pneumatization   121
8.5.1   Definition and Epidemiology   121
8.5.2   Pathogenesis   121
8.5.3   Clinical and Endoscopic Findings   121
8.5.4   Treatment Guidelines   122
8.5.5   Key Information to Be Provided by Imaging   122
8.5.6   Imaging Findings   122
8.6   Inverted Papilloma and Other
        Schneiderian Papillomas   122
8.6.1   Definition, Epidemiology, Pattern of Growth   122
8.6.2   Clinical and Endoscopic Findings   124
8.6.3   Treatment Guidelines   125
8.6.4   Key Information to Be Provided by Imaging   126
8.6.5   Imaging Findings   126
8.6.6   Follow-Up   131
8.7   Juvenile Angiofibroma   131
8.7.1   Definition, Epidemiology, Pattern of Growth   131
8.7.2   Clinical and Endoscopic Findings   132
8.7.3   Treatment Guidelines   132
8.7.4   Key Information to Be Provided by Imaging   133
8.7.5   Imaging Findings   133
8.7.6   Follow-Up   141
8.8   Pyogenic Granuloma
        (Lobular Capillary Hemangioma)   145
8.8.1   Definition, Epidemiology, Pattern of Growth   145
8.8.2   Treatment Guidelines   145
8.8.3   Key Information to Be Provided by Imaging   146
8.8.4   Imaging Findings   146
8.9   Unusual Benign Lesions   147
8.9.1   Pleomorphic Adenoma (Mixed Tumor)   147
8.9.2   Schwannoma   149
8.9.3   Leiomyoma   150
8.9.4   Paraganglioma   151
        References   152

R. Maroldi, Professor, MD; D. Farina, MD; A. Borghesi, MD
Department of Radiology University of Brescia, Piazzale
Spedali Civili 1, Brescia, 25123, Italy
M. Berlucchi, MD; D. Tomenzoli, MD; L. Pianta, MD
Department of Otorhinolaryngology University of Brescia,
Piazzale Spedali Civili 1, Brescia, 25123, Italy

8.1
Osteoma

8.1.1
Definition, Epidemiology, Pattern of Growth

Osteoma is a benign, slow-growing osteoblastic tumor, more commonly located in the outer table of the calvarium, the mandible, the paranasal sinuses, and occasionally in tubular bones (Samy and Mostafa 1971; Kransdorf et al. 1991; Sayan et al. 2002).

It is the most frequent benign tumor of the nose and sinonasal, since being found in 1% of patients who undergo plain sinus radiographs and in 3% of CT examinations obtained for sinonasal symptoms (Earwaker 1993). Osteoma usually presents between the third and sixth decade of life, with a male predominance of 1.5–2.6:1 (Metha and Grewal 1963; Atallah and Jay 1981). About 80% of osteomas occur in the frontal sinus, while ethmoid and maxillary sinus are affected in about 20% of cases (Earwaker 1993). Isolated cases of sphenoid osteoma have been observed (Fu and Perzin 1974).

Histologically, osteomas are divided into three categories: (1) the ivory or "eburnated" osteoma is composed of hard, dense bone, lacking a haversian system and containing only a minimal amount of fibrous tissue; (2) the osteoma spongiosum (mature osteoma) contains more trabecular tissue and often marrow component. It is surrounded by mature cancellous bone with small haversian systems; (3) the mixed osteoma contains both aspects of ivory and mature subtypes (Fu and Perzin 1974).

The etiology of the lesion is still unknown and speculative. Three main hypotheses have been proposed: (1) the embryologic theory, which postulates that osteoma arises at the junction between the embryonic cartilaginous ethmoid and the membranous frontal bones, does not explain the large number of osteomas located far from the fronto-ethmoid junction; (2) the traumatic theory identifies a previous trauma as the possible pathogenetic event; (3) the infective theory is related to the concomitant observation of osteoma and rhinosinusitis in about 30% of patients. Other theories consider osteomas osteodysplastic lesions, osteogenic hamartomas, embryonic bone rests, or as the result of sinus polyp ossification (Namdar et al. 1998).

Osteomas can occur in conjunction with Gardner's syndrome, which is characterized by the association of osteomas with intestinal polyposis and multiple soft tissue tumors, such as dermoid cysts and fibromas (Atallah and Jay 1981).

Osteomas of the paranasal sinuses are often asymptomatic and may be serendipitously detected on routine radiologic examinations. Furthermore, tumor growth is slow and occasionally characterized by a tendency to displace and compress the surrounding structures (about 10% of cases). Intracranial and intraorbital extent of sinus osteomas may occur as a late event (Rappaport and Attia 1994; Namdar et al. 1998; Huang et al. 2001).

8.1.2
Clinical and Endoscopic Findings

Frontal headache or facial pain, depending on tumor location, are the most frequently reported symptoms. Pain is presumably due to pressure caused by tumor expansion, to an acute or chronic sinusitis secondary to sinus ostium blockage, or to a secondary mucocele (Lieberman and Tovi 1984; Manaka et al. 1998). Nasal obstruction and mucopurulent rhinorrhea are rarely present.

Signs and symptoms of orbital or lacrymal pathway involvement (i.e., proptosis or exophthalmos, chemosis, diplopia, orbital pain, epiphora, decreased visual acuity, and even transient blindness) may be observed in large size lesions. Intracranial extension may be associated with complications such as CSF leak, meningitis, brain abscess, pneumocephalus, seizures, hemiparesis, and bitemporal quadrantanopsia (Bartlett 1971; Hartwidge and Varma 1984; Huneidi and Afshar 1989; Rappaport and Attia 1994).

In most cases, endoscopic evaluation of patients with osteoma is completely negative, the tumor being located inside a paranasal sinus. Displacement of nasal structures, such as the middle turbinate or the medial maxillary wall in case of an ethmoid or maxillary osteoma, respectively, may be observed. Direct visualization of the tumor is infrequent, occurring in large osteomas occupying the nasal fossa: the lesion appears as a firm mass covered by normal or atrophic mucosa.

8.1.3
Treatment Guidelines

Treatment of asymptomatic osteomas is controversial: some authors suggest tumor removal regardless of size, whereas others recommend a "wait and see" policy with serial CT scan controls (Savic and Djeric 1990; Brodish et al. 1999).

Namdar et al. (1998) suggested the following guidelines for treatment: in case of associated nasal obstruction or rhinosinusitis, medical therapy with antibiotics, decongestants, and steroids may be appropriate. Whenever medical therapy fails because of tumor location, the lesion is adjacent to frontal sinus ostium or more than 50% of the frontal sinus is occupied, or a noticeable increase in size has been documented by serial CT scans, surgery is recommended. Finally, chronic headache may be an indication for surgery when other causes are excluded.

Removal of the lesion may alternatively require a microendoscopic procedure or an external approach, in relation to tumor location, volume, and extension. Schick et al. (2001) precisely defined the limits and the indications for a microendoscopic removal: while most ethmoid osteomas can be resected endonasally, frontal osteomas are considered to be accessible whenever located medial to a virtual sagittal plane upward prolonging the lamina papyracea and originating from the inferior aspect of the posterior frontal sinus wall. Microendoscopic removal of frontal sinus osteomas can be achieved through Draf's type II or III frontal sinusotomy.

Tumor extension beyond the paranasal sinuses, or large osteomas which can not be entirely exposed through the nose must be removed via an external approach (SMITH and CALCATERRA 1989; NAMDAR et al. 1998; BRODISH et al. 1999; SCHICK et al. 2001). Osteoplastic frontal sinusotomy (with or without fat obliteration), with a coronal or uni-/bilateral brow incision, allows direct access to the frontal sinus and removal of osteomas with anterior and/or posterior wall involvement. Craniofacial resection has been described for the removal of giant fronto-ethmoid osteomas with intracranial complications (BLITZER et al. 1989).

8.1.4
Key Information to Be Provided by Imaging

- Location, extent, and site of origin
- Potential impairment of drainage pathways
- Extension beyond paranasal sinuses
- Position in respect to the lamina papyracea and inferior and posterior frontal sinus wall (endonasal accessibility)
- Presence of possible complications (intracranial and/or intraorbital)

8.1.5
Imaging Findings

Diagnosis of Osteoma is generally simple diagnosis, based on the detection – either on X-ray films or on CT scans – of a radiodense mass occupying the frontal sinus (more commonly) or, less frequently, the ethmoid or maxillary sinus (GILLMAN et al. 1997). According to the amount of mineralized bone within the lesion, osteomas may exhibit very high density, resembling cortical bone, or a gradually decreasing X-ray opacity/density to a "ground-glass" pattern (Fig. 8.1). All different patterns can be found at once in the same lesion (SOM and BRANDWEIN 1996). No enhancement is to be expected; nonetheless, contrast administration is normally unnecessary to obtain a diagnosis. MR is intrinsically inferior to CT in imaging osteomas, as both the low water content and the lack of mobile protons within osteomas result in very low signal intensity in all sequences. The possible presence of small amounts of fat tissue within the intertrabecular spaces may result in the detection of scattered hyperintense foci on both T1 and T2 sequences (RAO et al. 2001). The differential diagnosis includes osteoblastoma, osteosarcoma, and fibrous dysplasia, calcified hematoma being just an anecdotal alternative (HUANG and MISKO 1998). On CT, high density, well-defined borders, lack of contrast enhancement and lytic bone destruction, are generally sufficient clues to suggest a correct diagnosis. In addition, osteomas are generally confined to the sinus of origin. Obstruction of mucus drainage pathways (particularly the frontal recess) is the more frequent concern in sinonasal osteomas (Fig. 8.2). High quality CT multiplanar reconstructions – obtained with multidetector equipment – may be necessary to precisely identify the sinusal wall from which the lesion arises, to fully depict course and patency of

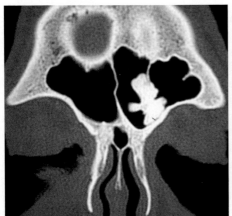 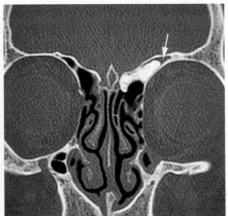

a   b

Fig. 8.1a,b. Frontal sinus osteomas. Plain CT on coronal plane, in two different patients. **a** A large frontal osteoma is detected, implanted on left sinus floor. No indirect signs of drainage impairment are observed. **b** The osteoma adheres to both floor and roof of frontal sinus in the most dependent part of the cavity. *Arrow* points to mucosal thickening or retained secretions secondary to sinus drainage blockage

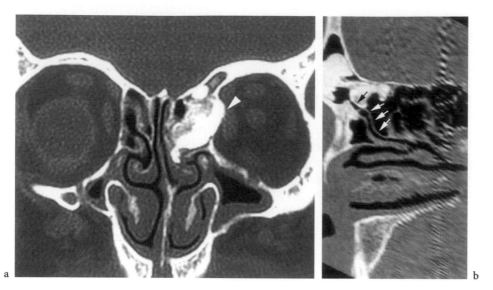

Fig. 8.2a,b. Fronto-ethmoidal osteoma. Plain CT on coronal (**a**) and sagittal reformatted plane (**b**). **a** A large fronto-ethmoidal osteoma exhibits a mixed pattern, ivory in its lateral part, ground glass in the medial portion. Lamina papyracea is encroached. The lesion contacts the medial rectus muscle (*arrowhead*). **b** Unexpectedly, sagittal reformation demonstrates patency of the frontal recess, all along its course (*black* and *white arrows*)

all sinus paths, and to correctly assess the integrity of thin bony walls such as the lamina papyracea or the cribriform plate.

8.1.6
Follow-Up

Osteomas do not show a propensity to recur after radical excision (SMITH and CALCATERRA 1989). Patients not undergoing surgery or having incomplete tumor removal require periodical radiologic evaluations (ATALLAH and JAY 1981; SPENCER and MITCHELL 1987; KOIUVNEN et al. 1997). The maximal rate of growth of osteoma is observed during the period of skeletal development: for this reason, growth of untreated or residual lesions is much slower when skeletal growth is completed.

8.2
Fibrous Dysplasia and Ossifying Fibroma

Fibrous dysplasia and ossifying fibroma are two clearly distinct diseases. For a long period, they have been considered as different varieties of the same disease, but since 1963, they have been differentiated into two separate entities (REED 1963). Fibrous

dysplasia is a developmental anomaly of the bone-forming mesenchyme with a defect in osteoblastic differentiation and maturation and the tendency of stabilize after puberty, whereas ossifying fibroma is a true benign neoplasm with varying aggressiveness depending on the clinical form (MARVEL et al. 1991). They will both be discussed in this chapter since they share very similar radiologic findings.

8.2.1
Definition, Epidemiology, Pattern of Growth

Fibrous dysplasia is a non-neoplastic, slowly progressing disorder of unknown etiology. The disease is characterized by resorption of normal bony tissue, which is replaced by fibrous tissue and immature woven bone histologically corresponding to different stages of bone metaplasia (SIMOVIC et al. 1996; COMMINS et al. 1998). Several causes (i.e., endocrine anomalies, trauma, defects of bone growth, development from a hamartoma) have been suggested to explain fibrous dysplasia pathogenesis (LICHTENSTEIN and JAFFE 1942; POUND et al. 1965; SMITH 1965), but to date none of them has been widely accepted.

Ossifying fibroma is a slow-growing benign neoplasm composed of a fibroblastic and osseous component (SHANMUGARATNAM 1991), which is considered to arise from mesenchymal blast cells giving origin to the periodontal ligament (HAMNER et al. 1968).

Both fibrous dysplasia and ossifying fibroma are more common in females than in males. Fibrous dysplasia is usually diagnosed within the first two decades of life (COMMINS et al. 1998; MURAOKA et al. 2001), whereas ossifying fibroma have been more frequently observed in the third and fourth decades (HAMNER et al. 1968; EVERSOLE et al. 1985), and a higher incidence has been reported in the black population (HARRISON and LUND 1993). The head and neck area is involved in 25% of cases of fibrous dysplasia (BRODISH et al. 1999); maxilla and mandible are the most frequently affected sites, followed by frontal, parietal, and occipital bones (NAGER et al. 1982). The molar and premolar periapical regions of the mandible and maxilla are the most frequently involved sites by ossifying fibroma (HAMNER et al. 1968; SCHMAMAN et al. 1970; WALDRON and GINSANTI 1973; EVERSOLE et al. 1985; HYAMS et al. 1988; SLOOTWEG et al. 1994; SU et al. 1997). The development of the lesion in the sinonasal tract distant from dental alveoli has been explained by the presence of primitive mesenchymal cell rests, ectopic periodontal rests, or by an incomplete migration of the medial part of the nasal anlage (KRAUSEN et al. 1977; FUJIMOTO et al. 1987).

Histologically, fibrous dysplasia may be divided into three groups (active form, potentially active form, inactive form) in relation to the number of mitoses, cellular matrix, and osseous component (STAMM et al. 2000). Sarcomatous transformation is a rare event, which occurs in about 0.5% of patients and is usually related to previous radiotherapy (SCHWARTZ and ALPERT 1964).

There are two main histological variants of ossifying fibroma: the classic and the cementiform or psammomatoid (SHANMUGARATNAM 1991). The latter is characterized by round calcific masses resembling psammomatoid bodies of meningiomas (SHANMUGARATNAM 1991).

From the histological point of view, fibrous dysplasia and ossifying fibroma have similar histological features but the former does not have a capsule and is characterized by a more immature bone without osteoblastic activity (HYAMS et al. 1988).

In 1968, RAMSEY et al. suggested classifying fibrous dysplasia into three forms: monostotic, polyostotic, and disseminated. The first one, which affects a single osseous site, is the most common type (accounting for 70% of cases) and generally regresses with puberty. Craniofacial involvement is usually unilateral and occurs in about 30% of patients. The polyostotic form is characterized by multiple lesions involving several bones and accounts for approximately 30% of cases. This type occurs earlier than the monostotic form and involves head and neck structures in 50% of patients. The disseminated form, also called McCune-Albright syndrome, is the most rare and prevalently involves young girls. It presents with multiple lesions and extraskeletal manifestations such as cutaneous and mucosal pigmentation, and endocrine abnormalities (i.e., sexual precocity, growth hormone, and prolactin hypersecretion) (PACINI et al. 1987).

A clinical variant of ossifying fibroma, called "juvenile ossifying fibroma," is more frequently observed in the sinonasal tract, where it predominantly affects male subjects (JOHNSON et al. 1991; EL-MOFTY 2002). It usually belongs to the cementiform type and is considered to have an aggressive biological behavior, mimicking a malignant neoplasm (MARVEL et al. 1991).

8.2.2
Clinical and Endoscopic Findings

Clinical features of fibrous dysplasia and ossifying fibroma are aspecific and determined by a submucosal slow expansion. A diagnostic delay of up to 10 years has been reported for ossifying fibroma (BOYSEN et al. 1979).

Even though painless facial and skull deformities are the most frequently observed signs, symptoms such as nasal obstruction, headache, epistaxis, anosmia, loosening of teeth, facial paralysis, hearing loss, trigeminal neuralgia-like pain, and recurrent rhinosinusitis due to drainage impairment may develop (BOLLEN et al. 1990; CAMILLERI 1991; FERGUSON 1994; SLOOTWEG et al. 1994; WENIG et al. 1995; REDAELLI DE ZINIS et al. 1996; CHONG and TANG 1997; COMMINS et al. 1998; MURAOKA et al. 2001; CHENG et al. 2002). Diplopia, proptosis, loss of visual acuity due to optic nerve compression, epiphora, limitation of ocular motility are other important symptoms and signs indicating an involvement of the orbit and/or of the lacrymal pathways (MOORE et al. 1985; OSGUTHORPE and GUDEMAN 1987; JOHNSON et al. 1991; SLOOTWEG et al. 1994; WENIG et al. 1995; REDAELLI DE ZINIS et al. 1996). Since both diseases display a submucosal pattern of growth, nasal endoscopy is often negative or shows a lesion covered by intact mucosa.

8.2.3
Treatment Guidelines

The management of fibrous dysplasia may be delayed when the patient is asymptomatic; vice versa, when clinical manifestations occur, surgical treatment is required. However, one should keep in mind that radical excision is not the first goal of surgery, which is instead meant to relieve symptoms. Selection of the surgical technique and extension of the resection depend on the site and size of the lesion, its closeness to vital structures (i.e., internal carotid artery, optic nerve, orbital cavity, middle and anterior cranial fossa), age of the patient, severity of signs and symptoms, and possibility of sarcomatous degeneration (KESSLER et al. 1998; STAMM et al. 2000). Although external approaches (SIMOVIC et al. 1996; COMMINS et al. 1998; MURAOKA et al. 2001) have been extensively used, recently some authors reported anecdotal cases treated through a more conservative transnasal microendoscopic approach (KESSLER et al. 1998; BRODISH et al. 1999; PASQUINI et al. 2002).

Radiotherapy is strongly contraindicated due to the risk of malignant transformation. Other factors, which should discourage its use, are a poor radiosensitivity and its negative effects on the growth centers in young patients.

Based on the concept that fibrous dysplasia is related to an excess of osteoclastic activity, some authors reported successful results using bisphosphonates, a well-known family of drugs that inhibit osteoclast reabsorption (LIENS et al. 1994; LANE et al. 2001).

Ossifying fibroma requires radical excision, which can be obtained by a simple microendoscopic approach (LONDON et al. 2002) or can require, in very large lesions, even an anterior craniofacial resection (REDAELLI DE ZINIS et al. 1996). Aggressive surgery is justified by the high percentage of recurrences, which has been estimated to account for approximately 30% in a large series of patients including all anatomic sites (JOHNSON et al. 1991). If only the ethmoid is considered, the overall recurrence rate is around 44% (REDAELLI DE ZINIS et al. 1996).

8.2.4
Key Information to Be Provided by Imaging

- Location of the disease (in fibrous dysplasia monostotic, polyostotic, and disseminated forms must be accurately differentiated)
- Assessment of lesion extent

- Relationships with adjacent structures, particularly with the orbit, internal carotid artery, optic nerve, cavernous sinus, middle and anterior cranial fossa
- Evidence of sarcomatous transformation (fibrous dysplasia)

8.2.5
Imaging Findings

Imaging findings of fibrous dysplasia reflect the pathophysiology of this lesion, (i.e., focal or complete replacement of medullary bone by woven fibroosseous tissue.) As a general rule, the cortex is unaffected by this process (KRANSDORF et al. 1990; SOM and LIDOV 1992).

The degree of mineralization of the tissue will determine radiographic and CT density of fibrous dysplasia. This may range from radiolucent, difficult to differentiate from a simple bone cyst (particularly in the monostotic form of the disease), to ground glass (equal proportions of fibrous and osseous tissue), or even sclerotic (predominance of dense osseous tissue) (KRANSDORF et al. 1990; WENIG et al. 1995) (Figs. 8.3, 8.4).

MR signal on SE T2 sequence is rather variable. Fibrous dysplasia has been reported as having overall hypointense signal and cystic/necrotic hyperintense areas (CASSELMAN et al. 1993; SOM and LIDOV 1992), but also hyper- or isointense signal as compared to subcutaneous fat tissue (UTZ et al. 1989). SE T1 signal is unanimously reported as hypointense (SOM and LIDOV 1992; UTZ et al. 1989; KRANSDORF et al. 1990); non-homogeneous enhancement may be obtained after contrast administration.

As the amount of fibrous tissue within the lesion progressively increases, expansile remodeling of the affected bone can occur (Fig. 8.5). In the maxillo-facial area, this may result in encroachment of optic canal and skull base foramina and fissures (STERLING et al. 1993), entailing the risk of potentially severe neurologic complications (COMMINS et al. 1998).

Imaging findings are usually insufficient to precisely discriminate between fibrous dysplasia and ossifying fibroma. As for fibrous dysplasia, CT density ranges between radiolucency (ENGELBRECHT et al. 1999), ground glass (STERLING et al. 1993), and sclerosis (MARVEL et al. 1991). Nonetheless, in most

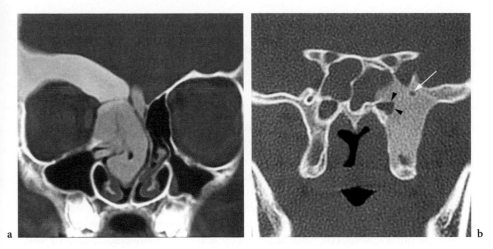

Fig. 8.3a,b. Fibrous dysplasia. Plain CT on coronal plane, in two different patients. **a** Lesion involves both the right frontal and ethmoid bone. Note expansion of crista galli and middle turbinate, the latter contralaterally displacing the nasal septum. **b** Monostotic form involves the sphenoid bone, expanding the left pterygoid root and laminae. Note initial narrowing of both foramen rotundum (*white arrow*) and vidian canal (*black arrowheads*), at its anterior opening

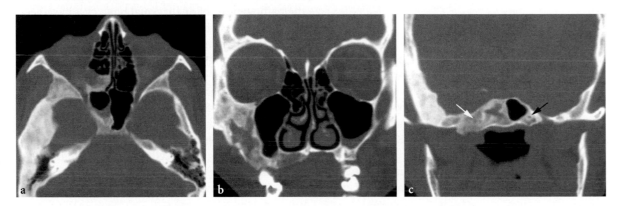

Fig. 8.4a–c. Fibrous dysplasia. Plain CT on axial (**a**) and coronal plane (**b,c**). Polyostotic form of the disease involves the temporal, sphenoid, frontal, maxillary, and palatine bone. Note the different degrees of mineralization of the expanded medullary cavities, ranging from ivory (temporal bone), to ground glass (sphenoid) and radiolucent (maxillary) appearance. Vidian canal, indicated by *black arrow* on the left, is not detected on the affected site (*white arrow*)

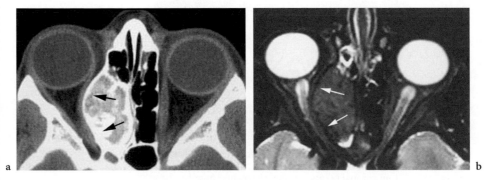

Fig. 8.5a,b. Fibrous dysplasia. Plain CT (**a**), SE T2 (**b**) on axial plane. **a** At CT, a high density ground glass lesion is detected in an 8-year-old boy with right proptosis. The right ethmoidal mass appears non-homogeneously hypointense on T2. The lesion abuts the right orbit, with no signs of invasion present (*arrows*)

cases ossifying fibroma is reported as a multiloculated lesion, bordered by a peripheral eggshell-like
dense rim (HAN et al. 1991). Whether the outer rim
is a proliferating part of the tumor or just reactive
hyperostosis is a matter of debate in the literature. At
MR, ossifying fibroma shows hyperintensity on T2
sequence, whereas its T1 pattern consists of intermediate-to-hyperintense signal in the central part
combined with hypointensity of the outer shell. The
latter strongly enhances after paramagnetic contrast administration (Fig. 8.6), a finding impossible
to appreciate at CT due to the bone-like density of
this component of the lesion.

Better than a density/signal pattern, the site of the
lesion may sometimes help to rule out a differential
diagnosis. Isolated sphenoid or temporal bone lesions as well as diffuse craniofacial involvement better apply to fibrous dysplasia, whereas the suspicion
of ossifying fibroma is raised in the presence of zygomatic or mandibular tumor. Fronto-ethmoid lesions
are, conversely, rather unpredictable (SOM and LIDOV
1992).

8.2.6
Follow-Up

Since complete resection of fibrous dysplasia is very
difficult to achieve and the recurrence rate ranges
from 25% to 75% (RAMSEY et al. 1968), it is mandatory to follow patients every 6 months during the
first year after surgery and, subsequently, every year.
Moreover, an ophthalmologic, neurologic, and endo-

crinologic evaluation at 6-month intervals is recommended in patients affected by McCune-Albright
syndrome (UZUN et al. 1999).

8.3
Aneurysmal Bone Cyst

8.3.1
Definition, Epidemiology, Pattern of Growth

Aneurysmal bone cyst is a benign bone lesion characterized by several sponge-like, blood- or serum-
filled, generally non-endothelialized spaces of various diameters. The first description dates back to the
early 1940s (JAFFE and LICHTENSTEIN 1942), but only
in 1950 was the term aneurysmal bone cyst introduced by LICHTENSTEIN (1950). However, the term
seems to be inaccurate, since the lesion is neither
a true aneurysm nor a cyst. Several hypotheses on
the pathogenesis of aneurysmal bone cyst have been
proposed. These include: (1) alterations of local osseous hemodynamics with elevated venous pressure
(LICHTENSTEIN 1950); (2) predisposing factors such
as trauma (LEVY et al. 1975); (3) local thrombosis
of veins and arterovenous malformations (BERNIER
and BHASKER 1958); (4) vascular alterations due to
a preexisting bony disorder (i.e., angioma, chondroblastoma, chondromyxoid fibroma, fibrosarcoma,
fibrous dysplasia, giant cell tumor, hemangioendothelioma, histiocytoma, nonossifying fibroma, non-
osteogenic fibroma, osteoblastoma, osteoclastoma,

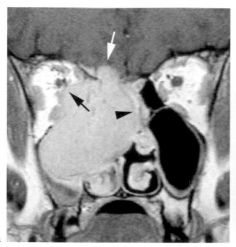
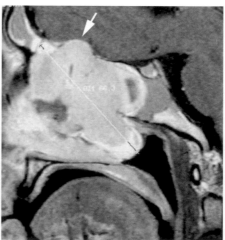

a   b

Fig. 8.6a,b. Ossifying fibroma. Gd-DTPA SE T1 on coronal (**a**) and sagittal (**b**) plane. Huge, brightly
enhancing ethmoido-maxillary mass encroaching both the nasal septum (*black arrowhead*) and
the anterior cranial fossa floor (*white arrow*). Medial orbital wall is laterally displaced (*black arrow*) but not invaded

osteosarcoma, unicameral bone cyst). (CITARDI et al. 1996; KRANSDORF and SWEET 1995; BURACZEWSKI and DABSKA 1971)

Aneurysmal bone cyst is slightly more frequent in females and develops in about 90% of patients during the first two decades of life (JAFFE and LICHTENSTEIN 1942; CALLIAUW et al. 1985). Most lesions involve long bone metaphyses, vertebrae, and pelvis, whereas the occurrence in the head and neck area is sporadic (2%). The mandible and maxilla are involved in 66% and 33% of cases, respectively, while rarely aneurysmal bone cyst has been observed in the orbitoethmoid complex (CITARDI et al. 1996; CHATEIL et al. 1997).

As described by BURACZEWSKI and DABSKA (1971), the development of aneurysmal bone cyst follows three different stages: the initial phase (I stage), which is characterized by osteolysis without peculiar findings; the growth phase (II stage), showing a rapid increase in size with osseous erosion and enlargement of involved bone associated with formation of a shell around the central part of the lesion; the stabilization phase (III stage), with a fully developed radiological pattern.

Histologically, aneurysmal bone cyst is classified into two variants. The classic form, which is the most common (about 95% of cases), is composed of blood-filled clefts among bony trabeculae associated with osteoid tissue in the stromal matrix (KERSHISNIK and BATSAKIS 1994). The solid form, which affects 5% of patients, is characterized by osteoid production, fibroblastic proliferation, and degenerated calcifying fibromyxoid elements (SANKERKIN et al. 1983).

8.3.2
Clinical and Endoscopic Findings

In the initial phase, the lesion may be asymptomatic or may cause aspecific symptoms. Subsequently, patients usually complain of local pain, nasal obstruction, epistaxis, headache, and progressive anosmia. Moreover, different ocular signs and symptoms (i.e., epiphora, recurrent dacryocystitis, blurry vision, proptosis, diplopia, alteration of the extraocular motility, central scotomas, decreased visual acuity, retroorbital headache, and even blindness) may occur (KIMMELMAN et al. 1982; SOM et al. 1991; PATEL et al. 1993; CITARDI et al. 1996; CHATEIL et al. 1997; SAITO et al. 1998; PASQUINI et al. 2002). Very rarely the lesion can present with meningitis and/or pneumocephalus due to intradural extension (SAITO et al. 1998).

Physical examination generally shows a submucosal expansile lesion with different location (maxilla, medial ocular canthus, frontal bone, cheek) depending on the site of origin (PATEL et al. 1993; CITARDI et al. 1996; SUZUKI et al. 2001).

Nasal endoscopy may reveal only a mild mucosal congestion of the lateral nasal wall. In other cases, it shows a fleshy mass in the nasal cavity or a pinkish bulging of the medial wall of the maxillary sinus with secondary deflection of the nasal septum (HADY et al. 1990; SOM et al. 1991; PATEL et al. 1993; PASQUINI et al. 2002).

8.3.3
Treatment Guidelines

Although several alternative options such as curettage with or without bone grafting, cryotherapy in association with surgery, intratumoral sclerotherapy, and local injection of calcitonin have been advocated, radical surgical excision must be considered the treatment of choice (KIMMELMAN et al. 1982; HADY et al. 1990; CHARTRAND-LEFEBVRE et al. 1996; CITARDI et al. 1996; DE MINTEGUIAGA et al. 2001). Whenever possible, performing radical surgery instead of curettage is mandatory since the recurrence rate after complete excision is indeed very low. Different surgical approaches ranging from minimally invasive endoscopic treatment (DE MINTEGUIAGA et al. 2001; PASQUINI et al. 2002) to external techniques (KIMMELMAN et al. 1982; HADY et al. 1990; SOM et al. 1991; PATEL et al. 1993) have been employed in relation to the site and extent of the lesion.

In view of the possible occurrence of post-irradiation sarcomas (TILLMAN et al. 1968), radiotherapy is contraindicated.

8.3.4
Key Information to Be Provided by Imaging

- Site, extent, and vascularization of the lesion
- Involvement of the surrounding structures (i.e. orbital cavity, cranial fossa)
- Concomitant presence of other osseous lesions

8.3.5
Imaging Findings

Imaging findings of aneurysmal bone cyst closely mirror the macroscopic structure of the lesion (i.e., multiple cavernous blood-filled spaces expanding and remodeling the host bone) (Som et al. 1991).

Conventional X-ray films demonstrate a well-defined lytic lesion, demarcated by a "ballooned" bony contour, probably reflecting new bone formation by the periosteum. In about 30% of cases, irregular densities can be seen within the lesion corresponding to calcified chondroid-like material (Kransdorf and Sweet 1995).

CT scan allows additional information such as focal cortical breaches and fluid-on-fluid levels (in up to 35% of cases) (Senol et al. 2002). Their identification requires, in some cases, a few minutes delay before scanning (to allow them to reform in the supine decubitus) and to display images with narrow window settings.

MR shows a well-defined expansile lesion demarcated by a thin rim and crossed by multiple internal septa. Both these display hypointense signal related to the presence of fibrous tissue. Fluid material retained within the cyst exhibits non-homogeneous signal, generally hypointense on T1 and hyperintense on T2. Nonetheless, focal areas of spontaneously hyperintense T1 signal are also described, reflecting the presence of different byproducts of hemoglobin (Hrishikesh et al. 2002). Fluid-on-fluid levels are much more commonly identified than on CT; they are thought to represent the layering of blood-tinged serous material above the unclotted liquid blood, laying in the dependent part of the cyst (Fig. 8.7).

After contrast administration, bright enhancement is observed exclusively along both peripheral rim and internal septa (De Minteguiaga et al. 2001).

Digital subtraction angiography also demonstrates the hypervascularity of the peripheral part of the lesion; however, this technique may play a more relevant role in the pre-treatment work-up. As significant blood loss may occur during surgery, preoperative embolization may grant easier resection of the lesion. Direct intraoperative sclerotherapy has also been reported (Chartrand-Lefebvre et al. 1996).

The differential diagnosis of aneurysmal bone cyst is rather complex, reflecting the controversy still existing about the real nature of this lesion. In fact, the propensity to create blood-filled spaces is shared by a list of extremely different lesions including fibrous dysplasia, chondromyxoid fibroma, non-ossifying fibroma, osteoblastoma, angioma, chondroblastoma, telangiectatic osteosarcoma. This observation has led several authors to consider aneurysmal bone cyst as a pathophysiologic change in a preexisting lesion, rather than a distinct entity (Kransdorf and Sweet 1995; Citardi et al. 1996). The main weak point of this theory is represented by the low rate of associated lesions ranging between 29% and 35%.

This could be interpreted as a progressive involution of the primary lesion that gradually looses its characteristic structure. Anyway, whenever an aneurysmal bone cyst is suspected, the main task of imaging is to accurately detect any coexisting bone change: in this regard, CT may be preferred to MR, particularly when areas with complex bone anatomy are assessed.

8.3.6
Follow-Up

Since treatment of aneurysmal bone cysts is associated with a 20% recurrence rate, most by (90%) occurring within 2 years, patients require a close endoscopic and radiological follow-up for at least 5 years after surgery (Ariel et al. 1992).

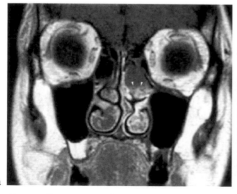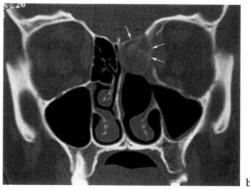

Fig. 8.7a,b. Aneurysmal bone cyst. Enhanced SE T1 (**a**) and plain post-surgery CT (**b**) on coronal plane. **a** A polypoid mass occupies the left ethmoid, the middle turbinate is medially displaced. Fluid–fluid level is present (*arrowheads*) with the inferior component exhibiting bright enhancement. **b** At 6 months after microendoscopic resection, submucosal recurrent lesion is associated with thickening and demineralization of lamina papyracea and fovea (*arrows*)

8.4
Sinonasal Mucocele

8.4.1
Definition, Epidemiology, Pattern of Growth

Mucocele may be defined as an accumulation of secretion products, desquamation, and inflammation within a paranasal sinus with expansion of its bony walls. The lesion is limited by a wall ("sac") made by respiratory mucosa with a pseudostratified columnar epithelium. According to LLOYD et al. (2000a), who reported data on 70 mucoceles, 89% of the lesions were located in the fronto-ethmoid area, while maxillary, ethmoid and sphenoid mucoceles were rarely observed. Mucocele more frequently occurs in the fourth and fifth decades of life, with approximately the same distribution in men and women.

The development of the lesion is thought to occur as the result of sinus ostium blockage. The accumulation of mucus creates a positive pressure inside the cavity (KASS et al. 1999), which might explain resorption of the surrounding bony walls. Nevertheless, these factors cannot be considered fully responsible for the process, since sinus occlusion can also result in chronic sinus atelectasis (KASS et al. 1997). According to WURSTER et al. (1986) and LUND et al. (1988), there is a dynamic process occurring at the interface between mucocele and bone, as suggested by high levels of bone re-absorbing factors such as PGE2, IL-1, and TNF, which have been demonstrated in the mucosa of the affected sinuses. Furthermore, histology more often demonstrates an active secretory columnar ciliated epithelium instead of a thin atrophic cuboidal epithelium, as would be expected from the positive pressure existing inside the lesion (LUND and MILROY 1991). As mucus continues to be produced, mucocele gradually expands, resulting in remodeling and/or erosion of the surrounding bone, with possible intraorbital and intracranial extension. Secondary infection (pyomucocele) can lead to a rapid expansion with significant risk of complications mostly involving the orbit.

Sinus ostia obstruction may be the consequence of chronic rhinosinusitis, allergic rhinitis, previous radiotherapy, trauma, scarring due to previous surgical procedures, or, more rarely, of sinonasal neoplasms. In recent years, some authors have alluded to a possible increase in the occurrence of mucoceles related to previous surgery (RAMBAUX et al. 2000); however, these data must be interpreted very cautiously.

8.4.2
Clinical and Endoscopic Findings

The clinical presentation of a mucocele varies in relation to the anatomical area involved. Occasionally, patients may present vague and non-specific complaints similar to those of chronic rhinosinusitis, but there are indeed symptoms and signs suggesting the diagnosis. When the frontal sinus is involved, frontal headache and proptosis may be the heralding manifestations; displacement of the ocular globe in a downward and outward direction may result in diplopia (IKEDA et al. 2000). If an erosion of the anterior or posterior wall of the frontal sinus is present, a Pott's puffy tumor or neurological symptoms may occur, respectively. When a mucocele arises in the ethmoid and/or sphenoid sinus the most frequent complaints are vertex or occipital headache, associated to various ophthalmologic symptoms (MORIYAMA et al. 1992; BENNINGER and MARKS 1995). Among these, one should bear in mind that sudden loss of vision may be the first symptom of a mucocele involving the sphenoid sinus. Finally, a lesion localized into the maxillary sinus may present with cheek pressure or pain, maxillary nerve hyperesthesia, dental pain, unilateral nasal obstruction, mucous or purulent rhinorrhea (BUSABA and SALMAN 1999).

At endoscopy, the appearance varies according to the phase of growth and to the site of the lesion. In fact, while in the intrasinusal phase no alterations are generally visible, expansion of the mucocele may lead to bony alterations of the lateral nasal wall, as anterior dislocation of the uncinate process, medialization of middle turbinate, bulging of the agger nasi cells or of the infundibular area. Furthermore, in a mucocele of the sphenoid sinus, a submucosal remodeling or a bulging in the sphenoethmoid recess or in the posterior ethmoid may be appreciated. In a purely frontal mucocele, endoscopy is usually negative.

8.4.3
Treatment Guidelines

Until the 1980s, mucocele was invariably treated by an external approach, which was meant not only to drain the mucus or pus collection, but also to completely remove the affected sinus mucosa. In 1989, KENNEDY et al. (1989) published a series of 18 sinus mucoceles treated by endoscopic marsupialization without recurrences after a mean follow up of 18 months. The philosophy behind microendoscopic operation is to marsupialize the lesion leaving untouched its epithelial-lined sac. Most surgeons are currently approaching mucoceles with a microendoscopic technique, which avoids any facial incision and gives similar results compared to transfacial operations (LUND 1998; BUSABA and SALMAN 1999; HARTLEY and LUND 1999; IKEDA et al. 2000; HAR-EL 2001; ICHIMURA et al. 2001).

However, a limited opening may not always warrant a steady drainage of mucocele, particularly in patients with a frontal localization who present one or more unfavorable conditions (diffuse polypoid rhinosinusitis, small frontal sinus, presence of abundant scar tissue due to previous surgery, facial trauma). In these cases, resorting to a type III drainage according to DRAF (1991), which involves the removal of the floor of both frontal sinuses together with the superior third of the nasal septum and drilling of the intrasinusal septum, may ensure a wider permanent drainage. Finally, mucoceles located in the far lateral extremity of a hyperpneumatized frontal sinus may be difficult to reach transnasally and require an external approach through an osteoplastic frontal sinusotomy. Whenever a mucocele is secondary to a tumor, selection of the surgical approach is obviously dictated by the nature, site, and extent of the tumor.

Diagnosis and treatment of a mucocele located in the sphenoid sinus and impairing visual acuity or causing visual loss must be considered an emergency, since only a prompt drainage within a few hours from the onset of symptoms may revert the deficit.

8.4.4
Key Information to Be Provided by Imaging

- Confirmation of the clinical diagnosis
- Assessment of the site and extension of the disease as well as of bony erosion entity (with special reference to orbital walls and skull base)
- Identification of anatomical variants, hyperostotic changes, or of a concomitant neoplasm causing the mucocele
- In case of frontal mucocele, information on the size of the sinus and the configuration of the frontal recess which can help in selecting the best surgical approach

8.4.5
Imaging Findings

Imaging plays a crucial role in defining the deep extension of mucoceles, particularly towards three important areas, orbit, anterior cranial fossa (up to 20%), and optic nerve canal (KOIKE et al. 1996). Sinus expansion with bulging of bony walls is the most typical presentation of mucocele (Fig. 8.8). Nonetheless, it must be emphasized that both bone defects and bulging usually involve all sinusal walls in lesions secondary to ostial obstruction, whereas they are more often focal in postoperative lesions. This is thought to be due to a compartmentalization of the sinusal cavity, occurring as a post-surgical change (HAN et al. 1995). As a consequence, post-surgical mucoceles, particularly in the ethmoid, may develop within a single isolated concameration without expanding all the walls. On MR, diagnosis can be suspected when

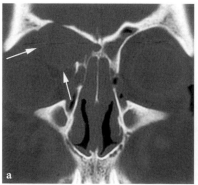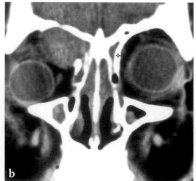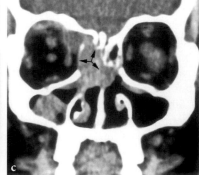

Fig. 8.8a–c. Mucocele. Plain CT on coronal plane (**a–c**). **a** Frontal sinus is expanded and remodeled, its floor is completely demineralized (*white arrows*). Inferolateral displacement of the ocular bulb can be observed. Retained secretions within sinus cavity (**b**) exhibit rather high density, reflecting desiccation. Scans acquired at the level of middle meatus (**c**) demonstrate an ethmoidal lesion destroying the medial orbital wall, nasal septum and ethmoid fovea (*black arrows*). The lesion impairs mucus drainage in the middle meatus and is, therefore, responsible for mucocele formation

signal a intensity differing from typical fluid and not solid is detected within a cell.

In fact, both CT and MR appearance of mucoceles largely depends on the composition of the entrapped material. At MR, the basic *expected* signal pattern of fluids (hyper T2, hypo T1) may be greatly altered by progressive dehydration and consequent increase of viscosity and protein concentration (Lim et al. 1999; Sievers et al. 2000). In detail, protein concentration within the range 20%–25% will result in hyperintensity at both T2 and T1. Further increase of concentration changes the signal pattern, which turns to hypointensity, respectively at 30% (T2) and 40% (T1) (Som et al. 1989) (Fig. 8.9). Similarly to the various signal patterns observed on MR, CT density ranges from fluid-like (cystic appearance) to progressively higher values as far as the entrapped material desiccates. Hypointense signal and high density on plain T1 can be observed also in the case of eosinophilic fungal rhinosinusitis (Van Tassel et al. 1989). After contrast administration, enhancement is observed exclusively at the periphery, along the thin mucosal layer, both at CT and MR (Lloyd et al. 2000a; Hejazi et al. 2001).

Anterior ethmoid mucoceles are more frequent than those arising from posterior ethmoid cells, probably because anterior ethmoid cells have smaller ostia, more easily obstructed in pathologic conditions. Ethmoid mucoceles tend to thin and remodel the adjacent lamina papyracea. They may also arise in cells resulting from the extensive pneumatization of adjacent structures, as in mucoceles developed within a concha bullosa.

Multiple mucoceles are infrequent, more often observed after facial fractures, complex facial surgery, and in patients with severe allergy (particularly in those with aspirin intolerance) (Price et al. 1981). Furthermore, an increased number of mucoceles secondary to endoscopic sinus surgery procedures has been reported (Raynal et al. 1999). These mucoceles tend to develop earlier (<22 months) than after open sinus surgery or trauma (<10 years). Different causes of sinus obstruction have been demonstrated by endoscopy and CT. Fronto-ethmoid mucoceles were caused by frontal recess occlusion due to fibrotic/osteogenic scar tissue, or anterior ethmoid synechia; maxillary sinus mucoceles were related to stenosis/occlusion of the ethmoid infundibulum because of uncinate process fragments or scar tissue. Besides, mucoceles of the maxillary sinus may develop after Caldwell-Luc procedures due to the entrapment of mucosa (Weber et al. 2000).

Although infrequent, sphenoid sinus mucoceles entail complex clinical problems, as they may erode the optic nerve canal, the sinusal wall separating from the cavernous sinus, or largely extend into a pneumatized pterygoid root. Expansion of the whole sphenoid sinus, remodeling, and focal erosion indicate the slow-growing development of a mucocele (Fig. 8.10). Signal patterns on MR and CT density may vary in relation to the protein content.

The differential diagnosis of mucocele is strictly related to the pattern of growth and site of origin of the lesion. In the early phase – not associated with sinus expansion and bone destruction – retention cyst, rhinosinusitis and polyposis should be considered. Though rather uncommon, the presence of intrasinusal calcifications could raise the suspect of non-invasive fungal rhinosinusitis (Sievers et al. 2000) (Fig. 8.11).

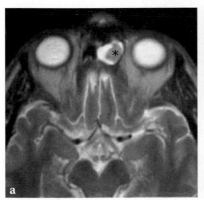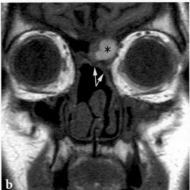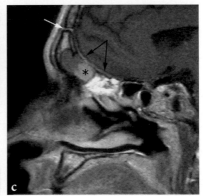

Fig. 8.9a–c. Post-surgical mucocele. MR SE T2 on axial plane (**a**), SE T1 on coronal plane (**b**), and enhanced SE T1 on sagittal plane (**c**). At 2 years after craniofacial resection for ethmoid adenocarcinoma, (**a**) MR demonstrates a mucocele occupying the left frontal sinus. **b** This is related to the presence of scar tissue impairing mucus drainage (*white arrows*). Note hypointensity on T2 and spontaneous T1 hyperintensity of the retained material in the inferior and inner portion of the mucocele (*asterisk*). **c** After contrast agent administration no enhancement of the mucocele or of the mucosa within frontal sinus is seen. Note regular and ossified margins of frontal sinusotomy (*white arrow*). Mild enhancement of the meningo-galeal complex is demonstrated at the level of the reconstructed anterior skull base floor (*black arrows*)

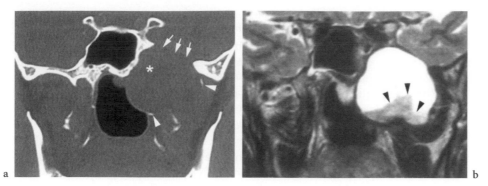

Fig. 8.10a,b. Mucocele. CT (**a**) and MR T2 (**b**), coronal plane. The lesion occupies and markedly expands the left sphenoid sinus. Bone remodeling is detected consisting of demineralization of the greater sphenoid wing (*arrows*), base of the pterygoid process (*asterisk*), and pterygoid laminae. Note the sharp margin of the residual part of the sphenoid wing, pointing out resorption rather than destruction. Eggshell calcifications are present at the periphery of the lesion (*white arrowheads*). Retained secretions show hypointense MR signal in the caudal part of the lesion (*black arrowheads*), probably due to dehydration and increase in protein content

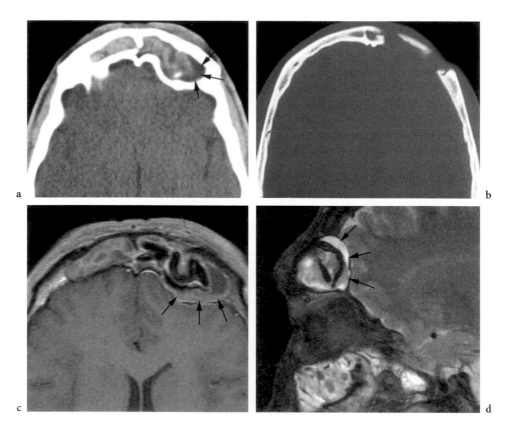

Fig. 8.11a–d. Fungal superinfection of residual cavity. Plain CT on axial plane (**a,b**), enhanced SE T1 on axial plane (**c**), fat-suppressed SE T2 on sagittal plane (**d**). At 3 years after craniotomic evacuation of a left frontal sinus mucocele, a residual cavity is demonstrated by both techniques, exhibiting expanded and remodeled bony walls. Retained material within the cavity shows spontaneous CT hyperdensity and hypointensity on all MR sequences in its central part. Findings are consistent with fungal superinfection. The peripheral rim lining the cavity (*arrows*) probably corresponds to the mucosal layer

Actually, in mycotic lesions these are more frequently seen in the central part of the sinus, whereas in a mucocele calcifications develop close to the mucosal layer (YOON et al. 1999).

A list of more critical differentials must be considered when extensive bone remodeling and destruction are observed, including necrotic squamous cell carcinoma, cystadenocarcinoma, plasmacytoma, and (for sphenoid sinus mucoceles) pituitary adenoma (SKOULAKIS et al. 1999; HEJAZI et al. 2001). At MR, enhancement pattern – better than T2 and plain T1 signal – helps to obtain the diagnosis: absent or exclusively peripheral contrast uptake enables one to predict mucocele with a sensitivity of up to 83%–93% and a specificity of up to 86%–95% (YOUSEM 1993; ATASOY et al. 2001).

8.4.6
Follow-Up

The follow up of patients treated through endonasal or open surgery for a mucocele entails a close clinical examination with endoscopic survey. Imaging is indicated when the patient presents ocular symptoms or when the cavity cannot be accessed or assessed (i.e., mucoceles previously located laterally in the frontal sinus, recurrence of nasal polyps).

8.5
Abnormal Sinus Pneumatization

8.5.1
Definition and Epidemiology

The observation of an abnormal pneumatization of a sinus, a condition first described by MEYES (1898), is a very rare event. According to the classification proposed by URKEN et al. (1987), three different categories are encompassed under the name of enlarged aerated sinuses: hypersinus, pneumosinus dilatans, and pneumocele. The first term refers to an abnormally aerated sinus which is increased in size but still within the range of normal limits and not associated with bony thinning or erosion. Pneumosinus dilatans is a sinus dilatation beyond the normal range but still with normal bony thickness. When focal bony erosion or diffuse thinning is detected, the definition of pneumocele is adopted. Some authors (CHAN et al. 1992) distinguish pneumocele from pneumatocele, the latter being characterized by the presence of air in

soft tissues. It is worth mentioning that this classification is not universally adopted, so that discrepancies in nomenclature may be encountered.

One or more paranasal sinuses can be involved at the same time. Frontal and sphenoid sinuses are most frequently involved (BACHOR et al. 1994), whereas the occurrence in the maxillary sinus and ethmoid is more rare.

Due to the infrequency of the disease, epidemiologic data are lacking. Nevertheless, the reported age of observation ranges between 12 and 72 years, with the highest peak of occurrence in the third and fourth decade (STRETCH and POOLE 1992; TELLADO et al. 2002)

8.5.2
Pathogenesis

Several hypotheses have been put forward to explain the occurrence of an abnormal sinusal pneumatization. According to some authors (BENEDIKT et al. 1991), a spontaneously drained mucocele could lead to this unusual dilation. One of the most credited theories is based on the existence of a valve obstructive mechanism, which could explain the intrasinusal entrapment of air with consequent pressure increase and sinus dilatation (WOLFENSBERGER 1984). However, this hypothesis does not explain why the abnormal pneumatization does not evolve in sinusitis; secretions and inflamed mucosa are in fact completely absent. Also, an alteration in bone turnover mechanism have been purposed (ROSENBERG 1994). In some cases a remodeling action on bony tissues due to a meningioma of the optic nerve (HIRST et al. 1979), or to a bone disease, such as fibrous dysplasia (LLOYD 1985) or Melnick-Needle syndrome (STRETCH and POOLE 1992), was considered the main pathogenetic factor. It seems appropriate to define these latter cases as "secondary" abnormal pneumatization, differentiating them from the "idiopathic" ones (TRIMARCHI et al. 2003).

8.5.3
Clinical and Endoscopic Findings

Signs and symptoms typical of abnormal paranasal sinus pneumatization are very different, according to the site of origin, the number of sinuses involved, and the entity of dilation. When the maxillary sinus is involved, facial pain, possibly increased by atmospheric pressure changes, nasal obstruction, facial deformity, are the most frequent presenting complaints (KOMORI and SUGISAKI 1988; BREIDHAL et al. 1997; MAURI et al. 2000; KARLIDAG et al. 2003; TRIMARCHI et al. 2003). Also hearing loss and ear pain (MORRISON et al. 1976), and enlargement of the swelling after exposure to sunlight have been detected (MAURI et al. 2000). Involvement of the lamina papyracea may lead to the onset of ocular disturbances, like eye ball displacement, diplopia or exophthalmos. In the presence of frontal sinus dilation, nasal obstruction, frontal headache, facial deformity, and eye ball displacement are frequently evident at diagnosis (ADAMS et al. 1998; KLOSSEK et al. 2000; WALKER and JONES 2002). Sphenoid abnormal pneumatization may present with visual disturbances (BACHOR et al. 1994; SKOLNICK et al. 2000), headache, pain in the proximity of the ocular bulb (ADAMS et al. 1998), abnormal secretion of pituitary hormones (REICHER et al. 1986). These clinical presentation modalities are sometimes hardly distinguishable from those typical of other expansile lesions.

At endoscopy, displacement of sinusal bony walls is commonly detected; conversely, no mucosal lesion is present. Nevertheless, facial deformities or sinusal wall displacement do not allow one to rule out a mass growing within the sinus and/or along a submucosal plane. The diagnosis of abnormal pneumatization is therefore based upon imaging evaluation.

8.5.4
Treatment Guidelines

The treatment of abnormal sinus pneumatization is surgery, which is meant to restore a normal ventilation of the sinus through a wide sinusotomy. Microendoscopic surgery, a minimally invasive approach, appears to be the most appropriate and effective option (TRIMARCHI et al. 2003). In maxillary localization, a wide meatotomy avoids further sinus enlargement and allows cessation of symptoms. When a cosmetic correction of facial deformity is required, an external approach may be necessary. A coronal approach for frontal sinus enlargement (KLOSSEK et al. 2000; TELLADO et al. 2002) or an infratemporal approach for maxillary enlargement and orbital involvement may be accomplished (TRIMARCHI et al. 2003). Bifrontal craniotomy has been attempted also with the aim to decompress optic nerves in case of sphenoid involvement (STRETCH and POOLE 1992).

8.5.5
Key Information to Be Provided by Imaging

- Demonstration that the expansile submucosal subcutaneus lesion is due to an abnormal pneumatization of a sinusal cavity
- Assessment of the actual size of the involved sinus(es)
- Precise definition of bony wall thickness, with special reference to the presence of areas of resorption (partial or complete)
- Involvement of critical areas (i.e., orbit, optic canal)
- Possible presence of lesions arising from bone or neoplasms associated with the abnormal pneumatization

8.5.6
Imaging Findings

Aberrant enlargement of a normally aerated sinus cavity is an obvious diagnosis, both at plain radiography and at CT. The latter provides additional information needed to differentiate pneumosinus dilatans from pneumocele and hypersinus (TRIMARCHI et al. 2003). According to URKEN et al.'s (1987) classification, pneumosinus dilatans is an abnormal sinus expansion that may cause deformity – such as frontal bossing – in the absence of any abnormality of bony sinus walls. Detection of focal or generalized thinning of sinus walls switches the diagnosis to pneumocele (Fig. 8.12). Hypersinus lacks both deformities and bone changes, as a consequence its diagnosis is based on the detection of sinus size exceeding statistically calculated normal limits.

The absence of inherent contrast between air and cortical bone (both hypointense on all sequences), restricts the role of MR in these conditions.

8.6
Inverted Papilloma and Other Schneiderian Papillomas

8.6.1
Definition, Epidemiology, Pattern of Growth

According to SHANMUGARATNAM (1991), inverted papilloma is an epithelial benign neoplasm com-

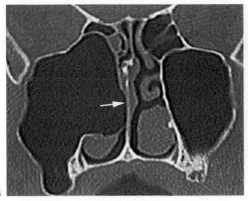
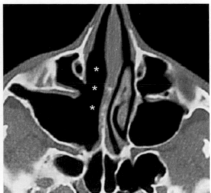

a   b

Fig. 8.12a,b. Pneumosinus dilatans. Plain CT on coronal plane (**a**) and, after surgery, on axial plane
(**b**). Abnormal enlargement of the right maxillary sinus, medially contacting the nasal septum
(*arrow*), no bone destruction is appreciated. After surgical resection of the medial maxillary sinus
wall and middle turbinate, normal caliber of the nasal fossa is restored (*asterisks*)

posed of invaginating crypts, thick ribbons or islands
of non-keratinizing squamous epithelium which may
alternate with or be covered by pseudostratified columnar (cylindrical) or ciliated respiratory epithelium. The infolding of the mucosa may result in the
presence of apparently discontinuous cell masses lying deep in the epithelial surface, but the basement
membrane is intact and may be shown to be continuous with that of surface epithelium.

Inverted papilloma originates from the schneiderian membrane, which is the ectodermally derived
mucosa that lines the nasal cavity and paranasal sinuses. The lesion is estimated to represent 0.4%–4.7%
of the surgically removed nasal tumors, with an incidence ranging from 0.6 to 1.5 cases per 100,000 inhabitants per year (BUCHWALD et al. 1995; OUTZEN et
al. 1996). Males are four to five times more frequently
affected than females (HYAMS 1971; PHILLIPS et al.
1990; WINTER et al. 2000). Inverted papilloma is prevalent in the fifth and sixth decades of life, although
isolated observations in the pediatric age group have
been reported (COOTER et al. 1998).

Even though its etiology is still unknown, recent
studies using in situ hybridization and polymerase
chain reaction have detected human papilloma virus
in up to 86% of the lesions (TANG et al. 1994). In particular, viral subtypes 6, 11, 16, and 18 were the most
frequently found (BRANDWEIN et al. 1989; FURUTA et
al. 1991; GAFFEY et al. 1996).

The lateral wall of the nasal fossa and the maxillary sinus are the most frequent sites of origin of inverted papilloma, whereas its exclusive localization
to the frontal (SHOHET and DUNCAVAGE 1996; CHEE
and SETHI 1999) or the sphenoid sinus (YIOTAKIS
et al. 2001a; LEE et al. 2003) is exceedingly rare. In

1971 HYAMS reported that in the majority of cases
with multiple site involvement the histologic findings suggested the spread to result from one single
lesion by metaplasia of the adjacent mucosa. In this
way, inverted papilloma could easily extend through
sinus ostia to the surrounding cavities without destroying the bony walls. Intracranial invasion is a
rare event, mostly noted in lesions recurring at the
level of the cribriform plate or ethmoid roof (VURAL
et al. 1999). Intraorbital extension may be observed
in lesions with extensive ethmoid involvement; however, the tumor usually laterally displaces the orbital
content without transgressing the periorbit (ELNER
et al. 1995; BAJAJ and PUSHKER 2002). The presentation of inverted papilloma is generally unilateral, but
bilateral involvement of the sinonasal tract has been
reported in a percentage of patients ranging from less
than 1% (PHILLIPS et al. 1990) to 9% (WEISSLER et
al. 1986).

The association between inverted papilloma and
squamous cell carcinoma, reported to be as high as
up to 56% (YAMAGUCHI et al. 1979), is likely to be
overestimated. In fact, recent accurate reviews of the
literature (PELAUSA and FORTIER 1992; MANSELL
and BATES 2000; KROUSE 2001) and data coming
from large series (HYAMS 1971; WEISSLER et al 1986;
KAPADIA et al. 1993) concur to indicate that the two
diseases are concomitantly diagnosed in 2% to 13%
of patients. A further 1%–1.5% of patients has been
shown to present a metachronous sinonasal malignant lesion (FECHNER and ALFORD 1968; WEISSLER
et al. 1986).

Staging systems have been developed for a range
of benign and malignant lesions of the nose and paranasal sinuses with the intent to guide selection of

surgical strategies and to allow comparison of treatment results. As mentioned by KROUSE (2000), several authors have developed staging systems for inverted papilloma very similar to those used for malignancies of the sinonasal tract. However, very recently two new staging systems specific for inverted papilloma have been introduced (KROUSE 2000; HAN et al. 2001) (Tables 8.1, 8.2).

8.6.2
Clinical and Endoscopic Findings

Although nonspecific, a well-established group of signs and symptoms is associated with inverted papilloma at initial presentation. Unilateral nasal obstruction and hyposmia are the predominant complaints when the lesion originates from the lateral nasal wall and fills the nasal fossa, while symptoms mimicking a sinus inflammatory disease, such as watery or mucopurulent rhinorrhea, headache, toothache, and facial pain are mostly reported when inverted papilloma involves the maxillary sinus. Less frequently, patients complain of additional symptoms such as diplopia, proptosis, epiphora and/or persistent headache and cerebrospinal fluid leak, which should suggest an extension of the lesion extending into the orbit and/or the anterior cranial fossa, respectively.

Endoscopic examination usually reveals a unilateral, pale, polypoid-like mass, covered by a papillary surface and protruding from the middle meatus (Fig. 8.13). More rarely the lesion occupies the supe-

Table 8.1. Staging system for inverted papilloma (Krouse)

T1 Tumor totally confined to the nasal cavity, without extension into the sinuses. The tumor can be localized to one wall or region of the nasal cavity, or can be bulky and extensive within the nasal cavity, but must not extend into the sinuses or into any extra nasal compartment. There must be no concurrent malignancy

T2 Tumor involving the ostiomeatal complex, and ethmoid sinuses, and/or the medial portion of the maxillary sinus, with or without involvement of the nasal cavity. There must be no concurrent malignancy

T3 Tumor involving the lateral, inferior, superior, anterior, or posterior walls of the maxillary sinus, the sphenoid sinus, and/or the frontal sinus, with or without involvement of the medial portion of the maxillary sinus, the ethmoid sinuses, or the nasal cavity. There must be no concurrent malignancy

T4 All tumors with any extra-nasal/extra-sinus extension to involve adjacent, contiguous structures such as orbit, the intracranial compartment, or the pterygomaxillary space. All tumors associated with malignancy

Table 8.2. Staging system for inverted papilloma (Han)

Group I Tumor involvement limited to the nasal cavity, lateral nasal wall, medial maxillary sinus, ethmoid sinus, and sphenoid sinus

Group II Same as group I except that tumor extends lateral to the medial maxillary wall

Group III Tumor extends to involve the frontal sinus

Group IV Tumor extends outside the sinonasal cavities (i.e., orbital or intracranial extension)

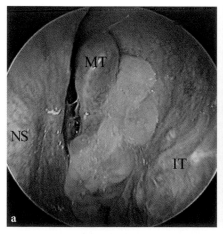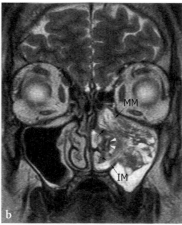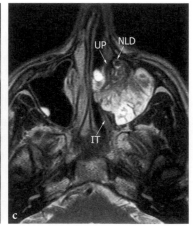

Figure 8.13 a-c. a Endoscopic view of inverted papilloma. Coronal (**b**) and axial (**c**) TSE T2 images show that only the small portion of the inverted papilloma protruding into the middle (*MM*) and inferior (*IM*) meati is actually demonstrated by endoscopy – *arrowheads* point to the inferior turbinate (**b**). Within the maxillary sinus, the main part appears hypointense compared with the bright signal of the thickened mucosa. *NLD*, nasolacrimal duct; *UP*, uncinate process; *MT*, middle turbinate; *IT*, inferior turbinate; *NS*, nasal septum

rior meatus. The concomitant presence of inflammatory polyps may be misleading and can cause a delay in establishing a proper diagnosis. Therefore, whenever the clinician is faced with a unilateral polypoid lesion, multiple biopsies are mandatory.

8.6.3
Treatment Guidelines

Surgery is unanimously considered the treatment of choice for inverted papilloma. Features repeatedly emphasized in the literature such as multicentricity, frequent association with squamous cell carcinoma, and high incidence of recurrences have prompted most of the authors to identify medial maxillectomy (by lateral rhinotomy or midfacial degloving) as the surgical technique of choice (Myers et al. 1990; Lawson et al. 1995; Outzen et al. 1996). However, the introduction in the early 1980s of microendoscopic surgery, along with the subsequent refinement of instrumentation and the increasing experience in endonasal surgery for inflammatory diseases, have led to successful results in the treatment of inverted papilloma even with more conservative techniques (Brors and Draf 1999; Lund 2000; Winter et al. 2000). According to Lund (2000), there is no single right or wrong surgical solution but rather a range of procedures from which a choice should be made in any individual case.

In our experience, based on the management of 47 patients (Tomenzoli et al. 2004), a microendoscopic approach is contraindicated when one of the following situations is present: extensive involvement of the frontal sinus; massive bone erosion (except for the medial wall of the maxillary sinus and the anterior wall of the sphenoid sinus); intradural invasion; intraorbital invasion; abundant scar tissue due to previous surgery; association with squamous cell carcinoma. Different microendoscopic resections may be adopted in relation to the site of origin and the extent of the lesion. When inverted papilloma is limited to the middle meatus, anterior and posterior ethmoid, and/or spheno-ethmoid recess, a type 1 resection, including anterior ethmoidectomy with clearance of the frontal recess, posterior ethmoidectomy, a large middle antrostomy, sphenoidotomy, partial or middle turbinectomy (according to tumor extent) is performed. In such a situation, an "en bloc" resection is easily obtained, making sure that the dissection is carried out in the subperiosteal plane.

Whenever the lesion extends from the middle meatus into the maxillary sinus or originates from the medial wall of the maxillary sinus, a type 2 resection is performed. In addition to all surgical steps of a type 1 resection, the operation includes a medial maxillectomy with or without section of the nasolacrimal duct, in relation to the anterior extent of the tumor.

Inverted papillomas that originate from or involve the posterolateral, anterior and/or inferior wall of the maxillary sinus are better managed through a type 3 resection, which corresponds to the technique indicated by Brors and Draf (1999) as an "endonasal Denker operation".

In patients undergoing a Type 2 or 3 resection, "en bloc" removal is rarely feasible due to the large extent of the lesion. Therefore, debulking of the nasal portion of the mass is first performed to subsequently focus on the most critical areas involved by the lesion, where dissection is always carried out in the subperiosteal plane. Drilling of the bone underlying the diseased mucosa is then performed to ensure surgical radicality.

In the era when transnasal resection without microendoscopic assistance was the only available technique, "recurrences" ranged from 40% (Oberman 1964) to 78% (Calcaterra et al. 1980). We concur with other authors (Hyams 1971; Lund 2000) that most of these "recurrences" were probably "residual" lesions, since the exposure offered by a transnasal approach did not guarantee an adequate radicality of the resection and "recurrent" lesions prevalently occurred at the same site of the primary (Lund 2000). By using external medial maxillectomy or microendoscopic dissection the occurrence of recurrences has dropped down to a prevalence ranging from 0% (Weissler et al. 1986) to 29% (Bielamowicz et al. 1993), and from 0% (Kamel 1995) to 33% (Stankiewicz and Girgis 1993), respectively.

Even though most recurrent inverted papillomas present within 2 years following treatment, late recurrences may also occur. Therefore, it is mandatory to prospectively follow patients with endoscopic controls every 4 months during the first postoperative year and subsequently every 6 months for at least 4 years. In contrast to other benign diseases such as juvenile angiofibroma, which requires radiologic evaluation for early detection of recurrent submucosal lesions (Nicolai et al. 2003), imaging should be obtained only in patients with clear endoscopic evidence of disease or with a complete stenosis of sinus ostium/a precluding a full endoscopic sinus inspection. In the latter situation, imaging evaluation is aimed not only at detecting recurrent lesions, but also to diagnose possible sequelae such as mucocele.

8.6.4
Key Information to Be Provided by Imaging

- Information on the nature of the lesion
- Sites involved by the lesion
- Presence and location of bony erosion
- Possible association of inverted papilloma with a malignant neoplasm

8.6.5
Imaging Findings

In general, there are two clinical settings in which imaging is faced with the diagnosis of inverted papilloma, namely the evaluation of a unilateral nasal obstruction or the assessment of the local spread of a lesion already identified by the endoscopic examination (LEHNERDT et al. 2001; WOODRUFF and VRABEC 1994).

In the first case, there is a high probability that the lesion is detected on a screening CT for rhinosinusitis, while in the second one the patient is more frequently imaged by MR.

Almost all inverted papillomas are unilateral. Bilateral involvement has been reported; it is more likely related to the perforation of the nasal septum rather than to an actual multifocal origin (YOUSEM et al. 1992; DAMMANN et al. 1999).

The imaging features typical of inverted papilloma are based on the site of origin, the pattern of changes of the lateral nasal wall framework, and – respectively – the *lobulated surface contour* on CT and the *striated inner pattern* on MR.

Most inverted papillomas arise from both surfaces of the lateral nasal wall, i.e., the nasal and maxillary. Those originating from the middle meatus spread early into the maxillary sinus (SAVY et al. 2000) via remodeling and destruction of its very thin or dehiscent medial bony wall. Those originating from the maxillary sinus tend to fill the cavity and further gain access into the nasal cavity via the accessory ostium or via the physiologic ostium.

On CT, high densities within the inverted papilloma are shown in up to 50% of cases; more frequently they appear multiple and discrete. It has been demonstrated by SOM and LIDOV (1994) that in most cases they represent residual bone included within the lesion rather than calcifications (Figs. 8.14, 8.15). Nevertheless, displacement and remodeling of sinusal walls may be observed at the same time (Fig. 8.16).

The peculiar macroscopic arrangement of inverted papilloma is characterized by the alternation of quite

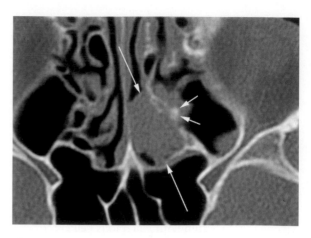

Fig. 8.14 At CT, an inverted papilloma arising from left superior turbinate (*long arrows*) fills the superior meatus, and abuts the ground lamella of the middle turbinate that shows irregular sclerotic changes (*short arrows*)

regular parallel folds made of a highly cellular metaplastic epithelium and of an underlying less cellular stroma. On CT examination, when surrounded by air, these folds give inverted papilloma its typical lobulated contour, which is consistent with the endoscopic appearance of a polypoid lesion with several microdigitations on its surface (DAMMANN et al. 1999). MR does more, because the inner macroscopic arrangement is demonstrated as a septate striated pattern or a convoluted cerebriform pattern both on T2 and contrast-enhanced T1 (YOUSEM et al. 1992; OJIRI et al. 2000). Thus, on T2 these parallel folds of inverted papilloma appear as thick striations of hyperintense signal alternate with thinner ones, closer to fat intensity. The thinner striations have been correlated with the metaplastic epithelium, while the thicker ones have been considered to correspond to the less cellular edematous stroma. On contrast-enhanced T1, the stroma shows a strong enhancement while the thinner epithelium has a lesser enhancement (Fig. 8.17).

This pattern was described by YOUSEM et al. (1992) in 5/10 patients while, recently, OJIRI et al. (2000) demonstrated the striated appearance in 8/10 patients on both T2 and contrast-enhanced T1.

In our experience of 20 inverted papillomas (their size ranging from 1 to 6 cm) the pattern was demonstrated in all studies on contrast-enhanced T1, while on T2 it was detectable only for lesions more than 3 cm in size (MAROLDI et al. 2004). One possible explanation for the increasing observation of this finding could be the improved spatial resolution. In fact, YOUSEM et al. (1992) acquired images with a 256 matrix, OJIRI et al. (2000) obtained slices of 3-mm of

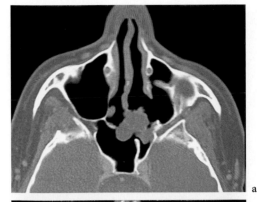

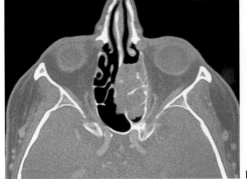

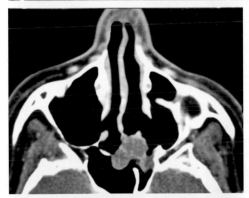

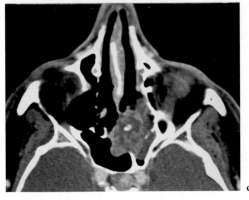

Fig. 8.15a–d. Inverted papilloma of left posterior ethmoid sinus. At CT, the lesion extends into both sphenoid sinuses. Lobulated contours are well detectable on bone-window images (**a,b**). Non-homogeneous density and irregular bone densities are more evident on soft-tissue windows (**c,d**)

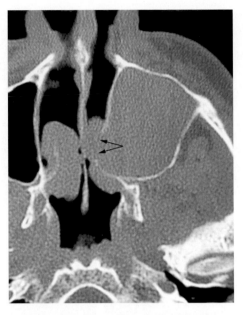

Fig. 8.16. At CT, a maxillary sinus inverted papilloma fills the whole paranasal cavity and displaces all sinusal walls. Focal remodeling and thinning of the posterior aspect of medial sinus wall is seen (*arrows*), suggesting the extent through the posterior fontanelle area, a path of lesser resistance

thickness. Our protocol entails 512 matrix with a 210-mm FOV on axial planes; slices of 2–3 mm of thickness are used, therefore providing a higher resolution (MAROLDI et al. 2004).

The combined use of thin slices and multiple planes of examination makes it possible to recognize that the geometry of the lesion (i.e., the orientation of the septa) depends on the growth along least resistance areas (Fig. 8.18). Moreover, this *striated appearance* is particularly evident in those narrow spaces (i.e., ethmoid infundibulum, fontanelle, meatus) where the lesion is constricted by adjacent structures. In effect, the cerebriform convoluted pattern can be resolved by this examination technique in a complex combination of several parallel or fan-shaped groups of folds (exiting/entering holes/fissures), merging the concept of striated septa with the one of curvilinear convoluted cerebriform pattern. In addition, it is sometimes feasible to identify the site of origin – or the path of growth – by tracing back the quite parallel septa to their center. Besides showing a high sensitivity, this pattern proves to be highly predictive of inverted papilloma. In our series it was actually observed only in two malignant tumors: in both cases pathologic examination of the surgical specimen demonstrated areas consistent with inverted

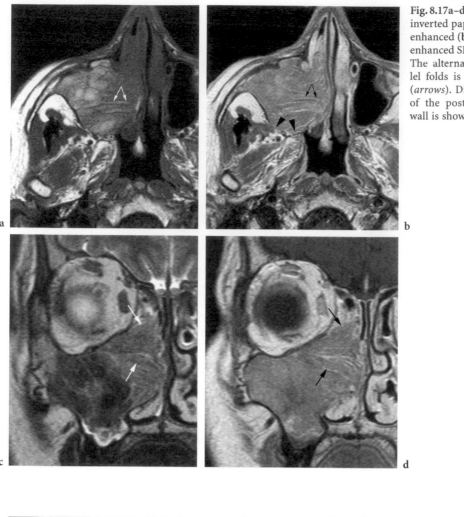

Fig. 8.17a–d. Striated inner pattern of inverted papilloma on MR. Plain (**a**) and enhanced (**b**) axial SE T1, TSE T2 (**c**) and enhanced SE T1 (**d**) on the coronal plane. The alternation of quite regular parallel folds is detectable on all sequences (*arrows*). Displacement and remodeling of the posterolateral maxillary sinusal wall is shown (*arrowheads*)

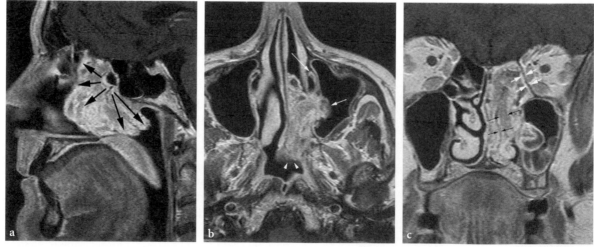

Fig. 8.18a–c. Inverted papilloma arising from the left middle turbinate, SE T1 enhanced sagittal (**a**), axial (**b**), and coronal (**c**) planes. **a** Because the path of least resistance is on the sagittal plane, the striated parallel septations turn into a fan-like pattern detectable on the sagittal SE T1 enhanced image (*arrows*). **b** The lesion extends into the ethmoid infundibulum and protrudes into the maxillary sinus (*short arrow*). Posteriorly, it projects through the choana (*arrowheads*). Uncinate process (*long arrow*). **c** On the coronal plane, the striated appearance results from the parallel orientation of the septa (*black arrows*). Integrity of left lamina papyracea/periorbita is shown (*white arrows*)

papilloma where MR showed the pattern (Fig. 8.19) (MAROLDI et al. 2004). Conversely, foci of squamous cell carcinoma within the inverted papilloma require the histological examination to be identified (YOUSEM et al. 1992).

8.6.5.1
Differential Diagnosis

Inverted papilloma arising from the maxillary sinus has to be distinguished from antrochoanal polyp, fungus ball, and from malignant neoplasms (SAVY et al. 2000).

The antrochoanal polyp, though exhibiting a similar pathway of extent, is usually diagnosed in adolescents, rather than in adults, and shows a homogeneous cystic content. Nevertheless, its *variant* – i.e., the angiomatous polyp – may be more difficult to differentiate. In fact, a strangled antrochoanal polyp passing through a constrictive ostium generally shows a more complex signal pattern. Its constricted mucosal folds and vessels resemble linear and parallel/fan-shaped

structures exiting the ostium (Fig. 8.20). Moreover, the intranasal portion of the sinochoanal polyp exhibits bright enhancement, probably due to stasis. If a mainly cystic intra-sinusal component is present, an angiomatous polyp is more probable.

On CT, fungus balls may show findings comparable to those of inverted papilloma, namely remodeling and destruction of the medial antral wall and discrete densities within the lesion. They are easily differentiated on MR because almost totally hypointense on T2 sequences.

Generally, squamous cell carcinomas – being the most frequent antral malignant lesion – are characterized by a more extensive destruction of the bony walls, and do not show the striated pattern on MR.

The differential diagnosis is more complex for inverted papilloma presenting as a unilateral nasal mass. Of course, sinonasal polyposis typically involves both nasal cavities; therefore the detection of a unilateral polypoid lesion in the adult raises the suspicion of inverted papilloma among other benign and malignant neoplasms.

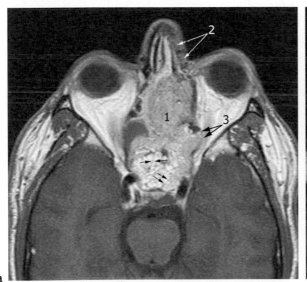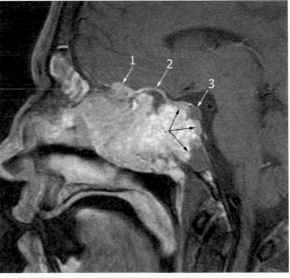

a   b

Fig. 8.19a,b. Enhanced SE T1 on axial (**a**) and sagittal (**b**) planes. **a** Squamous cell carcinoma of the left ethmoid (*1*) with erosion of left nasal bone (*2*), displacement and remodeling of left lamina papyracea/periorbita (*3*). The posterior part of the lesion (*black arrows*), located in the sphenoid sinus, shows more intense enhancement. Thin hypointense and parallel linear densities, arranged in a roughly septation pattern, can be detected within the tumor (*short black arrows*). Pathologic examination of the specimen demonstrated foci of IP in this area. On sagittal plane (**b**), two different sites of anterior cranial fossa floor abnormalities are demonstrated. Anteriorly, extradural intracranial neoplastic invasion (*1*) is suggested by the presence of enhancing tissue extending through the bone/periosteum, covered by thickened enhancing dura. A few millimeters posteriorly, the fluid signal intensity of a mucocele secondary to the more lobulated component (*black arrows*) remodels both the planum sphenoidalis (*2*) and the roof/posterior wall of the sphenoid sinus (*3*)

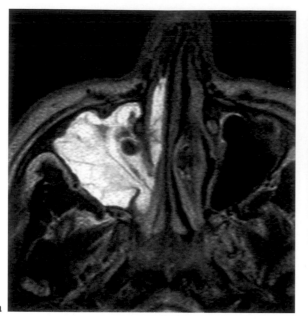
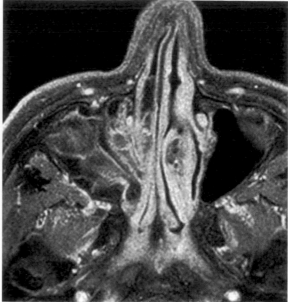

Fig. 8.20a,b. Angiomatous polyp of the right maxillary sinus, TSE T2 and enhanced VIBE on the axial plane

8.6.5.2
Pathways of Spread

There are two problems to solve when assessing the extent of inverted papilloma: to distinguish it from intrasinusal-retained secretions, and to define its relationship with both the orbit and the skull base (Yousem et al. 1992; Savy et al. 2000). MR can adequately answer both issues (Oikawa et al. 2003).

Three relevant aspects regarding inverted papilloma pathways of spread have to be outlined: adjacent bony structures are destroyed by mean of pressure erosion; extension into adjacent sinusal cavities occurs through a centrifugal pattern; involvement of skull base is, usually, late, being observed after several failed surgical exccisions. As most inverted papillomas arise from the lateral nasal wall or from the maxillary sinus, they grow centrifugally into the ethmoid labyrinth and later into the sphenoid or the frontal sinus (Fig. 8.21). Thinning and bowing of adjacent bony structures and of the nasal septum is frequent (approximately 80%–90%).

Erosion is common at the level of the lateral nasal wall or of the turbinates (more than 80%); it is also seen in nearly 50% of cases at the level of the ethmoid. Extensive erosion of the lamina papyracea or of the cribriform plate is more often associated with a coexistent squamous cell carcinoma (Dammann et al. 1999).

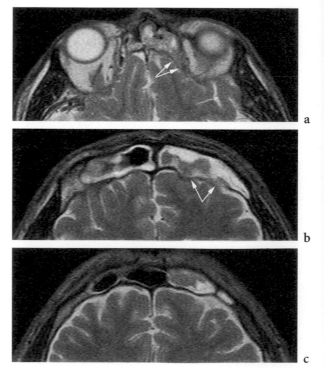

Fig. 8.21a–c. Inverted papilloma of left frontal sinus, TSE T2 on the axial plane. The lesion has lobulated contours, intermediate signal intensity, clearly distinguished from surrounding retained hyperintense mucus. Focal areas of posterior wall erosion are demonstrated [*arrows* on (a) and (b)]

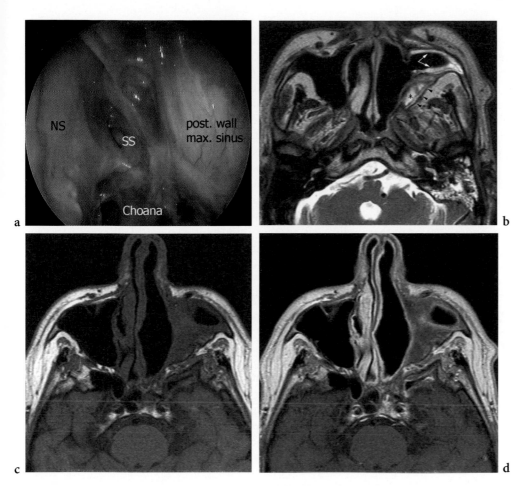

Fig. 8.22a–d. Post-microendoscopic removal of left nasal wall inverted papilloma. Endoscopy (**a**), TSE T2 (**b**), plain (**c**) and enhanced (**d**) SE T1 on the axial plane. **a** Endoscopy shows complete healing of the nasal fossa and posterior maxillary sinus wall, which is characterized by mild bulging. **b** On T2 sequence, the bulging corresponds to submucosal thickened connective tissue – due to previous surgery – showing intermediate signal (*asterisk*). Thickened hyperintense mucosa invests the zygomatic recess of left maxillary sinus (*white arrows*). Periosteal thickening of posterolateral antral wall presents with a double layer pattern (*arrowheads*). **c** On the axial plane, obtained a few millimeters cranial, scar tissue partially fills the maxillary sinus. **d** After GD-DTPA administration minimal enhancement of the scar tissue is shown. *SS*, sphenoid sinus; *NS*, nasal septum

8.6.6
Follow-Up

At the end of surgical treatment in almost all inverted papillomas the removal of middle turbinate, medial maxillary sinus and anterior sphenoid sinus walls creates a wide cavity easy to access at endoscopy during the follow-up (DAMMANN et al. 1999; PETIT et al. 2000) (Fig. 8.22).

For this reason, imaging is indicated mainly to define the extent of a recurrent inverted papilloma, particularly to demonstrate its relationship with the skull base or the orbit. Of course, recurrences located deep in the frontal sinus can be detected by imaging only. The same diagnostic criteria used to identify the primary inverted papilloma apply to relapsing lesions. Also in this setting, MR provides a sensitivity superior to CT (PETIT et al. 2000).

8.7
Juvenile Angiofibroma

8.7.1
Definition, Epidemiology, Pattern of Growth

Juvenile angiofibroma is a lesion composed of vascular and fibrous elements in varying proportion, which accounts for 0.5% of all head and neck tumors and typically occurs in adolescent males. Recent immunohistochemical and electron microscopy studies suggest that the lesion must be considered a vascular malformation (or hamartoma) instead of a tumor (SCHICK et al. 2002). The point of origin is identified by some authors in the area of the sphenopalatine foramen, while others, based on the results of CT or MR imaging, indicate that the lesion takes origin in the pterygopalatine fossa, at the aperture of the vidian canal. Juvenile angiofibroma has the peculiar tendency to grow in the submucosal plane into the nasopharynx, along the vidian canal into the basisphenoid, and laterally towards the pterygopalatine and infratemporal fossa. Another important feature of juvenile angiofibroma is the early invasion of the cancellous bone of the pterygoid root; from here, the lesion can extend laterally to involve the greater wing of the sphenoid bone. Intracranial extension mainly occurs into the middle cranial fossa along the maxillary nerve into the parasellar region and the cavernous sinus; another pattern involves growth through the inferior and the superior orbital fissures. Erosion of the anterior skull base is seldom observed. It is noteworthy that most of the lesions with intracranial extension are extradural; only very rare instances of juvenile angiofibromas crossing the dura have been documented in the literature (DANESI et al. 2000).

8.7.2
Clinical and Endoscopic Findings

Nasal obstruction and epistaxis are the typical symptoms of juvenile angiofibroma; their occurrence in a young male should always arouse the suspicion of such a disease. Additional symptoms such as diplopia, cheek swelling, and headache can be reported by patients with advanced lesions extending into the superior orbital fissure, the infratemporal fossa, and the cranial fossa, respectively. The endoscopic finding of a smooth-surfaced, clearly vascularized, expansile lesion growing behind the middle turbinate is another important element highly suggestive for juvenile angiofibroma (Fig. 8.23). Since epidemiologic and endoscopic findings are so typical, biopsy is almost unanimously considered contraindicated, since it carries a considerable and undue risk of hemorrhage.

8.7.3
Treatment Guidelines

Even though several methods (i.e., embolization, cryotherapy, hormonal therapy, chemotherapy) have been proposed for the treatment of juvenile angiofibroma, surgery is commonly considered the main-

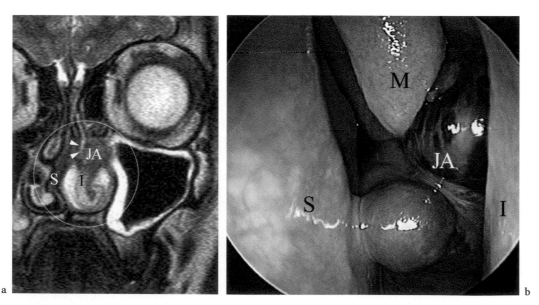

Fig. 8.23a,b. Juvenile angiofibroma (*JA*). **a** Coronal TSE T2 shows a hypointense mass filling the left nasal cavity. It projects among nasal septum (*S*), middle (*arrowheads*) and inferior (*I*) turbinates. Retained fluid within the obstructed nasal cavity appears as hyperintense signal surrounding the inferior turbinate. **b** Endoscopy demonstrates a bluish and vascularized polyp. *I*, Inferior turbinate; *M*, middle turbinate; *S* nasal septum

stay. Radiotherapy has also been shown to be effective in isolated institutions; however, the observation of a few cases of radioinduced tumors, as well as the possible alterations of maxillary growth, bring the validity of this treatment into question.

Since many years, transfacial techniques (through a lateral rhinotomy or a midfacial degloving) and the infratemporal approach are considered the best options. More recently, the rapid spread of endonasal techniques using endoscopes or both a microscope and endoscopes has prompted many surgeons to treat even small and intermediate-size juvenile angiofibromas with such a conservative approach with apparently satisfactory results. Even in our experience, juvenile angiofibromas involving the nasopharynx, the nasal cavities, the sphenoid, the ethmoid, the maxillary sinus, and/or the pterygomaxillary fossa can be managed successfully through endoscopic surgery (NICOLAI et al. 2003). Lesions extending into the infratemporal fossa and/ or the cavernous sinus frequently require an external approach. The head and neck surgeon is therefore faced with a wide spectrum of surgical techniques that can be selected in the single patient mainly in relation to the size and the extent of the lesion. An informed consent to switch intraoperatively to an external procedure should always be obtained from the patient.

8.7.4
Key Information to Be Provided by Imaging

- Confirmation of the suspected nature of the disease
- Extent of the lesion, with specific emphasis on orbit, infratemporal fossa, intracranial (cavernous sinus, ICA, dura) and intraosseous involvement
- Pattern of vascularization (unilateral vs. bilateral; recruitment of internal carotid artery branches)

8.7.5
Imaging Findings

The diagnosis of juvenile angiofibroma on CT and MR is based on three features: the site of origin of the lesion (LLOYD et al. 2000b); its hypervascular appearance after contrast enhancement (SCHICK and KAHLE 2000); and its pattern of growth.

First, as juvenile angiofibroma arises close to the sphenopalatine foramen – either just on its submucosal aspect or from the adjacent pterygopalatine fossa – it usually presents as a mass expanded medially into the nasal cavity, and eroding the root of the pterygoid process.

It has been suggested that the actual site of origin should be a recess of the pterygopalatine fossa behind the sphenopalatine ganglion, at the exit aperture of the vidian canal (Fig. 8.24). The evidence that up to 96% of the 72 juvenile angiofibromas in the series of Lloyd caused enlargement or erosion of the anterior part of the vidian canal should support this hypothesis.

Second, as juvenile angiofibroma mainly consists of a vascular histological component, the administration of contrast agent – either iodinated or paramagnetic – causes a strong and usually quite homogeneous, enhancement on CT or MR T1 sequences (Fig. 8.25). Moreover, the diagnosis of juvenile angiofibroma on MR is suggested by the presence – on both T1 and T2 sequences – of several signal voids within the lesion, indicating major intra-lesion vessels (Fig. 8.26).

As the mass increases in size, enlargement of the internal maxillary artery can be directly detected by CT or MR. Cystic changes are rare; those reported have been correlated to spontaneous or post-chemotherapy tumor regression (SCHICK and KAHLE 2000) (Fig. 8.27).

Third, bone involvement by juvenile angiofibroma consists either of bone remodeling – for example the thinning and anterior displacement of the postero-superior antral wall – and bone erosion, typically at the level of the pterygoid root. In the latter case, access to the cancellous content of the sphenoid bone enables the juvenile angiofibroma to extend deeply into the medullary spaces of the basisphenoid or, even, to replace the diploe of the greater wing of the sphenoid (LLOYD et al. 1999). Although bone erosion can be more easily shown by CT, MR is adequate in demonstrating cortical erosion and cancellous replacement by tumor (Fig. 8.28).

Therefore, the typical juvenile angiofibroma is diagnosed by CT or MR with almost total certainty, making pre-operative biopsy unnecessary. Juvenile angiofibroma arising outside the lateral margins of the posterior nares is very rare. Approximately 50 cases have been reported in the literature, the maxillary sinus being the commonest atypical site (SCHICK and KAHLE 2000).

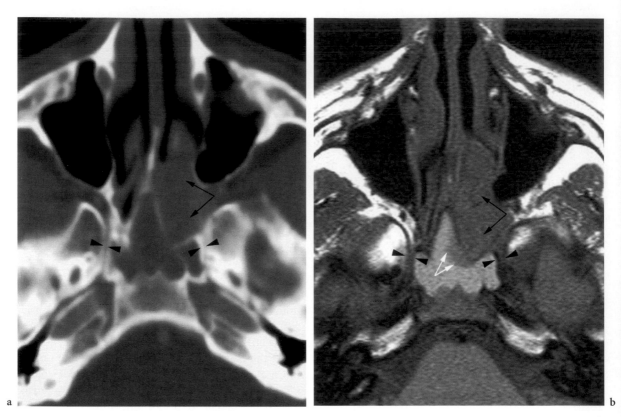

a   b

Fig. 8.24a,b. Juvenile angiofibroma. Plain CT (**a**), and plain SE T1 (**b**) in the axial plane (same patient as in Fig. 8.23). Both techniques demonstrate a lesion arising from the medial aspect of the left pterygopalatine fossa in the region of the sphenopalatine foramen (*black arrows*). The exit aperture of the pterygoid/vidian canal is markedly enlarged, whereas its posterior portion is normal (*arrowheads*). Chronically retained secretions fill the sphenoid sinus, being hyperintense on T1 sequence because of the increased protein concentration. MR shows a small part of the juvenile angiofibroma abutting the sinusal lumen (*white arrows*). Reactive sclerosis of the left pterygoid root spongiosa is demonstrated on both techniques

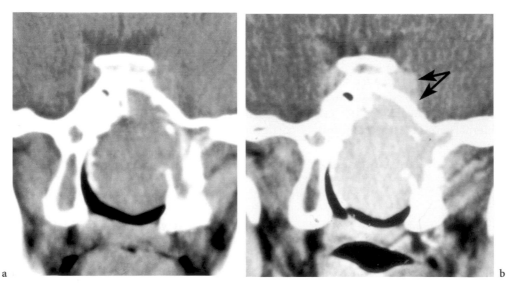

a   b

Fig. 8.25a,b. Juvenile angiofibroma: pattern of enhancement. CT before (**a**) and after (**b**) contrast administration, coronal plane. After contrast injection a bright and quite uniform enhancement is observed. Intracranial extent at the cavernous sinus level appears equally as a hyperdense nodule (*arrows*). The epicenter of juvenile angiofibroma is located at the sphenopalatine foramen

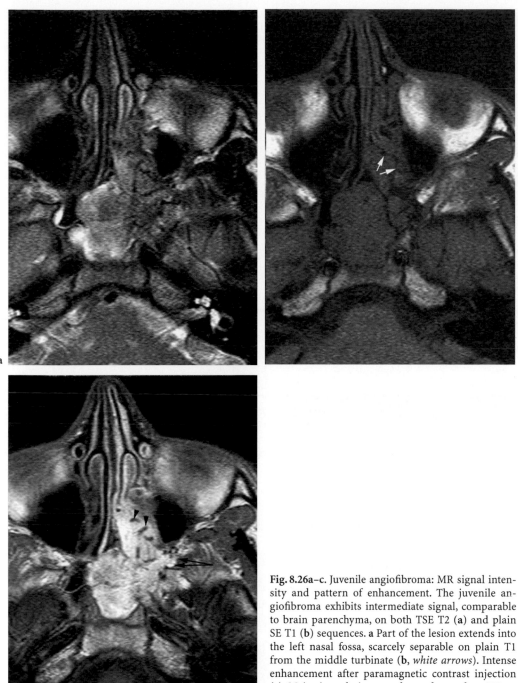

Fig. 8.26a–c. Juvenile angiofibroma: MR signal intensity and pattern of enhancement. The juvenile angiofibroma exhibits intermediate signal, comparable to brain parenchyma, on both TSE T2 (**a**) and plain SE T1 (**b**) sequences. **a** Part of the lesion extends into the left nasal fossa, scarcely separable on plain T1 from the middle turbinate (**b**, *white arrows*). Intense enhancement after paramagnetic contrast injection (**c**). Major intra-lesion vessels are detected on MR as serpiginous flow voids (*arrowheads*). A small part of juvenile angiofibroma abuts the left pterygopalatine fossa (*black arrows*)

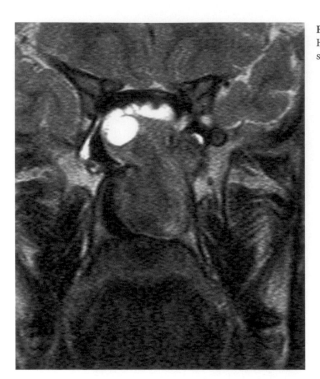

Fig. 8.27 Juvenile angiofibroma. TSE T2, coronal plane. Hyperintensity of the intra-sphenoidal component of the lesion reflects spontaneous cystic changes

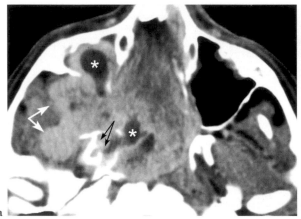

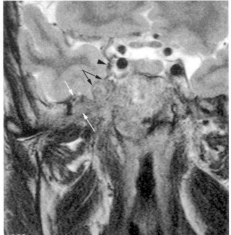

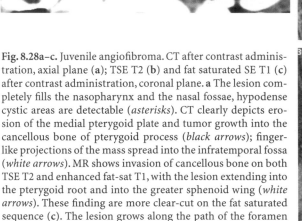

Fig. 8.28a–c. Juvenile angiofibroma. CT after contrast administration, axial plane (**a**); TSE T2 (**b**) and fat saturated SE T1 (**c**) after contrast administration, coronal plane. **a** The lesion completely fills the nasopharynx and the nasal fossae, hypodense cystic areas are detectable (*asterisks*). CT clearly depicts erosion of the medial pterygoid plate and tumor growth into the cancellous bone of pterygoid process (*black arrows*); finger-like projections of the mass spread into the infratemporal fossa (*white arrows*). MR shows invasion of cancellous bone on both TSE T2 and enhanced fat-sat T1, with the lesion extending into the pterygoid root and into the greater sphenoid wing (*white arrows*). These finding are more clear-cut on the fat saturated sequence (**c**). The lesion grows along the path of the foramen rotundum (*black arrows*) and, submucosally, along the under surface of sphenoid bone (*black arrowheads*), without invading cavernous sinus (*single black arrowhead* in **b**)

8.7.5.1
Pathways of Spread

Of course, the pathways of spread of juvenile angiofibroma will influence the choice of the surgical approach (Fig. 8.29).

Owing to its nature, juvenile angiofibroma tends to grow along the paths of least resistance, causing displacement of adjacent soft tissues, rather than invasion. Adherence can be present, particularly when the lesion contacts the dura, but dural or brain infiltration is rare (DANESI et al. 2000; SCHOLTZ et al. 2001).

Its peculiar dual pattern of bone involvement (remodeling and destruction) is likely to result from two different mechanisms of interaction between juvenile angiofibroma and bony structures. Displacement of the periosteal invested cortical surfaces causes remodeling and thinning, with only late breakthrough and destruction, whereas the direct growth of juvenile angiofibroma along perforating arteries into the cancellous root of the sphenoid lets the lesion extend into the medullary content of the sphenoid (floor of sphenoid sinus, greater wing). This could explain why the vidian canal (invested by a periosteal layer), though the closest to the growing lesion, shows more frequently enlargement of its anterior third, rather

than destruction. Moreover, further posterior extension into the canal is infrequent, and usually observed in advanced lesions.

Due to the knowledge of the elementary interactions of juvenile angiofibroma with surrounding structures and its constant site of origin, the patterns of spread are highly predictable (LLOYD et al. 2000b; SCHICK and KAHLE 2000).

From its site of origin in the pterygopalatine fossa, the juvenile angiofibroma extends medially into the nasal cavity and nasopharynx – the areas of least resistance – via enlargement and erosion of the sphenopalatine foramen. Growth of tumor anteriorly indents the postero-superior maxillary sinus wall, resulting in anterior bowing of the sinusal wall, the so-called antral sign, described by Holman and Miller on lateral plain X-ray (LLOYD and PHELPS 1986) (Fig. 8.30) .

The lateral extent, via an enlarged pterygo-maxillary fissure, gives rise to infratemporal fossa spread. Extension into this space is demonstrated by detecting the "finger-like projections" of the enhancing juvenile angiofibroma characterized by sharp and lobulated margins (Fig. 8.31). In this area, the least resistant structure consists of the fat tissue between the pterygoid muscles, usually splayed.

From the pterygo-maxillary fissure, the lesion can also access the apex of the orbit through the inferior orbital fissure, and further extends into the middle cranial fossa via the superior orbital fissure (Fig. 8.32).

Posterior spread from pterygopalatine fossa is almost certainly the most dangerous for the patient because it enables the juvenile angiofibroma to penetrate the cancellous bone of the root of pterygoid process. From this site, juvenile angiofibroma extends both medially, into the floor of the sphenoid sinus, and laterally, into the greater wing (LLOYD et al. 1999). As the center of growth of the intrasinusal component of juvenile angiofibroma is located at the intersection between the floor and the lateral wall, there is evidence to suggest that the intrasinusal extension comes from the root of the pterygoid, rather than being due to upward extension from the choana. Lateral spread allows the juvenile angiofibroma to replace the diploe of the greater wing, usually with late erosion of the inner table.

The key to detecting the diploic invasion consists of differentiating its medullary content from the lesion on the basis of CT density and MR signal. On CT, this is achieved by the strong enhancement of juvenile angiofibroma within the diploe. On MR, the optimal discrimination is obtained by combining a plain T1 with a post-contrast T1 with or without fat

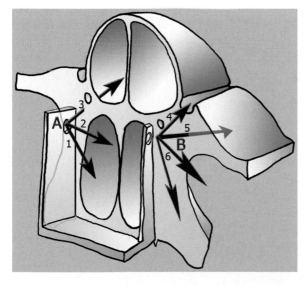

Fig. 8.29. Pathways of spread of juvenile angiofibroma. *A*, extent through the sphenopalatine foramen into the nasal fossa (*1*) and – via the choana – into the nasopharynx (*2*); through the erosion of the sphenoid sinus floor into the sphenoid sinus (*3*). *B*, extent from the pterygopalatine fossa along the foramen rotundum (actually a groove or a complete bone canal) (*4*), into the cancellous bone of the greater wing of the sphenoid (*5*), and into the masticator space (*6*)

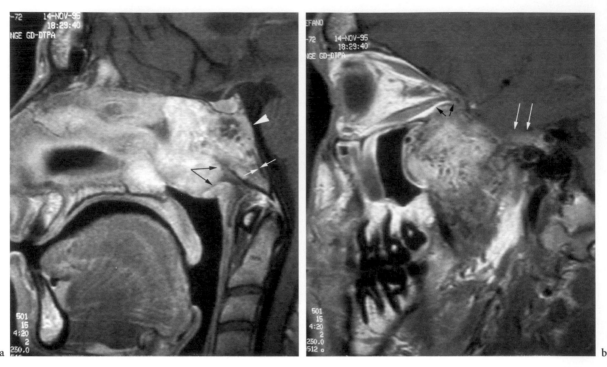

Fig. 8.30a,b. Juvenile angiofibroma. SE T1 after contrast administration, sagittal plane. **a** The lesion infiltrates the medullary bone of clivus, the intracranial cortical boundary being detectable only in its inferior part (*white opposing arrows*). Reactive thickening of the adjacent dura of prepontine cistern (*white arrowhead*). Submucosal growth along the undersurface of the sphenoid bone is appreciated (*black arrows*). **b** The lesion indents the posterior wall of the maxillary sinus, reaches the inferior orbital fissure (*black arrows*) and spreads along the foramen rotundum (*white arrows*)

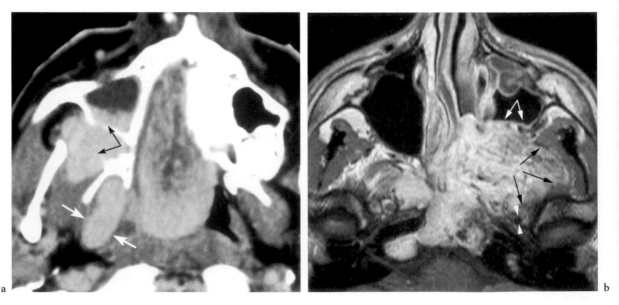

Fig. 8.31a,b. Juvenile angiofibroma. CT (**a**) and SE T1 (**b**) after contrast administration, both in the axial plane. **a** Finger-like projections of the juvenile angiofibroma grow into the infratemporal fossa. The posterior wall of the maxillary sinus is remodeled and interrupted (*black arrows*). A small part of the lesion extends posteriorly to the pterygoid plates (into the pterygoid fossa) along the medial pterygoid muscle (*white arrows*). **b** The enhancing juvenile angiofibroma occupies the left masticator space (*black arrows*). Laterally it borders the temporalis muscle, posteriorly it reaches the foramen ovale. An enlarged middle meningeal artery is detected (*white arrowheads*). Remodeling of posterolateral maxillary sinus wall is seen (*white arrows*)

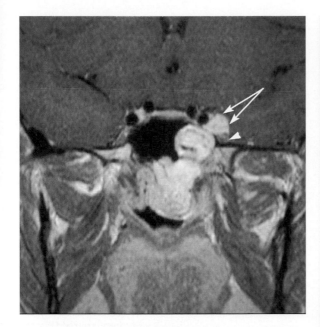

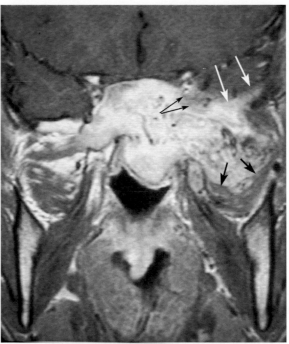

Figure 8.32. Juvenile angiofibroma. Enhanced SE T1 in the coronal plane. The juvenile angiofibroma invades the sphenoid sinus through the floor. A second component reaches the cavernous sinus (*white arrows*) through the foramen (groove) rotundum, running above the maxillary nerve (*arrowhead*)

Fig. 8.33. Juvenile angiofibroma. Enhanced SE T1 in the coronal plane. The juvenile angiofibroma completely replaces the cancellous bone of both the left pterygoid root and the greater sphenoid wing. The inferior orbital fissure is reached through a defect of the lateral wall of sphenoid sinus (*thin black arrows*). Intracranial growth is appreciated along the floor of middle cranial fossa (*white arrows*). The extracranial component of the lesion invades the infratemporal fossa. The lateral pterygoid muscle is inferiorly displaced (*thick black arrows*)

saturation (Fig. 8.33). The latter makes it possible to easily distinguish the hyperintense enhanced juvenile angiofibroma from the suppressed signal of the normal bone marrow. An alternative option to reduce marrow signal on T1 sequences consists of decreasing the TR and selecting thinner sections: while the signal of bone marrow greatly diminishes, juvenile angiofibroma maintains its hyperintensity. Replacement of the cancellous structure of the clivus can be observed in advanced lesions that completely fill the sphenoid sinuses and displace both the lateral walls and the roof.

Juvenile angiofibroma shows two different types of intracranial invasion: extent along a canal, and spread through bone destruction. It is interesting to note that even medium size lesions may gain access into the middle cranial fossa by growing along the foramen rotundum, and running lateral to the cavernous sinus to reach the anterior aspect of the Meckel's cave. Generally, the second pattern occurs when huge lesions break through the inner table of the greater wing or the lateral sphenoid sinus walls.

Regardless of the pattern of intracranial access, infiltration of the dura is very rare. In fact, it has been recently reported that even when cross sectional imaging suggests cavernous sinus invasion or internal carotid artery involvement, a dissection plane can

be found in most cases, making complete removal feasible (DANESI et al. 2000).

8.7.5.2
Angiography

Surgical resection is currently the most widely accepted treatment for juvenile angiofibroma. Due to its high vascularization, surgical removal can sometimes be difficult because of significant intraoperative hemorrhage, resulting in incomplete resection and higher rate of persistence. Pre-operative embolization was introduced in 1972 to obtain lesion devascularization and facilitate complete excision of the tumor (ROBERSON et al. 1972). Nowadays, the availability of intra-arterial digital subtraction angiography, microcatheters, and embolic agents – such as PVA particles – makes superselective embolization of feeders easier and safer (VALAVANIS and CHRISTOFORIDIS 2000). Though some authors questioned the usefulness of this procedure, as in their experience no significant difference in surgical bleeding was observed, there is increasing evidence that embolization is a safe and effective method to reduce intra-operative blood loss (SINILUOTO et al. 1993; MOULIN et al. 1995; LI et al. 1998). Nevertheless, the shrinkage of lesion achieved by embolization has been indicated as a contributory cause to incomplete excision of juvenile angiofibroma by McCOMBE et al. (1990).

At present, the role of angiography is to provide a detailed map of feeders, demonstrating the recruitment of internal carotid artery, vertebral or contralateral external carotid artery branches, and to obtain preoperative devascularization.

According to LASJAUNIAS et al. (1980), the angiographic findings of juvenile angiofibroma consist of moderate enlargement of feeding arteries, intense "parenchymal" blush, absence of large arteriovenous shunts, or early venous return (Fig. 8.34).

The pattern of arterial feeders recruited is predictable in most cases. It is strictly related to the pathways of spread, but not to the actual size of the lesion, though most large lesions are multi-compartmental. In our experience of 15 patients treated by exclusive endonasal excision, there was no correlation between the volume of juvenile angiofibroma and the number of feeding vessels (NICOLAI et al. 2003). However, recruitment of internal carotid artery, vertebral branches was significantly more frequent among lesions with several external carotid artery feeders. Notably, though internal carotid artery feeders

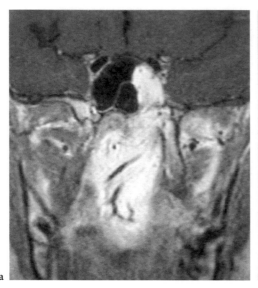
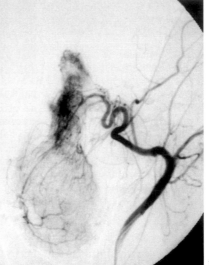

Fig. 8.34a,b. Juvenile angiofibroma. Enhanced SE T1 in the coronal plane (a); intra-arterial DSA (b). a On MR, the lesion shows a prevalent endoluminal growth within the nasopharynx. Upwards extension in the pterygoid root and within the sphenoid sinus is also appreciated. b DSA demonstrates vascular feeders arising from the distal part of the sphenopalatine artery; a more prominent blush is observed at the level of the nasal part of the lesion

a   b

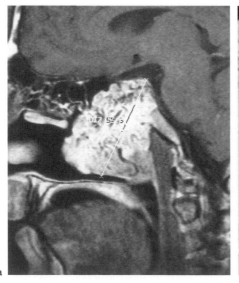
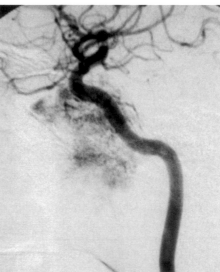

Fig. 8.35a,b. Juvenile angiofibroma. Enhanced SE T1 in the sagittal plane (a); intra-arterial DSA (b). a The lesion fills the sphenoid sinus. Infiltration of the clivus is demonstrated by the encroachment of both its cortical layers and replacement of the medullary content. b DSA demonstrates the several subtle feeders from the internal carotid artery, not embolized

a   b

were demonstrated in approximately 47% of cases (Fig. 8.35), intracranial extent was present only in 13%.

During the last decade the availability of small particles and microcatheters has made it possible to reach even peripheral small branches of the external carotid artery, preserving adjacent normal vessels from being devascularized by the more proximal occlusion obtained by Gelfoam or Spongel embolization (Fig. 8.36). In fact, the goal of embolization is to achieve vessel occlusion at the capillary level. Consequently, polyvinyl-alcohol particles with a minimal size of 150 µm have been suggested, as significant arteriovenous shunts have been demonstrated for particles of 50 µm or less by nuclear medicine techniques (SCHROTH et al. 1996).

The rate of minor and major complications for embolization of external carotid artery branches is negligible, approximately 4% (UNGKANONT et al. 1996).

It is evident that the major challenge to angiography regards the management of juvenile angiofibroma vascularization by internal carotid artery feeders. Advanced lesions with intracranial extent have been successfully excised after pre-operative embolization of external carotid artery branches with acceptable blood loss, despite involvement of the internal carotid artery branches in the blood supply. Devascularization by direct tumor puncture and embolization, advocated by CASASCO et al. (1999), entails an unacceptable risk of major neurologic complications. Balloon occlusion and sacrifice of the internal carotid artery is required in rare cases (CASASCO ct al. 1999).

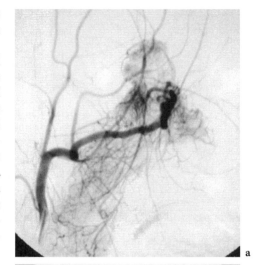

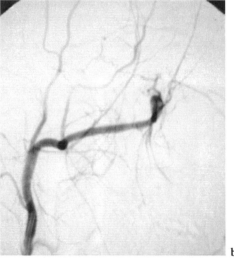

Fig. 8.36a,b. Juvenile angiofibroma. DSA, before (**a**) and after (**b**) embolization. The juvenile angiofibroma is fed by terminal branches of the sphenopalatine artery, it occupies the nasal fossa and the nasopharynx; upwards it extends into the sphenoid sinus, downwards it reaches the superior part of the oropharyngeal lumen. Embolization permits complete devascularization of the mass

8.7.6
Follow-Up

There are two different types of persistent lesions: those left intentionally because their resection would require unacceptable neural damage, and those left due to intraoperative oversight (Figs. 8.37, 8.38). In both cases, proper management mandates a precise assessment of site, size, and extent of the lesion.

Recurrences are a peculiar characteristic of juvenile angiofibroma. In fact, most authors doubt this theory and consider more likely the hypothesis of incomplete excision leaving lesion remnants (ANDREWS et al. 1989; CHAGNAUD et al.1998; LLOYD et al. 2000b;).

To support this hypothesis is the fact that most persistent lesions occur within months or a few years of primary treatment and more commonly are found in anatomical areas difficult to reach at surgery. This presumption is consistent with CHAGNAUD et al. (1998) who demonstrated that lesion remnants were already detectable at the first follow-up with cross sectional imaging.

Persistent lesions are more frequent when the primary juvenile angiofibroma invades the infratemporal fossa, sphenoid sinus, pterygoid root, clivus, and cavernous sinus (HERMAN et al. 1999; HOWARD et al. 2001). According to McCOMBE et al. (1990), "recurrences" are also related to primary juvenile angiofibroma size, being more frequent in large lesions.

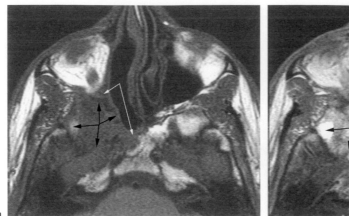
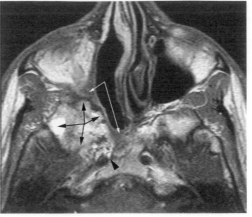

Fig. 8.37a,b. Follow-up of juvenile angiofibroma. SE T1 before (**a**) and after (**b**) contrast administration, axial plane. At 4 years after incomplete surgical resection a residual submucosal lesion is detected within the greater wing of sphenoid bone (*black arrows*). **b** After contrast administration, the lesion shows the typical enhancement of juvenile angiofibroma. Posteriorly it is in close contact with the carotid canal (*black arrowhead*). Only a smooth re-epithelized mucosa is visible from the nasal fossa (*white arrows*)

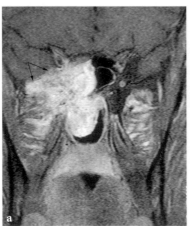
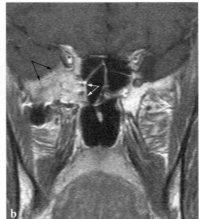
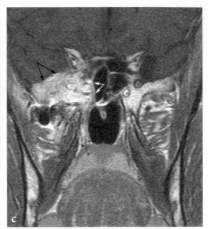

Fig. 8.38a–c. Juvenile angiofibroma. Same patient as in Fig. 8.37. Enhanced T1 sequences in the coronal plane. Pretreatment examination for planning sub-total resection of the residual juvenile angiofibroma (**a**). Follow-up study after 13 months (**b**) and 18 months (**c**) after surgery. During surgery, a part of the lesion was intentionally left within the greater wing of the sphenoid bone, due to its relevant lateral extension and due to middle cranial fossa extradural invasion. Both the superior (*black arrows*) and medial (*white arrows*) limits of the lesion appear rather concave on preoperative and first follow-up MR examination, whereas 18 months after surgery their surface results more or less convex. This change in shape indicates progression of the lesion

Depending on the clinical condition (known or high-risk remnant lesion vs low-risk), follow-up will be scheduled: every few months for known remnants/high risk patients and every 6 months during the first year, then yearly, for the others, respectively (CHAGNAUD et al. 1998; ROGER et al. 2002). In the first case, the goal of imaging is to detect changes in size of known remnants in order to decide the proper treatment strategy or to identify lesions arising from potential sites of

persistence. In the second case, follow-up should be extended until adulthood, even though date supporting this strategy have not been provided yet.

Of course, unexpected persistent lesions show the same imaging characteristics as the primitive ones (Fig. 8.39), but their detection may be hampered by postoperative changes. These consist of altered bony and soft structures, due to surgical resection, healing, and chronic inflammatory re-

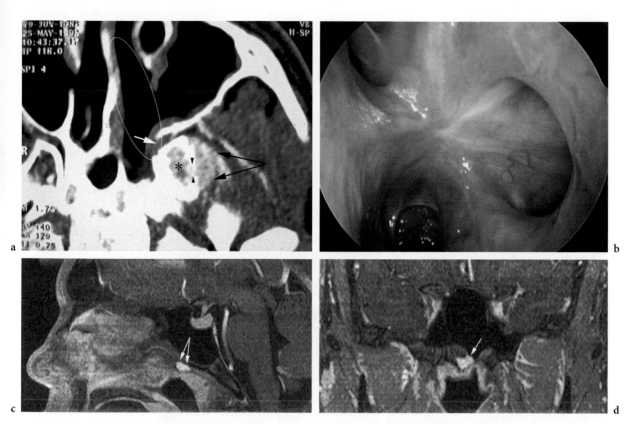

Fig. 8.39a–d. Recurrent/persistent juvenile angiofibromas in two different patients. CT after contrast administration, axial plane (a); endoscopic view (b); enhanced VIBE sequence in sagittal and coronal planes (c,d). a A thin plaque of non-enhancing scar tissue is detected at the level of sphenopalatine foramen (*white arrow*). The submucosal relapse (*black arrows*) has its epicenter at the pterygoid root level where the medullary bone is replaced by the enhanced juvenile angiofibroma (*asterisk*). Erosion of pterygoid bony boundaries is seen (*arrowheads*). The encircled area corresponds to the endoscopic view (b), which does not show any abnormality. c,d In a different patient, a relapsing juvenile angiofibroma is detected 2 years after endonasal surgery (*arrows*) located submucosally within residual sphenoid sinus floor

action of the sinonasal mucosa (CHAGNAUD et al. 1998).

Bony defects of the sinonasal framework and skull base mainly depend both on the specific surgical approach and on the extent of the erosion caused by juvenile angiofibroma.

However, some constant postoperative findings appear to be the partial or total excision of the posterior, and medial antral walls, of the pterygoid root and of the floor of the sphenoid sinus, detectable in almost half of the patients, regardless of the surgical approach (Fig. 8.40).

The scar tissue replacing the site previously occupied by juvenile angiofibroma – pterygopalatine fossa, inferior orbital fissure, infratemporal fossa – appears usually hypointense on both T1 and T2 and does not enhance on CT or MR after contrast agent administration. Conversely, enhancement is shown either by the thickened inflamed sinonasal mucosa or by lesion remnants. Of course, inflammatory mucosal changes appear hyperintense also on T2 sequences, whereas juvenile angiofibroma has intermediate signal intensity. In addition, signal voids may be observed, their detection probably depending on the overall size of the persistent juvenile angiofibroma.

Nevertheless, it is not infrequent to image enhancing submucosal areas filling previous site(s) of the lesion. Serial examinations appear necessary to effectively estimate their growth, a finding that should be consistent with residual lesions (Fig. 8.41). However, known lesion remnants – left in place during surgery – may not show increase in size (DESCHLER et al. 1992). Angiography has been advocated to obtain a definite diagnosis, but it is hampered by false positive results (BREMER et al. 1986).

Owing to this limitation, and because the surgical treatment of small residuals – particularly those intracranially located – is rather controversial, the role

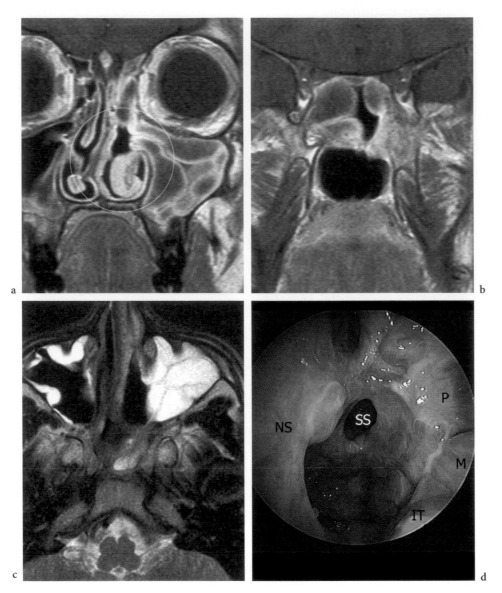

Fig. 8.40a–d. Juvenile angiofibroma: postsurgical changes after endonasal surgery, normal findings. Enhanced SE T1 in the coronal plane (**a,b**), TSE T2 in the axial plane (**c**), endoscopic view (**d**). Thickening of the mucosal layer of both maxillary and sphenoid sinuses and ballooning of the mucosa (with liquid content) is quite a common finding in early postoperative examinations. The encircled area corresponds to the endoscopic view. *NS*, nasal septum; *SS*, sphenoid sinus; *P*, mucosa investing the posterior maxillary sinus wall; *M*, inferior border of the widened maxillary ostium; *IT*, inferior turbinate

of angiography remains unclear (CHAGNAUD et al. 1998).

In effect, small submucosal residuals may be demonstrated by imaging modalities in otherwise asymptomatic patients with negative endoscopy. To adopt a proper treatment strategy, it would be necessary to know more about their spontaneous evolution: recurrent symptoms, regression of residual lesion, or

persistent asymptomatic, residual complications. Moreover, spontaneous regression of juvenile angiofibroma residues has been reported (STANSBIE and PHELPS 1986; DOHAR and DUVALL 1992).

A systematic postoperative imaging follow-up is, consequently, suggested. The use of MR is preferable because it avoids further radiation exposure of the young patients.

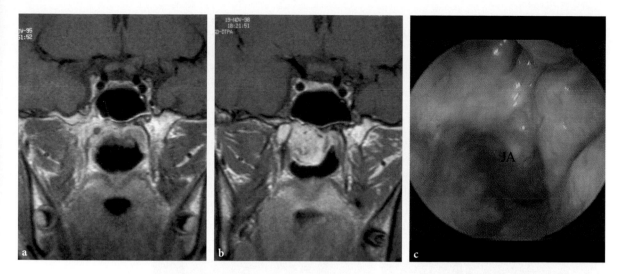

Fig. 8.41a–c. Recurrent/persistent juvenile angiofibroma (*JA*). SE T1 after contrast administration, coronal plane (**a,b**); endoscopic view (**c**). **a** Normal postsurgical MR findings are demonstrated in the first follow-up examination. **b** Patient did not follow a regular imaging and clinical follow-up. He presented 3 years after surgery showing a recurrent/persistent lesion at the level of the pterygoid root (**b**) with a prevalently exophytic pattern of growth, detectable on endoscopic examination (**c**)

8.8
Pyogenic Granuloma
(Lobular Capillary Hemangioma)

8.8.1
Definition, Epidemiology, Pattern of Growth

First reported in the nineteenth century by PONCET and DOR (1897) with the term of botryomycoma, pyogenic granuloma is a benign, rapidly growing lesion, characterized by a lobular proliferation of capillaries (MILLS et al. 1980), also known with several other names (i.e., telangiectatic granuloma, granuloma pedunculatum, infected granuloma). Even though the term "pyogenic granuloma" is the most commonly used, it does not address the true nature of the lesion, which is neither the result of a bacterial infection nor a true granuloma (EL-SAYED and AL-SERHANI 1997).

In 1980, the synonym "lobular capillary hemangioma" was proposed as an adequate term to indicate a lesion which consists of capillaries arranged in lobules and separated by a loose connective tissue stroma, often infiltrated by inflammatory cells (MILLS et al. 1980).

Lobular capillary hemangioma mainly affects the female population, with a peak incidence in the third decade (range: 11–65 years) (LEYDEN and MASTER 1973; EL-SAYED and AL-SERHANI 1997). The lesion may involve skin and mucosa, most often in the oral cavity, where the lips are more frequently affected (about 38% of patients). Sinonasal localization ranges from 7% to 29%, the anterior portion of the nasal septum and the turbinates being the most frequently involved areas (JAFEK et al. 1977; MILLS et al. 1980).

The pathogenesis of the lesion is still unclear. Nasal trauma and hormonal imbalances have been postulated as possible etiologic factors (LANCE et al. 1992). The second hypothesis seems to play a role in a variant of lobular capillary hemangioma known as granuloma gravidarum, which usually appears on the gingival mucosa during pregnancy (MILLER et al. 1999).

8.8.2
Treatment Guidelines

The ideal treatment for lobular capillary hemangioma is radical surgery, which in most cases can be performed through a microendoscopic approach even in very extensive lesions. Other alternative treatments (i.e., electrocoagulation, cryotherapy, Nd:YAG laser) have been successfully employed (MAYER 1962; LEOPARD 1975; POWELL et al. 1994). Routine use of preoperative microembolization, which was suggested to improve bleeding control in oral lesions (FORMAN and GOLDBERG 1990), does not seem routinely justified for sinonasal localizations.

8.8.3
Key Information to Be Provided by Imaging

- Site, size, and vascularization of the lesion

8.8.4
Imaging Findings

Pyogenic granuloma has no distinctive imaging features. CT shows a soft tissue density mass with lobulated contours more commonly arising from the nasal septum (SIMO et al. 1998) (Fig. 8.42). Sinus opacification can be observed when the mass impairs any of the mucus drainage pathways. Bony remodeling is usually observed, while bony destruction has been described in a single case (LANCE et al. 1992).

On MR, pyogenic granuloma exhibits intermediate to bright signal on T2 and hypointense signal on T1 sequences (Fig. 8.43). Relevant enhancement is observed after either Gd-based or iodine contrast administration (EL-SAYED and AL-SERHANI 1997). Angiography demonstrates the presence of several arteries converging into the lesion.

The differential diagnosis should be restricted to highly vascularized sinonasal masses: hemangioma, hemangiopericytoma, juvenile angiofibroma, paraganglioma and vascularized metastases (kidney, thy-

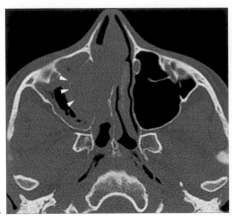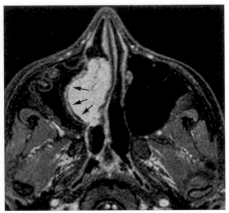

Fig. 8.42a,b. Pyogenic granuloma. Plain CT, enhanced VIBE, axial plane. A polypoid mass occupies the right nasal fossa, indenting the medial maxillary sinus wall. This appears almost completely demineralized on CT (*white arrowheads*), whereas MR shows permeation of a residual hypointense periosteal layer (*black arrows*). CT density is unremarkable, bright and uniform enhancement is demonstrated on Gd-DTPA VIBE sequence

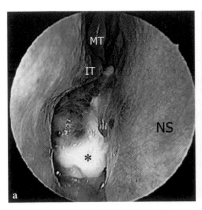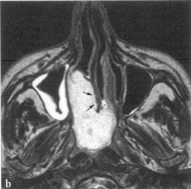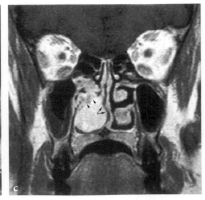

Fig. 8.43a–c. Pyogenic granuloma. Endoscopy (a), TSE T2 (b) on axial plane, enhanced T1 on coronal plane (c). a Endoscopy of the right nasal fossa shows a pale polypoid mass completely filling the inferior meatus and displacing superiorly the inferior turbinate (*IT*). *NS*, nasal septum; *MT*, middle turbinate. The lobular capillary hemangioma has a hyperintense signal on T2 sequence, it turns around the septum to extend into the contralateral choana. At surgery, the lesion was demonstrated to arise from posterior nasal septum (*arrows*). c On the enhanced coronal T1 image a focal irregularity on the right surface of the nasal septum (*arrows*) is seen. The inferior turbinate is displaced superiorly (*arrowheads*)

roid, lung, breast). Unfortunately, among these, exclusively juvenile angiofibroma holds pathognomonic features (site of origin, presence of intralesional vascular flow voids, age, and male sex of patients). As a consequence, pyogenic granuloma can be suspected only by matching imaging findings and clinical history (female sex, age in the range 20–40 years, pregnancy, site of origin of the lesion).

8.8.4.1
Differential Diagnosis with Cavernous Hemangioma

On CT, cavernous hemangioma may be very difficult to be suspected. Plain study can detect a unilateral hypodense mass, that may be associated with destruction of the sinusal bony walls, showing poor to mild, non-homogeneous enhancement (LOH et al. 1994; KIM et al. 1995; DUFOUR et al. 2001). On MR, cavernous hemangioma usually shows intermediate T1 and hyperintense T2 signal, prior to contrast administration (Fig. 8.44). The enhancement is remarkable. Signal voids corresponding to enlarged vessels may also be detected within the lesion. Angiography further defines the vascular supply to the mass. Preoperative embolization has been recommended to prevent uncontrollable hemorrhage (KILDE et al. 2003).

The differential diagnosis includes capillary hemangioma (pyogenic granuloma), hemangioendothelioma, angiosarcoma, and Kaposi's sarcoma. Most

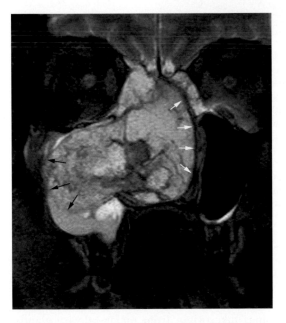

Fig. 8.44. Cavernous hemangioma. TSE T2 fat-sat coronal plane. In the right nasal fossa a large hemangioma extends deeply into the maxillary sinus (*black arrows*) and displaces the nasal septum contralaterally (*white arrows*)

cavernous hemangiomas arise from the maxillary sinus (KULKARNI et al. 1989), while capillary hemangioma more frequently is seen at the nasal septum (IWATA et al. 2002; KILDE et al. 2003) and is characterized by a dense enhancement on both CT and MR. Furthermore, adjacent bony structures are usually remodeled rather than eroded (DILLON et al. 1991).

8.9
Unusual Benign Lesions

A large spectrum of unusual benign lesions taking origin from minor salivary glands (i.e., pleomorphic adenoma, monomorphic adenoma) (COMPAGNO and WONG 1977; CANO CUENCA et al. 2000; LONDON et al. 2002) and soft tissues (i.e., benign fibrous histiocytoma, hemangioma, inflammatory myofibroblastic tumor, leiomyoma, myxoma, paraganglioma, schwannoma) (GREGOR and LOFTUS-COLL 1994; BASAK et al. 1998; SUYSAL et al. 2001; BLOOM et al. 2001; KILDE et al. 2003; CAKMAK et al. 2003; KETABCHI et al. 2003) has been reported in the sinonasal tract (Fig. 8.45).

The predominant symptom is unilateral nasal obstruction, which is mostly related to the presence of a polypoid or sessile lesion of variable macroscopic appearance. When the lesion entirely fills the nasal cavity, determination of the site of origin can be very difficult even resorting to endoscopic examination.

Information provided by imaging rarely suggests the histologic diagnosis, but it is essential to discriminate between liquid vs. solid content of the lesion, together with the degree of vascularization. Moreover, imaging may detect connection or extension to the anterior cranial fossa.

Apart from the very rare lesions extending intracranially (NICOLAI et al. 1996), benign tumors are generally amenable with microendoscopic surgery.

Since most of the aforementioned lesions share the same epidemiologic, clinical and radiologic profile, as well as the same treatment guidelines, only pleomorphic adenoma, schwannoma, leiomyoma, and paraganglioma, which are more frequently observed in the sinonasal tract, will be discussed in detail.

8.9.1
Pleomorphic Adenoma (Mixed Tumor)

With more than 100 cases reported in the literature (COMPAGNO and WONG 1977; FREEMAN et al.

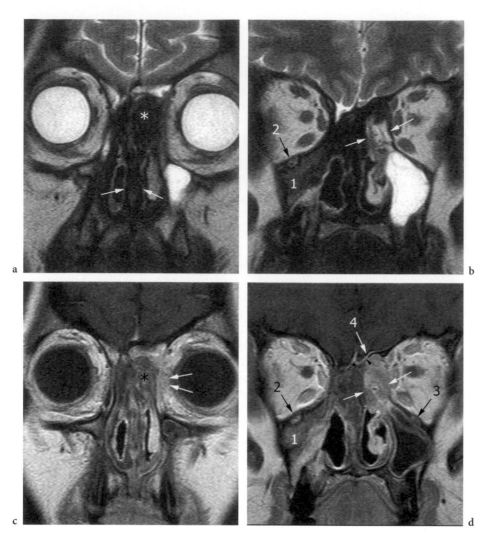

Fig. 8.45a–d. Myofibroblastic inflammatory tumor. TSE T2 (**a**) and enhanced T1 (**b**) on coronal plane. **a** On left side, the ethmoid is occupied by an hypointense mass (*asterisk*) abutting the adjacent lamina papyracea. Extensive thickening of the nasal septum due to spread of lesion is demonstrated (*arrows*). Retained secretions within frontal sinus are characterized by bright signal. **b** Posteriorly, the mass shows intermediate signal intensity (*white arrows*), it causes blockage of left maxillary sinus. On the opposite side, the maxillary sinus is partially filled by signal intensity consistent with lesion (*1*). Thickening of anterior infraorbital canal is present (*2*). **c** Same level as (**a**) after Gd-DTPA: non-homogeneous enhancement of the left ethmoid (*asterisk*) and septal lesions is shown. Effacement of intraorbital fat is also present (*arrows*). **d** Same level as (**b**) after Gd-DTPA: enhancement of the lesion extending into right maxillary sinus is demonstrated (*1*). Compared to the left side (*3*), the right infraorbital nerve presents perineural thickening and enhancement (*2*). Focal interruption of hypointense periosteal/bony layer (*arrowhead*) of the left fovea is associated with enhanced thickened dura (*4*)

1990; PRAGER et al. 1991; LIAO and CHONG 1993; WAKAMI et al. 1996; GOLZ et al. 1997; JASSAR et al. 1999; MAKEIEFF et al. 1999; FACON et al. 2002), pleomorphic adenoma is the most common benign tumor of the sinonasal tract after osteoma and inverted papilloma. Histologically, the neoplasm displays a pleomorphic architecture, being made up of luminal-type ductal epithelial cells, myoepithelial cells and tissue of mucoid, myxoid, or chondroid appearance (SHANMUGARATNAM 1991). Most pleomorphic adenomas take origin from major salivary glands, whereas only about 10% affect minor salivary glands, more commonly of the hard and soft palate (PRAGER et al. 1991; LIAO and CHONG 1993). The tumor may rarely occur in other sites such as the lacrimal gland, larynx, pharynx, sinonasal tract, and trachea. Data from two major reviews of patients with pleomorphic adenoma of the sinonasal area (COMPAGNO and WONG 1977; WAKAMI et al. 1996) clearly identify the nasal septum as the most frequently affected site, followed by the maxillary sinus. Pleomorphic adenoma usually affects patients in the fifth decade of life, with a slight female predominance. At present, no one of the histogenetic hypotheses (i.e., misplaced embryogenic ectodermal epithelial cells, residual of the vomeronasal organ, fully developed salivary gland tissue) postulated to explain the origin of the lesion from the nasal septum is fully accepted (STEVENSON 1932; MATTHEW et al. 1944; EVANS and CRUICKSHANK 1970). Strangely enough, fewer minor salivary glands are present in the septal submucosa than in other sinonasal anatomic areas (WALLACE et al. 1990).

A recurrence rate of 10% after surgical treatment has been specifically reported for sinonasal localizations by COMPAGNO and WONG (1977). According to the authors, this low recurrence rate might be related to the histologic profile of sinonasal pleomorphic adenoma, which presents more cells and less myxoid stroma than the major salivary gland counterpart. Distant metastases and malignant degeneration have been rarely observed (FREEMAN et al. 1990; CHO et al. 1995).

8.9.1.1
Imaging Findings

Sinonasal pleomorphic adenoma generally appears as a well-defined soft tissue mass, most commonly arising from the nasal septum (PISANI et al. 1998) (Fig. 8.46). Bone destruction is unexpected, unless malignant transformation has occurred (YIOTAKIS et al. 2001b). Ossification has been described in an isolated report (LEE et al. 1992).

As for lesions arising in more typical sites (such as the parotid gland), MR findings consist of T2 hyperintensity, low to intermediate T1 signal and non-homogeneous enhancement (YIOTAKIS et al. 2001b; UNLU et al. 2003).

Nonetheless, none of the above-mentioned features support a definitive diagnosis.

8.9.2
Schwannoma

According to the WHO classification (SHANMUGARATNAM 1991), schwannoma is a benign tumor taking origin from Schwann cells. Even though this tumor has been in the past indicated with other synonyms such as neurilemmoma, neurinoma, neurolemmoma, neuroma, perineural fibroblastoma, peripheral fibromatosis, peripheral glioma and schwannoglioma, schwannoma nowadays is universally considered the most adequate term. From a macroscopic standpoint, schwannomas are well encapsulated, gelatinous, or cystic lesions.

Schwannoma frequently occurs in the head and neck area (25%–45%), but only about 4% of the lesions involve the sinonasal tract (YOUNIS et al. 1991; DONNELLY et al. 1992). In this region, the ethmoid complex is the more frequently affected site, followed by the maxillary sinus, nasal septum, and sphenoid

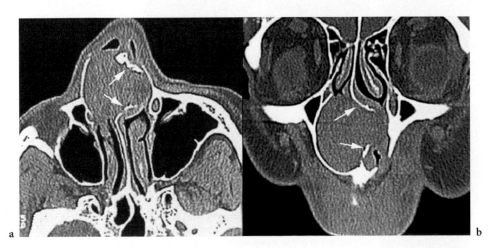

Fig. 8.46a,b. Pleomorphic adenoma. Plain CT on axial (**a**) and coronal plane (**b**). Non-homogeneous soft tissue mass centered on the anterior part of the septum and occupying both nasal vestibules. Both displacement and erosion of the septum are demonstrated (*arrows*). (Courtesy of Castelnuovo, MD and Di Giulio, MD, Pavia, Italy)

sinus (Berlucchi et al. 2000). Most cases occur between the second and fifth decade of life (range: 6–78 years); there is no specific association with sex or race (Higo et al. 1993). Even though some schwannomas of the sinonasal tract are associated with Von Recklinghausen's disease, the neoplasm usually occurs in the solitary form (Oi et al. 1993).

The risk of malignant transformation is very low; however an increase in patients affected by Von Recklinghausen's disease (about 10%–15% of cases) has been observed (Butugan et al. 1993).

8.9.2.1
Imaging Findings

CT and MR appearance of sinonasal schwannomas is rather nonspecific. Remodeling and interruption of adjacent bony structures are frequent findings, which may be present alone or in association (Fujiyoshi et al. 1997) (Fig. 8.47). MR findings reflect the histologic features of the lesion. In detail, the prevalence of Antoni A component (highly cellular) results in intermediate signal on both T1 and T2. On the other hand, whenever an Antoni B pattern is predominant, schwannomas exhibit a more cystic appearance. In fact, in these cases, T2 hyperintensity is observed,

due to the presence of intercellular loose myxoid stroma. Contrast uptake is variable and often non-homogeneous (Bando et al. 1992; Sarioglu et al. 2002, Cakmak et al. 2003; Quesada et al. 2003). No enhancement is observed in cystic areas of Antoni B schwannomas (Sarioglu et al. 2002). Intracranial extension has been reported in few cases (Fujiyoshi et al. 1997).

8.9.3
Leiomyoma

Leiomyoma is a benign myogenic neoplasm which may sporadically occur in the sinonasal area (Zijlker and Visser 1989; Nall et al. 1997). From the histological standpoint, it is classified into the following subtypes: vascular, nonvascular, and epithelioid, also known as leiomyoblastoma (Batsakis 1978). In the former type, the lesion seems to arise from vessel walls. In the second type, neoplastic cells are generally spindle-shaped and associated with lengthened blunt-ended nuclei and eosinophilic cytoplasm. In the epithelioid form, the cells are round or polygonal, with clear or eosinophilic cytoplasm (Shanmugaratnam 1991).

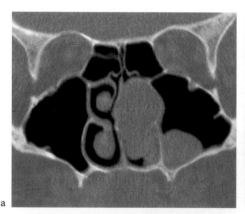
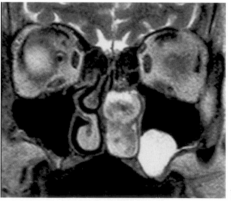
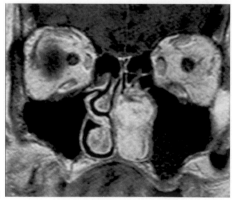

Fig. 8.47a–c. Benign schwannoma. Plain CT (**a**), SE T2 (**b**), Gd-DTPA SE T1(**c**), coronal plane. A soft tissue mass occupies the left nasal fossa. Mild displacement of the nasal septum is observed, in the absence of bone destruction. Bright contrast enhancement might reflect the relative prevalence of Antoni *A* component in the histology of the lesion

HACHISUGA et al. (1984), in a large series of 562 patients affected by leiomyoma, observed only five cases of sinonasal involvement. NICOLAI et al. (1996), in a review of the literature, identified about 30 instances of well-documented sinonasal leiomyomas. The neoplasm usually affects subjects between the fifth and sixth decade of life, with a slight predominance for females.

The rarity of such a lesion in the sinonasal tract may be explained by the paucity of vascular smooth muscle fibers, which are considered the elements of origin (BATSAKIS 1978; MCCAFFREY et al. 1978;). According to other theories, the lesion could stem from aberrant undifferentiated mesenchymal cells or from piloerector or sweat gland muscles (BATSAKIS 1978; BARR et al. 1990).

8.9.3.1
Imaging Findings

Both the lack of specificity of CT or MR findings and the extreme rarity of sinonasal leiomyoma make an imaging based diagnosis nearly impossible. As an aggressive pattern of growth has sometimes been described for this benign lesion – including bone destruction and orbit encroachment (HARCOURT and GALLIMORI 1993; TROTT et al. 1994) – the main role of imaging is to precisely define the deep extension of the lesion.

8.9.4
Paraganglioma

Paraganglioma is a benign neoplasm made up of cells originating from the neural crest and later migrating together with ganglionic cells of the autonomic nervous system. Histologically, the lesion is characterized by nests of epithelioid cells (Zellballen), surrounded by a capillary network (SHANMUGARATNAM 1991). Other terms such as glomus tumor, chemodectoma and apudoma have been used, but at present paraganglioma is the recommended name. Paragangliomas are commonly divided into adrenal (i.e., pheochromocytomas) and extra-adrenal in relation to the site of origin. The latter group includes cervicofacial paragangliomas, which rarely secrete catecholamines and therefore are classified as non-chromaffin. Most cases take origin in the temporal bone (glomus jugulare and glomus tympanicum), above the bifurcation of the carotid artery (carotid body), and from the nodose ganglion (glomus intravagale) (LACK et al. 1977), whereas localization in the sinonasal tract is exceedingly rare, with approxi-

mately 30 cases reported in the literature (KETABCHI et al. 2003). In this area, the lesion more frequently involves the ethmoid and the middle turbinate; furthermore, there is a slight predominance in females and in the fifth decade of life (KETABCHI et al. 2003).

As in other anatomic sites, paraganglioma of the sinonasal tract may display an aggressive behavior and an infiltrating growth pattern (WELKOBORSKY et al. 2000). According to a recent review of the literature (KETABCHI et al. 2003), six patients with paraganglioma of the sinonasal tract presented distant or regional metastases. Increased mitotic figures, necrosis, vascular invasion, aneuploidy and a high proliferation rate may be important indicators for identifying lesions with a potentially aggressive biological behavior (SHANMUGARATNAM 1991; WELKOBORSKY et al. 2000)

8.9.4.1
Imaging Findings

Sinonasal paragangliomas exhibit no distinctive imaging feature. On both CT and MR sinonasal paragangliomas appear as markedly enhancing lesions; bone destruction can be observed (MYSSIOREK 2001) (Fig. 8.48). The differential diagnosis is therefore restricted to highly vascularized lesions, such as lobular capillary hemangioma, hemangiopericytoma, schwannoma, and metastases (particularly from kidney, breast, and thyroid cancer).

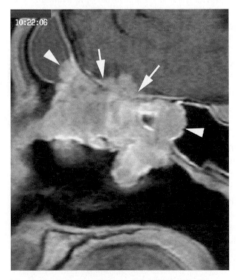

Fig. 8.48. Paraganglioma. Gd-DTPA SE T1 on sagittal plane. Brightly enhancing ethmoid lesion eroding the anterior cranial fossa floor. Note encroachment of the hyperintense signal of the dura (*arrows*), indicating intradural extension. The lesion also invades both the frontal and sphenoid sinus (*arrowheads*)

References

Adams WM, Jones RI, Chavda SI et al (1998) Pneumosinus dilatans: a discussion of four cases and the possible aetiology. Rhinology 36:40–42

Andrews JC, Fisch U, Valavanis A et al (1989) The surgical management of extensive nasopharyngeal angiofibromas with the infratemporal fossa approach. Laryngoscope 99:429–437

Ariel M, De Dios V, Bond JR et al (1992) Aneurysmal bone cyst: a clinicopathologic study of 238 cases. Cancer 69:2921–2931

Atasoy C, Ustuner E, Erden I et al (2001) Frontal sinus mucocele: a rare complication of craniofacial fibrous dysplasia. Clin Imaging 25:388-391

Attallah N, Jay MM (1981) Osteomas of the paranasal sinus. J Laryngol Otol 95:291–304

Bachor E, Weber R, Kahle R et al (1994) Temporary unilateral amaurosis with pneumosinus dilatans of the sphenoid sinus. Skull Base Surg 4:169–175

Bajaj MS, Pushker N (2002) Inverted papilloma invading the orbit. Orbit 21:155–159

Bando K, Obayashi M, Tsuneharu F (1992) A case of subfrontal schwannoma. No Shinkei Geka 20:1189–1194

Barr GD, More IAR, McCallum HM (1990) Leiomyoma of the nasal septum. J Laryngol Otol 104:891–893

Bartlett JR (1971) Intracranial complications of frontal and ethmoid osteomas. Br J Surg 58:607–609

Basak S, Mutlu C, Erkus M et al (1998) Benign fibrous histiocytoma of the nasal septum. Rhinology 36:133–135

Batsakis JG (1978) Tumors of the head and neck: clinical and pathological considerations, 2nd edn. Williams & Wikins, Baltimore

Benedikt RA, Brown DC, Roth MK et al (1991) Spontaneous drainage of an ethmoidal mucocele: a possible cause of pneumosinus dilatans. AJNR Am J Neuroradiol 12:729–731

Benninger MS, Marks S (1995) The endoscopic management of sphenoid and ethmoid mucoceles with orbital and intracranial extension. Rhinology 33:157–161

Berlucchi M, Piazza C, Blanzuoli L et al (2000) Schwannoma of the nasal septum: a case report with review of the literature. Eur Arch Otorhinolaryngol 257:402–405

Bernier JL, Bhasker SN (1958) Aneurysmal bone cyst of mandibula. Oral Surg 11:1018

Bielamowicz S, Calcaterra TC, Watson D (1993) Inverting papilloma of the head and neck: the UCLA update. Otolaryngol Head Neck Surg 109:71–76

Blitzer A, Kalmon D, Conley J (1989) Craniofacial resection of ossifying fibromas and osteomas of the sinuses. Arch Otolaryngol Head Neck Surg 115:1112–1115

Bloom DC, Finley JC Jr, Broberg TG et al (2001) Leiomyoma of the nasal septum. Rhinology 39:233–235

Bollen E, Vielvoye J, Van Dijk JG et al (1990) Trigeminal neuralgia-like pain in an aged woman with fibrous dysplasia of the skull. Headache 30:277–279

Boysen ME, Olving JH, Vatne K et al (1979) Fibro-osseous lesions of the cranio-facial bones. J Laryngol Otol 93:793–807

Brandwein M, Steinberg B, Thung S et al (1989) Human papillomavirus 6/11 and 16/18 in Schneiderian inverted papillomas. In situ hybridiziation with human papillomavirus RNA preobes. Cancer 63:1708–1713

Breidahl AF, Szwajkun P, Chen YR (1997) Pneumosinus dilatans of the maxillary sinus: a report of two cases. Br J Plast Surg 50:33–39

Bremer JW, Neel HB 3rd, DeSanto LW et al (1986) Angiofibroma: treatment trends in 150 patients during 40 years. Laryngoscope 96:1321–1329

Brodish BN, Morgan CE, Sillers MJ (1999) Endoscopic resection of fibrous-osseous lesions of the paranasal sinuses. Am J Rhinol 13:111–116

Brors D, Draf W (1999) The treatment of inverted papilloma. Curr Opin Otolaryngol Head Neck Surg 7:33–38

Buchwald C, Franzmann MB, Tos S (1995) Sinonasal papillomas: a report of 82 cases in Copenhagen Country, including a longitudinal epidemiological and clinical study. Laryngoscope 105:72–79

Buraczewski J, Dabska M (1971) Pathogenesis of aneurysmal bone cyst. Cancer 28:597–604

Busaba NY, Salman SD (1999) Maxillary sinus mucoceles: clinical presentation and long-term results of endoscopic surgical treatment. Laryngoscope 109:1446-1449

Butugan O, Grazel SS, de Almeida ER et al (1993) Schwannoma of the nasal septum: report of the two cases. Rev Laryngol 114:33–36

Cakmak O, Yavuz H, Yucel T (2003) Nasal and paranasal sinus schwannomas. Eur Arch Otorhinolaryngol 260:195–197

Calcaterra TC, Thompson JW, Paglia DE (1980) Inverting papillomas of the nose and paranasal sinuses. Laryngoscope 90:53–60

Calliauw L, Roels H, Caemaert J (1985) Aneurysmal bone cysts in the cranial vault and base of skull. Surg Neurol 23:193–198

Camilleri AE (1991) Craniofacial fibrous dysplasia. J Laryngol Otol 105:662–666

Cano Cuenca B, Gimenez Vaillo F, Perez Climent F et al (2000) Mucinous cystadenoma of a minor salivary gland of the nasal fossa. An Otorrinolaringol Ibero Am 27:469–476

Casasco A, Houdart E, Biondi A et al (1999) Major complications of percutaneous embolization of skull-base tumors. AJNR Am J Neuroradiol 20:179–181

Casselman JW, De Jonge I, Neyt L et al (1993) MRI in craniofacial fibrous dysplasia. Neuroradiology 35:234–237

Chagnaud C, Petit P, Bartoli J et al (1998) Postoperative follow-up of juvenile nasopharyngeal angiofibromas: assessment by CT scan and MR imaging. Eur Radiol 8:756–764

Chan FL, Chow SK, Sham JST (1992) Infratemporal pneumatocele arising from maxillary sinus. Clin Radiol 45:27–30

Chartrand-Lefebvre C, Dubois J, Roy D et al (1996) Direct intraoperative sclerotherapy of an aneurysmal bone cyst of the sphenoid. AJNR Am J Neuroradiol 17:870–872

Chateil JF, Dousset V, Meyer P et al (1997) Cranial aneurysmal bone cysts presenting with raised intracranial pressure: report of two cases. Neuroradiology 39:490–494

Chee LWJ, Sethi DS (1999) The endoscopic management of sinonasal inverted papillomas. Clin Otolaryngol 24:61–66

Cheng C, Takahashi H, Yao K et al (2002) Cemento-ossifying fibroma of maxillary and sphenoid sinuses: case report and literature review. Acta Otolaryngol Stockh (Suppl) 547:118–122

Cho KJ, el-Naggar AK, Mahanupab P et al (1995) Carcinoma ex-pleomorphic adenoma of the nasal cavity: a report of two cases. J Laryngol Otol 109:677–679

Chong VF, Tang LH (1997) Maxillary sinus ossifying fibroma. Am J Otolaryngol 18:419–424

Citardi MJ, Janjua T, Abrahams JJ et al (1996) Orbitoethmoid aneurysmal bone cyst. Otolaryngol Head Neck Surg 114:466–470

Commins DJ, Tolley NS, Milford CA (1998) Fibrous dysplasia and ossifying fibroma of the paranasal sinuses. J Laryngol Otol 112:964–968

Compagno J, Wong RT (1977) Intranasal mixed tumours (pleomorphic adenomas): a clinicopathologic study of 40 cases. Am J Clin Pathol 68:213–218

Cooter MS, Charlton SA, Lafreniere D et al (1998) Endoscopic management of an inverted nasal papilloma in a child. Otolaryngol Head Neck Surg 118:876–879

Dammann F, Pereira P, Laniado M et al (1999) Inverted papilloma of the nasal cavity and the paranasal sinuses: using CT for primary diagnosis and follow-up. AJR Am J Roentgenol 172:543–548

Danesi G, Panizza B, Mazzoni A et al (2000) Anterior approaches in juvenile nasopharyngeal angiofibromas with intracranial extension. Otolaryngol Head Neck Surg 122:277–283

De Minteguiaga C, Portier F, Guichard JP et al (2001) Aneurysmal bone cyst in the sphenoid bone: treatment with minimally invasive surgery. Ann Otol Rhinol Laryngol 110:331–334

Deschler DG, Kaplan MJ, Boles R (1992) Treatment of large juvenile nasopharyngeal angiofibroma. Otolaryngol Head Neck Surg 106:278–284

Dillon WP, Som PM, Rosenau W (1991) Hemangioma of the nasal vault: MR and CT features. Radiology 180:761–765

Dohar JE, Duvall AJ 3rd (1992) Spontaneous regression of juvenile nasopharyngeal angiofibroma. Ann Otol Rhinol Laryngol 101:469–471

Donnelly M, Al-Seder MH, Blayney AW (1992) Benign nasal schwannoma. J Laryngol Otol 106:1011–1015

Draf W (1991) Endonasal micro-endoscopic frontal sinus surgery: the Fulda concept. Op Tech Otolaryngol Head Neck Surg 4:234–240

Dufour H, Fesselet J, Metellus P et al (2001) Cavernous hemangioma of the sphenoid sinus: case report and review of the literature. Surg Neurol 55:169–173; discussion 173

Earwaker J (1993) Paranasal sinus osteomas: A review of 46 cases. Skeletal Radiol 22:417–423

El-Mofty S (2002) Psammomatoid and trabecular juvenile ossifying fibroma of the craniofacial skeleton: two distinct clinicopathologic entities. Oral Surg Oral Med Oral Pathol Oral Radiol Endod 93:296–304

Elner VM, Burnstine MA, Goodman ML et al (1995) Inverted papillomas that invade the orbit. Arch Ophthalmol 113:1178–1183

El-Sayed Y, Al-Serhani A (1997) Lobular capillary haemangioma (pyogenic granuloma) of the nose. J Laryngol Otol 111:941–945

Engelbrecht V, Preis S, Hassler W et al (1999) CT and MRI of congenital sinonasal ossifying fibroma. Neuroradiology 41:526–529

Evans RW, Cruickshand AH (1970) Major problems in pathology. Epithelial tumors of the salivary glands. Saunders WB, Philadelphia

Eversole LR, Leider AS, Nelson K (1985) Ossifying fibroma: a clinicopathologic study of sixty-four cases. Oral Surg Oral Med Oral Pathol 60:505–511

Facon F, Paris J, Ayache S et al (2002) Adènome plèomorphic des fosses nasals: une localisation à la cloison inter sinuso nasale. Rev Laryngol Otol Rhinol 123:103–107

Fechner RE, Alford DO (1968) Inverted papilloma and squamous carcinoma. An unusual case. Arch Otolaryngol 88:507–512

Ferguson BJ (1994) Fibrous dysplasia of the paranasal sinuses. Am J Otolaryngol 15:227–230

Forman D, Goldberg HI (1990) Microembolization and resection of a highly vascular pyogenic granuloma. J Oral Maxillofac Surg 48:415–418

Freeman SB, Kennedy KS, Parker GS et al (1990) Metastasizing pleomorphic adenoma of the nasal septum. Arch Otolaryngol Head Neck Surg 116:1331–1333

Fu YS, Perzin KH (1974) Non-epithelial tumors of the nasal cavity, paranasal sinuses, and nasopharynx: a clinicopathologic study. Cancer 33:1289–1305

Fujimoto Y, Katoh M, Miyata M et al (1987) Cystic cemento-ossifying fibroma of the ethmoidal cells. J Laryngol Otol 101:946–952

Fujiyoshi F, Kajiya Y, Nakajo M (1997) CT and MR imaging of nasoethmoid schwannoma with intracranial extension. AJR Am J Roentgenol 169:1754–1755

Furuta Y, Shinohara T, Sano K et al (1991) Molecular pathologic study of human papillomavirus infection in inverted papilloma and squamous cell carcinoma of nasal cavities and paranasal sinuses. Laryngoscope 101:79–85

Gaffey MJ, Frierson HF, Weiss LM et al (1996) Human papillomavirus and Epstein-Barr virus in sinonasal Schneiderian papillomas. An in situ hybridization and polymerase chain reaction study. Am J Clin Pathol 106:475–482

Gillman GS, Lampe HB, Allen LH (1997) Orbitoethmoid osteoma: case report of an uncommon presentation of an uncommon tumor. Otolaryngol Head Neck Surg 117: S218–220

Golz A, Ben-Arie Y, Fradis M (1997) Pleomorphic nasoseptal adenoma. J Otolaryngol 26:399–401

Gregor RT, Loftus-Coll B (1994) Myxoma of the paranasal sinuses. J Laryngol Otol. 108:679–681

Hachisuga T, Hashimoto O, Enjoji A (1984) Angioleiomyoma: a clinicopathological reappraisal of 562 cases. Cancer 54:126–130

Hady MR, Ghanaam B, Hady MZ (1990) Aneurysmal bone cyst of the maxillary sinus. J Laryngol Otol 104:501–503

Hamner JE, Scofeild HH, Cornyn J (1968) Benign fibro-osseous jaw lesions of periodontal membrane origin. Cancer 22:861–878

Han JK, Smith TL, Loehrl T et al (2001) An evolution in the management of sinonasal inverting papilloma. Laryngoscope 111:1395–1400

Han MH, Chang KH, Lee CH et al (1991) Sinonasal psammomatoid ossifying fibromas: CT and MR manifestations. AJNR Am J Neuroradiol 12:25–30

Han MH, Chang KH, Lee CH et al (1995) Cystic expansile masses of the maxilla: differential diagnosis with CT and MR. AJNR Am J Neuroradiol 16:333–338

Harcourt JP, Gallimore AP (1993) Leiomyoma of the paranasal sinuses. J Laryngol Otol 107:740–741

Har-El G (2001) Endoscopic management of 108 sinus muceles. Laryngoscope 111:2131–2134

Harrison D, Lund VJ (1993) Tumours of the Upper Jaw. London, Churchill Livingstone

Hartley BE, Lund VJ (1999) Endoscopic drainage of pediatric paranasal sinus mucoceles. Int J Pediatr Otorhinolaryngol 50:109–111

Hartwidge C, Varma TR (1984) Intracranial aeroceles as a

complication of frontal sinus osteoma. Surg Neurol 24:401–404

Hejazi N, Witzmann A, Hassler W (2001) Ocular manifestations of sphenoid mucoceles: clinical features and neurosurgical management of three cases and review of the literature. Surg Neurol 56:338–343

Herman P, Lot G, Chapot R et al (1999) Long-term follow-up of juvenile nasopharyngeal angiofibromas: analysis of recurrences. Laryngoscope 109:140–147

Higo R, Yamasoba T, Kikuchi S (1993) Nasal neurinoma: case report and review of literature. Auris Nasus Larynx 20:297–301

Hirst LW, Miller NR, Allen GS (1979) Sphenoidal pneumosinus dilatans with bilateral optic nerve meningiomas. J Neurosurg 51:402–407

Howard DJ, Lloyd G, Lund V (2001) Recurrence and its avoidance in juvenile angiofibroma. Laryngoscope 111:1509–1511

Hrishikesh KA, Narlawar RS, Deasi SB et al (2002) Case report: Aneurysmal bone cyst of the ethmoid bone. Br J Radiol 75:916–918

Huang HM, Liu CM, Lin KN et al (2001) Giant ethmoid osteoma with orbital extension, a nasoendoscopic approach using an intranasal drill. Laryngoscope 111:430–432

Huang PC, Misko G (1998) Imaging quiz case 1. Osteoma of the ethmoidal sinus. Arch Otolaryngol Head Neck Surg 124:602, 604–605

Huneidi A, Afshar F (1989) Chronic spontaneous tension pneumocephalus due benign frontal osteoma. Br J Neurosurg 3:389–392

Hyams VJ (1971) Papillomas of the nasal cavity and paranasal sinuses. A clinicopathological study of 315 cases. Ann Otol Rhinol Laryngol 80:192–206

Hyams VJ, Batsakis JG, Michaels L (1988) Tumors of the upper respiratory tract and ear. Washington, Armed Forces Institute of Pathology

Ichimura K, Ohta Y, Maeda YI et al (2001) Mucoceles of the paranasal sinuses with intracranial extension. Postoperative course. Am J Rhinol 15:243–247

Ikeda K, Takahashi C, Oshima T et al (2000) Endonasal endoscopic marsupialization of paranasal sinus mucoceles. Am J Rhinol 14:107–111

Iwata N, Hattori K, Nakagawa T et al (2002) Hemangioma of the nasal cavity: a clinicopathologic study. Auris Nasus Larynx 29:335–339

Jafek BW, Wood RP 2nd, Dion M (1977) Granuloma pyogenicum. Ear Nose Throat J 56:228–233

Jaffe HL, Lichtenstein L (1942) Solitary unicameral bone cyst with emphasis on the roentgen picture, the pathologic appearance, and the pathogenesis. Arch Surg 44:1004–1025

Jassar P, Stafford ND, MacDonald AW (1999) Pleomorphic adenoma of the nasal septum. J Laryngol Otol 113:483–485

Johnson LC, Yousefi M, Vinh TN et al (1991) Juvenile active ossifying fibroma: its nature, dynamics and origin. Acta Otolaryngol Stockh (Suppl) 488:1–40

Kamel RH (1995) Transnasal endoscopic medial maxillectomy in inverted papilloma. Laryngoscope 105:847–853

Kapadia SB, Barnes L, Pelzman K et al (1993) Carcinoma ex oncocytic schneiderian (cylindrical cell) papilloma. Am J Otolaryngol 14:332–338

Karlidag T, Yalcin S, Kaygusuz I et al (2003) Bilateral pneumosinus dilatans of the maxillary sinuses. Br J Oral Maxillofac Surg 41:122–123

Kass ES, Fabian RL, Montgomery WW (1999) Manometric study of paranasal sinus mucoceles. Ann Otol Rhinol Laryngol 108:63–66

Kass ES, Salman S, Rubin PA et al (1997) Chronic maxillary atelectasis. Ann Otol Rhinol Laryngol 106:109–116

Kennedy DW, Josephson JS, Zinreich SJ et al (1989) Endoscopic sinus surgery for mucoceles: a viable alternative. Laryngoscope 99:885–895

Kershisnik M, Bataskis JG (1994) Aneurysmal bone cysts of the jaws. Ann Otol Rhinol Laryngol 103:164–165

Ketabchi S, Massi D, Santoro R et al (2003) Paraganglioma of the nasal cavity: a case report. Eur Arch Otorhinolaryngol 260:336–340

Kilde JD, Rhee JS, Balla AA et al (2003) Hemangioma of the sphenoid and ethmoid sinuses: two case reports. Ear Nose Throat J 82:217–221

Kim HJ, Kim JH, Hwang EG (1995) Bone erosion caused by sinonasal cavernous hemangioma: CT findings in two patients. AJNR Am J Neuroradiol 16:1176–1178

Kimmelman CP, Potsic WP, Schut L (1982) Aneurysmal bone cyst of the sphenoid in a child. Ann Otol Rhinol Laryngol 91:339–341

Kessler A, Berenholz LP, Segal S (1998) Use of intranasal endoscopic surgery to relieve ostiomeatal complex obstruction in fibrous dysplasia of the paranasal sinuses. Eur Arch Otorhinolaryngol 255:454–456

Klossek JM, Dufour X, Toffel P et al (2000) Pneumosinus dilatans: a report of three new cases and their surgical management. Ear Nose Throat J 79:48–51

Koike Y, Tokoro K, Chiba Y et al (1996) Intracranial extension of paranasal sinus mucocele: two case reports. Surg Neurol 45:44–48

Koiuvnen P, Lopponen H, Fors AP et al (1997) The growth rate of osteomas of the paranasal sinuses. Clin Otolaryngol 22:111–114

Komori E, Sugisaki M (1988) Ectopic pneumosinus maxillary dilatans. A case report. J Craniomaxillofac Surg 16:240–242

Kransdorf MJ, Moser RP Jr, Gilkey FW (1990) Fibrous dysplasia. Radiographics 10:519–537

Kransdorf MJ, Stull MA, Gilkcy FW et al (1991) Osteoid osteoma. Radiographics 11:671–696

Kransdorf MJ, Sweet DE (1995) Aneurysmal bone cyst: concept, controversy, clinical presentation, and imaging. AJR Am J Roentgenol 164:573–580

Krausen AS, Gulman S, Zografakis G (1977) Cementomas. II. Aggressive cemento-ossifying fibroma of the ethmoid region. Arch Otolaryngol Head Neck Surg 103:371–373

Krouse JH (2000) Development of a staging system for inverted papilloma. Laryngoscope 110:965–968

Krouse JH (2001) Endoscopic treatment of inverted papilloma: safety and efficacy. Am J Otolaryngol 22:87–99

Kulkarni MV, Bonner FM, Abdo GJ (1989) Maxillary sinus hemangioma: MR and CT studies. J Comput Assist Tomogr 13:340–342

Lack EE, Cubilla AL, Woodruff JM et al (1977) Paragangliomas of the head and neck region. Cancer 39:397–409

Lance E, Schatz C, Nach R et al (1992) Pyogenic granuloma gravidarum of the nasal fossa: CT features. J Comput Assist Tomogr 16:663–664

Lane JM, Khan SN, O'Connor WJ et al (2001) Bisphosphonate therapy in fibrous dysplasia. Clin Orthop Rel Reser 382:6–12

Lasjaunias P, Picard L, Manelfe C et al (1980) Angiofibroma of the nasopharynx. A review of 53 cases treated by embolisation. The role of pretherapeutic angiography. Pathophysiological hypotheses. J Neuroradiol 7:73–95

Lawson W, Ho BT, Shaari CM et al (1995) Inverted papilloma: a report of 112 cases. Laryngoscope 105:282–288

Lee JT, Bhuta S, Lufkin R et al (2003) Isolated inverting papilloma of the sphenoid sinus. Laryngoscope 113:41–44

Lee KC, Chan JK, Chong YW (1992) Ossifying pleomorphic adenoma of the maxillary antrum. J Laryngol Otol 106:50–52

Lehnerdt G, Weber J, Dost P (2001) Die einseitige verschattung der nasennebenhöhlen im CT oder MRT – Hinweis für einen seltenen histologischen befund. Laryngorhinootologie 80:141–145

Leopard PJ (1975) Cryosurgery, and its application to oral surgery. Br J Oral Surg 13:128–152

Levy WM, Miller AS, Bonakdarpour A et al (1975) Aneurysmal bone cyst secondary to other osseous lesions: report of 57 cases. Am J Clin Pathol 63:1–8

Leyden JJ, Master GH (1973) Oral cavity pyogenic granuloma. Arch Dermatol 108:226–228

Li JR, Qian J, Shan XZ et al (1998) Evaluation of the effectiveness of preoperative embolization in surgery for nasopharyngeal angiofibroma. Eur Arch Otorhinolaryngol 255:430–432

Liao BS, Chong E (1993) Septal pleomorphic adenoma masquerading as squamous cell carcinoma. Ear Nose Throat J 72:781–782

Lichtenstein L (1950) Aneurysmal bone cyst: A pathological entity commonly mistaken for giant cell tumor and occasionally for hemangioma and osteogenic sarcoma. Cancer 3:279–289

Lichtenstein L, Jaffe HL (1942) Fibrous dysplasia of bone. Arch Pathol 33:777–781

Lieberman A, Tovi F (1984) A small osteoma of the frontal sinus causing headaches. J Laryngol Otol 98:1147–1149

Liens D, Delmas PD, Meunier PJ (1994) Long term effects of intravenous pamidronate in fibrous dysplasia of bone. Lancet 343:953–954

Lim CC, Dillon WP, McDermott MW (1999) Mucocele involving the anterior clinoid process: MR and CT findings. AJNR Am J Neuroradiol 20:287–290

Lloyd G, Lund VJ, Savy L et al (2000a) Optimum imaging for mucoceles. J Laryngol Otol 114:233–236

Lloyd G, Howard D, Lund VJ et al (2000b) Imaging for juvenile angiofibroma. J Laryngol Otol 114:727–730

Lloyd G, Howard D, Phelps P et al (1999) Juvenile angiofibroma: the lessons of 20 years of modern imaging. J Laryngol Otol 113:127–134

Lloyd GA (1985) Orbital pneumosinus dilatans. Clin Radiol 36:381–386

Lloyd GA, Phelps PD (1986) Juvenile angiofibroma: imaging by magnetic resonance, CT and conventional techniques. Clin Otolaryngol 11:247–259

Loh LE, Ho KH, Thoo A et al (1994) Hemangioma of the ethmoidal sinuses. Singapore Med J 35:211–214

London SD, Schlosser RJ, Gross CW (2002) Endoscopic management of benign sinonasal tumors: a decade of experience. Am J Rhinol 16:221–227

Lund VJ (1998) Endoscopic management of paranasal sinus mucocoeles. J Laryngol Otol 112:36–40

Lund VJ (2000) Optimum management of inverted papilloma. J Laryngol Otol 114:194–197

Lund VJ, Milroy CM (1991) Fronto-ethmoidal mucocoeles: a histopathological analysis. J Laryngol Otol 105:921–923

Lund VJ, Wilson H, Sajeda M et al (1988) Prostaglandin synthesis in the pathogenesis of fronto-ethmoidal mucocoeles. Acta Otolaryngol (Stockh) 106:145–151

Makeieff M, Youssef B, Gardiner Q et al (1999) Adénome plèomorphe de la cloison nasale. A propos d'un cas. Ann Otolaryngol Chir Cervicofac 116:368–371

Manaka H, Tokoro K, Sakata K et al (1998) Intradural extension of mucocele complicating frontoethmoid sinus osteoma: case report. Surg Neurol 50:453–456

Mansell NJ, Bates GJ (2000) The inverted schneiderian papilloma: a review and literature report of 43 new cases. Rhinology 38:97–101

Maroldi R, Farina D, Palvarini L et al (2004) MRI findings of inverted papilloma: differential diagnosis with malignant sinonasal tumors. Am J Rhinol in press

Marvel JB, Marsh MA, Catlin FI (1991) Ossifying fibroma of the mid-face and paranasal sinuses: diagnostic and therapeutic considerations. Otolaryngol Head Neck Surg 104:803–808

Matthew S, Ersner MD, Saltzman M (1944) A mixed tumor of the nasal septum. Report of a case. Laryngoscope 54:287–296

Mauri M, de Oliveira CO, Franche G (2000) Pneumosinus dilatans of the maxillary sinus. Ann Otol Rhinol Laryngol 109:278–280

Mayer I (1962) Electrocoagulation of oral lesions. Oral Surg 16:522–528

McCaffrey TV, McDonald TJ, Unni KK (1978) Leiomyoma of the nasal cavity. J Laryngol Otol 92:817–819

McCombe A, Lund VJ, Howard DJ (1990) Recurrence in juvenile angiofibroma. Rhinology 28:97–102

Metha BS, Grewal GS (1963) Osteoma of the paranasal sinuses along with a case of an orbito-ethmoid osteoma. J Laryngol Otol 77:601–610

Meyes J (1898) Pneumosinus dilatans. Nederlands Tijdsschrift voor Geneeskunde 11:143

Miller FR, D'Agostino MA, Schlack K (1999) Lobular capillary hemangioma of the nasal cavity. Otolaryngol Head Neck Surg 120:783–784

Mills SE, Cooper PH, Fechner RE (1980) Lobular capillary hemangioma: the underlying lesion of pyogenic granuloma. A study of 73 cases from the oral and nasal mucous membranes. Am J Surg Pathol 4:470–479

Moore AT, Buncic JR, Muro IR (1985) Fibrous dysplasia of the orbit in childhood. Clinical features and management. Ophthalmology 92:12–20

Morrison MD, Tchang SP, Maber BR (1976) Pneumocele of the maxillary sinus. Report of a case. Arch Otolaryngol 102:306–307

Moriyama H, Hesaka H, Tachibana T et al (1992) Mucoceles of ethmoid and sphenoid sinus with visual disturbance. Arch Otolaryngol Head Neck Surg 118:142–146

Moulin G, Chagnaud C, Gras R et al (1995) Juvenile nasopharyngeal angiofibroma: comparison of blood loss during removal in embolized group versus nonembolized group. Cardiovasc Intervent Radiol 18:158–161

Muraoka H, Ishihara A, Kumagai J (2001) Fibrous dysplasia with cystic appearance in maxillary sinus. Auris Nasus Larynx 28:103–105

Myers EN, Fernau JL, Johnson JT et al (1990) Management of inverted papilloma. Laryngoscope 100:481–490

Myssiorek D (2001) Head and neck paragangliomas: an overview. Otolaryngol Clin North Am 34:829–836

Nager GT, Kennedy DW, Kopstein E (1982) Fibrous dysplasia: a review of the disease and its manifestations in the temporal bone. Ann Otol Rhinol Laryngol Suppl 92:1–52

Nall AV, Stringer SP, Baughman RA (1997) Vascular leiomyoma of the superior turbinate: first reported case. Head Neck 19:63–67

Namdar I, Edelstein DR, Huo J et al (1998) Management of osteomas of the paranasal sinuses. Am J Rhinol 12:393–398

Nicolai P, Berlucchi M, Tomenzoli D et al (2003) Endoscopic surgery for juvenile angiofibroma: when and how. Laryngoscope 113:775–782

Nicolai P, Redalli de Zinis LO, Facchetti F et al (1996) Craniofacial resection for vascular leiomyoma of the nasal cavity. Am J Otolaryngol 17:340–344

Oberman HA (1964) Papillomas of the nose and paranasal sinuses. Am J Clin Pathol 42:245–258

Oi H, Watanabe Y, Shojaku H et al (1993) Nasal septum neurinoma. Acta Otolaryngol (Stockh) Suppl 504:151–154

Oikawa K, Furuta Y, Oridate N et al (2003) Preoperative staging of sinonasal inverted papilloma by magnetic resonance imaging. Laryngoscope 113:1983–1987

Ojiri H, Ujita M, Tada S et al (2000) Potentially distinctive features of sinonasal inverted papilloma on MR imaging. AJR Am J Roentgenol 175:465–468

Osguthorpe JD, Gudeman SK (1987) Orbital complications of fibrous dysplasia. Otolaryngol Head Neck Surg 97:403–405

Outzen KE, Grontveld A, Jorgensen K et al (1996) Inverted papilloma: incidence and late results of surgical treatment. Rhinology 34:114–118

Pacini F, Perri G, Bagnolesi P et al (1987) McCune-Albright syndrome with gigantism and hyperprolactinemia. J Endocrinol Invest 10:417–420

Pasquini E, Ceroni Compadretti G, Sciarretta V et al (2002) Transnasal endoscopic surgery for the treatment of fibrous dysplasia of maxillary sinus associated to aneurysmal bone cyst in a 5-year-old child. Int J Pediatr Otorhinolaryngol 62:59–62

Patel BC, Sabir DI, Flaharty PM et al (1993) Aneurysmal bone cyst of the orbit and ethmoid sinus. Arch Ophthalmol 111:586–587

Pelausa EO, Fortier MAG (1992) Schneiderian papilloma of the nose and paranasal sinuses: the University of Ottawa experience. J Otolaryngol 21:9–15

Petit P, Vivarrat-Perrin L, Champsaur P et al (2000) Radiological follow-up of inverted papilloma. Eur Radiol 10:1184–1189

Phillips PP, Gustafson RO, Facer GW (1990) The clinical behavior of inverting papilloma of the nose and paranasal sinuses: report of 112 cases and review of the literature. Laryngoscope 100:463–469

Pisani P, Dosdegani R, Ramponi A et al (1998) Adenoma pleomorfo del setto nasale. Acta Otorhinolaryngol Ital 18:30–33

Poncet A, Dor L (1897) Botryomycose humaine. Rev Chir (Paris) 18:966

Pound E, Pickrell K, Hunger W et al (1965) Fibrous dysplasia of the maxilla. Ann Surg 161:406–410

Powell JL, Bailey CL, Coopland AT et al (1994) Nd:YAG laser excision of a giant gingival pyogenic granuloma of pregnancy. Lasers Surg Med 14:178–183

Prager DA, Weiss MH, Buchalter WL et al (1991) Pleomorphic adenoma of the nasal cavity. Ann Otol Rhinol Laryngol 100:600

Price HI, Batnitzky S, Karlin CA et al (1981) Multiple paranasal sinus mucoceles. J Comput Assist Tomogr 5:122–125

Quesada JL, Enrique A, Lorente J et al (2003) Sinonasal schwannoma treated with endonasal microsurgery. Otolaryngol Head Neck Surg 129:300–302

Rambaux P, Bertrand B, Eloy P et al (2000) Endoscopic endonasal surgery for paranasal sinus mucoceles. Acta Otorhinolaryngol Belg 54:115–122

Ramsey HE, Strong EW, Frazel EL (1968) Fibrous dysplasia of the craniofacial bones. Am J Surg 116:542–547

Rao VM, Sharma D, Madan A (2001) Imaging of frontal sinus disease. Concepts, interpretation and technology. Otolaryngol Clin North Am 34:23–39

Rappaport JM, Attia EL (1994) Pneumocephalus in frontal sinus osteoma. J Otolaryngol 23:430–436

Raynal M, Peynegre R, Beautru R et al (1999) Mucocèles sinusiennes et iatrogénie chirurgicale. Ann Otolaryngol Chir Cervicofac 116:85–91

Redaelli de Zinis LO, Ansarin M, Galli G et al (1996) Approccio chirurgico transbasale-subfrontale in un caso di fibroma ossificante etmoidale. Gior Pat Chir Cr Fa 2:42–45

Reed RJ (1963) Fibrous dysplasia of bone: a review of 25 cases. Arch Pathol 75:480–495

Reicher MA, Bentson JR, Halbach VV et al (1986) Pneumosinus dilatans of the sphenoid sinus. AJNR Am J Neuroradiol 7:865–868

Roberson GH, Biller H, Sessions DG et al (1972) Presurgical internal maxillary artery embolization in juvenile angiofibroma. Laryngoscope 82:1524–1532

Roger G, Tran Ba Huy P, Froehlich P et al (2002) Exclusively endoscopic removal of juvenile nasopharyngeal angiofibroma: trends and limits. Arch Otolaryngol Head Neck Surg 128:928–935

Rosenberg AE (1994) Skeletal system and soft tissues tumors. In: Cotran RS, Kumar V, Robbins SL (eds) Robbins pathologic basis of disease, 5th edn. WB Saunders, Philadelphia, pp 1213–1271

Saito K, Fukuta K, Takahashi M et al (1998) Benign fibroosseous lesions involving the skull base, paranasal sinuses, and nasal cavity. J Neurosurg 88:1116–1119

Samy LL, Mostafa H (1971) Osteoma of the nose and paranasal sinuses with a report of 21 cases. J Laryngol Otol 85:449–469

Sankerkin NG, Mott MG, Roylance J (1983) An unusual intraosseous lesion with fibroblastic, osteoclastic, osteoblastic, aneurysmal and fibromyxoid elements: "solid" variant of aneurysmal bone cyst. Cancer 51:2278–2286

Sarioglu S, Ozkal S, Guneri A et al (2002) Cystic schwannoma of the maxillary sinus. Auris Nasus Larynx 29:297–300

Savic D, Djeric DR (1990) Indications for surgical treatment of osteomas of the frontal and ethmoid sinuses. Clin Otolaryngol 15:397–404

Savy L, Lloyd G, Lund VJ et al (2000) Optimum imaging for inverted papilloma. J Laryngol Otol 114:891–893

Sayan NB, Ucok C, Karasu HA et al (2002) Peripheral osteoma of the oral and maxillofacial region: a study of 35 new cases. J Oral Maxillofac Surg 60:1299–1301

Schick B, Plinkert PK, Prescher A (2002) Die vaskulare komponente: gedanken zur entstehung des Angiofibroms. Laryngorhinootologie 81:280–284

Schick B, Kahle G (2000) Radiological findings in angiofibroma. Acta Radiol 41:585–593

Schick B, Steigerwald C, El Tahan AER et al (2001) The role of endonasal surgery in the management of frontoethmoid osteoma. Rhinology 39:66–70

Schmaman A, Smith I, Ackerman LV (1970) Benign fibro-osseous lesions of the mandible and maxilla: a review of 35 cases. Cancer 26:303–312

Scholtz AW, Appenroth E, Kammen-Jolly K et al (2001) Juvenile nasopharyngeal angiofibroma: management and therapy. Laryngoscope 111:681–687

Schroth G, Haldemann AR, Mariani L et al (1996) Preoperative embolization of paragangliomas and angiofibromas. Measurement of intratumoral arteriovenous shunts. Arch Otolaryngol Head Neck Surg 122:1320–1325

Schwartz DR, Alpert MA (1964) The malignant transformation of fibrous dysplasia. Am J Med Sci 274:35–54

Senol U, Karaali K, Akyuz M et al (2002) Aneurysmal bone cyst of the orbit. AJNR Am J Neuroradiol 23:319–321

Shanmugaratnam K (1991) Histological typing of tumours of the upper respiratory tract and ear. Springer-Verlag, Berlin Heidelberg New York

Shohet JA, Duncavage JA (1996) Management of the frontal sinus with inverted papilloma. Otolaryngol Head Neck Surg 114:649–652

Sievers KW, Greess H, Baum U et al (2000) Paranasal sinuses and nasopharynx CT and MRI. Eur J Radiol 33:185–202

Simo R, De Carpentier J, Rejali D et al (1998) Paediatric pyogenic granuloma presenting as a unilateral nasal polyp. Rhinology 36:136–138

Simovic S, Klapan I, Bumber Z et al (1996) Fibrous dysplasia in paranasal cavities. ORL J Otorhinolaryngol Relat Spec 58:55–58

Siniluoto TM, Luotonen JP, Tikkakoski TA et al (1993) Value of pre-operative embolization in surgery for nasopharyngeal angiofibroma. J Laryngol Otol 107:514–521

Skolnick CA, Mafee MF, Goodwin JA (2000) Pneumosinus dilatans of the sphenoid sinus presenting with visual loss. J Neuroophthalmol 20:259–263

Skoulakis CE, Velegrakis GA, Doxas PG et al (1999) Mucocele of the maxillary antrum in an eight-year-old boy. Int J Pediatr Otorhinolaryngol 47:283–287

Slootweg PJ, Panders AK, Nikkels PGJ (1994) Juvenile ossifying fibroma: an analysis of 33 cases with emphasis on histopathological aspects. J Oral Pathol 23:385–388

Smith JF (1965) Fibrous dysplasia of the jaws. Arch Otolaryngol 81:592–603

Smith ME, Calcaterra TC (1989) Frontal sinus osteoma. Ann Otol Rhinol Laryngol 98:896–900

Som PM, Brandwein M (1996) Sinonasal cavities: inflammatory diseases, Tumors, fractures, and postoperative findings. In: Som PM, Curtin HD (eds) Head and neck imaging. Mosby Year Book, St. Louis, pp 227–229

Som PM, Dillon WP, Fullerton GD et al (1989) Chronically obstructed sinonasal secretions: observations on T1 and T2 shortening. Radiology 172:515–520

Som PM, Lidov M (1992) The benign fibroosseous lesion: its association with paranasal sinus mucoceles and its MR appearance. J Comput Assist Tomogr 16:871–876

Som PM, Lidov M (1994) The significance of sinonasal radiodensities: ossification, calcification, or residual bone? AJNR Am J Neuroradiol 15:917–922

Som PM, Schatz CJ, Flaum EG et al (1991) Aneurysmal bone cyst of the paranasal sinuses associated with fibrous dysplasia: CT and MR findings. J Comput Assist Tomogr 15:513–515

Soysal V, Yigitbasi OG, Kontas O et al (2001) Inflammatory myofibroblastic tumor of the nasal cavity: a case report and review of the literature. Int J Pediatr Otorhinolaryngol 61:161–165

Spencer MG, Mitchell DB (1987) Growth of a frontal sinus osteoma. J Laryngol Otol 101:726–728

Stamm AC, Watashi CH, Malheiros PF et al (2000) Micro-endoscopic surgery of benign sino-nasal tumors. In: Stamm AC, Draf W, eds. Micro-endoscopic surgery of paranasal sinuses and the skull base. Springer, Berlin Heidelberg New York, pp 489–514

Stankiewicz JA, Girgis SJ (1993) Endoscopic surgical treatment of nasal and paranasal sinus inverted papilloma. Otolaryngol Head Neck Surg 109:988–995

Stansbie JM, Phelps PD (1986) Involution of residual juvenile nasopharyngeal angiofibroma (a case report). J Laryngol Otol 100:599–603

Sterling KM, Stollman A, Sacher M et al (1993) Ossifying fibroma of sphenoid bone with coexistent mucocele: CT and MRI. J Comput Assist Tomogr 17:492–494

Stevenson HN (1932) Mixed tumor of the septum. Ann Otol Rhinol Laryngol 41:563–570

Stretch JR, Poole MD (1992) Pneumosinus dilatans as the aetiology of progressive bilateral blindness. Br J Plast Surg 45:469–473

Su L, Weathers DR, Waldron CA (1997) Distinguishing features of focal cemento-osseous dysplasia and cemento-ossifying fibromas. II. A clinical and radiologic spectrum of 316 cases. Oral Surg Oral Med Oral Pathol Oral Radiol Endod 84:540–549

Suzuki F, Fukuda S, Yagi K et al (2001) A rare aneurysmal bone cyst of the maxillary sinus: a case report. Auris Nasus Larynx 28:131–137

Tang AC, Grignon DJ, MacRae DL (1994) The association of human papillomavirus with Schneiderian papillomas: a DNA in situ hybridization study. J Otolaryngol 23:292–297

Tellado MG, Mendez R, Lopez-Cedrun JL et al (2002) Pneumosinus dilatans of the frontal and ethmoidal sinuses: case report. J Craniomaxillofac Surg 30:62–64

Tillman BP, Dahlin DC, Lipscomb PR et al (1968) Aneurysmal bone cyst: an analysis of ninety nine cases. Mayo Clin Proc 43:478–495

Tomenzoli D, Castelnuovo P, Pagella F et al (2004) Different endoscopic surgical strategy in the management of inverted papilloma of the sinonasal tract: experience with 47 patients. Laryngoscope 114:193–200

Trimarchi M, Lombardi D, Tomenzoli D et al (2003) Pneumosinus dilatans of the maxillary sinus: a case report and review of the literature. Eur Arch Otorhinolaryngol 260:386–389

Trott MS, Gewirtz A, Lavertu P et al (1994) Sinonasal leiomyomas. Otolaryngol Head Neck Surg 111:660–664

Ungkanont K, Byers RM, Weber RS et al (1996) Juvenile nasopharyngeal angiofibroma: an update of therapeutic management. Head Neck 18:60–66

Unlu HH, Celik O, Demir MA et al (2003) Pleomorphic adenoma originated from the inferior nasal turbinate. Auris Nasus Larynx 30:417–420

Urken ML, Som PM, Lawson W et al (1987) Abnormally large

frontal sinus. II. Nomenclature, pathology and symptoms. Laryngoscope 97:606–611

Utz JA, Kransdorf MJ, Jelinek JS et al (1989) MR appearance of fibrous dysplasia. J Comput Assist Tomogr 13:845–851

Uzun C, Adali MK, Koten M et al (1999) McCune-Abright syndrome with fibrous dysplasia of the paranasal sinus. Rhinology 37:122–124

Valavanis A, Christoforidis G (2000) Applications of interventional neuroradiology in the head and neck. Semin Roentgenol 35:72–83

Van Tassel P, Lee YY, Jing BS et al (1989) Mucoceles of the paranasal sinuses: MR imaging with CT correlation. AJR Am J Roentgenol 153:407–412

Vural E, Suen JY, Hanna E (1999) Intracranial extension of inverted papilloma: an unusual and potentially fatal complication. Head Neck 21:703–706

Wakami S, Muraoka M, Nakai Y (1996) Two cases of pleomorphic adenoma of the nasal cavity. Nippon Jibiinkoka Gakkai Kaiho 99:38–45

Waldron CA, Ginsanti JS (1973) Benign fibro-osseous lesions of the jaws: a clinical-radiologic-histologic review of sixty-five cases. II. Benign fibro-osseous lesions of periodontal ligament origin. Oral Surg Oral Med Oral Pathol 35:340–350

Walker JL, Jones NS (2002) Pneumosinus dilatans of the frontal sinuses: two cases and a discussion of its aetiology. J Laryngol Otol 116:382–385

Wallace RD, Ardent MD, Irene RT (1990) Pathologic quiz case 1. Pleomorphic adenoma. Arch Otolaryngol Head Neck Surg 116:486–488

Weber R, Keerl R, Draf W (2000) Endonasale endoskopische chirurgie von kieferhöhlenmukozelen nach Caldwell-Luc operation. Laryngorhinootologie 79:532–535

Weissler MC, Montogmery WW, Turner PA et al (1986) Inverted papilloma. Ann Otol Rhinol Laryngol 95:215–221

Welkoborsky HJ, Gosepath J, Jacob R et al (2000) Biologic characteristic of paragangliomas of the nasal cavity and paranasal sinuses. Am J Rhinol 14:419–426

Wenig BM, Vinh TN, Smirniotopoulos JG et al (1995) Aggressive psammomatoid ossifying fibromas of the sinonasal region: a clinicopathologic study of a distinct group of fibro-osseous lesions. Cancer 76:1155–1165

Winter M, Rauer RA, Gode U et al (2000) Invertierte papillome der nase und ihrer nebenhöhlen. Langzeitergebnisse nach endoskopischer endonasaler resektion. HNO 48:568–572

Wolfensberger M (1984) Zur pathogenese des pneumosinus maxillaris dilatans. HNO 32:518–520

Woodruff WW, Vrabec DP (1994) Inverted papilloma of the nasal vault and paranasal sinuses: spectrum of CT findings. AJR Am J Roentgenol 162:419–423

Wurster CF, Levine TM, Sisson GA (1986) Mucocele of the sphenoid sinus causing sudden onset of blindness. Otolaryngol Head Neck Surg 94:257–259

Yamaguchi KT, Shapsay SM, Incze JS et al (1979) Inverted papilloma and squamous cell carcinoma. J Otolaryngol 8:171–178

Yiotakis I, Psarommatis I, Manolopoulos L et al (2001a) Isolated inverted papilloma of the sphenoid sinus. J Laryngol Otol 115:227–230

Yiotakis I, Dinopoulou D, Ferekidis E et al (2001b) Pleomorphic adenoma of the nose. Rhinology 39:55–57

Yoon JH, Na DG, Byun HS et al (1999) Calcification in chronic maxillary sinusitis: comparison of CT findings with histopathologic results. AJNR Am J Neuroradiol 20:571–574

Younis RT, Gross CW, Lazar RH (1991) Schwannomas of the paranasal sinuses. Arch Otolaryngolo Head Neck Surg 117:677–680

Yousem DM (1993) Imaging of sinonasal inflammatory disease. Radiology 188:303–314

Yousem DM, Fellows DW, Kennedy DW et al (1992) Inverted papilloma: evaluation with MR imaging. Radiology 185:501–505

Zijlker TD, Visser R (1989) A vascular leiomyoma of the ethmoid. Report of case. Rhinology 27:129–135

9 Malignant Neoplasms

Roberto Maroldi, Davide Lombardi, Davide Farina, Piero Nicolai,
and Ilenia Moraschi

CONTENTS

9.1 Malignant Neoplasms: General Remarks *159*
9.1.1 Epidemiology *159*
9.1.2 Pattern of Growth and Clinical Evaluation *160*
9.1.2.1 Maxillary Sinus *160*
9.1.2.2 Ethmoid *161*
9.1.2.3 Sphenoid Sinus *161*
9.1.2.4 Frontal Sinus *161*
9.1.3 Endoscopic Appearance *162*
9.1.4 Staging Systems *162*
9.1.5 Treatment Guidelines and Outcome *163*
9.1.6 Key Information to Be Provided by Imaging *164*
9.1.7 Imaging Strategies. Key Findings *165*
9.1.7.1 Imaging to Assess the Patterns of Growth of
Maxillary Sinus Neoplasms *166*
9.1.7.2 Imaging to Assess the Pattern of Growth of
Naso-Ethmoidal Neoplasms *170*
9.2 Adenoid Cystic Carcinoma *177*
9.2.1 Definition, Epidemiology, Pattern of Growth *177*
9.2.2 Clinical and Endoscopic Findings *177*
9.2.3 Treatment Guidelines and Outcome *177*
9.2.4 Key Information to Be Provided by Imaging *178*
9.2.5 Imaging Findings *178*
9.2.5.1 Imaging to Assess Perineural Spread *179*
9.3 Sinonasal Neuroectodermal Tumors *185*
9.3.1 Olfactory Neuroblastoma *185*
9.3.1.1 Definition, Epidemiology, Pattern of Growth *185*
9.3.1.2 Clinical and Endoscopic Findings *185*
9.3.1.3 Staging Systems *185*
9.3.1.4 Treatment Guidelines and Outcome *186*
9.3.1.5 Key Information to Be Provided by Imaging *187*
9.3.1.6 Imaging Findings *187*
9.3.2 Sinonasal Neuroendocrine Carcinoma and
Sinonasal Undifferentiated Carcinoma *188*
9.3.2.1 Definition, Epidemiology, Pattern of Growth *188*
9.3.2.2 Clinical and Endoscopic Findings *189*
9.3.2.3 Treatment Guidelines and Outcome *189*
9.3.2.4 Key Information to Be Provided by Imaging *190*
9.3.2.5 Imaging Findings *190*
9.3.3 Ewing's Sarcoma *190*
9.3.3 1 Definition, Epidemiology, Pattern of Growth *190*
9.3.3.2 Clinical and Endoscopic Findings *191*
9.3.3.3 Treatment Guidelines and Outcome *191*
9.3.3.4 Key Information to Be Provided by Imaging *192*
9.3.3.5 Imaging Findings *192*
9.4 Melanoma *193*
9.4.1 Definition, Epidemiology, Pattern of Growth *193*
9.4.2 Clinical and Endoscopic Findings *194*
9.4.3 Treatment Guidelines and Outcome *194*
9.4.4 Key Information to Be Provided by Imaging *195*
9.4.5 Imaging Findings *195*
9.5 Soft Tissue, Cartilaginous, and Bone Sarcomas *196*
9.5.1 Definition, Epidemiology, Pattern of Growth *196*
9.5.2 Clinical and Endoscopic Findings *197*
9.5.3 Treatment Guidelines and Outcome *197*
9.5.4 Key Information to Be Provided by Imaging *199*
9.5.5 Imaging Findings *199*
9.6 Hemangiopericytoma *204*
9.6.1 Definition, Epidemiology and Pattern of Growth *204*
9.6.2 Clinical and Endoscopic Findings *205*
9.6.3 Treatment Guidelines and Outcome *205*
9.6.4 Key Information to Be Provided by Imaging *205*
9.6.5 Imaging Findings *205*
9.7 Lymphoproliferative Neoplasms *205*
9.7.1 Definition, Epidemiology, Pattern of Growth *205*
9.7.2 Clinical and Endoscopic Findings *207*
9.7.3 Treatment Guidelines and Outcome *208*
9.7.4 Key Information to Be Provided by Imaging *208*
9.7.5 Imaging Findings *208*
9.8 Secondary Tumors *211*
9.8.1 Definition, Epidemiology, Pattern of Growth *211*
9.8.2 Clinical and Endoscopic Findings *211*
9.8.3 Treatment Guidelines *211*
9.8.4 Imaging Findings *212*
References *213*

9.1
Malignant Neoplasms: General Remarks

9.1.1
Epidemiology

Malignant neoplasms of the sinonasal tract are quite rare, since they account for only 1% of all malignancies (Tufano et al. 1999; Rinaldo et al. 2002b), with an annual incidence of 0.5–1 new cases/100,000 inhabitants. Although infrequent, sinonasal neoplasms include a variety of histotypes, a distinctive feature which reflects the peculiar density in this area of different anatomic structures.

R. Maroldi, MD, Professor; D. Farina, MD; I. Moraschi, MD
Department of Radiology University of Brescia, Piazzale
Spedali Civili 1, Brescia, BS, 25123, Italy
D. Lombardi, MD; P. Nicolai, MD, Professor; L. Pianta, MD
Department of Otorhinolaryngology University of Brescia,
Piazzale Spedali Civili 1, Brescia, BS, 25123, Italy

Sinonasal tract malignancies account for 2–3% of all head and neck cancers; up to 80% of cases are maxillary sinus carcinomas (LE et al. 1999; TIWARI et al. 2000). Of the remaining tumors, most arise from the ethmoid sinus (WAX et al. 1995; CANTÙ et al. 1999a). More rarely the nasal fossa is the site of origin of malignancies. Malignant tumors originating within the sphenoid or the frontal sinus are exceedingly rare.

In the maxillary sinus, the most frequent histotype is squamous cell carcinoma, which accounts for up to 73% of all malignancies (TIWARI et al. 2000). Other histotypes, such as adenocarcinoma, adenoid cystic carcinoma, mucoepidermoid carcinoma are less frequently observed.

As far as ethmoid malignancies are concerned, adenocarcinoma, squamous cell carcinoma, and olfactory neuroblastoma are the most common histotypes. However, the prevalence of the different malignant tumors in the literature is extremely variable (WAX et al. 1995; SHAH et al. 1997; LUND et al. 1998; CANTÙ et al. 1999a; BRIDGER et al. 2000; BHATTACHARYYA 2002).

The carcinogenic effect of some factors like exposure to wood and leather dust in the development of ethmoid adenocarcinoma is well recognized (CANTÙ et al. 1999a). Other etiological factors, such as nickel and chrome refining processes, have been linked to the development of squamous cell and anaplastic carcinoma (GOLDENBERG et al. 2001). In contrast, tobacco and alcohol, do not seem to be associated with an increased risk for sinonasal tract malignancies (GOLDENBERG et al. 2001).

9.1.2
Pattern of Growth and Clinical Evaluation

During the early phase of growth, sinonasal tract malignancies are characterized by the absence of symptoms or by the presence of mild and nonspecific complaints. In a review performed by TUFANO et al. (1999), the mean duration of symptoms was 20 months. Consequently, diagnosis is mostly achieved when the disease is locally advanced (PAULINO et al. 1998) and the tumor has already involved adjacent structures such as hard palate, nasal fossa, masticatory space, premaxillary soft tissues, skin, orbit, or anterior cranial fossa. At this stage, signs and symptoms become more typical and related to specific pathways of spread.

For these reasons, symptoms of sinonasal tract malignancies will be discussed according to *topographic* criteria, with the intent to describe the typical pre-

sentation for each anatomic subsite. Squamous cell carcinoma and adenocarcinoma will be considered as tumors typically affecting the maxillary sinus and the ethmoid, respectively. Peculiar signs and symptoms for specific histotypes will be instead discussed in the dedicated sections.

9.1.2.1
Maxillary Sinus

Unilateral nasal obstruction, due to the extension of the lesion into the nasal fossa through the ethmoidal infundibulum or by the erosion of the medial bony wall, is often the presenting complaint of a maxillary sinus carcinoma (MIYAGUCHI et al. 1990). Epistaxis and nasal discharge may be associated. Another frequent heralding symptom is facial pain, which may be localized to the orbit, the cheek, or the tooth, according to the local extent of the tumor (MIYAGUCHI et al. 1990).

Other signs and symptoms are related to the growth of the neoplasm according to different pathways. Anterior extension beyond the bony wall is suggested by a premaxillary swelling, which can be observed in up to 41.7% of patients (PAULINO et al. 1998). Progression of the disease into the soft tissues may lead to skin fixation and ulcer. A lesion extending towards the orbit may be associated with symptoms related to involvement of the infraorbital nerve, such as pain, paresthesia and/or anesthesia of the skin covering the upper lip, the nasal pyramid, and the premaxillary region. When the mass pushes and dislocates the ocular bulb, proptosis and diplopia may appear. It is worth remembering that diplopia may also be a sign of extrinsic ocular muscles infiltration. Epiphora is caused by compression or infiltration of the lacrimal pathways or by an abnormal stimulation of the vidian nerve. Posterior extension towards the pterygopalatine fossa is suggested by ipsilateral tooth and facial pain due to maxillary nerve involvement; major palatine nerve involvement is associated with hemi-palate paresthesia and pain. Xerophthalmia suggests infiltration of the sphenopalatine ganglion. Trismus due to extension of the lesion into the masticatory space is usually a sign of an advanced-stage disease. The extension towards the underlying alveolar process may be accompanied by tooth protrusion and eventual unhealed tooth extraction (PAULINO et al. 1998). Hard palate involvement is suggested by a submucosal swelling or by the appearance of an ulcerated lesion.

At presentation, cervical node metastases may be detected in 3% to 20% of patients; regional metastases develop in 7.3% to 28.9% of patients after treatment (RINALDO et al. 2002b). The occurrence of lymph node metastases is more common in tumors with oral cavity involvement (KIM et al. 1999a; CANTÙ et al. 2002). Levels I, II, and III are the most frequently involved, whereas the prevalence of retro-lateral-pharyngeal node metastases is not well established (CANTÙ et al. 2002; RINALDO et al. 2002b).

9.1.2.2
Ethmoid

Early predominant symptoms and signs of ethmoid malignancies are nasal obstruction and/or epistaxis (WAX et al. 1995); nasal discharge may be also present at diagnosis. When the nasal septum has been infiltrated and the contralateral nasal fossa has been filled by the tumor, bilateral nasal obstruction is detected (BILLER et al. 1989; SALVAN et al. 1998). Pain, either for direct neural infiltration or for the occurrence of an acute obstructive sinusitis caused by the tumor itself, may be the heralding symptom in about 11% of patients (LUND et al. 1998); the first trigeminal branch is the most frequently involved.

Though ocular complaints may reveal the existence of an ethmoid malignancy, their occurrence can be observed also when the lamina papyracea has been compressed and displaced but not yet invaded. Most ethmoid cancers, when diagnosed, abut the lamina papyracea. Once it has been eroded, there is still a barrier that prevents orbital fat invasion: the periosteum investing the orbital bones (KRAUS et al. 1990; SALVAN et al. 1998). Tumor extent through the periosteum may be micro- or macroscopic. In the first case, signs and symptoms of intraorbital extension are usually absent. Conversely, spread through the posterior lamina papyracea is associated with orbital signs like periorbital swelling, extrinsic ocular muscle impairment, orbital displacement, proptosis, or visual disturbance. Epiphora and recurrent dacryocystitis should suggest the possibility of an anterior ethmoidal adenocarcinoma infiltrating the lacrimal pathway.

Superior extension into the anterior cranial fossa through the ethmoid roof is observed in up to 50% of cases of ethmoid cancers (BRIDGER and BALDWIN 1989; KRAUS et al. 1990; WAX et al. 1995). Subsequent involvement of the olfactory tract may cause hypo- or anosmia. However, the same symptoms may occur also in presence of a neoplasm interfering with the air flow in proximity of the olfactory epithelium (WAX et al. 1995). Tumor extent beyond the ethmoid bony roof may cause dural dis-

placement, and eventually infiltration, either micro- or macroscopic. When the mass is extradural or has only a microscopic dural infiltration, all signs and symptoms suggestive for CNS involvement, apart for headache, could be absent. Massive transdural growth, with possible brain infiltration, may be instead associated with cerebrospinal fluid leakage, mental confusion and seizures.

Less frequently the tumor extends posteriorly towards the sphenoid, pterygopalatine fossa, and middle cranial fossa or into the optic canal through the posterior medial orbital wall (CHEESMAN et al. 1986).

Cervical node metastases are observed in less than 3% of patients with adenocarcinoma. A higher incidence, up to 46%, is associated with undifferentiated carcinoma (CANTÙ et al. 2002).

9.1.2.3
Sphenoid Sinus

The occurrence of a sphenoid sinus malignancy is extremely rare, accounting for 2% of all sinonasal tract malignancies (OSGUTHORPE 1994; WESTERVELD et al. 2001). The limited endoscopic accessibility and the absence of specific symptoms account for a late diagnosis. The most frequent presenting complaint is occipital headache. From the sinus the tumor can extend towards the nasopharynx, causing posterior epistaxis and/or nasal obstruction. Lateral extension causes cavernous sinus invasion, with possible impairment of the first and second trigeminal branches, the third, fourth, and sixth cranial nerves. Superior extension, across to the sinus roof, may cause optic nerve or optic chiasm infiltration with subsequent visual disturbances. Proptosis can be observed when the orbital apex has been invaded.

9.1.2.4
Frontal Sinus

Frontal sinus malignancies account for 2% of all sinonasal tract neoplasms (OSGUTHORPE 1994). During the early phases of growth, the lesion is associated with sinusitis-like symptoms, such as frontal headache, nasal discharge, and occasional epistaxis; frontal swelling may also be present. Subsequently, the tumor may extend superiorly and/or posteriorly to involve the anterior cranial fossa, giving origin to seizures, visual disturbances or mental confusion. If the neoplasm extends into the orbit, proptosis with inferior dislocation of the ocular bulb and extrinsic ocular muscle impairment may appear.

9.1.3
Endoscopic Appearance

Endoscopic evaluation of a sinonasal tract mass is not completely reliable neither in defining local extension nor in suggesting the histology. At endoscopy, in fact, only the portion of the lesion occupying the nasal fossa may be examined (Fig. 9.1). Moreover, the appearance of a malignant tumor, which usually consists of a polypoid, fleshy mass, with irregular surface, possible ulcers and superficial hemorrhages, is quite nonspecific. A submucosal pattern of growth can be observed in some non-epithelial tumors, like chondrosarcoma or lymphomas. However, other lesions, such as osteomas, fibrous dysplasia, and pneumosinus dilatans may show a similar endoscopic appearance.

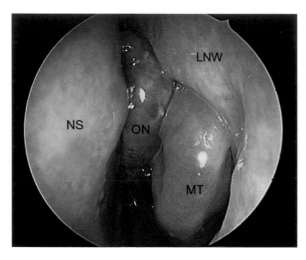

Fig. 9.1. Endoscopic view of an olfactory neuroblastoma (*ON*) presenting as a polypoid mass possibly arising from the ethmoid and projecting into the nasal fossa between nasal septum (*NS*) and middle turbinate (*MT*). Lateral nasal wall (*LNW*). Corresponding MR image of this patient in Fig. 9.25

9.1.4
Staging Systems

A classification for maxillary sinus cancer was already reported in the first edition of the Manual for Cancer Staging of the American Joint Committee on Cancer (AJCC) in 1977; however, only in 1987, a common classification was adopted from both the AJCC and the Union Internationale Contre le Cancer (UICC). Conversely, even though some independent classification for staging ethmoid cancer had been proposed (ELLINGWOOD and MILLION 1979; ROUX et al. 1991), only in 1997 was an official staging system specific

for the ethmoid site published. Approximately at the same time, an original classification for ethmoid cancer was developed by CANTÙ et al. (1997) (Table 9.1), with the intent to better stratify patients survival according to the extent of the tumor to adjacent anatomic areas. By analyzing a cohort of 123 patients undergoing craniofacial resection, they demonstrated with their classification a progressive worsening of the prognosis from T2 to T4 categories, a finding which was not observed when using 1997 AJCC-UICC classification (CANTÙ et al. 1999b).

The most recent update of AICC and UICC (SOBIN and WITTEKING 2002) (Table 9.2–9.3) classification has introduced some important modifications. First of all, the second site of paranasal sinuses (the first one being the maxillary sinus) has been defined as "naso-ethmoidal complex", which includes two different regions, the ethmoid sinuses and the nasal cav-

Table 9.1. Classification of malignant ethmoid tumors at the Istituto Nazionale per lo Studio e la Cura dei Tumori

T1	Tumor involving the ethmoid and nasal cavity, sparing the most superior ethmoid cells
T2	Tumor with an extension to or erosion of the cribriform plate, with or without erosion of the lamina papyracea and without extension into the orbit
T3	Tumor extending into the anterior cranial fossa extradurally and/or into the anterior two thirds of the orbit, with or without erosion of the anteroinferior wall of the sphenoid sinus, and/or involvement of the maxillary and/or frontal sinus
T4	Tumor with intradural extension, and/or involving the orbital apex, the sphenoid sinus, the pterygoid plate, the infratemporal fossa, or the skin

Table 9.2. AJCC-UICC staging system for maxillary sinus tumors (2002)

T1	Tumor limited to maxillary sinus mucosa with no erosion or destruction of bone
T2	Tumor causing bone erosion or destruction including extension into the hard palate and/or middle nasal meatus, except extension to posterior wall of maxillary sinus and pterygoid plates
T3	Tumor invades any of the following: bone of the posterior wall of the maxillary sinus, subcutaneous tissues, floor or medial wall of orbit, pterygoid fossa, ethmoid sinuses
T4a	Tumor invades anterior orbital contents, skin of cheek, pterygoid plates, infratemporal fossa, cribriform plate, sphenoid or frontal sinuses
T4b	Tumor invades any of the following: orbital apex, dura, brain, middle cranial fossa, cranial nerves other than maxillary division of trigeminal nerve (V_2), nasopharynx, or clivus

Table 9.3. AJCC-UICC staging system for nasal cavity and ethmoid sinus tumors (2002)

T1	Tumor restricted to any one subsite, with or without bony invasion
T2	Tumor invading two subsites in a single region or extending to involve an adjacent region within the naso-ethmoidal complex, with or without bony invasion
T3	Tumor extends to invade the medial wall or floor of the orbit, maxillary sinus, palate, or cribriform plate
T4a	Tumor invades any of the following: anterior orbital contents, skin of nose or cheek, minimal extension to anterior cranial fossa, pterygoid plates, sphenoid or frontal sinuses
T4b	Tumor invades any of the following: orbital apex, dura, brain, middle cranial fossa, cranial nerves other than (V2), nasopharynx, or clivus

ity. The former is divided in right and left, while four subsites (septum, floor, lateral wall, and vestibule) made up the latter. Secondarily, a better stratification of patients in regards to invasion of the orbit (anterior part vs. apex) and of the anterior skull base (bone, dura, and brain) has been provided. This has led to the division of T4 lesions into two different sub-categories (T4a and T4b), with the aim to separate resectable from unresectable tumors.

9.1.5
Treatment Guidelines and Outcome

As anticipated, squamous cell carcinoma and adenocarcinoma are the most frequently encountered malignant tumors of the maxillary sinus and of the naso-ethmoid complex, respectively. Therefore, treatment guidelines as herein reviewed specifically apply to such tumors and to other histotypes requiring a similar treatment planning, while alternative treatment schedules for specific tumors will be discussed in the dedicated sections.

Malignant tumors of the maxillary sinus are generally diagnosed at an advanced stage, since the symptoms during the early phase of growth are vague and somewhat nonspecific. This means that most of the lesions we are faced with have already extended beyond the limits of the maxillary sinus, invading the nasal fossa, ethmoid, orbit, palate, pterygopalatine and infratemporal fossa, cheek, and/or skull base.

Since recurrences at the primary site are the main cause of treatment failure, any effort should be done to properly eradicating the primary lesion. The application of this principle is made currently easier by the tremendous improvement of reconstructive techniques, which allow a satisfactory rehabilitation of functional deficits and aesthetic defects.

There is general consensus that early lesions (T1-T2) require surgery, which according to the location and extent of the lesion as delineated by imaging and intraoperative confirmed, can varies from different types of partial maxillectomies (i.e., inferior maxillectomy, medial maxillectomy, subtotal maxillectomy) to radical maxillectomy (See Chapter 5). Even though there is no definitive proof that postoperative radiotherapy may be beneficial in improving the local control rate of early lesions, its use seems to be indicated whenever at the examination of the surgical specimen poor prognostic findings such as positive margins, high-grade, perineural spread, or vascular invasion are detected.

Locally advanced lesions (T3-T4) of the maxillary sinus are best treated by a combination of surgery and radiotherapy. A radical maxillectomy extended to the adjacent anatomic structures involved by the tumor (premaxillary subcutaneous tissues, skin of the cheek, infratemporal and pterygopalatine fossa, pterygoid plates, ethmoid) is indicated for most T3 lesions.

Along the years the philosophy of management in patients with orbit involvement has evolved from a very aggressive ablative surgery towards a more conservative approach. There is indeed convincing evidence in the literature that sparing orbital content whenever the periorbita is not transgressed by the tumor does not compromise the local control rate of the disease (CARRAU et al. 1999). In this setting, partial resection of the periorbita with frozen sections to precisely assess the deep extent of invasion and reconstruction with fascia lata are recommended. Invasion of the orbital fat or muscles through the periorbita requires instead clearance of the orbit (IMOLA and SCHRAMM 2002), which is associated with a good local control of the disease when the anterior half of the orbit is invaded, whereas involvement of the apex invariably carries a high risk of local recurrence with subsequent intracranial invasion.

The question whether radiotherapy should be administered before or after surgery has not received a definitive answer; however, the general trend is nowadays in favor of postoperative treatment.

An alternative modality of treatment for advanced lesions of the maxillary sinus is the so-called trimodal therapy, which was introduced back in the 1970s by SATO et al (1970) and has been progressively refined down the years (ICHIMURA et al. 1998; NIBU et al. 2002). A combination of "conservative surgery", radiation therapy and regional chemotherapy has been used with the intent to minimize the sequelae of aggressive surgery while providing at the same time a satisfactory local control of the disease. Patients treated with this scheme have experienced a 5-year survival rate of up to 76% (NISHINO et al. 2000).

In a large series of maxillary sinus cancers, 61.7% of which were squamous cell carcinoma, advanced T stage, presence of nodal metastases, high grade of the tumor, and increasing age of the patient were found to negatively affect the prognosis (BHATTACHARYYA 2003).

Guidelines for cancer of the naso-ethmoidal complex are quite similar to those for maxillary sinus cancer, surgery with adjuvant postoperative radiotherapy for high-risk patients (extent to critical areas; unfavorable histological findings) being the cornerstone treatment.

During the last decade there has been growing interest in exploring the possibilities of microendoscopic surgery in the management of selected malignant lesions of the naso-ethmoidal complex (DRAF et al. 2000; STAMMBERGER et al. 1999; GOFFART et al. 2000; KUHN et al. 2001, ROH et al. 2004). Even though definitive criteria are far to be established, preliminary results suggest that there are indeed lesions which may be amenable to endonasal removal. In our opinion, indications can not be strictly correlated to T category, but a more detailed analysis of the different situations of tumor extent is required. The size of the tumor is not "per se" a contraindication; for instance, large polypoid lesions simply filling the nasal fossa, with a very limited insertion on any turbinate, the septum, or the lateral wall of the nasal fossa are an excellent indication for microendoscopic surgery. Even involvement of the mucosa lining the lamina papyracea does not preclude an endonasal resection, since the entire lamina papyracea and even a portion of the periorbita can be easily removed with the tumor. Lesions growing into the maxillary sinus through the lateral nasal wall but not directly involving the other walls of the sinus can also be managed trans-nasally. Conversely, whenever tumor extends anteriorly and encroaches the lacrimal pathways, lacrimal bone, and/or nasal bones an external approach, preferably through a lateral rhinotomy, is mandatory. In the tumors invading the mucosa covering the ethmoid roof or the cribriform plate our personal preference is for combining a transnasal microendoscopic approach with a subfrontal extradural craniotomy (anterior craniofacial resection), to obtain a safer superior margin of resection. Intuitively, also more advanced lesions involving the anterior skull base and the dura are managed by a similar approach, which requires

an intradural resection whenever the dura is in close contact or it is clearly infiltrated by the tumor and therefore needs to be included in the surgical specimen. It is worth mentioning that the introduction of anterior craniofacial resection in the treatment of malignant neoplasms of the naso-ethmoidal complex with a critical superior extension has considerably changed the prognosis of these tumors. In fact, in a recent retrospective multicentric study analyzing 1307 patients who underwent anterior craniofacial resection, PATEL et al. (2003) observed a 53% 5-year recurrence-free survival rate. Histology of the tumor, the extent of intracranial extension, and the status of surgical margins were independent significant predictors of both recurrence-free and disease-specific survival (PATEL et al. 2003).

Even for malignant tumors of the naso-ethmoidal complex, isolated successful experiences with an alternative treatment schedule have been reported. KNEGT et al. (2001) treated a series of 62 patients with adenocarcinoma of the naso-ethmoidal complex with surgical debulking, periodical topical applications of a 5-fluorouracil emulsion, with or without postoperative radiotherapy obtaining an 87% 5-year disease-free survival rate.

When dealing with ethmoid cancer, advanced T stage and histology are considered the most important factors influencing survival, whereas nodal metastasis, due to small incidence, has an unclear effect on survival (BHATTACHARYYA 2002).

In our opinion, surgery is contraindicated in patients with extensive involvement of the brain, encasement of the internal carotid artery, or extension of the lesion to the cavernous sinus and/or to the optic chiasm, who are better treated by a combination of radiotherapy and chemotherapy.

9.1.6
Key Information to Be Provided by Imaging

- Discrimination between tumor and fluid collections/mucoceles.
- Involvement of maxillary sinus:
  - Is there any bone erosion of sinusal walls? (Medial, anterior, postero-lateral walls? Inferior recess? Orbital floor?)
  - Is there any invasion of the nasal fossa?
  - Is there any invasion of the lacrimal pathways?
  - Is there any invasion of pre-antral soft tissues?
  - Is there any invasion of masticatory space/infratemporal fossa? If positive, are pterygoid muscles, mandibular nerve invaded?

- Is there any invasion of the pterygopalatine fossa?
- Is there any perineural spread?
- Is there any invasion of the alveolar process and/or of the hard palate?
- Is there any invasion of the lateral nasopharyngeal wall?
- Involvement of the orbit and lacrimal pathways:
  - Is the periorbita intact or transgressed?
  - If the periorbita is transgressed, does the tumor invade the anterior and/or posterior segment of the orbital content?
  - Are the superior orbital fissure and/or the optic canal invaded?
  - Are the lacrimal pathways invaded?
- Involvement of the anterior skull base:
  - Is the tumor in contact with the anterior skull base floor? Where is the contact area located (Ethmoid roof? Cribriform plate? Roof of the sphenoid sinus? Postero-superior wall of the frontal sinus?)
  - Is there any bony erosion?
  - Is dura transgressed?
  - Is brain invaded?
- Involvement of the middle cranial fossa:
  - Is the tumor in contact with the middle cranial fossa floor? Where is the contact area located? (Roof of the infratemporal fossa? Root of the pterygoid process? Lateral wall of the sphenoid sinus?)
  - Is there any bony erosion?
  - Is dura transgressed?
  - Is brain invaded?
  - Is there any sign of perineural spread?
- Involvement of the nasal septum, contralateral extent, nasal bones.
- Involvement of the anterior, inferior and posterior wall of the sphenoid sinus, nasopharynx, and/or clivus
- Involvement of the frontal sinus:
  - Is there any bone erosion of sinusal walls? (Anterior? Superior? Posterior? Medial?)

9.1.7
Imaging Strategies. Key Findings

Sinonasal malignant neoplasms are generally imaged by CT or MR in two different clinical situations. The first scenario includes patients with nasal symptoms, thus arising the suspect of chronic rhinosinusitis, but unresponsive to medical therapy, whereas the second one consists in the request of assessing the local extent of a tumor already detected by clinical examination.

Because CT is considered the technique of choice in the clinical workup of chronic rhinosinusitis, it will be the first imaging technique used to examine patients with nasal or sinusal masses mimicking symptoms of chronic rhinosinusitis or causing blockage of one or more sinusal cavities. It is worth remembering that the detection of a unilateral nasal obstruction on CT (BARNES 1986; WOODRUFF and VRABEC 1994) should prompt, even in the absence of bone remodeling or destruction, a diagnosis alternative to chronic rhinosinusitis (i.e., the presence of a nasal mass). In this setting, two different strategies are available to the radiologist. The first consists in the administration of iodinated contrast agent. Generally, a relevant enhancement of the mucosa lining both the nasal structures and the sinusal walls will be obtained, whereas the secretions entrapped within a blocked sinus will not change their density. Therefore, it will be possible to separate retained secretions from the mass - its degree of enhancement varying according to several elements, as histotype, inflammation, and necrosis. Conversely, the differentiation between the mass and the enhanced mucosa lining the nasal structures may be very difficult or impossible.

Because of this limitation in contrast resolution of CT, the second strategy consists in submitting the patient to MR. In fact, the discrimination of tumor from adjacent nasal structures and retained secretions results more feasible by combining T2, plain and enhanced T1 sequences.

A thorough delineation of tumor extent towards sinonasal bony framework, orbit, intracranial content, cranial nerves, and vessels as well as detailed assessment of neoplastic involvement of structures and spaces adjacent to the sinonasal tract is the second step in the diagnostic work-up.

As local spread of nasal and paranasal neoplasms depends on their site of origin, the imaging features of the two main patterns of growth (i.e., maxillary and naso-ethmoidal tumors) are considered in detail.

Because most maxillary sinus tumors are squamous cell carcinoma and most naso-ethmoidal tumors are adenocarcinoma, these two histotypes are used to illustrate the pattern of spread of epithelial neoplasms arising in these sites. Some peculiar aspects of the pattern of growth and signal/density abnormalities of the adenoid cystic carcinoma and non-epithelial tumors, as olfactory neuroblastoma, lymphomas, and sarcomas will be discussed in detail.

9.1.7.1
Imaging to Assess the Patterns of Growth of Maxillary Sinus Neoplasms

Progressive growth of maxillary sinus malignant neoplasms leads to extra-sinusal spread through the invasion of one or more of its five bony walls: *medial, anterior, postero-lateral, inferior (alveolar recess), and roof* (Fig. 9.2). According to the direction of tumor growth, different implications regarding treatment and prognosis will result.

Invasion of the *medial wall* is certainly the less critical pathway of spread as it leads to intra-nasal extent where the lesion has to grow further prior to involve critical structures, usually via ethmoid sinus invasion. Nonetheless, once the tumor reaches the choana and spreads along its lateral surface, there is the risk of nasopharyngeal wall invasion with pos-

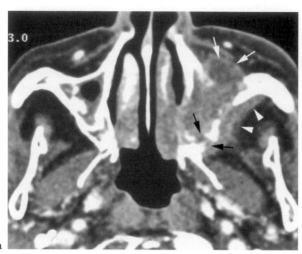
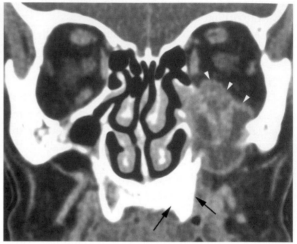

Fig. 9.2a,b. Squamous cell carcinoma of left maxillary sinus. On post-contrast CT images the lesion shows slight heterogeneous enhancement. On the axial plane (**a**) the tumor is shown to invade the anterior (*white arrows*), the postero-lateral (*arrowheads*), and the medial sinusal walls. Invasion of the pterygopalatine fossa is present (*black arrows*). On the coronal plane (**b**) intraorbital invasion with involvement of the inferior rectus muscle is detected (*arrowheads*). Marked sclerosis of the alveolar process (*black arrows*) suggests reactive changes or intramedullary spread

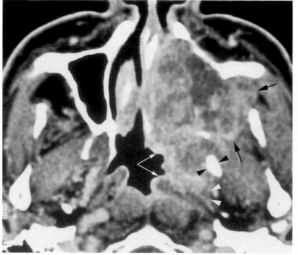
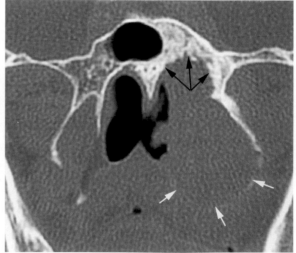

Fig. 9.3a,b. Squamous cell carcinoma of left maxillary sinus. On post-contrast CT in the axial plane (**a**), extensive involvement of the masticator space (*black arrows*) with a residual bone fragment of the pterygoid laminae (*black arrowheads*) is demonstrated. In addition, tumor invades the left nasopharyngeal wall and the pre-styloid compartment of the parapharyngeal space (*white arrowheads*). Invasion of the pterygoid process with both erosion and sclerotic changes is shown (*black arrows*) in the coronal plane (**b**). The left pterygoid canal is not detectable. Downward extent is associated with remodeling and lateral displacement of the lateral pterygoid lamina (*white arrows*)

sible involvement of the opening of the Eustachian tube (Fig. 9.3)

Because in the area of posterior fontanellae (behind natural sinusal ostium) the medial wall is thin and very often dehiscent, in some cases its neoplastic invasion can be suggested on CT by the extent of the mass into the nasal cavity, rather than by bone destruction. Conversely, invasion of the anterior portion of the medial wall may be directly demonstrated by bone erosion, eventually extended to the horizontal portion of the uncinate process and to the inferior concha. Particular attention has to be placed to the lacrimal pathways because their involvement – like the invasion of pre-antral soft tissues through the *anterior wall* - contraindicates the surgical approach with midfacial degloving.

Tumor extent toward the *alveolar process* and into the *hard palate* should be evaluated by means of coronal (or sagittal) images (Fig. 9.2b, 9.4). A critical pathway of spread may be observed when the posterior portion of the alveolar process is invaded, as the neoplasm may involve the buccinator muscle and/or the maxillary tuberosity, from which it may access the pterygomandibular raphe.

Certainly, the two most critical bony boundaries are the *postero-lateral wall*, a pathway to spread into the masticator space and pterygopalatine fossa, and the *maxillary sinus roof* – i.e., the orbital floor – because its involvement leads to orbital invasion. In both settings, the main goal of imaging is to assess the integrity of the bony-periosteal barrier (Fig. 9.2b, 9.4).

As most malignant maxillary sinus tumors are squamous cell carcinomas, this histotype is used to describe the expected MR signal intensity of neoplasms in this site. Because of its highly cellular composition, squamous cell carcinoma has usually homogeneous intermediate-to-low signal intensity on T2 sequences and moderate-to-relevant enhancement after contrast agent administration (Som et al. 1989) (Fig. 9.5).

The first step in the assessment of neoplastic extent is the evaluation of the relationship of maxillary sinus tumor with the sinusal walls. The sinusal walls contacting the neoplasm may present various signal patterns on imaging studies, ranging from inflammatory changes to abnormalities indicating neoplastic invasion.

On CT, *chronic inflammatory* abnormalities of the bony walls may be either due to long standing mucus drainage impairment or represent reactive changes induced by tumor contact. They appear as asymmetric thickening of sinusal walls. On MR, both T2 and T1 sequences show thicker hypointense sinusal walls, even though focal areas of signal hyperintensity may be observed (Maroldi et al. 1996) (Fig. 9.5b). The presence of a double shape, due to a hypointense line parallel to the outer surface of the wall, represents periosteal thickening. Inflammatory changes of the sinusal mucosa are frequently associated. They usu-

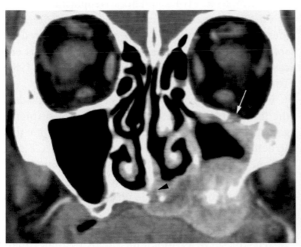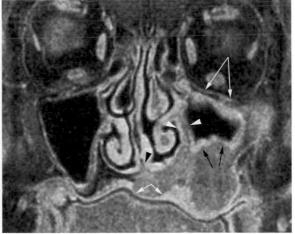

a b

Fig. 9.4a,b. Squamous cell carcinoma of left maxillary sinus, post-contrast coronal multislice CT (**a**) and VIBE (**b**). Both techniques demonstrate the sub-periosteal and sub-mucosal spread of tumor, which is covered by residual mucosa both in the maxillary sinus (*black arrows*) and in the left nasal fossa floor. The precise extent of submucosal spread into the hard palate is clearly defined by MR (*short white arrows*). Both CT and MR show invasion of the bony nasal septum (*black arrowhead*). Whereas on CT the medial left maxillary sinus wall appears undetectable, as the mineralized component is reabsorbed, its residual bony framework is still detectable on MR (*white arrowheads*). On CT, enlargement of the infraorbital foramen is shown (*white arrow on* **a**). At this level, MR shows regular and smooth thickening of the periorbita (*long white arrows on* **b**)

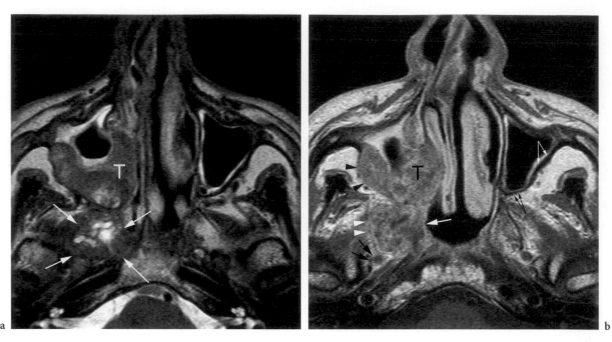

Fig. 9.5a,b. Squamous cell carcinoma of right maxillary sinus. **a** On TSE T2 the tumor (*T*) has heterogeneous hypointense intensity signal, lower than fluid and mucosa within the sinus. Apart for the invasion of pterygopalatine fossa and pterygoid process (*arrows*), the path of neoplastic spread progresses posteriorly (**b**) with involvement of masticator space (*white arrowheads*) where tumor abuts the mandibular nerve (*black thick arrows*). While part of the lesion is still confined by the posterolateral wall (*black arrowheads*), invasion of the choana with spread into the lateral nasopharyngeal wall is present (*white thick arrows*). Thickening of left maxillary sinus walls is particularly evident along the postero-lateral wall (*white thin arrows*), where focal hyperintense areas are also present (*black thin arrows*)

ally appear as diffuse and lobulated thickening, hypodense on CT, homogeneously hyperintense on T2 sequences, hypointense on plain T1. After contrast agent administration, the thin superficial mucosal layer enhances – a finding more easily demonstrated on MR – whereas the liquid content within the submucosa does not (SOM et al. 1988).

Among the different patterns of bone changes due maxillary sinus neoplasms, remodeling may be observed, even though less frequently than cortical destruction, permeative bone invasion with subperiosteal and submucosal spread (Fig. 9.4), which may be more thoroughly mapped by MR (see Chapter 4).

9.1.7.1.1
Imaging Findings of Pterygopalatine Fossa, Root of Pterygoid Process, and Cavernous Sinus Invasion

Fat tissue surrounding nerves and vessels inside fossae and fissures is a key point to assess neoplastic invasion, both on CT and MR. As an example of this, the sphenopalatine artery is a useful landmark to early detect neoplastic involvement of the pterygopalatine fossa. The artery appears as a twisted signal void surrounded by fat tissue on both T1 and TSE T2 sequences, easily detectable in all planes. After contrast agent administration, it can be demonstrated as an enhanced vessel on axial and coronal high resolution CT or enhanced VIBE sequences. Neoplastic invasion of the pterygopalatine fossa is suspected whenever the fat tissue surrounding the vessel is replaced by soft tissue density/intensity and/or the vessel is encased or not recognizable (WOODRUFF et al. 1986; TOMURA et al. 1999) (Fig. 9.6).

Once the pterygopalatine fossa has been invaded, the tumor may progress toward the adjacent pterygoid process of the sphenoid bone, and from this structure further spread intracranially. On CT and MR imaging, the *pterygoid process* is a key anatomic structure to detail the actual extent of neoplastic tissue not only for its strategic position but also for its complex architecture (YU et al. 2000). In fact, both its cortical and medullary bone components are traversed - or serve as floor - for canals (Vidian canal) and grooves (foramen rotundum) along which run nerves surrounded by tiny vessels and fat. When tumor invades the pterygoid process, cortical destruction, intra-medullary growth, and permeative invasion are patterns that may be observed, on occasion simultaneously (Fig. 9.3b). Conversely, sclerosis of its

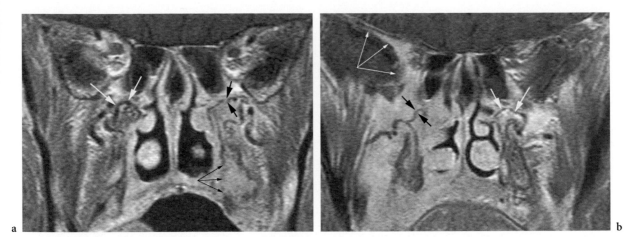

Fig. 9.6a,b. Adenoid cystic carcinoma of left (**a**) and right (**b**) maxillary sinus with pterygopalatine fossa invasion on enhanced coronal T1 images. **a** Normal right pterygopalatine artery is indicated by *white arrows*. On left side fat surrounding the ptery-gopalatine artery is replaced by solid tissue (*short black arrows*). Invasion of medial pterygoid plate is detectable (*long black arrows*). **b** Tumor arises from right side, solid enhancing tumor tissue surrounds the pterygopalatine artery (*black arrows*). *Short white arrows indicate normal* pterygopalatine artery on left side. Invasion of the superior orbital fissure with spread along the sphenoid wing is demonstrated (*long white arrows*)

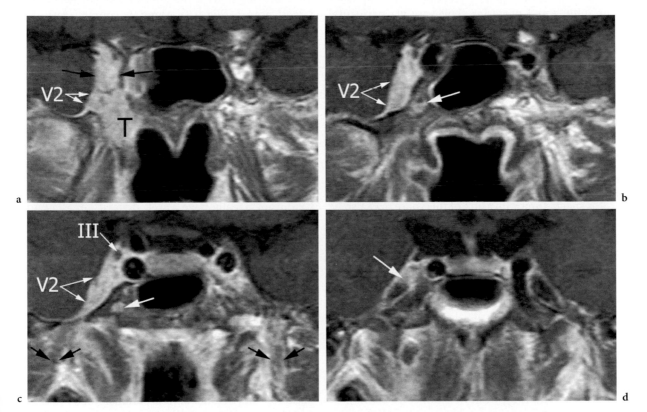

Fig. 9.7a-d. Cavernous sinus invasion by adenoid cystic carcinoma arising from right maxillary sinus. **a–d** Coronal enhanced T1 images (**a–d**) show tumor (*T*) invading (**a**) the pterygoid process and superior orbital fissure (*black arrows*) with perineural spread along the maxillary nerve (*V2*). Perineural spread along vidian nerve is suggested by enlargement of the vidian canal filled by enhancing tissue which surrounds a thin, hypointense, and probably compressed nerve (*white arrow on* **b** *and* **c**). Sclerotic changes in the diploic bone of the right sphenoid are indicated by replacement of the normal fat content by hypointense signal. The invaded right cavernous sinus appears enlarged, with a more convex lateral outline on **b** and **c**. Intracavernous tumor tissue splays the third cranial nerve (*III*) from internal carotid artery (**c**). **d** Tumor reaches the Meckel cave (*white arrow*), whose walls are thickened compared with the contralateral. Mandibular branch of trigeminal nerve (*black arrows on* **c**)

medullary bone component does not always indicate neoplastic bone involvement, apart for adenoid cystic carcinoma and lymphoma (YASUMOTO et al. 2000). Once the osseous structure of the pterygoid process is replaced by tumor, intracranial spread may occur via the cavernous sinus (superiorly) or the foramen lacerum (posteriorly).

The MR findings of cavernous sinus invasion include enlargement and lateral bulging of the sinus and replacement of the hyperintense venous signal by the intermediate tumor tissue on either coronal and axial T2 or enhanced T1 sequences (LAINE et al. 1990). Neoplastic encasement of the internal carotid artery at the cavernous sinus may be detected by MR, either on TSE T2 or T1 sequences. Reliable signs of vessel infiltration include enhancement of the thickened vessel wall and encasement of the internal carotid artery greater than two thirds of its circumference (KOMIYAMA 1990; COTTIER et al. 2000)

In addition to bone penetration, maxillary tumor extending into the pterygopalatine fossa may enter the middle and posterior skull base via perineural spread along maxillary and vidian nerves, respectively, or may directly invade the orbit via the superior orbital fissure (MAROLDI et al. 1997).

CT and MR findings indicating perineural spread are discussed in detail in section 9.2.1

9.1.7.1.2
Masticator Space Invasion

Neoplastic growth beyond the postero-lateral wall of the maxillary sinus gives tumor access into the masticator space. Tumor invasion of this space may also be caused by spread from the pterygopalatine fossa via the pterygomaxillary fissure. Effacement of fat and invasion of structures belonging to the space are the findings to be demonstrated by imaging. Important anatomical landmarks are the pterygoid muscles, the internal maxillary and middle meningeal arteries, the mandibular nerve and the inferior alveolar nerve. They are better visualized by MR than by CT (PALING et al. 1987). Detection of normal signal intensity of pterygoid muscles or of a residual fat layer surrounding the nerves helps to rule out neoplastic infiltration (MATZKO et al. 1994; CURTIN 1998) (Fig. 9.3, 9.5).
A combination of axial and coronal high resolution TSE T2 and enhanced T1 are recommended to precisely demonstrate both normal structures and subtle abnormal findings within masticator space. Particularly, one should carefully evaluate the relationship between tumor tissue invading the space and the mandibular nerve, as the latter may pro-

vide a direct route through middle skull base floor via perineural spread or foramen ovale invasion. Furthermore, the mandibular nerve - and foramen ovale - serve as landmarks for separating the masticator space from the adjacent prestyloid compartment of parapharyngeal space, the middle layer of the deep cervical fascia – separating the two spaces - being not detectable by imaging techniques.

The mandibular nerve may be identified on CT and MR axial planes starting at the foramen ovale where it should be evaluated by mean of thin slices (MARSOT-DUPUCH et al. 1990). At this level, it appears as a hypointense oval structure on TSE T2, partially surrounded by enhanced signal on 0.5 mm VIBE sequences, probably reflecting the presence of a perineural vascular plexus besides the accompanying accessory meningeal artery (WILLIAMS 1999). After exiting the foramen, its separation into three branches may be appreciated only on VIBE thin partitions, whereas standard TSE T2 and T1 usually permit detecting at least the inferior alveolar nerve, its largest branch (Fig. 9.8). Along its course inferiorly directed toward the opening of the mandibular canal, the inferior alveolar nerve can be identified running medially both to the lateral (nerve's superior tract) and to the medial (nerve's inferior tract) pterygoid muscles.

9.1.7.2
Imaging to Assess the Pattern of Growth of Naso-Ethmoidal Neoplasms

Neoplasms arising from ethmoid sinus or nasal cavity do not usually have a well defined *bony box* to completely fill before extending through its walls to become symptomatic, as in maxillary sinus neoplasms. Unilateral or bilateral nasal obstruction, possibly leading earlier to endoscopic or CT examination, is more frequently observed than in maxillary tumors (Fig. 9.9). Therefore, imaging findings may range from the detection of a nasal polypoid lesion to the demonstration of a large naso-ethmoidal mass abutting the bony framework of a complex *bony box* including in its boundaries the lamina papyracea, the lacrimal pathways, the medial maxillary wall, the nasal septum, and the anterior cranial fossa floor. In addition, naso-ethmoidal tumors may extend into the frontal sinus and involve nasal bones – anteriorly – or into the sphenoid sinus – posteriorly. Less frequently, the nasopharynx or the soft palate are invaded via the choana.

More often than in maxillary sinus tumors, a naso-ethmoidal neoplasm has already invaded the

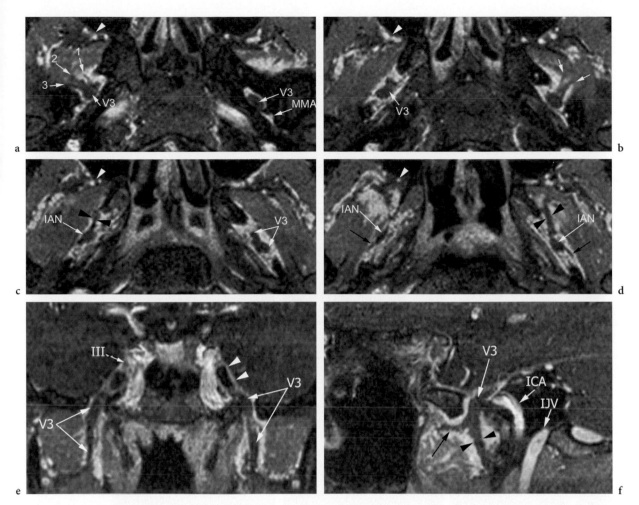

Fig. 9.8a–f. Mandibular nerve demonstrated on 0.5 mm enhanced VIBE images. **A–d** Four different axial levels show the course and some of the major branches of the mandibular nerve (*V3*). The left mandibular nerve (**a**) is imaged at the level of the foramen ovale, the right immediately below, where three branches are detectable, probably accounting for medial pterygoid (*1*), temporomasseteric (*2*), and middle deep temporal (*3*) nerves. Middle meningeal artery (*MMA*) **b** Two branches of the mandibular nerve are imaged on left side, while on right side the morphology of the nerve changes to give off (**c**) a large anterior trunk (*black arrowheads*), more clearly demonstrated on left side (*black arrowheads on* **d**), which is probably the lingual nerve. **d** Inferior alveolar nerve (*IAN*) is the largest trunk of the nerve; it gives off other small branches (*black arrows on* **d**). Right pterygopalatine artery (*white arrowheads on* **a–d**). **e** Coronal MPR shows the mandibular nerve (*V3*) surrounded by enhancing venous plexus. Meckel cave (*arrowheads*) and third cranial nerve (*III*) within the cavernous sinus are shown. **f** The sagittal MPR shows part of the extracranial course of the mandibular nerve (*V3*): lingual nerve (*black arrow*); inferior alveolar nerve (*arrowheads*); internal carotid artery (*ICA*); internal jugular vein (*IJV*)

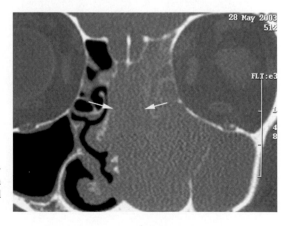

Fig. 9.9. Adenocarcinoma of left nasal fossa. Coronal plane CT demonstrates a soft tissue mass occupying the left nasal cavity. Erosion of the perpendicular plate and lateral displacement of the medial wall of the left maxillary sinus suggest the presence of a tumor

contralateral nasal fossa and ethmoid at diagnosis (Fig. 9.10).

Small lesions may be very difficult to demonstrate with imaging techniques. Moreover, their precise site of origin may become apparent only at surgery, particularly when the nasal fossa is completely filled by tumor.

Regarding orbital invasion, recent evidence in the medical literature supports a more conservative approach on condition that the periorbita is not invaded,

as in this occurrence the eye can be spared without increasing local recurrences or survival and adequate postoperative function can be maintained (ROUX et al. 1997; IMOLA and SCHRAMM 2002). Therefore, the first priority of imaging consists in assessing the integrity of the periorbita (CURTIN and RABINOV 1998). In case of ambiguous findings of orbital invasion on imaging studies, it will be necessary to clearly inform the patient about the potential need of orbital clearance, although only intra-operative mapping of

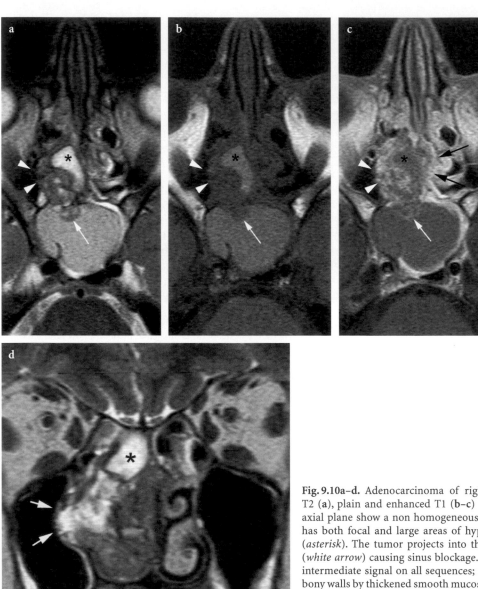

Fig. 9.10a–d. Adenocarcinoma of right ethmoid sinus. TSE T2 (**a**), plain and enhanced T1 (**b–c**) images obtained in the axial plane show a non homogeneous soft tissue mass which has both focal and large areas of hyperintensity on TSE T2 (*asterisk*). The tumor projects into the right sphenoid sinus (*white arrow*) causing sinus blockage. Dehydrated mucus has intermediate signal on all sequences; it is separated from the bony walls by thickened smooth mucosa. The adenocarcinoma causes focal displacement of the medial wall of the right maxillary sinus (*arrowheads*). Nasal septum invasion with contralateral extent is better shown on enhanced T1 (*black arrows*). On coronal plane (**d**) the tumor causes focal bulging of the medial wall of right maxillary sinus (*arrows*). Cribriform plate is normal, suggesting possible endonasal approach

the orbital wall(s) - with gross examination and frozen sections - provides clear-cut information. In this setting, it should be noticed that the negative predictive value of MR (MAROLDI et al. 1996) is higher than its positive predictive value, recently reported to be about 80% by EISEN et al. (2000) (Fig. 9.11).

The second priority of imaging consists in assessing the relationship between the lesion and the anterior cranial fossa floor. Findings provided by CT and MR are relevant in predicting the need for craniofacial resection. Coronal TSE T2 sequences are indicated to assess the integrity of the hypointense interface between sinonasal and intracranial structures, which corresponds to bone/periosteum independently from the grade of bone mineralization (Fig. 9.12–9.16). Enhanced SE T1 on sagittal and coronal planes are particularly useful to *grade* intracranial extent (Fig. 9.17) , and to differentiate between extra-dural and trans-dural invasion (EL-BELTAGI et al. 2002; ISHIDA et al. 2002) (see chapter 4).

In evaluating the relationship between a naso-ethmoidal tumor mass and orbit/anterior cranial fossa floor, one should consider that these structures are mostly made by thin osseous layers, easily displaced and remodeled, particularly the lamina papyracea and the cribriform plate. However, displacement and

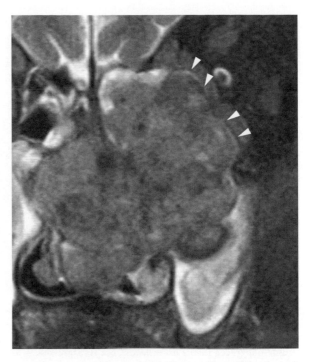

Fig. 9.11. Large adenocarcinoma arising from left ethmoid, invading both nasal fossae and left maxillary sinus. On fat sat coronal T2 marked displacement and remodeling of left lamina papyracea is shown. A residual hypointense, continuous, interface separates tumor from orbital content indicating that the lesion is confined by the periorbita (*arrowheads*)

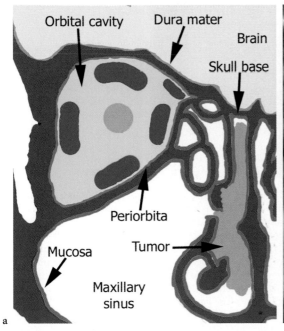

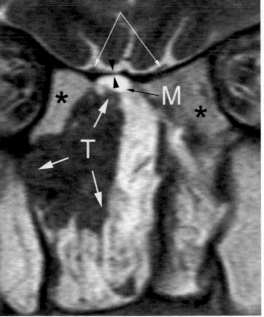

Fig. 9.12. a Schematic drawing of a naso-ethmoidal mass non-contacting the ethmoid roof. In this setting, if the histological type does not contraindicate surgery, micro-endoscopic endonasal approach is feasible. **b** Adenocarcinoma (intestinal type) of right ethmoid (*T*) separated from the ethmoid roof by a small mucocele (*M*), which causes focal remodeling of the planum sphenoidale (*arrowheads*). Olfactory tracts (*long white arrows*); fluid retention within both posterior ethmoid sinuses (*asterisks*)

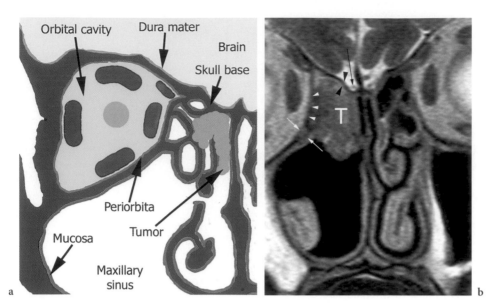

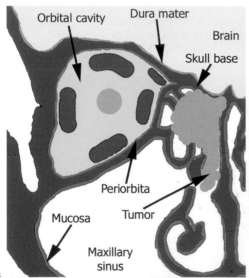

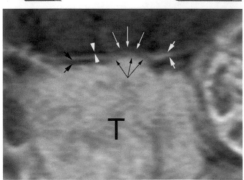

Fig. 9.13. a Schematic drawing of a naso-ethmoidal mass contacting the ethmoid roof. In this setting, if the histological type does not contraindicate surgery, micro-endoscopic endonasal approach is feasible. **b** Recurrent adenocarcinoma of right ethmoid abutting the lamina cribrosa and the fovea ethmoidalis (*black arrowheads*), whose signal is normal. The tumor also abuts the lamina papyracea (*white arrowheads*), not transgressed. A focal area of neoplastic involvement is seen in the inferior aspect of the lamina papyracea (*thin white arrows*). A residual hypointense signal still separates tumor from intraorbital fat, possibly consisting with non-invaded periorbita. Definitive intraoperative assessment is necessary

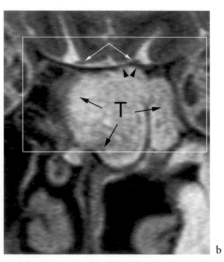

Fig. 9.14a–c. a Schematic drawing of a naso-ethmoidal mass partially *eroding* the ethmoid roof. In this setting, if the histological type does not contraindicate surgery, micro-endoscopic endonasal approach is feasible. Definitive intraoperative assessment is necessary. **b** Recurrent adenocarcinoma (intestinal type) of left ethmoid extended into the sphenoid sinus (*T*). Focal thinning of the hypointense interface corresponding to the planum sphenoidale (*arrowheads*) indicates partial erosion of bone by the tumor, still confined by the bone/periosteal barrier. Olfactory tracts (*white arrows*). The area included in the *white box* is magnified on an enhanced T1 image (**c**). The different signals of the bone/periosteal layer (*short black arrows*), thickened dura (*white short arrows*), and CSF (*arrowheads*) are shown in detail. When compared with TSE T2, the residual bone/periosteal layer appears thinner because it enhances. The dura overlying the focal bulging is homogeneously thickened (*white arrows*) and has signal intensity slightly lower than the underlying tumor and enhancing periosteum

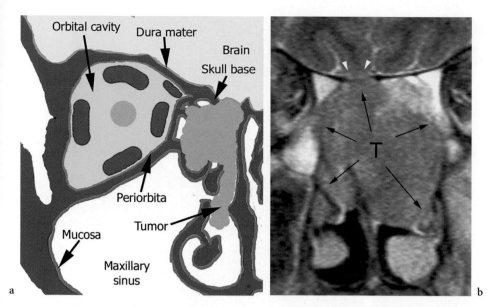

Fig. 9.15. a Schematic drawing of a naso-ethmoidal mass with intracranial extradural extent. In this setting, if the histological type does not contraindicate surgery, anterior cranial resection is required. **b** Naso-ethmoidal squamous cell carcinoma (*T*) causes focal invasion of the planum sphenoidale where the CSF signal is effaced. Tumor extends intracranially (*arrowheads*)

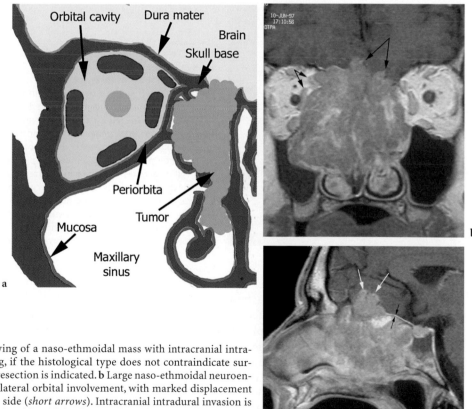

Fig. 9.16. a Schematic drawing of a naso-ethmoidal mass with intracranial intradural extent. In this setting, if the histological type does not contraindicate surgery, anterior craniofacial resection is indicated. **b** Large naso-ethmoidal neuroendocrine carcinoma with bilateral orbital involvement, with marked displacement of orbital muscles on right side (*short arrows*). Intracranial intradural invasion is also present (*long arrows*). Breaking of the dura, replaced by tumor signal (*white arrows*), is better shown on the sagittal enhanced T1 image (**c**). Adjacent thickened dura (*black arrows*)

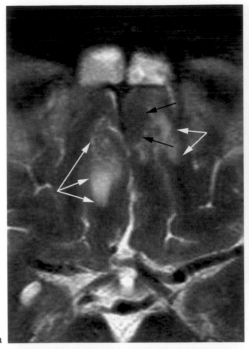

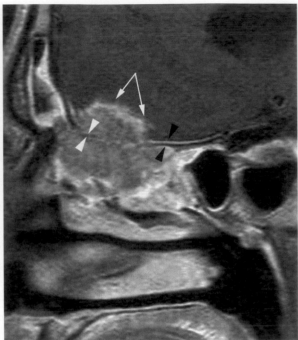

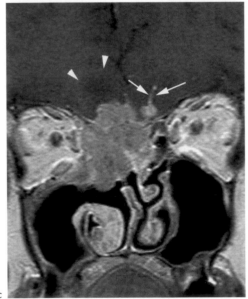

Fig. 9.17a–c. Adenocarcinoma of right ethmoid sinus with intracranial intradural invasion. **a** On axial T2, bilateral edema of the olfactory lobe (*white arrows*) raises the suspect of cerebral invasion. On left side, an oval area with signal lower that the edematous surrounding brain tissue effaces the bright signal of CSF - close to the left aspect of the crista galli (*black arrows*). Post-contrast sagittal images (**b**) demonstrate invasion of the anterior skull base floor (*white arrowheads*) with intracranial spread and upwards displacement of an irregularly thickened dura (*white arrows*). Posterior to the area of intracranial invasion the dura is regularly thickened suggesting reactive change. **c** Linear enhancement into the sulci (*arrows*) on both olfactory lobes is consistent with leptomeningeal invasion. The ill-defined hypointensity surrounding the tumor invading the right olfactory groove indicates brain invasion and edema

remodeling is not exclusively related to tumor growth, as it may occur also in case of a mucocele secondary to mucus drainage blockage by a neoplasm.

Furthermore, intestinal-type adenocarcinoma, which is one of the most frequently encountered naso-ethmoidal malignancies, has a proper fluid component mimicking a mucocele (Fig. 9.10, 9.11b). Therefore, in presence of a naso-ethmoidal mass, any solid tissue within a mucocele-like lesion should raise the suspect of intestinal-type adenocarcinoma.

Conversely, true mucoceles should be differentiated from fluid-content areas of this specific histotype.

Meticulous attention should be paid to the evaluation of lacrimal system, particularly if epiphora is present, as imaging is highly accurate in predicting neoplastic invasion (89%) (EISEN et al. 2000). CT and MR findings indicating lacrimal pathways involvement are: dilation of the lacrimal sac, lacrimal bone and/or nasolacrimal duct walls erosion, and abnormal signal within the duct replacing its normal mucosa.

9.2
Adenoid Cystic Carcinoma

9.2.1
Definition, Epidemiology, Pattern of Growth

Adenoid cystic carcinoma accounts for 1% of all head and neck malignancies; it occurs more frequently in minor than in major salivary glands. In the head and neck, the sinonasal tract is the most common localization for adenoid cystic carcinoma of the minor salivary glands (KIM et al. 1999b). The majority of the lesions occur in middle-aged patients; there are very few cases below the age of 20 and over the age of 80.

Histologically, three patterns with different distribution are recognized: cribriform, tubular, and solid. Arrangement of tumor cells according to a "Swiss cheese" pattern is the distinctive hallmark of cribriform lesions, which are the most frequently observed.

Adenoid cystic carcinoma is a slow-growing but aggressive malignancy, with a peculiar tendency for local perineural invasion and spread along major nerves as well as along periosteal planes and for distant metastases, which are rare at diagnosis (5%), but occur during the course of the disease in over 50% of patients. Distant localizations mainly involve lungs, brain, and liver and may present even 15–20 years after the initial diagnosis. Regional metastases are instead uncommon (5%), not only at presentation but also as a late event. Overall, only a minority of patients is definitively cured on the long term.

9.2.2
Clinical and Endoscopic Findings

Due to their slow and silent growth, most adenoid cystic carcinomas of the sinonasal tract are diagnosed at a locally advanced stage (WISEMAN et al. 2002). Apart from the usual signs and symptoms associated with malignancies of the sinonasal tract, persistent pain in the trigeminal territory is a finding occurring in 20% of patients, which should prompt the physician to rule out the presence of an adenoid cystic carcinoma with nerve involvement.

At endoscopy, the lesion usually appears as a mass covered by an apparently normal mucosa, with a lobulated surface and a color varying from white to gray. Very rarely, adenoid cystic carcinoma presents as a polypoid mass. Macroscopically, it is very difficult to assess the extent of submucosal growth.

9.2.3
Treatment Guidelines and Outcome

Surgery is the mainstay of treatment for adenoid cystic carcinoma. Fulfilling the oncologic principle of achieving clear margins is more difficult in this tumor than in other malignant lesions, due to its insidious submucosal and subperiosteal growth as well as to the tendency to spread along named nerves even far from the site of the lesion. Therefore, the surgeon should be aware of the need to check the radical tumor removal with multiple frozen sections and, possibly, to extend the resection to obtain clear margins. This principle is even more relevant in the sinonasal tract, where, for instance, adenoid cystic carcinoma may invade the sphenopalatine fossa and spread intracranially along the maxillary and vidian nerves. Post-operative radiotherapy is commonly indicated, particularly in sinonasal localizations, with the intent to treat residual microscopic disease. A 66 Gy dose is recommended whenever multiple margins are positive or there is extensive soft tissue involvement (GARDEN et al. 1995).

Overall and disease-free survival of patients with adenoid cystic carcinoma typically declines along the years. In a recent report strictly focused on sinonasal localizations, WISEMAN et al. (2002) found a 5-year, 10-year, and 15-year overall survival of 65%, 55%, and 28%, respectively. Interestingly enough, sinonasal primaries have a poorer prognosis when compared with primaries in the major salivary glands and oral cavity/oropharynx (KHAN et al. 2001).

Treatment with radiation alone is indicated for unresectable lesions or recurrences. Fast neutron radiotherapy has been shown to give a better local-regional control of the disease than photon beam radiotherapy (GRIFFIN et al. 1988). Encouraging results have been obtained with this technique as a post-operative adjunct even in patients who had undergone only surgical "debulking" (DOUGLAS et al. 2000). However, base of the skull invasion has still a negative impact on both local-regional control and survival (DOUGLAS et al. 2000). Very recently, SCHULZ-ERTNER et al. (2004) have reported a good local-regional control on unfavorable adenoid cystic carcinomas with combined photon and carbon ion radiotherapy.

Adenoid cystic carcinoma is considered a chemoinsensitive tumor, so that chemotherapy is only in very rare instances indicated as a first-line treatment. However, encouraging results in the management of recurrent adenoid cystic carcinoma have been reported by using a combination of vinorelbine and cisplatin (AIROLDI et al. 2001).

Unlike other malignant tumors of the head and neck, patients with adenoid cystic carcinoma may survive for years with distant metastases, which can be even resected in carefully selected patients. Therefore, the presence at diagnosis of secondary lesions does not "per se" exclude to treat the primary with a curative intent.

Advanced T stage (Spiro and Huvos 1992; Khan et al. 2001; Mendenhall et al. 2004) and positive margins (Garden et al. 1995; Prokopakis et al. 1999) have been shown to have a negative impact on local control of the disease. More controversial results have been reported instead on histological subtype (Khan et al. 2001) and local microscopic perineural invasion (Vrielinck et al. 1988; Prokopakis et al. 1999). According to Garden et al. (1995) perineural involvement was an adverse prognostic factor only when perineural spread along a major (named) nerve was present.

Considering the natural history of adenoid cystic carcinoma, periodic follow up evaluations, adjusted for stage of the disease and response to treatment, should be extended far longer than the traditional 5-year period.

9.2.4
Key Information to Be Provided by Imaging

- Assessment of critical extent (particular attention should be paid to detect perineural and subperiosteal spread) and volume of the primary lesion (see section 9.1.6)
- Presence of distant metastases

9.2.5
Imaging Findings

Imaging findings of adenoid cystic carcinoma depend on its particular pattern of growth which is characterized by early submucosal spread eventually leading to subperiosteal bone invasion, *permeative invasion* of adjacent connective spaces containing fat tissue and muscles, and by perineural spread. In addition, adenoid cystic carcinoma has a peculiar natural history, consisting of a protracted clinical course with a slow but relentless rate of growth, the occurrence of multiple recurrences, and late distant metastases (Kim et al. 1994; Fordice et al. 1999).

The sinonasal tract may be either the site of origin of the neoplasm or it may be invaded by a lesion arising from adjacent sites, more often the hard palate

(Kuhel et al. 1992; Beckhardt et al. 1995; Ginsberg and DeMonte 1998). MR is the imaging technique of choice, as its superior contrast resolution enables to early detect signal changes due to the peculiar patterns of growth of this histotype.

However, both the CT density and the signal intensity on MR studies are non-specific and do not permit to differentiate adenoid cystic carcinoma from other malignancies (Fig. 9.18). Not even the signal intensity of adenoid cystic carcinoma on T2 sequences ensures to distinguish the solid subtype from the cribriform one (Yousem et al. 2000), although initial reports suggested (Sigal et al. 1992).

Nevertheless, adenoid cystic carcinoma may be suspected on imaging studies when a submucosal lesion is associated with findings indicating perineural spread, particularly if the neoplasm is located in the postero-inferior aspect of maxillary sinus and close to the hard palate (Maroldi et al. 1999).

Though perineural spread along named nerves may be thoroughly delineated by MR, there are two less evident patterns of spread that require dedicated techniques of study and meticulous images analysis: subperiosteal bone invasion and extent into fat spaces. Both patterns arise from the tendency of adenoid cystic carcinoma to invade fat and bone similarly to lymphomas (i.e., with permeative rather than

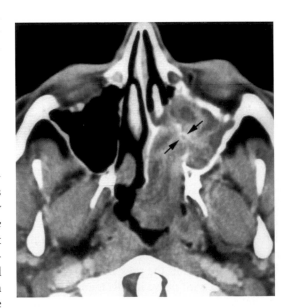

Fig. 9.18 Adenoid cystic carcinoma of left maxillary sinus. Postcontrast CT shows a mass with a pattern of growth similar to an antrochoanal polyp: the tumor extends from maxillary sinus into the nasopharynx. Nonhomogeneous enhancement and the association of erosion and sclerosis of the residual maxillary sinus wall suggest a tumor

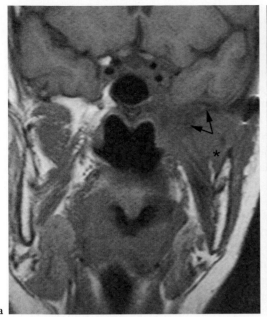
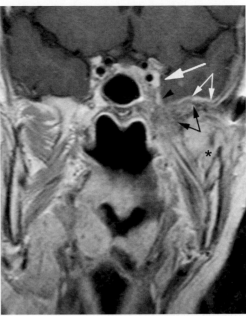

a   b

Fig. 9.19a,b. Recurrent adenoid cystic carcinoma primary arising from left maxillary sinus, treated by surgery and radiation therapy 6 years before. The patient complained of periorbital pain for two months on left side, and had left exophthalmos. **a** Coronal plain T1 shows replacement of fat tissue within the masticator space (*asterisk*) without displacement of adjacent pterygoid muscles. In addition, nonhomogeneous hypointensity replaces the bone marrow signal of left sphenoid bone (*arrows*) (pterygoid process, greater wing, anterior clinoid, and sphenoid sinus floor). The cortical lining of these bony structures is not detectable. **b** Administration of contrast agent causes enhancement of neoplastic tissue permeating the masticator space, of pterygoid muscles – which maintain their organization in bundles. Enhancement of the diploic bone of the sphenoid (up to the left clinoid) is consistent with extensive lymphomatous-like invasion. Perineural spread is demonstrated by nodular thickening and enhancement of the third nerve (*thick white arrow*) and maxillary nerve (*arrowhead*). Irregular meningeal thickening is present along middle cranial fossa floor (*thin white arrows*)

expansive growth. As a result, even extensive replacement of fat by the hypointense tumor may be associated with few *mass-effect* signs on plain SE T1. In fact, muscles and vessels appear *encased* by tumor, which shows bright enhancement after contrast agent administration (Fig. 9.19).

Moreover, plain SE T1 are particularly useful to detect bone marrow replacement by tumor. One should carefully search for focal/diffuse hypointense areas within medullary/diploic bone of the maxillae – particularly the alveolar process - and sphenoid – mostly the pterygoid root, the greater and lesser wings -. If these abnormal areas are hypointense also on TSE T2 and enhance on fat-sat T1 sequences, permeative invasion associated with sclerotic changes is suggested. Though CT may reveal medullary bone sclerosis, its intrinsic contrast resolution is insufficient to detect bone marrow enhancement. Nevertheless, subperiosteal bone invasion and fat tissue infiltration by adenoid cystic carcinoma may be suspected on high resolution CT whenever the technique shows subtle

areas of cortical bone erosion, particularly if associated with sclerosis and fat tissue effacement.

Although imaging may reveal the occurrence of these two patterns of growth and detail the gross, macroscopic, extent of neoplasm, very often adenoid cystic carcinoma is characterized by extensive and unexpected submucosal microscopic spread that either imaging techniques or careful surgical examination fail to detect, being demonstrated only by random biopsies.

9.2.5.1
Imaging to Assess Perineural Spread

Tumor extent along the peripheral nerve stroma (neural sheath) – via endoneurium, perineurium, or perineural lymphatics – is defined as *perineural spread*. Although this process occurs more frequently in a *centripetal* direction, toward the skull base foramina, perineural spread can extend along the opposite direction (i.e., centrifugal).

Perineural spread should not be confused with perineural invasion, which is the microscopic demonstration of tumor cells surrounding very small nerves branches, namely a process beyond detectability of radiologic imaging techniques, which is associated with increased risk of local recurrence and decreased survival when a major nerve is involved.

Though adenoid cystic carcinoma is very frequently associated with perineural spread, other malignant neoplasms of the head and neck may show this pattern of growth. Among them are squamous cell carcinomas arising from either the skin or the mucosal epithelium, desmoplastic melanoma of the skin, lymphoma, and virtually any salivary gland carcinoma.

The frequency of perineural spread in adenoid cystic carcinoma is highly variable in the different series reported in literature (15-60%) (VRIELINCK et al. 1988; YOUSEM et al. 2000). It is important to note that neurological signs and symptoms (dull pain, paresthesia) are not a reliable clue for early diagnosis of perineural spread. In fact, asymptomatic patients may account for up to 30-45% (SUR et al. 1997; CALDEMEYER et al. 1998; TOMURA et al. 1999). Moreover, tumor size or histological subtype should not be considered predictors of perineural extension as already observed by VAN DER WAL et al. (1990). As a result, imaging plays a prominent role in the detection of subclinical spread of adenoid cystic carcinoma along nerve structures.

A key issue to improve perineural spread detection with imaging consists in selecting technical parameters that maximize both spatial and contrast resolution. While on CT few parameters have to be tailored to this purpose – as the choice of small FOV, thin slices (1-3 mm) and high-resolution bone algorithm – more variations are possible on MR. Apart from increasing spatial resolution similarly to CT (small FOV and thin slices), improved contrast resolution is strongly recommended, particularly by mean of fat-saturated T1 sequences after contrast agent administration. In our experience, 3D VIBE sequences provide an excellent solution by obtaining high resolution fat-saturated images in an acceptable study time.

On this sequence, the normal nerve is hypointense, clearly detectable where it is surrounded by enhanced venous plexus, for example along bony grooves and canals – like the inferior alveolar nerve within the mandibular canal, the vidian, maxillary and mandibular nerves through respective foramina, or the hypoglossal nerve at the condylar canal. In addition, the enhanced hyperintense pterygoid plexus

helps in identifying the branching of the hypointense mandibular nerve into its major trunks, outside the skull base foramina (Fig. 9.20).

The purpose of high resolution MR imaging is to demonstrate even subtle signal changes of the nerve itself and/or to detect asymmetric thickening of the enhanced signal surrounding the nerve.

In fact, at histology perineural spread is characterized by a chain of events that MR enables to detect earlier than CT. The progressive accumulation of neoplastic cells around a nerve leads to an increase of its diameter, more frequently segmental. A further step consists in the destruction of the blood-nerve barrier: when this occurs, extravasation of contrast material may be observed, resulting in asymmetric nerve enhancement. In most cases these changes are beneath the threshold of CT detection. As the nerve enlarges, foramina/fissures through which it courses are remodeled, widened and, finally, eroded (CURTIN et al. 1985; WOODRUFF et al. 1986; CURTIN 1998). Therefore CT findings of perineural spread include widening/erosion of foramina/canals and asymmetric enhancement within the same foramina/canals (Fig. 9.21, 9.22). Also in this setting MR is superior to CT, as it enables to detect the neoplastic infiltration of medullary bone (Fig. 9.19).

Once tumor cells invade the perineural spaces, they can grow either along a centrifugal direction (to the periphery) or centripetally (towards skull base, Meckel's cave, and cavernous sinus) (VRIELINCK et al. 1988). On enhanced SE T1 and CT images, this is reflected by the replacement of the fluid signal of Meckel's cave by solid and enhancing tissue and by the increase of the convexity of the lateral border of cavernous sinus.

Chronic atrophy of masticator, tongue or oral floor muscles should be considered an indirect sign of perineural spread: in such cases CT and T1 weighted images show degeneration of denervated muscles, in which muscular tissue has been variably replaced by fat tissue (Fig. 9.23). Also acute and subacute denervation changes are detectable by MR (FISCHBEIN et al. 2001). They can be suspected in the presence of hyperintense T2 signal, abnormal contrast enhancement and increased muscular size, which is secondary to expansion of the extracellular space. As far as the process progresses to a chronic state, key findings of denervation are represented by fatty replacement and volume loss of the muscle.

Two factors may be advocated to explain MR false negative results, namely the presence of skip lesions and the resurfacing phenomenon (GINSBERG et al. 1996; GINSBERG 1999; RICE 1999; GINSBERG 2002).

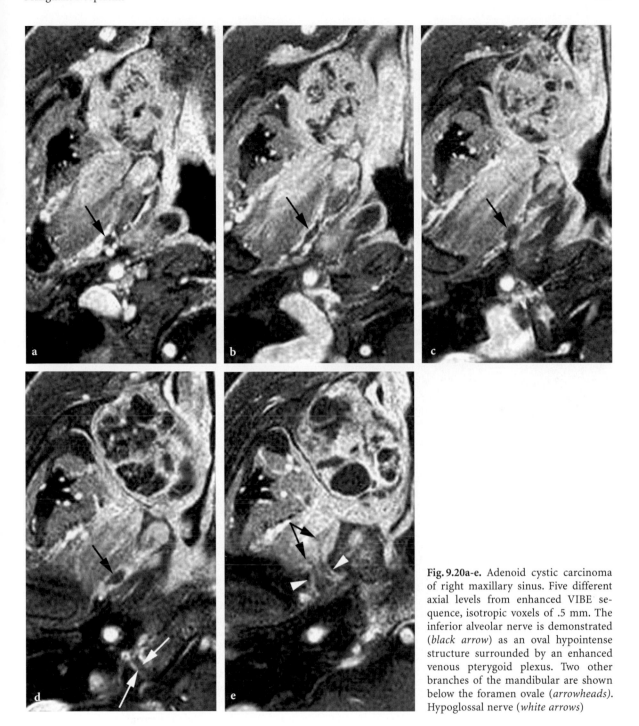

Fig. 9.20a-e. Adenoid cystic carcinoma of right maxillary sinus. Five different axial levels from enhanced VIBE sequence, isotropic voxels of .5 mm. The inferior alveolar nerve is demonstrated (*black arrow*) as an oval hypointense structure surrounded by an enhanced venous pterygoid plexus. Two other branches of the mandibular are shown below the foramen ovale (*arrowheads*). Hypoglossal nerve (*white arrows*)

Actually, microscopic tumor nests along the course of a nerve are undetected because below the threshold of MR imaging (PARKER and HARNSBERGER 1991; CALDEMEYER et al. 1998). Therefore, MR may show a discontinuity of perineural spread along the course of a nerve (skip lesions) as well as resurfacing of tumor immediately distal to a foramen or canal (resurfacing phenomenon). The last is secondary to compression of nerve and perineural tumor by the surrounding bone. For these reasons, nerve structures should be carefully scrutinized, both at preoperative MR and during surgery, along their entire course to decrease the risk of underestimation of tumor extension (MAROLDI et al. 1999).

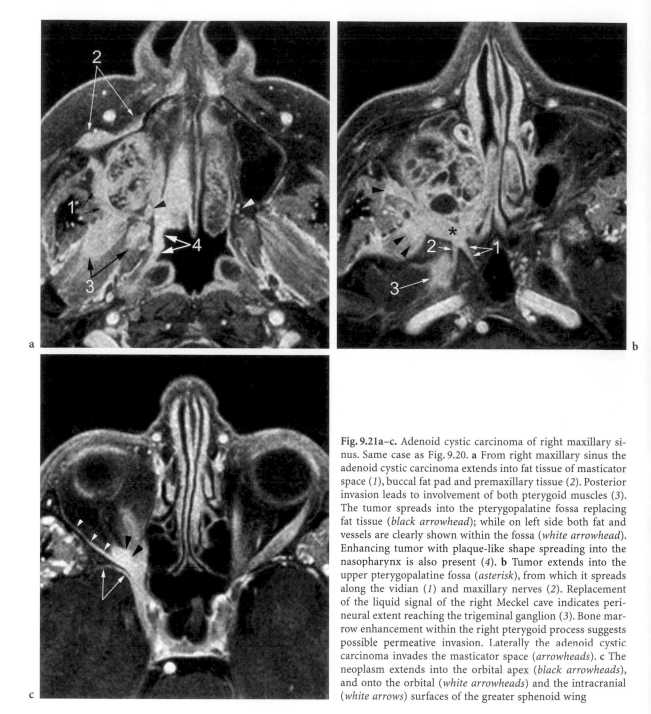

Fig. 9.21a–c. Adenoid cystic carcinoma of right maxillary sinus. Same case as Fig. 9.20. **a** From right maxillary sinus the adenoid cystic carcinoma extends into fat tissue of masticator space (*1*), buccal fat pad and premaxillary tissue (*2*). Posterior invasion leads to involvement of both pterygoid muscles (*3*). The tumor spreads into the pterygopalatine fossa replacing fat tissue (*black arrowhead*); while on left side both fat and vessels are clearly shown within the fossa (*white arrowhead*). Enhancing tumor with plaque-like shape spreading into the nasopharynx is also present (*4*). **b** Tumor extends into the upper pterygopalatine fossa (*asterisk*), from which it spreads along the vidian (*1*) and maxillary nerves (*2*). Replacement of the liquid signal of the right Meckel cave indicates perineural extent reaching the trigeminal ganglion (*3*). Bone marrow enhancement within the right pterygoid process suggests possible permeative invasion. Laterally the adenoid cystic carcinoma invades the masticator space (*arrowheads*). **c** The neoplasm extends into the orbital apex (*black arrowheads*), and onto the orbital (*white arrowheads*) and the intracranial (*white arrows*) surfaces of the greater sphenoid wing

In addition, false positive MR findings may occur when nerve enhancement is detected. Actually, the blood-nerve barrier may be disrupted in several conditions such as inflammation (this may hamper post-surgical and post-RT evaluation), demyelination, axonal degeneration, ischemia and trauma (NEMZEK et al. 1998).

Beyond identifying the presence of perineural spread, MR is also expected to provide a precise map of all neural structures involved in each patient. NEMZEK et al. (1998) obtained an accuracy of 63% for the complete mapping of perineural spread. In their series MR underestimation was in most cases related to the presence of skip lesions.

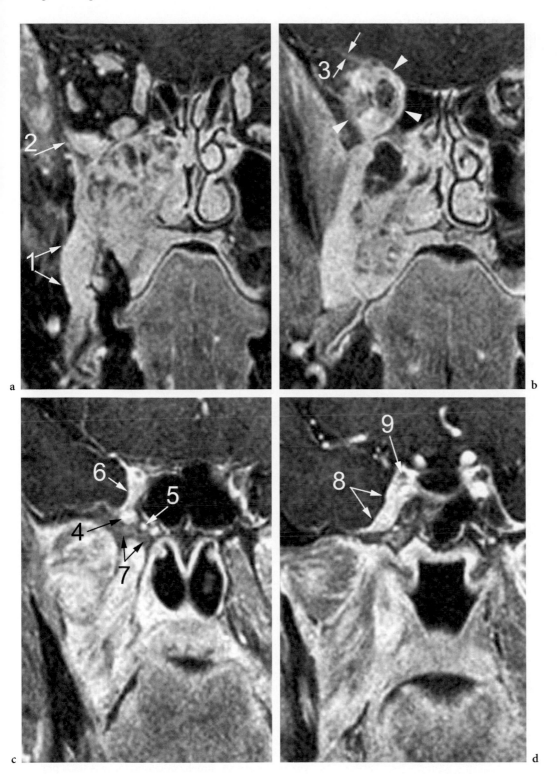

Fig. 9.22a–d. Adenoid cystic carcinoma of right maxillary sinus. Same case as Figs. 9.20 and 9.21. **a** Coronal VIBE shows invasion of right hard palate, lateral extent into the buccinator muscle insertion (*1*). Subperiosteal intraorbital invasion lateral to the infraorbital nerve appears as a round soft tissue mass (*2*). The intraorbital component reaches the apex (*arrowheads on* **b**). Enhancement along the greater wing of the sphenoid is present (*3*). **c** Perineural spread along maxillary nerve (*4*) and vidian nerve (*5*) and in the inferior portion of cavernous sinus (*6*). Abnormal enhancement of the pterygoid process (*7*). Tumor spreads into Meckel cave (*8*), and cavernous sinus, which shows a more convex lateral outline. Abnormal signal of the third cranial nerve is also present (*9*)

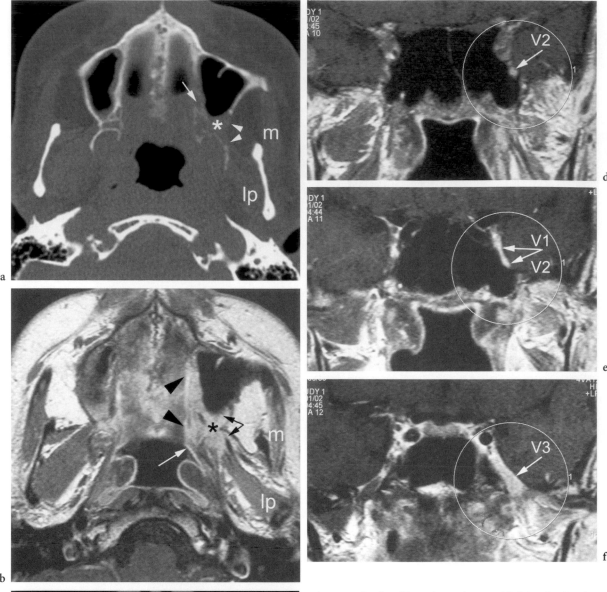

Fig. 9.23a–f. Adenoid cystic carcinoma of left hard palate invading the maxillary sinus. The young patient complained of left face paresthesias for about one year. **a-b** Plain CT and enhanced axial MR obtained at the level of the hard palate show permeative erosion of the pterygoid laminae (*arrowheads on CT, black arrows on MR*). The epicenter of tumor is located at the inferior portion of the pterygopalatine fossa (*asterisk*). **a** On CT, enlargement and subtle erosion of the opening of the greater palatine canal is demonstrated (*white arrow*). **b** Enhancement along the medial maxillary sinus wall indicates invasion on MR (*arrowheads*). Tumor reaches the nasopharynx (*white arrow*). Atrophy of masticator muscles is present. Masseter muscle (*m*); lateral pterygoid muscle (*lp*). **c** At the level of the upper pterygopalatine fossa, a more extensive erosion of its bony boundaries is present with destruction of the vertical lamina of the palatine bone (*white arrow*), and of the pterygoid process (*black arrows*). **d-f** Surgery proved perineural spread along left maxillary nerve (*V2*), ophthalmic nerve (*V1*), and mandibular nerve (*V3*)

9.3
Sinonasal Neuroectodermal Tumors

9.3.1
Olfactory Neuroblastoma

9.3.1.1
Definition, Epidemiology, Pattern of Growth

Olfactory neuroblastoma or esthesioneuroblastoma is a rare neuroectodermal malignant tumor which accounts for 5% of all malignancies of the sinonasal tract (DULGUEROV et al. 2001). Even though it has been reported to occur at any age, from 3 to 88 years, the lesion typically displays a bimodal distribution with two main peaks, in the second and the sixth decade of life (WALCH et al. 2000).

There is nowadays convincing evidence that olfactory neuroblastoma arises from olfactory epithelium (SERVENIUS et al. 1994; CARNEY et al. 1995), which covers the cribriform plate, the superior third of the nasal septum, and the upper part of the superior and middle turbinates. However, the lesion can be occasionally detected in other adjacent areas, as the nasopharynx and the paranasal sinuses (KAIREMO et al. 1998). Olfactory epithelium is made up of three types of cells: olfactory neurosensory cells, sustentacular supporting cells, and basal reserve cells. Olfactory neuroblastoma is thought to take origin from the basal progenitor cells (DULGUEROV et al. 2001).

Based only upon light microscopic features, it would be sometimes very difficult to differentiate olfactory neuroblastoma from other sinonasal malignant neoplasms, such as sinonasal undifferentiated carcinoma, neuroendocrine carcinoma, rhabdomyosarcoma, plasmacytoma, malignant melanoma, and some non-Hodgkin's lymphoma (LUND and MILROY 1993). Diagnosis is therefore supported by using an adequate panel of immunohistochemical studies; positivity for neuron specific enolase, synaptophysin, chromogranin, S-100 protein, neurofilaments are usually detected.

Olfactory neuroblastoma is a slow-growing but aggressive malignancy, characterized by a tendency to early spread along the olfactory phyla into the anterior cranial fossa and to give origin to regional and distant metastases.

Cervical nodes are the most frequently involved metastatic site; secondary localization to bone, lung, pleura, liver, spinal epidural space can also be observed (SHEEHAN et al. 2000).

9.3.1.2
Clinical and Endoscopic Findings

Due to the slow growth and the high vascularization of the tumor, unilateral nasal obstruction and epistaxis are the most frequent presenting complaints (DULGUEROV et al. 2001). Additional signs and symptoms are usually suggestive for an advanced-stage tumor. Olfactory neuroblastoma may also produce vasopressin, thus causing the syndrome of inappropriate antidiuretic hormone secretion (OSTERMAN et al. 1986; AHWAL et al. 1994), characterized by hyponatremia without edema and increased urinary sodium loss (VASAN et al. 2004).

Palpable cervical nodes may be present at diagnosis. According to LEVINE et al. (1999), the rate of patients with nodal metastasis increases from 6% to 25% when the entire clinical history of patients is considered. These data are in keeping with those from RINALDO et al. (2002a) and FERLITO et al. (2003), who extensively reviewed the literature and found an overall rate of lymph node metastases (synchronous and metachronous) from olfactory neuroblastoma of approximately 23%. At endoscopy, olfactory neuroblastoma appears as a broad-based, highly vascularized mass, with polypoid appearance. It usually has an irregular, lobulated surface and a color varying from gray to red (WALCH et al. 2000). Particularly in the early stages, the mass is typically confined to the olfactory cleft, but more advanced lesions frequently extend through the upper part of the nasal septum to involve both nasal fossae.

9.3.1.3
Staging Systems

Different staging systems based on the extension of the lesion (KADISH et al. 1976; DULGUEROV and CALCATERRA 1992) have been specifically proposed for olfactory neuroblastoma (Table 9.4, 9.5).

The main source of criticism towards Kadish classification is that it groups together in the C category situations with a different impact on prognosis as, for example, skull base involvement and widespread disease. DULGUEROV and CALCATERRA (1992) provided a more reliable prognostic stratification of patients, by creating a T4 category for patients with brain involvement. However, their staging system is strictly focused on the local extent of the tumor and does not take into account regional as well as distant metastases.

Moreover, HYAMS (1982) developed a histopathological grading system, based on six parameters

Table 9.4. Kadish staging system (1976)

Stage	Features
A	Tumor confined to the nasal cavity
B	Tumor confined to the nasal cavity, involving one or more paranasal sinuses
C	Tumor extending beyond the nasal cavity and paranasal sinuses. Includes involving of the orbit, skull base, intracranial cavity, cervical lymph nodes and distant metastatic sites

Table 9.5. Dulguerov and Calcaterra staging (1992)

Stage	Features
T1	Tumor involving the nasal cavity and/or paranasal sinuses, sparing the most superior ethmoidal cells
T2	Tumor involving the nasal cavity and/or paranasal sinuses, including the sphenoid, with extension to and erosion of the cribriform plate
T3	Tumor extending into the orbit or protruding into the anterior cranial fossa
T4	Tumor involving the brain

related to growth pattern and to other histological findings (lobular architecture, mitotic index, nuclear polymorphism, presence of rosettes, fibrillary matrix, and necrosis). Lesions can be classified in four grades, from 1 to 4, according to the increasing cellular dedifferentiation.

9.3.1.4
Treatment Guidelines and Outcome

According to the results of a recent meta-analysis (DULGUEROV et al. 2001), the combination of surgery and radiotherapy was associated with the highest 5-year survival rate (65%). In particular, the management of olfactory neuroblastoma has been radically changed by the introduction of anterior craniofacial resection, which has the advantage to ensure an adequate margin of excision even at the level of the anterior cranial fossa. This approach, followed by postoperative radiotherapy, is currently considered the gold standard for lesions without gross brain infiltration. In case of advanced-stage disease or of a poorly differentiated olfactory neuroblastoma, patients should instead undergo chemotherapy, either alone or combined with surgery and/or radiotherapy (LEVINE et al. 1999). Cisplatin, doxorubicin, etoposide, and vincristine have been used in different combinations (EICH et al. 2001; SIMON et al. 2001; LUND

et al. 2003). However, platinum-based regimens seem to be associated with the best responses (SHEEHAN et al. 2000).

In recent years, promising results in the management of selected cases of olfactory neuroblastoma mostly limited to the naso-ethmoidal complex have been reported with the use of a micro-endoscopic approach (STAMMBERGER et al. 1999; CASIANO et al. 2001; CAKMAK et al. 2002). Postoperative stereotactic radiotherapy has been added with the intent to optimize the local control of the disease and, at the same time, to minimize the morbidity (WALCH et al. 2000). Additional experience with a long postoperative follow up is certainly warranted to definitively establish the role of such an alternative approach.

The presence of cervical node metastasis requires an adequate neck dissection and/or radiotherapy (according to the treatment selected for the primary lesion). Since an extremely variable rate of cervical metastases is reported in the literature, elective treatment is a matter of debate. As a matter of fact, it seems reasonable to assess the status of retropharyngeal as well as of cervical lymph nodes by imaging studies and to treat the neck only in those patients who have positive nodes.

Local recurrence, which occurs in 17%-30% of patients, is the most frequent cause of treatment failure, whereas regional recurrence and distant metastases may account for up to 20% and 4%, respectively (LUND et al. 2003). While local and regional recurrences are amenable to salvage treatment in 33-50% and one third of patients, respectively, distant metastases almost invariably carry an ominous prognosis (DULGUEROV et al. 2001).

A very peculiar finding to keep in mind with olfactory neuroblastoma is that local recurrences may occur even many years after treatment. In the paper by LUND ct al. (1998), 5-year actuarial survival was 62%, but at 10 year survival dropped down to 47%. The high rate of late recurrences explain why in olfactory neuroblastoma patients follow up surveillance must be extended for at least 10 years.

Prognosis of olfactory neuroblastoma is correlated not only to the extension of the lesion, but also to Hyams's histopathologic grade (MIYAMOTO et al. 2000). Other factors having an impact on survival are the presence of metastatic lymph nodes (KOKA et al. 1998) and shrinkage of the lesion after chemotherapy (MCELROY et al. 1998; MORITA et al. 1993).

9.3.1.5
Key Information to be Provided by Imaging

- Assessment of critical extents and volume of the primary lesion (see section 9.1.6)
- Presence of lymph node metastases
- Presence of distant metastases

9.3.1.6
Imaging Findings

The imaging features of olfactory neuroblastoma are nonspecific. Nevertheless, this neoplasm should be suspected when a mass is detected in the superior nasal cavity, causing either remodeling or destruction of adjacent bony structures, and erosion of the cribriform plate or of the fovea ethmoidalis (SOM et al. 1986; WOODHEAD and LLOYD 1988; LI et al. 1993; DERDEYN et al. 1994; SCHUSTER et al. 1994; PICKUTH et al. 1999).

In fact, because olfactory neuroblastoma arises from the olfactory epithelium, most cases have the epicenter in the uppermost nasal cavity or in the adjacent ethmoid cells.

The signal characteristics of olfactory neuroblastoma - both density and intensity - overlap those of other neoplasms in the nasal cavity (SCHUSTER et al. 1994; PICKUTH et al. 1999) (Fig. 9.24). Calcifications within the mass have been reported to be frequently observed on CT (SOM and LIDOV 1994). However, as SOM and LIDOV (1994) pointed out, such densities very often cannot be differentiated from residual bone, which is a common finding among several malignancies. Inverted papillomas and chondroid tumors can calcify as well.

Due to its high vascularization, olfactory neuroblastoma shows either homogeneous or heterogeneous intense enhancement (SCHUSTER et al. 1994). Actually, a dense blush is detectable on angiography.

Though infrequent, two additional elements are useful to suggest the diagnosis of olfactory neuroblastoma: the presence of a marginal tumor cyst within the intracranial part and hyperostosis of adjacent bone. The cysts have not a true lining because they are composed of compressed tumor and fibrous tissue. Their content consists of hemorrhagic, degenerated mucoid material, and necrotic tumor. In a series of 54 lesions (neoplastic and inflammatory) with gross intracranial extent, marginal tumor cysts have been observed only in olfactory neuroblastoma (3 out of 5) (SOM et al. 1994).

An exuberant osteoblastic reaction has been described to be associated with olfactory neuroblastoma in few cases. Conversely, less specific bone changes such as remodeling – particularly bowing of sinusal walls - and erosion are more common (REGENBOGEN et al. 1988).

9.3.1.6.1
Pathways of Spread

Because endoscopy accurately delineates the intranasal extent, the key point of imaging studies is to

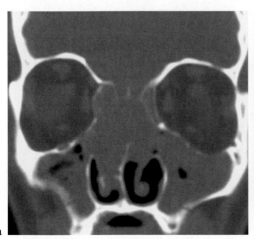 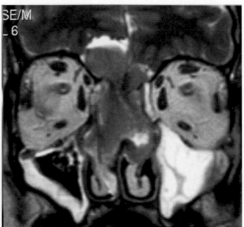

a   b

Fig. 9.24a,b. Olfactory neuroblastoma. **a** Coronal CT shows a soft tissue mass with its epicenter within the right ethmoid, associated with contralateral invasion and remodeling of right lamina papyracea. **b** On coronal T2 sequence the epicenter is more precisely located close to the lamina cribrosa. While on CT the lamina cribrosa appears regular, MR demonstrates that the tumor extends into the anterior cranial fossa with bilateral involvement and with an associated cystic lesion on right side. The olfactory neuroblastoma has a low- to intermediate signal

demonstrate the precise relationship of olfactory neuroblastoma with the skull base, the orbit, and to detail the intracranial extent. Of course, the assessment of intrasinusal invasion is also important.

At an early stage, olfactory neuroblastoma can be totally confined within the nasal cavity or the ethmoid, without contacting the roof. More frequently, the lesion abuts the cribriform plate or the fovea ethmoidalis. In this setting, imaging is required to assess the degree of anterior skull base involvement (Fig. 9.25). Absence of changes of the bony interface on CT does not reliably exclude subtle intracranial spread. MR is ideally suited for this, because it shows even small neoplastic projections that travel through the sieve-like openings across the fenestrations of the cribriform plate, whereas positivity on CT requires bone destruction (LI et al. 1993).

Unfortunately, even MR may fail, most frequently because of overestimation, particularly when dealing with focal abnormalities of the anterior cranial floor. However, it achieves a superior confidence in the planning of an exclusively endonasal approach, though intraoperative mapping (with frozen sections) is necessary (LLOYD et al. 2000).

Advanced lesions tend to spread into the anterior cranial fossa floor and into the contralateral nasal cavity through the destruction of the nasal septum.

9.3.2
Sinonasal Neuroendocrine Carcinoma and Sinonasal Undifferentiated Carcinoma

9.3.2.1
Definition, Epidemiology, Pattern of Growth

Sinonasal neuroendocrine carcinoma and sinonasal undifferentiated carcinoma are two rare and aggressive malignancies, which have been only in recent years recognized and categorized. They share the prevalent site of origin (i.e., superior part of the nasal cavity, upper ethmoid) as well as some imaging, clinical and histological features. Both the identification and the distinction of the two histotypes require an evaluation of the immunohistochemical profile (SMITH et al. 2000), which is otherwise essential for the differentiation from other malignant neoplasms such as olfactory neuroblastoma, lymphoma, Ewing's sarcoma, and melanoma.

Sinonasal neuroendocrine carcinoma, first identified by SILVA et al. (1982), is supposed to take origin from submucosal glands (SMITH et al. 2000). Most neuroendocrine carcinomas occur in the lung, but an extra pulmonary origin from several anatomic areas is possible (WESTERVELD et al. 2001). In the head and neck, the most common site of origin is the larynx, with only a few cases involving the sinonasal tract. The immunohistochemical profile shows positivity

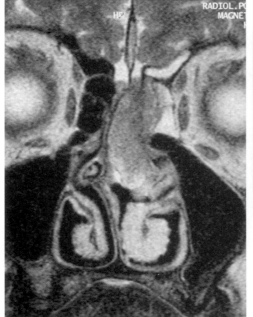
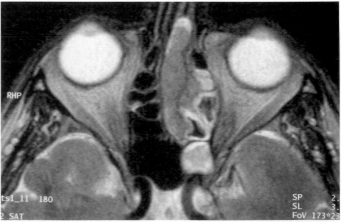

Fig. 9.25a,b. Olfactory neuroblastoma arising from left ethmoid. The perpendicular plate is displaced towards the left, the mass projects inferiorly down to the level of the horizontal middle turbinate. Laterally, the tumor spreads through the vertical lamella of the middle turbinate. The lesion contacts both the horizontal and vertical laminae of the cribriform plate. **b** Blockage of the small left sphenoid sinus results in mucus filling. Permeated invasion of the ethmoid cells is present

for neuroendocrine markers such as neuron specific enolase, chromogranin A, synaptophysin and also for other markers as Cam 5.2 and AE1:AE3; conversely, S-100 and neurofilaments are usually negative (PEREZ-ORDONEZ et al. 1998). Although the neoplasm has been described at any age between 16 and 77 years, the prevalent distribution is in the fifth and sixth decade (PEREZ-ORDONEZ et al. 1998; SMITH et al. 2000).

First described by FRIERSON et al. (1986), sinonasal undifferentiated carcinoma consists of undifferentiated cells supposed to derive from schneiderian epithelium or nasal ectoderm (GREGER et al. 1990). The immunohistochemical evaluation shows positivity for cytokeratin, epithelial membrane antigens, and possible positivity for neuron specific enolase, whereas vimentin and S-100 protein are usually negative (GORELICK et al. 2000). Sinonasal undifferentiated carcinoma is usually diagnosed in the sixth decade of life, with a range between 31 and 81 years (MUSY et al. 2002).

Due to their aggressiveness, both sinonasal neuroendocrine and undifferentiated carcinoma tend to early involve adjacent bony structures, with invasion of soft tissue, orbit and anterior cranial fossa (KIM et al. 2004).

9.3.2.2
Clinical and Endoscopic Findings

Clinical manifestations of sinonasal neuroendocrine and undifferentiated carcinoma are nonspecific, though suggestive for a rapidly growing neoplasm. Therefore, involvement of multiple sinonasal structures as well as extension into the orbit and/or the cranial cavity are not infrequently detected at presentation (MUSY et al. 2002).

Paraneoplastic hypersecretion of ACTH and calcitonin have been reported in two cases of sinonasal neuroendocrine carcinoma (KAMEYA et al. 1980); more recently, also a syndrome of inappropriate antidiuretic hormone secretion has been diagnosed in association with a neuroendocrine carcinoma (VASAN et al. 2004).

In sinonasal undifferentiated carcinoma, cervical node metastases are detected at diagnosis in a rate of patients ranging between 13% (MUSY et al. 2002) and 50% (SMITH et al. 2000), whereas distant spreading is present in up to 31% (JENG et al. 2002).

9.3.2.3
Treatment Guidelines and Outcome

Surgery with platinum-based postoperative chemotherapy should be considered the treatment of choice for sinonasal neuroendocrine carcinomas with limited local extent (PEREZ-ORDONEZ et al. 1998). According to GALERA-RUIZ et al. (2001b), advanced lesions are best treated by a regimen similar to that of small cell lung cancer, which includes a combination of chemotherapy (cisplatin + etoposide) and radiotherapy. Differently, in the experience of Memorial Sloan Kettering Cancer Center, a good response was obtained with platinum-based neoadjuvant chemotherapy and radiotherapy followed by surgery (PEREZ-ORDONEZ et al. 1998). A similar combination of chemotherapy, radiotherapy, and possibly subsequent surgery has been proposed by FITZEK et al. (2002). In case of disseminated disease, platinum-based chemotherapy is the treatment of choice. Radiotherapy may also have a role in the palliation of non resectable lesions.

Even though local recurrence is the most common cause of treatment failure, regional and distant spreading (especially to the brain and spine) may also occur (SMITH et al. 2000). In the series from PEREZ-ORDONEZ et al. (1998), after a 37-month follow up, only one patient (16.7%) affected by sinonasal neuroendocrine carcinoma was free of disease, one (16.7%) died for local recurrence and distant metastases, and the remaining four (66.6%) were alive with disease (local and/or distant recurrence).

Due to the aggressiveness of sinonasal undifferentiated carcinoma and to its high probability of systemic spreading, almost all authors concur on the need of a treatment which should include a combination of radiotherapy and chemotherapy. By contrast, the role of surgery is controversial.

Some authors (GORELICK et al. 2000; MUSY et al. 2002; KIM et al. 2004) have proposed an integrated therapeutic protocol which included surgery. The choice of this therapeutic protocol is supported by either the detection in the majority of patients of viable neoplastic cells within the field of irradiation (MUSY et al. 2002) and by the observation of a better survival when surgery was added to chemotherapy with radiation (KIM et al. 2004). In the paper by MUSY et al. (2002), the overall 2-year survival for patients affected by sinonasal undifferentiated carcinoma was 47%; when stratified by treatment modality, survival was as high as 64% for patients who underwent craniofacial resection and 25% for those who did not. However, some bias related to treatment selection in relation to the stage of the lesion might have influenced the results. More recently, RISCHIN et al. (2004) reported promising results in the treatment of locally advanced sinonasal undifferentiated carcinoma with a regimen of neoadjuvant chemotherapy (5-fluorouracil and platinum) followed by concurrent chemo-radiation. With this protocol, they achieved a 2-year disease-free and overall survival of 43% and 64%, respectively. Surgery should be reserved only for those patients with residual resectable disease.

Local-regional and distant metastases develop in a high rate of patients (63% and 50%, respectively), prevalently within two years from treatment (KIM et al. 2004).

9.3.2.4
Key Information to Be Provided by Imaging

- Assessment of critical extents and volume of the primary lesion (see section 9.1.6)
- Presence of lymph node metastases
- Presence of distant metastases

9.3.2.5
Imaging Findings

Sinonasal neuroendocrine carcinoma is not associated with distinctive CT or MR imaging features (KANAMALLA et al. 2000). On CT, it may appear as a well-defined and homogeneous soft tissue mass. Bone remodeling and/or bone destruction may also be noted. Expansion of sinusal walls, rather than destruction, could be a useful indicator that the tumor is not a conventional squamous cell carcinoma. In the series of KANAMALLA et al. (2000), no evidence of intra-tumoral calcification was found. A single report in the literature described partially calcified low density naso-ethmoidal neuroendocrine carcinoma with intracranial extension (MANOME et al. 1990). On MR, the lesion has been described to appear hypointense on T1 images and heterogeneously hyperintense on T2. It shows minimal heterogeneous enhancement after contrast agent administration (KANAMALLA et al. 2000) (Fig. 9.16).

The biological aggressiveness of undifferentiated carcinoma often results in large, rapidly growing lesions with extensive bone destruction and invasion of adjacent structures. Lesions tend to arise in the ethmoid and superior nasal cavity, as they probably derive from schneiderian epithelium or nasal ectoderm. Intracranial and intraorbital invasion are frequent. In the series of PHILLIPS et al. (1997), the imaging features of undifferentiated carcinoma were not specific. On CT, tumor usually did not show calcifications and enhanced variably. It appeared isointense to skeletal muscles on T1, iso- to hyperintense on T2 with non-homogeneous enhancement after contrast agent administration (Fig. 9.26).

9.3.3
Ewing's Sarcoma

9.3.3 1
Definition, Epidemiology, Pattern of Growth

Ewing's sarcoma, a tumor arising within bone marrow, is included in the group of primitive neuroectodermal tumors, which encompasses three different subtypes: 1) neuroblastoma 2) central nervous system tumors like medulloblastoma 3) peripheral neuroectodermal tumors like Ewing's sarcoma (BATSAKIS et al. 1996).

Even though two variants (skeletal and extra-skeletal) of Ewing's sarcoma are traditionally recognized, it is sometimes difficult to separate the two entities (MILLS and FECHNER 1989).

Ewing's sarcoma is usually found in long bones of the extremities in children and young white adults, with a peak incidence in the second decade (HOWARTH et al. 2004). There is a constant male predominance (HOWARTH et al. 2004). It is considered the second most common pediatric bone tumor, with an incidence of 3 new cases per 1,000,000 inhabitants per year (PAULUSSEN et al. 2001).

Head and neck area is rarely involved either by skeletal (HOWARD and DANIELS 1993) and extra-skeletal subtype (VACCANI et al. 1999; BOOR et al. 2001), with the mandible and the skull being the preferential sites of origin (SIEGAL et al. 1987). Sinonasal tract involvement is extremely rare, with about 50 cases reported in the English literature. Most of them were observed in the maxillary sinus, whereas less than 10 cases each involved the ethmoid and the nasal fossa. Race, gender and age features are similar to those reported for lesion with a skeletal localization, even though the lesion may occur at an older age.

The pathogenesis of the tumor is still unclear; however, a specific chromosomal translocation (t11:22) (q24:q12), which is present in up to 90% of cases (VACCANI et al. 1999), is considered to play an important role.

Ewing's sarcoma has a slow growth but also a high tendency to develop distant metastases, more frequently to lungs, bone and bone marrow (BURDACH et al. 2003).

Histological diagnosis of Ewing's sarcoma is based on identification of the aforementioned specific chromosomal translocation (YOSHIDA et al. 1997) and immunohistochemical profile (positivity for S-100 protein, CD99, FLI-1). Intracytoplasmic glyco-

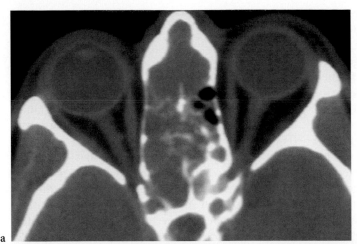

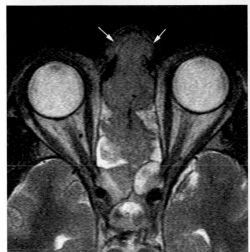

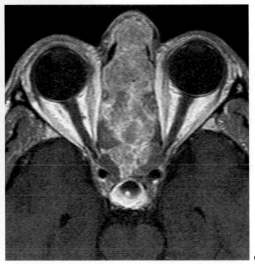

Fig. 9.26a–c. Sinonasal undifferentiated carcinoma arising within the right ethmoid. **a** Axial CT shows irregular and diffuse erosion of ethmoid cells. Fat sat TSE T2 (**b**)and enhanced T1 (**c**) obtained at the same level of CT show a low intensity mass invading both ethmoid sinuses, partially surrounded by fluid, and the nasal bones. Enhancement is rather heterogeneous

gen is found in up to 90% of cases (PAS and PAS-d positivity) (COTRAN et al. 1989; VACCANI et al. 1999). Differential diagnosis includes other small cell tumors, such as hemangiopericytoma, olfactory and primitive neuroblastoma, small cell osteosarcoma, mesenchymal chondrosarcoma, some non-Hodgkin lymphomas, rhabdomyosarcoma, and undifferentiated carcinoma.

9.3.3.2
Clinical and Endoscopic Findings

Ewing's sarcoma shares similar clinical presentation and endoscopic appearance with other sinonasal neoplasms. Since Ewing's sarcoma in its skeletal variant has an osseous origin, pathologic fracture of nasal bones may be the presenting complaint (HOWARTH et al. 2004). Pain, which is the most frequent symptom in long bones localization, is less frequently observed in head and neck area.

Sinonasal lesions are associated with a lower rate of regional and distant dissemination than the skeletal counterpart. At diagnosis, distant metastases are detected in 15%-30% of patients (JOHNSON and POMEROY 1975).

9.3.3.3
Treatment Guidelines and Outcome

Prognosis of Ewing's sarcoma has radically changed with the advent of chemotherapy, which includes different regimens based on vincristine, adriamycin, doxorubicin, and cyclophosphamide or ifosfamide with or without etoposide (WEXLER et al. 1996). Chemotherapy is currently used in a neoadjuvant setting, followed by radiotherapy. Surgery is indicated for residual or recurrent lesions. More aggressive protocols include also adjuvant chemotherapy.

Some authors instead proposed multimodality regimens including surgery (VACCANI et al. 1999).

Treatment protocol was modulated according to the extension of the lesion and to its response to chemotherapy (VACCANI et al. 1999). Whenever a patient with a resectable lesion showed a good response to chemotherapy, surgery was performed. Conversely, in presence of an unresectable lesion and/or of a poor response to systemic therapy, radiation therapy was delivered. Nevertheless, in all patients chemotherapy was prolonged for the full course of the treatment (30-48 weeks). Radiotherapy is also useful in cases not amenable of complete surgical excision, unless unacceptable morbidity (DUNST et al. 1991). Whenever metastatic disease is detected at diagnosis, palliative protocols including chemotherapy and radiotherapy are available.

High doses chemotherapy and/or total body radiation therapy and possibly bone marrow transplant can give a chance of control to patients with distant metastases (HOROWITZ et al. 1993).

Unfavorable prognostic factors are trunk localization, high tumor volume, low response to chemotherapy, and development of distant metastases (HAYES et al. 1989; EVANS et al. 1991; PICCI et al. 1993; VLASAK and SIM 1996). The latter, in particular, has shown to significantly decrease 5-year survival (HOWARTH et al. 2004), which drops from 65% to 30% (WOOD et al. 1990).

9.3.3.4
Key Information to Be Provided by Imaging

- Assessment of critical extents and volume of the primary lesion (see section 9.1.6)
- Presence of lymph node metastases
- Presence of distant metastases

9.3.3.5
Imaging Findings

On CT, Ewing's sarcoma arising from sinonasal tract osseous structures or skull base is characterized by permeative destruction of bone, usually associated with a large soft tissue component and no calcification, reflecting the aggressive nature of the tumor (HARMAN et al. 2003).

On MR, Ewing's sarcoma usually has a homogeneous hypo- to hyperintense signal on T2 sequences, though hemorrhagic and necrotic areas within soft tissues can result in a more heterogeneous pattern and often appear hyperintense on T2 sequences (HANNA et al. 1994; SINGH et al. 2002) (Fig. 9.27). Whereas CT more easily demonstrates the erosion of the thin lamellae of the ethmoid, MR is superior in detecting bone marrow invasion and grading intracranial extent (HARMAN et al. 2003). Sclerotic changes of the diploic bone have been described on MR by FREEMAN et al. (1988).

The combination of patient's age with the presence of an intra- and extraosseous mass without calcifications can suggest the diagnosis of Ewing's sarcoma (Fig. 9.28).

Few extraosseous sinonasal tract Ewing's sarcomas have been reported. Many of them arose from nasal cavity structures and presented as a nonspecific polypoid mass (PONTIUS and SEBEK 1981; LANE and IRONSIDE 1990; CSOKONAI et al. 2001; AFERZON et al. 2003).

Chest CT, bone marrow aspirate, and/or bone scintigraphy with technetium 99m, thallium 201, or gallium 67 are helpful in detecting distant metastases at presentation and in post treatment follow up (FLETCHER 1991; VACCANI et al. 1999). Also FDG-

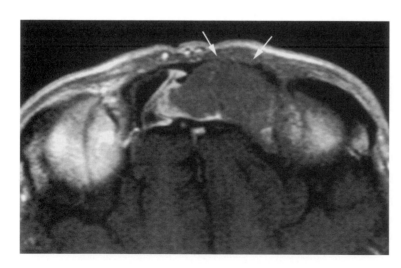

Fig. 9.27 Ewing sarcoma arising in an adult male from the left frontal sinus. On postcontrast T1 sequence the mass has slight enhancement, its signal rather low compared with the surrounding thickened sinusal mucosa. Erosion of the anterior wall is demonstrated (*white arrows*)

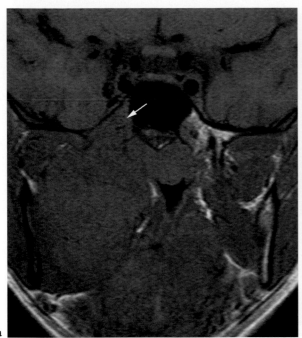
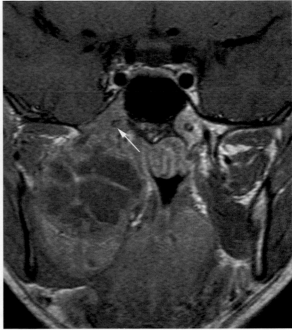

a

b

Fig. 9.28a,b. Ewing sarcoma arising in an adolescent female from pterygoid process. The extra-osseous component of tumor is prevalent, with extensive invasion of the masticator space. On plain T1 coronal plane (a) the signal of the lesion is similar to pterygoid muscles. This hypointense signal – which replaces the diploic bone within pterygoid (*white arrow on* a) - shows enhancement after contrast agent administration (b) indicating the presence of intraosseous neoplastic tissue. Cortical lining of the vidian canal is unchanged (*white arrow*)

PET has been purposed instead of scintigraphy in the diagnostic work-up. Laboratory tests able to arise a suspicion of metastases (lactate dehydrogenase, reverse transcription PCR) can be also used for staging or during follow-up (SORENSEN et al. 1993; VLASAK and SIM 1996).

9.4
Melanoma

9.4.1
Definition, Epidemiology, Pattern of Growth

Melanoma is composed by a proliferation of melanocytes, which derive from the neural crest and subsequently migrate into the skin and mucosal surfaces with an ectodermal origin (RAMOS et al. 1990; MANOLIDIS and DONALD 1997; LUND et al. 1999; PANDEY et al. 1999). Malignant melanoma is usually divided in two categories (cutaneous and mucosal), which, despite a common cytological derivation, differ for biologic behavior. Mucosal melanoma, which is more aggressive, is more rarely observed than the

cutaneous counterpart (BATSAKIS et al. 1998; PATEL et al. 2002b; MEDINA et al. 2003). In the head and neck region, sinonasal tract and oral cavity are the most frequently involved areas (MEDINA et al. 2003). Sinonasal malignant melanoma is quite an uncommon observation, accounting for less than 1% of all melanomas and for 2–8% of all the malignancies of the nose and paranasal sinuses (TRAPP et al. 1987; KINGDOM and KAPLAN 1995; LUND et al. 1999). It is more frequent in Caucasians and it usually occurs in patients around the age of 50 or older, even though, in a small rate (10-20%), also younger people may be affected (RINALDO et al. 2001; PATEL et al. 2002b). The most frequent sites of origin of sinonasal malignant melanoma are the nasal septum, the lateral nasal wall, the middle and inferior turbinates (LUND 1993; MANOLIDIS and DONALD 1997; MEDINA et al. 2003). Nevertheless, also paranasal sinuses, in particular maxillary and ethmoid, nasal vestibule and floor of the nasal cavity may be affected (LUND 1993). Localization into the sinonasal tract may also occur as a result of an ocular melanoma invading the sinonasal tract or of a metastatic spreading from distant sites (TRAPP et al. 1987; PATEL et al. 2002b). The great majority of patients present with a tumor confined to the primary site, albeit locally advanced (Stage I); far uncommon is the observation at diagnosis of regional (Stage II) or distant metastases (Stage III) (MANOLIDIS and DONALD 1997; PATEL et al. 2002b). Due to the large size of the lesion at presentation, to the possible presence of multiple neoplastic foci and amelanotic areas (MANOLIDIS and DONALD 1997; LUND et al. 1999), the real site of origin and the extent of the lesion are sometimes difficult to assess.

Differential diagnosis is usually with olfactory neuroblastoma, some non-Hodgkin lymphomas, plasmacytoma, Ewing's sarcoma, rhabdomyosarcoma, small cell undifferentiated carcinoma; in the cases without typical histological features, diagnosis may be supported by the immunohistochemical profile (i.e., positivity for S-100 protein, vimentin, and for HMB-45) (STERN and GUILLAMONDEGUI 1991; LUND et al. 1999; RINALDO et al. 2001).

9.4.2
Clinical and Endoscopic Findings

Clinical manifestations of mucosal malignant melanoma are quite nonspecific. Metastases to cervical lymph nodes are detected in a 5.7% to 18.7% of patients (MANOLIDIS and DONALD 1997; PATEL et al. 2002b), mostly at the submandibular and upper jugular levels. Distant metastases, in particular to lung and brain, are found in 3.1% to 14% of patients (STERN and GUILLAMONDEGUI 1991; BATSAKIS et al. 1998; RINALDO et al. 2001).

At endoscopy, mucosal melanoma appears as a polypoid lesion, with areas of necrosis or superficial hemorrhages (RINALDO et al. 2001). Its color varies from pink to brownish (MATIAS et al. 1988) or grayish. This may reflect the different grades of pigmentation of the lesion; poorly pigmented or not pigmented tumors may account for up to one third of all the cases (RINALDO et al. 2001).

9.4.3
Treatment Guidelines and Outcome

The mainstay for treatment of mucosal malignant melanoma is surgical excision. Oncological radicality may be reached only by a complete removal of the lesion; in order to reduce the risk of local recurrence, it is essential to ensure wide, free surgical margins (RINALDO et al. 2001). Several approaches are avail-

able, depending principally on the extent and on the localization of the tumor. As the tumor, at diagnosis, is often great in size, with possible extension to the surrounding structures, such as orbit and/or cranial cavity, external approaches (i.e. transfacial and transcranial) should be considered the first choice (LUND et al. 1999). Mucosal melanoma, due to its aggressiveness and possible multifocality, has more restrictive indications for purely endoscopic resection than other malignant tumors. Surgery, either external or endoscopic, may be also a valid tool for palliative treatment of non-resectable lesions (RINALDO et al. 2001). Invasion of the brain, of the optic chiasm and/or distant metastases contraindicate a surgical treatment.

In presence of cervical metastases, a tailored neck dissection, in relation to the dimension, the extent and the number of nodes, must be planned. Elective neck dissection is generally not indicated, even though the availability of PET scan and sentinel lymph node biopsy in the pre-treatment diagnostic work-up may change this orientation in the future (MEDINA et al. 2003).

The role of post-operative radiotherapy is controversial, despite some reports which advocate the use of radical (GILLIGAN and SLEVIN 1991) or adjuvant radiotherapy (STERN and GUILLAMONDEGUI 1991). However, recent studies (LUND et al. 1999; PATEL et al. 2002b) suggest that there is no evidence of the efficacy of post-operative radiotherapy in mucosal malignant melanoma.

The high aggressiveness of mucosal malignant melanoma is reflected by a high rate of local, regional and distant failure, which accounts for 50%, 20% and 40%, respectively (PATEL et al. 2002b). Tumor thickness rather than free surgical margins appears to affect local recurrence rate (KINGDOM and KAPLAN 1995). Moreover, tumor thickness greater than 5 mm, advanced clinical stage, vascular invasion at histology, and development of distant metastases have a negative prognostic impact on treatment outcome (PATEL et al. 2002b).

Malignant mucosal malignant melanoma is associated with a poor survival. By reviewing 21 papers, PATEL et al. (2002b) found a mean 5-year disease–specific survival of 17%. According to several authors (KINGDOM and KAPLAN 1995; LUND et al. 1999), follow up should be extended beyond the usual 5-year period, since the natural history of malignant melanoma is also characterized by a tendency to develop late recurrences.

9.4.4
Key Information to Be Provided by Imaging

- Assessment of critical extents and volume of the primary lesion (see section 9.1.6)
- Presence of lymph node metastases
- Presence of distant metastases

9.4.5
Imaging Findings

CT appearance of sinonasal melanomas is nonspecific. Density values and enhancement pattern do not provide key information. Bone destruction is observed in most malignant tumors. The site of origin may offer more substantial clues for the differential diagnosis whenever the lesion arises from the anterior nasal septum or middle/inferior turbinates (AZIZI et al. 2001).

MR findings largely depend upon the histological features of the lesion (Fig. 9.29). Melanotic melanomas exhibit a peculiar pattern - consisting of hypointense signal on T2 and spontaneous hyperintensity on T1 – as the result of paramagnetic properties of melanin. More in detail, paramagnetic effect could be due either to metal ions bound to melanin, or to free radicals formation. Conversely, amelanotic variant displays a less specific pattern: hyperintense on T2, hypointense on plain T1.

According to YOUSEM et al. (1996), melanin concentration, rather than the classification as mela-notic or amelanotic, plays a role in producing the typical MR pattern. In fact, a T1 hyperintense/T2 hypointense signal is highly frequent (87.5% of cases) when melanin-containing cells within the lesion exceed 10%. The same pattern is rather or totally unexpected in lesions with less than 10% or no melanin-containing cells (14.3% and 0% of cases, respectively).

Though intratumoral hemorrhage may be identified in up to 42% of cases, this does not seem to affect MR signal. In YOUSEM's et al. (1996) series, in fact, on plain T1 sequence 3/7 of non-hemorrhagic melanotic melanomas were hyperintense, whereas 2/5 hemorrhagic amelanotic melanomas were not.

Contrast enhancement ranges between mild to moderate, its degree being difficult to define in spontaneously hyperintense lesions.

The differential diagnosis of lesions with a hyperintense signal on T1 includes hemorrhagic areas in primary sinonasal lesions (hemangioma, juvenile angiofibroma), hyperproteinaceous secretions in mucoceles, fat-containing lesions, hemorrhagic metastases (from lung, kidney, thyroid, breast primaries). A more precise diagnosis can be suggested matching imaging findings with the clinical history and the endoscopic appearance.

MR findings of amelanotic melanoma are nonspecific as they are shared by a longer and wider list of different lesions, including squamous cell carcinoma, adenocarcinoma, minor salivary glands neoplasms, olfactory neuroblastoma, and fibroosseous lesions.

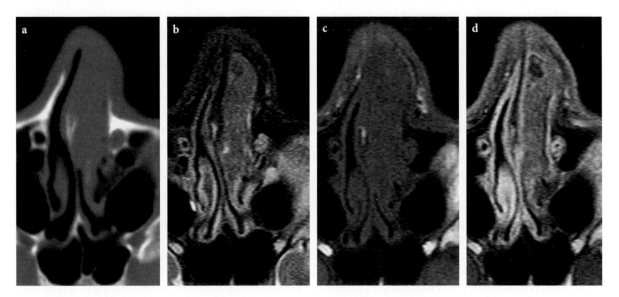

Fig. 9.29a–d. Melanoma of the left nasal cavity. Axial CT (**a**), TSE T2 (**b**), unenhanced (**c**), and enhanced (**d**) T1. The tumor presents as a polypoid mass, filling the nasal cavity, without specific signal features

9.5
Soft Tissue, Cartilaginous, and Bone Sarcomas

9.5.1
Definition, Epidemiology, Pattern of Growth

A great variety of histological subtypes taking origin from soft tissues, cartilage and bone is grouped together under the term of *sarcomas*. They account for about 1% of all malignancies of the head and neck region and for up to 15% of sinonasal tract tumors (SERCARZ et al. 1994). Among head and neck sarcomas, those arising from the sinonasal tract are affected by the worst prognosis, probably due to a delay in diagnosis and the proximity to critical structures, such as skull base and orbit (SERCARZ et al. 1994).

Even though sarcomas are characterized by different biological behavior, metastatic pattern and treatment outcome, they display a similar pattern of local growth (CARRAU et al. 1994). They tend to grow along anatomic planes (fascias, muscles and bones), showing a compressive pattern. At the periphery of the lesion, a pseudocapsule, made up of normal tissue, tumor cells, and an inflammatory response induced by the neoplasm itself, is appreciable (PELLITTERI et al. 2003). The pathogenesis is still unknown; nevertheless, factors such as exposure to ionizing radiations, industrial pollution, traumas, fibrous and bony dysplasia are supposed to have a role (CARRAU et al. 1994; SERCARZ et al. 1994).

We will focus our discussion on rhabdomyosarcoma, chondrosarcoma, osteosarcoma, and leiomyosarcoma which are the most frequently encountered sarcomas of the sinonasal tract.

Rhabdomyosarcoma originates from primitive mesenchymal tissue expressing myogenic differentiation; satellite cells associated with skeletal muscle embryogenesis are the possible elements of origin (HICKS and FLAITZ 2002). Even though three histological subtypes of the tumor are recognized (embryonal, alveolar, and pleomorphic), in a small percentage of patients it is impossible to classify the lesion (CALLENDER et al. 1995). The embryonal subtype is the most frequently found in the pediatric age, followed by the alveolar and the pleomorphic, which is otherwise more common in the adult population (CARRAU et al. 1994; HICKS and FLAITZ 2002). Differential diagnosis is with Ewing's sarcoma, neuroblastoma, lymphomas, and small cell neuroendocrine carcinoma. In some cases diagnosis is based

upon the immunohistochemical profile; positivity of markers like actin, desmin, MyoD-1 may suggest the diagnosis. Rhabdomyosarcoma is the most frequent soft tissue sarcoma in the pediatric age, accounting for up to 75% of all child sarcomas and for 6% of all pediatric cancers; head and neck district is the most commonly involved (37% of cases) (CALLENDER et al. 1995). Occurrence of head and neck rhabdomyosarcoma in adults is instead rare. In fact, no more than 10% of all soft tissues tumors and 1% of all neoplasms in the sinonasal district are rhabdomyosarcomas (CALLENDER et al. 1995; HICKS and FLAITZ 2002). Conversely, sinonasal tract localization is present in about 8% of all adult age rhabdomyosarcomas (CARRAU et al. 1994).

Chondrosarcomas are malignant tumors with a cartilaginous origin. The most frequent sites of origin are long bones and pelvis (GADWAL et al. 2000); an extra-skeletal origin is reported in less than 1% of all cases. Chondrosarcomas account for up to 10% of primary bone tumors. About 10% of all chondrosarcomas occurs in the head and neck region, where maxillary sinus is the most frequently involved site (DOWNEY et al. 2001; COPPIT et al. 2002). The lesion is commonly diagnosed in the sixth decade, without gender predominance (CARRAU et al. 1994); the pediatric population is rarely affected.

Histologically, chondrosarcomas are divided into three grades (Grade 1: well differentiated; Grade 2: intermediate differentiated; Grade 3: poorly differentiated), according to the degree of cellularity, nuclear size and atypia, mitotic activity (COPPIT et al. 2002). Detection of an aggressive growth pattern on cross sectional imaging helps to distinguish a benign chondroma from a Grade 1 chondrosarcoma in case of limited biopsy material.

Based on histogenesis, chondrosarcomas are classified in primary (originating from undifferentiated perichondrial cells), secondary (taking origin from altered cells of a chondroma or cartilaginous exostosis), and mesenchymal (stemming from primitive mesenchymal cells) (DOWNEY et al. 2001). Mesenchymal type is a variant credited with the highest biologic aggressiveness and metastasizing potential (KNOTT et al. 2003).

Chondrosarcoma is usually characterized by a slow growth, with a natural tendency to displace and deform the surrounding structures, rather than to infiltrate and destroy them (GIGER et al. 2002). However, this indolent lesion may have a fatal outcome due to compression and invasion of adjacent vital structures (ROSENBERG et al. 1999). Grading and tumor size show a significant correlation with local and systemic aggressiveness (CARRAU et al. 1994).

Osteosarcoma is a rare malignant tumor taking origin from bony tissue, which mainly involves long bones (GADWAL et al. 2001). Overall incidence is 1:100,000 inhabitants per year (HA et al. 1999). Only a small rate of osteosarcomas, ranging from 4% to 13%, has a craniofacial localization (HA et al. 1999; GADWAL et al. 2001). In this area, mandible (45%) and maxilla (38%) are the most commonly involved sites (KASSIR et al. 1997). Moreover, osteosarcoma accounts for 0.5%-1% of all sinonasal tract tumors (PARK et al. 2003). Interestingly, the mean age of patients with head and neck osteosarcoma ranges between 26 and 40 years; therefore, most patients are 10 to 15 years older than those with osteosarcoma arising from appendicular skeleton (HA et al. 1999). The occurrence in the pediatric age is instead very rare, with only a few case reports and small series reported in the literature (GADWAL et al. 2001). Apparently, the lesion is not associated with gender predominance.

Bone abnormalities and diseases as Paget's disease, fibrous dysplasia, myositis ossificans, other hereditary pathologies like retinoblastoma, Li-Fraumeni syndrome have been suggested as specific risks factors (ODA et al. 1997). Moreover, the high risk of occurrence of osteosarcoma after radiotherapy or chemotherapy for other malignancies is well documented (GALERA-RUIZ et al. 2001a).

According to the cellular pattern of differentiation, osteosarcoma is usually classified in three subtypes: osteoblastic, chondroblastic, and fibroblastic (JUNIOR et al. 2003). No significant correlation between histological subtype and prognosis has been observed.

If the grade of differentiation is taken into account, also osteosarcoma may be divided in Grade I (well differentiated), Grade II (intermediate differentiated), and Grade III (poorly differentiated). In the head and neck region, intermediate- and high grade lesions are the most frequently found (AUGUST et al. 1997; JUNIOR et al. 2003). Osteosarcoma has a local aggressiveness, with a remarkable tendency to infiltrate and involve surrounding soft tissues (HA et al. 1999).

Leiomyosarcoma accounts for approximately 7% of all soft tissue sarcomas and occurs more frequently in the gastrointestinal tract and uterus. Sinonasal tract localization is rare, with about 40 cases reported in the literature (LIPPERT et al. 1996).

9.5.2
Clinical and Endoscopic Findings

Sarcomas of the sinonasal tract, especially low-grade lesions, may silently grow for a long period of time. Symptoms may be present for as long as 46 months before the lesion is diagnosed (PATEL et al. 2002a); they are frequently related to the extension into the surrounding spaces, which causes eye ball displacement, amaurosis, trigeminal numbness, or dentition disruption (GADWAL et al. 2001; PATEL et al. 2002a). At endoscopy, the most common appearance of sarcomas is that of a submucosal mass.

Sarcomas display a local aggressiveness and a propensity to metastasis which are correlated with the degree of differentiation rather than with histology (PELLITTERI et al. 2003). Lymph node metastases are rare and typically associated with high-grade tumors. Reported rates range from 3 to 8%, with the exception of some specific histotype, such as rhabdomyosarcoma (PELLITTERI et al. 2003). Conversely, distant metastases can occur also in low-grade neoplasms, even though with a lower rate than the high-grade counterpart (PELLITTERI et al. 2003).

9.5.3
Treatment Guidelines and Outcome

Treatment of sarcomas depends on several factors related to either the tumor (histological subtype, grade of differentiation, stage and size) or the patient (age, performance status).

Rhabdomyosarcoma, due to the local aggressiveness and to the tendency to early metastasis, must be treated with a multimodality treatment. When only surgery with or without radiotherapy were available for the treatment of this neoplasm, 5-year survival rate was around 10% (CALLENDER et al. 1995). The advent of chemotherapeutic protocols (including vincristine, adriamycin, cyclophosphamide, dactinomycin) in association with radiotherapy and, when required, with surgery has dramatically improved the overall and disease-free survival of the disease. According to such therapeutic guidelines, for example, CALLENDER et al. (1995) found a 5-year local-regional control and an overall survival of 88% and 60%, respectively. Another important observation from their study was that the control of distant spreading and 10-year disease-specific survival were significantly higher (72% *vs.* 24% and 82% *vs.* 36%, respectively) in patients who had received chemotherapy for at least 1 year when compared to patients who did not (CALLENDER et al. 1995). The high risk for nodal metastases makes comprehensive radiotherapy of the neck mandatory. Indications for surgery are quite limited and include excision of small, easily resectable residual or recurrent lesions or palliative resections.

Presence of distant metastases, meningeal extension, adult age, alveolar or unclassified subtype, incomplete resection are considered negative prognostic factors (CALLENDER et al. 1995; SERCARZ et al. 1994).

Rhabdomyosarcoma is characterized by a high, e local, regional, and distant recurrence rate. This is the reason why a "systemic" approach to the disease is mandatory also during post-treatment follow-up. The occurrence of local relapse should be accurately ruled out either clinically and by MR. When the sinonasal tract is considered, a relatively high risk of early relapse/recurrence along meningeal planes and then into the brain parenchyma is worth being underlined. Therefore, periodic MR evaluation (every three months for the first year and then every six months) should be considered mandatory, especially for those lesions encroaching or approximating the skull base. With the specific aim of detecting meningeal or cerebral parenchyma diffusion, PET scans do not show a satisfactory diagnostic accuracy, due to the high metabolic activity of the brain. Conversely, PET is essential in revealing the presence of systemic diffusion of the disease. Cervical node metastases, another frequent pattern of failure for rhabdomyosarcoma, may be detected by US of the neck.

Chondrosarcoma is amenable to surgical excision with a high success rate (SERCARZ et al. 1994). The tendency to present in the well differentiated form (Grade I) explains why chondrosarcoma is the head and neck soft tissues malignant tumor with the best prognosis. Overall 5-year survival, combined for the different grades, may vary from 44% to 81% (DOWNEY et al. 2001).

Surgery must ensure wide clear surgical margins. In presence of small lesions without skull base or orbital involvement, especially if located at the level of nasal septum, an endoscopic resection may be safely accomplished (MATTHEWS et al. 2002). Radiotherapy or chemotherapy should be performed whenever positive margins, which are the most important

prognostic factor together with grading, are detected. In fact, the rate of relapse in presence of positive margins is as high as 65% (MARK et al. 1993). Radio- and/or chemotherapy may also be used in case of recurrences or with a palliative intent.

Chondrosarcoma does not usually display a very aggressive behavior and local recurrence is the most common cause of death. Nevertheless, 20% of patients, especially with a high-grade lesion or mesenchymal subtype, develop distant metastases, being the lung the most affected site. The observation of late recurrences explains the need for a prolonged follow-up.

The treatment for *osteosarcoma* must be based upon wide, aggressive surgical excision, with special attention paid to achieve negative margins. Positive margins, in fact, are an indeed negative prognostic factor (KASSIR et al. 1997; PATEL et al. 2002a). Neoadjuvant chemotherapy should be administrated to patients with high-grade tumors or with lesions unlikely to be completely excised. Adjuvant radiotherapy should be reserved to those cases in which surgery was unable to ensure a complete resection (PATEL et al. 2002a). Following these therapeutic criteria, 5-year overall, disease-specific, and recurrence-free survival of 70%, 75%, and 70%, may be observed (PATEL et al. 2002a). These data are consistent with those obtained at the University of Washington (ODA et al. 1997).

The most common pattern of failure for osteosarcoma is local recurrence, which may be more frequent in patients with positive surgical margins or with tumors greater than 4 cm in size (PATEL et al. 2002a). Distant recurrence is instead rare, with rates commonly ranging between 13% and 23% (VAN Es et al. 1997; BENNETT et al. 2000; PATEL et al. 2002a).

The aggressiveness of *leiomyosarcoma* requires a complete surgical excision followed by radiotherapy, in spite of limited radiosensitivity (KECK et al. 2001). In presence of small, easily resectable lesions, surgery alone may be considered curative (KURUVILLA et al. 1990). Radio- and chemotherapy should also be a valid option whenever palliation is required (BATRA et al. 2001). According to BATRA et al. (2001), leiomyosarcoma is characterized by a poor prognosis, with a 20% 5-year overall survival; recurrences may develop in up to 55% of patients. According to some other authors, the occurrence of the neoplasm within the paranasal sinuses rather than into the nasal cavity would be associated with a higher risk of recurrence (KURUVILLA et al. 1990). Local recurrence is the most common pattern of failure.

9.5.4
Key Information to Be Provided by Imaging

- Assessment of critical extents and volume of the primary lesion (see section 9.1.6)
- Presence of lymph node metastases
- Presence of distant metastases

9.5.5
Imaging Findings

As in several other expansile lesions of the sinonasal tract, many patients with a sarcoma may have undergone CT as the first imaging study. CT is particularly valuable in case of osteogenic sarcoma because it better defines the bony components of this malignant tumor (LEE et al. 1988). However, for most patients with soft tissue sarcomas, MR is the study of choice. It provides excellent definition of the relationship between tumor and neurovascular structures.

Imaging studies should be obtained before biopsy or exploration of the tumor, because surgery may blur the boundary between tumor and adjacent structures. When the internal carotid artery is thought to be at risk, MR angiography may help to detect arterial involvement. The diagnostic workup should include at least chest radiography, to rule out lung metastasis.

In most soft tissue sarcomas, cross sectional imaging findings are nonspecific and do not permit to distinguish among the different histotypes or even differentiate sarcomas from epithelial malignancies. However, in some lesions the presence of peculiar imaging features – combined with clinical and demographic findings – helps to suggest the proper diagnosis.

Unlike soft tissue sarcomas, the diagnosis of those arising from cartilage or bone may be easier due to specific imaging features related to the presence of cartilaginous or osteoid matrix, to peculiar intratumoral calcifications, or to periosteal reaction.

On CT, most *rhabdomyosarcomas* appear as poorly defined, homogeneous (HAGIWARA et al. 2001; LEE et al. 1996; SOHAIB et al. 1998) or non homogeneous (LATACK et al. 1987) solid masses, distorting soft tissues, destroying bone and extending into surrounding spaces. After contrast agent administration, enhancement is generally similar to adjacent muscles (LEE et al. 1996; LATACK et al. 1987). Necrosis is an uncommon finding; hemorrhage or calcifications are generally not present (LEE et al. 1996; HAGIWARA et al. 2001).

On T2 images, tumor signal is usually higher than muscles and fat (YOUSEM et al. 1990; HAGIWARA et al. 2001), and very often heterogeneous (GINSBERG 1992) (Fig. 9.30). On T1, rhabdomyosarcomas appear isointense or slightly hyperintense than adjacent muscles. All tumors enhance. In some rhabdomyosarcoma multiple enhanced rings - resembling bunches of grapes - may be demonstrated. This has been described by HAGIWARA et al. (2001) to be characteristic of *botryoid embryonal rhabdomyosarcomas*. This peculiar MR finding (*botryoid sign*) is probably related to the mucoid rich stroma covered by a thin layer of tumor cells (HAGIWARA et al. 2001).

MR imaging seems to be better than CT for initial and follow up examination of rhabdomyosarcoma because of its multiplanar capability and ability to define the extent of lesion (LEE et al. 1996).

A part for the botryoid sign, several malignant tumors of the head and neck show similar finding. Lymphoma is different from rhabdomyosarcoma in its multifocal involvement and it is less often associated with invasion and destruction of adjacent bone. Liposarcomas usually have a component of fat density or intensity. Chordoma, chondrosarcoma, and osteosarcoma often have calcifications (LEE et al. 1996). Squamous cells carcinoma, which has imaging findings similar to rhabdomyosarcoma, mainly occurs in adults. Although rhabdomyosarcoma has a predilection for children less than 15 years, NAKHLEH et al. (1991) reported a series of young adults (age ranging from 18 to 36 years) who had either embryonal or alveolar rhabdomyosarcoma of the head and neck. Therefore, the diagnosis of rhabdomyosarcoma should be considered in a young adult with an invasive soft tissue mass in the sinonasal tract.

Sinonasal tract *chondrosarcomas* may arise in tissues known to be formed of cartilage, as the nasal septum, or in bones that ossify in cartilage, as the sphenoid, the junction of the sphenoid with the perpendicular plate of the ethmoid, and with the vomer (RASSEKH et al. 1996). A possible explanation for chondrosarcomas arising from sinuses that do not contain cartilage at any stage of their development, as the maxilla, is that the tumor arises from connective cells which possess the capacity to form chondroblasts or osteoblasts (JONES 1973). It is interesting to observe that in the maxilla, chondrosarcoma more frequently develops in the walls, unlike the osteosarcoma that tends to arise from the alveolar ridge (LEE and VAN TASSEL 1989).

Imaging findings distinctive of chondrosarcoma are optimally obtained by a combination of CT and MR (LLOYD et al. 1992). Owing to its slow-growing

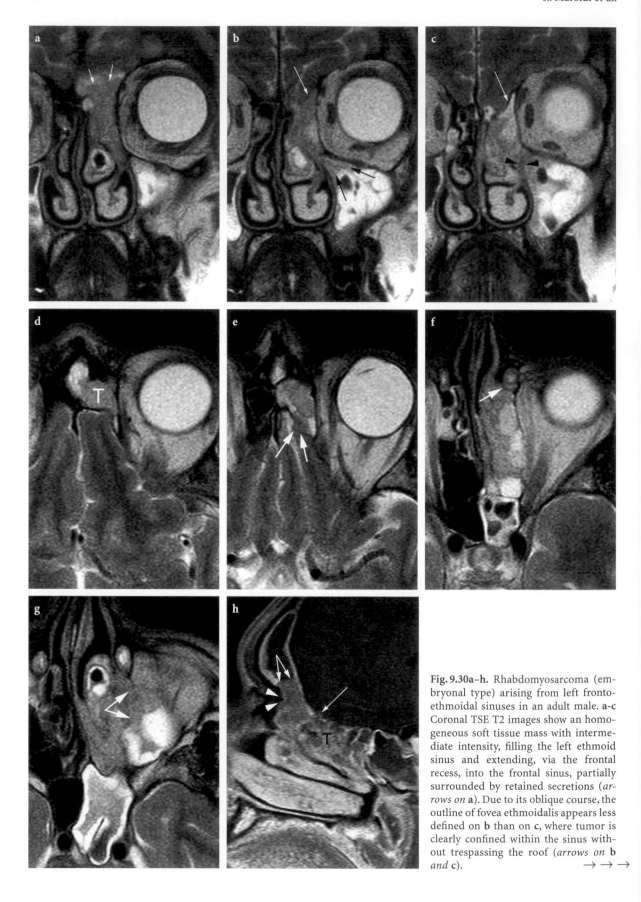

Fig. 9.30a–h. Rhabdomyosarcoma (embryonal type) arising from left fronto-ethmoidal sinuses in an adult male. **a-c** Coronal TSE T2 images show an homogeneous soft tissue mass with intermediate intensity, filling the left ethmoid sinus and extending, via the frontal recess, into the frontal sinus, partially surrounded by retained secretions (*arrows on* **a**). Due to its oblique course, the outline of fovea ethmoidalis appears less defined on **b** than on **c**, where tumor is clearly confined within the sinus without trespassing the roof (*arrows on* **b** *and* **c**).
→ → →

nature and location in symptom-insensitive structures, sinonasal tract chondrosarcoma tends to present a considerable size at the time of diagnosis (LEE and VAN TASSEL 1989). On CT, chondrosarcoma usually is shown as a lobulated soft tissue mass eroding the bone and extending into adjacent soft tissues. The transitional zone is sharp, without periosteal reaction (LEE and VAN TASSEL 1989). Chondroid matrix within the tumor has a density lower than cancellous bone, although denser areas corresponding to local-

ized bone ossification can be present (CHEN et al. 2002). When intratumoral calcifications are present, their nodular, plaque- or ring-like shape usually is a distinctive feature (LEE and VAN TASSEL 1989; LLOYD et al. 1992; RASSEKH et al. 1996) (Fig. 9.31).

At CT, the differential diagnosis is from other sinonasal tumors which present as a soft tissue mass with bone destruction and calcifications. Chondroma, osteochondroma and osteoblastoma have high density internal areas, but these lesions tend not to invade

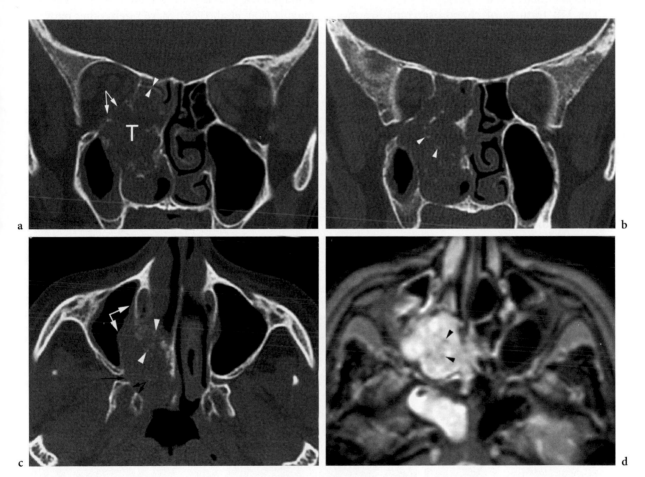

Fig. 9.31a–d. Chondrosarcoma of right naso-ethmoidal area. On coronal CT (**a-b**), the tumor both displaces (*arrowhead on* **a**) and invades adjacent structure (ar*rows*). **b** Several small intratumoral densities, half-ring-like (*arrowheads*) can be recognized. On axial CT (**c**), invasion of maxillary sinus (*white arrows*), vertical lamella of the palatine bone (*long black arrow*), and pterygoid process (*short black arrows*) is shown. Intratumoral calcifications (*arrowheads*). **d** On T2 axial image, the chondrosarcoma has heterogeneous hyperintense signal with hypointense small areas corresponding to intratumoral calcifications (*arrowheads*)

Fig. 9.30a–h. (Continued) Tumor extends into the middle meatus and the ethmoidal infundibulum (*black arrows on* **b**) causing blockage of maxillary sinus, and invades its medial wall (*arrowheads*). On axial TSE T2 images (**d-g**) the portion of tumor within the left frontal sinus (*T*) is shown to abut the posterior wall (*white arrows on* **e**). The tumor invades also the posterior ethmoid cells causing blockage of the left sphenoid sinus (**f**). Anteriorly the lesion reaches the nasolacrimal duct (*arrow on* **f**). Invasion of middle meatus and maxillary sinus is seen on **g** (*arrows*). On sagittal enhanced T1 (**h**) the rhabdomyosarcoma (*T*) has mild, quite homogeneous enhancement. The extent within the frontal sinus is clearly defined as the signal of tumor differs from both fluid retention and mucosa thickening (*short arrows*). At the level of frontal sinus ostium, the lesion contacts a thick and prominent bony "beak" (*arrowheads*). A focal area of intracranial extent is demonstrated (*long arrow*)

the bone (RASSEKH et al. 1996). Inverted papilloma can present with high densities in up to 50% of cases; more frequently multiple and discrete, in most cases they represent residual bone rather than calcifications (SOM and LIDOV 1994). Meningioma can have a similar appearance, but it tends to cause hyperostosis in the adjacent bone, rather than spotty calcifications. Osteosarcoma may resemble a chondrosarcoma with dense calcifications, but the calcifications are usually more diffuse and ill defined or linear with a "sunray" appearance (LLOYD et al. 1992).

The MR features of chondrosarcoma are more characteristic, they reflect the presence of an internal chondroid avascular matrix surrounded by a more vascularized peripheral growing tissue. On T2 weighted sequences, the chondroid matrix is hyperintense because of high water content, while ossified or cartilage areas appear hypointense (GEIRNAERDT et al. 1993). The administration of contrast agent results in enhancement of the vascularized peripheral rim and of several curvilinear septa that correspond to fibrovascular tissue components. A sharp demarcation between the enhancing rim or fibrovascular septa and the avascular chondroid matrix is usually observed. Other non-enhancing areas can be related to the presence of mucoid or necrosis.

Mesenchymal chondrosarcoma has a predilection for head and neck. In the sinonasal tract, skeletal le-sions more commonly involve the maxilla. The presence of a bimorphic pattern on histology - a highly vascularized mesenchymal component surrounding cartilage islands - accounts for the relevant and inhomogeneous *lobular* enhancement on both CT and MR, mostly peripheral with a central low vascularized area. Arc- or ring-like, stippled and dense calcifications can be present (SHAPEERO et al. 1993; CHIDAMBARAM and SANVILLE 2000).

Most non radiation-induced *osteosarcomas* of the sinonasal tract arise from the inferior aspect of the maxilla (LEE et al. 1988), More rarely, other paranasal sinuses are the primary site (PARK et al. 2004). An abnormal soft tissue mass with bone destruction is usually demonstrated by cross sectional imaging. Whereas CT is superior to MR in detecting tumor matrix mineralization – which occurs in up to 75% of the cases - and osteoid matrix calcification (LEE et al. 1988), MR is even more effective in demonstrating the intramedullary and extra osseous tumor components on both T1- and T2-weighted images (BOYKO et al. 1987) (Fig. 9.32). When periosteal reaction is present, the typical *sunburst* appearance is better shown by thin-slice CT scans (OOT et al. 1986) (Fig. 9.33). Totally periosteal growth of a sphenoid sinus osteosarcoma with intracranial extent and absence of wall destruction has been recently described (HAYASHI et al. 2000).

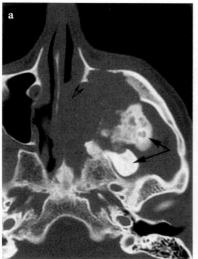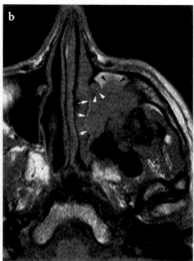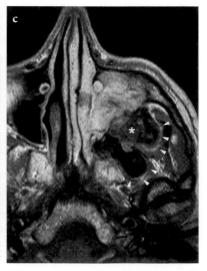

Fig- 9.32a–c. Osteosarcoma of left maxillary sinus. On axial CT (**a**), tumor presents as a soft tissue mass with large, irregular high densities at its posterior boundary corresponding to two nodules with different degree of tumor matrix mineralization (*thick arrows*). Medial maxillary wall is not recognizable. Erosion of nasolacrimal duct is shown (*thin arrows*). On unenhanced axial T1 image (**b**), a clear separation of tumor from intrasinusal hyperintense mucus is shown (*black arrowheads*). The medial maxillary sinus wall is displaced and distorted (*short arrows*). Invasion of nasolacrimal duct is present (*black arrowheads*). **c** After contrast agent administration, not only the intrasinusal portion enhances, but also the lesser mineralized nodule (*usterisk*). In addition, a soft tissue plaque-like enhancement is demonstrated surrounding the mineralized nodules (*arrowheads*)

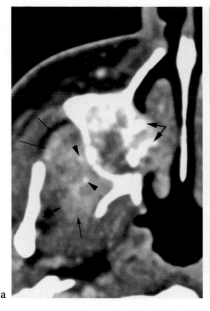

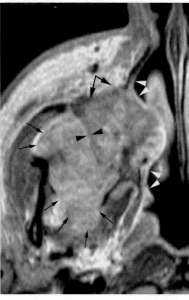

a

b

Fig. 9.33a,b. Osteosarcoma of the right maxillary sinus. a CT shows that the tumor displaces the medial maxillary sinus wall with extensive periosteal reaction (*thick arrows*). Masticator space is invaded (*thin arrows*). Scattered intra-tumoral high densities are seen (*arrowheads*). b Enhanced T1 image demonstrates the submucosal spread of tumor (*white arrowheads*), invasion of the anterior (*short arrows*) and postero-lateral (*black arrowheads*) walls. Detailed map of masticator space spread is also shown (*long arrows*)

Although most sinonasal tract *leiomyosarcomas* have been reported to arise from nasal cavity structures - such as the septum, the vestibule, the turbinates , and the choana – they can also origin from the paranasal sinuses and the hard palate (TANAKA et al. 1998; SUMIDA et al. 2001; BATRA et al. 2001; KECK et al. 2001). Cross sectional imaging findings are nonspecific. In addition, the pattern of growth of the lesion may range from a non aggressive polypoid mass to a destructive lesion. On CT, leiomyosarcoma appears as a nonhomogeneous soft tissue bulky lesion (BATRA et al. 2001), that remodels or invades the

bone and shows slight to moderate enhancement. As in other locations in the body, the tumor is frequently associated with extensive necrotic or cystic changes and does not contain calcifications (TANAKA et al. 1998) (Fig. 9.34).

On MR, the tumor has been reported to present homogeneous intermediate signal on T1 weighted images and minimally inhomogeneous intermediate to slightly high signal on T2 weighted images compared to muscle. Moderate and inhomogeneous enhancement has been described (TANAKA et al. 1998) (Fig. 9.35).

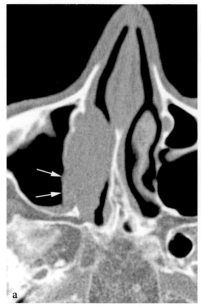

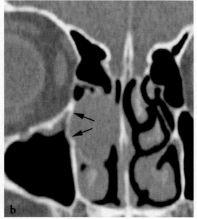

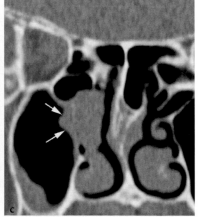

a

b

c

Fig. 9.34a–c. Leiomyosarcoma of right nasal fossa. a CT shows a soft tissue polypoid mass extending along lateral nasal wall and possibly invading the medial maxillary sinus wall (*arrows*). b-c Coronal CT images show remodeling (*black arrows*) and possible invasion of the medial maxillary sinus wall. (suggested by focal thickening on the sinusal surface of the wall) (*white arrows*)

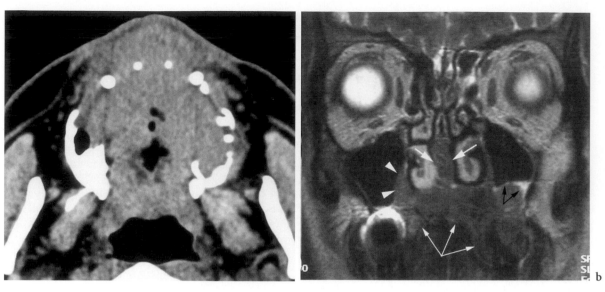

Fig. 9.35a,b. Leiomyosarcoma of hard palate with extensive erosion of bone on axial CT (**a**). The mass is characterized by upwards extent into the nasal cavity with submucosal spread into the nasal septum (*thick white arrows*), right medial maxillary sinus wall (*arrowheads*), and left maxillary sinus (*black arrows*). Bilateral involvement of hard palate by the hypointense tumor signal is seen (*thin white arrows*)

9.6
Hemangiopericytoma

9.6.1
Definition, Epidemiology and Pattern of Growth

Hemangiopericytoma is a mesenchymal tumor originating from Zimmermann's pericytes (i.e. extravascular cells surrounding small vessels) (ZIMMERMAN 1923; SERRANO et al. 2002). Hemangiopericytoma, first described in 1942 (STOUT and MURRAY 1942), accounts for only 1% of all vascular neoplasms and for 3-5% of sarcomas (BATSAKIS 1979). The most frequently involved sites are the lower limbs and trunk (ENZINGER and SMITH 1976). The rate of head and neck involvement ranges between 15% and 25%, with sinonasal tract localization present in 5% of patients (BATSAKIS 1979); ethmoid, nasal cavity, and sphenoid are the preferential sites of origin (SERRANO et al. 2002).

Over 120 cases of sinonasal hemangiopericytomas have been reported in the English literature, with age at presentation ranging between 4 and 80 years (mean 55) (CATALANO et al. 1996). An exceptional case of congenital hemangiopericytoma had also been described (GOTTE et al. 1999). No gender predominance is reported (HERVÉ et al. 1999).

Etiology of such a neoplasm remains unknown, even though trauma, steroid therapy and altered hormone secretions are considered predisposing factors (REINER et al. 1990; CASTELNUOVO et al. 2003). Some authors (CATALANO et al. 1996), in fact, have hypothesized that previous facial traumas, found in two out of seven patients with sinonasal hemangiopericytoma, could have led to an abnormal capillary and pericyte proliferation.

Hemangiopericytoma usually does not display a particularly aggressive pattern of growth, producing obstructive symptoms at presentation, even though tendency to bone erosion, with consequent intracranial and/or intraorbital extension, has been observed (HEKKENBERG et al. 1997).

Hemangiopericytoma of the sinonasal tract are characterized by a less aggressive biologic behavior, if compared to those affecting other sites, such as the pelvis (CATALANO et al. 1996).

In fact, malignant transformation with regional or distant spreading are rarely observed. The reason is not clear, even though some speculations have been put forward. According to some authors (CATALANO et al. 1996), paranasal sinus hemangiopericytomas may be discovered before than in other sites (i.e. pelvis), due to an earlier clinic presentation.

Differential diagnosis includes benign and malignant lesions, such as lobular capillary hemangioma, leiomyoma, hemangiomas, solitary fibrous tumor, synovial sarcoma, mesenchymal chondrosarcoma and other soft tissue tumors, olfactory neuroblastoma, Ewing's sarcoma, non-Hodgkin lymphomas.

9.6.2
Clinical and Endoscopic Findings

Clinical presentation is consistent with a slowly-growing and indolent mass. At endoscopy, the lesion commonly appears as a polypoid, soft, tan-colored, easily bleeding mass.

9.6.3
Treatment Guidelines and Outcome

Wide surgical excision is the mainstay of treatment of sinonasal hemangiopericytomas (CASTELNUOVO et al. 2003). In order to minimize intraoperative bleeding, a preoperative selective embolization may be effective (CATALANO et al. 1996; SERRANO et al. 2002), but it should not be routinely indicated (HEKKENBERG et al. 1997). The most accepted surgical approaches for sinonasal hemangiopericytomas are the external ones, such as lateral rhinotomy, midfacial degloving, craniofacial resection, infratemporal routes. In recent years, however, also endonasal endoscopic resection for selected lesions has been successfully adopted (BHATTACHARYYA et al. 1997; SERRANO et al. 2002; CASTELNUOVO et al. 2003).

Radiotherapy should be reserved to patients with advanced and/or unresectable lesions, whereas chemotherapy appears reliable only with the aim of palliation, in presence of systemic spreading. Adjuvant radiotherapy may be also used in presence of incomplete surgical resection (HERVÉ et al. 1999).

Prognosis appears to be significantly influenced only by tumor stage at diagnosis and completeness of surgical resection (CATALANO et al. 1996). Moreover, local recurrence and metastatic potential are significantly lower in paranasal sinuses than in other sites. In the literature review performed at Mount Sinai Hospital, overall recurrence rate, in most cases due to incomplete surgical resection, reached 18% (22 out of 119 cases), distant metastases occurred in 2.5% (3/119), whereas 4 patients (3.3%) died of the disease (CATALANO et al. 1996). By comparing these data to those regarding axial-skeletal hemangiopericytomas, it is possible to highlight the different biologic aggressiveness. Non-sinusal lesions, in fact, are characterized by higher local recurrence, distant metastases, and mortality rate (up to 50%, 65%, and 60%, respectively) (CATALANO et al. 1996; HEKKENBERG et al. 1997). Recurrences may occur even 17 years after treatment, so that follow-up should be prolonged, possibly for a life-long period (CATALANO et al. 1996; HERVÉ et al. 1999).

9.6.4
Key Information to Be Provided by Imaging

- Assessment of critical extents and volume of the primary lesion (see section 9.1.6)

9.6.5
Imaging Findings

Most sinonasal tract hemangiopericytomas occur in the nasal cavity and in the maxillary sinus (HERVÉ et al. 1999). Imaging features of are nonspecific. On CT hemangiopericytoma appears as an expansile, soft tissue mass, which may be large and associated with bone remodeling or erosion (MAFEE 1993). Calcifications may be present, enhancement ranges from moderate to relevant. On MR, hemangiopericytoma is intermediate to hyperintense on T2, low to intermediate on T1, and has a moderate to marked enhancement following contrast agent administration (SERRANO et al. 2002) (Fig. 9.36).

9.7
Lymphoproliferative Neoplasms

9.7.1
Definition, Epidemiology, Pattern of Growth

Lymphoproliferative neoplasms include a variety of different lesions originating from lymphoid cells. The main lymphoproliferative neoplasms are Hodgkin and non-Hodgkin lymphomas, which originate from lymphocytes; they differ for etiopathogenetic factors, pattern of growth, and prognosis.

Lymphomas account for 3% to 5% of all malignancies, and up to 60% of cases are non-Hodgkin lymphomas (QURAISHI et al. 2000). Hodgkin lymphoma develops within lymph nodes and may then spread, in a quite predictable fashion, through lymphatic channels to contiguous lymph node chains and then to other structures. Non-Hodgkin's lymphomas, which are classified into B and T-NK subtypes according to lymphocytic phenotype, may originate from lymph nodes or, in a quite consistent percentage of cases (20-40%), from an extranodal site (FAJARDO-DOLCI et al. 1999). Non-Hodgkin lymphomas may be characterized by a dissemination of the disease, with involvement also of nodal and extranodal sites far from the original site.

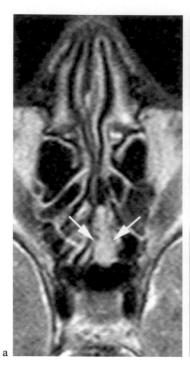 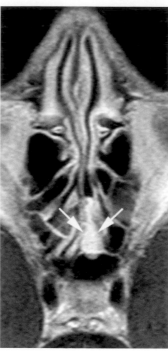

a   b

Fig. 9.36a,b. Hemangiopericytoma of left ethmoid sinus. Axial TSE T2 (**a**) and enhanced T1 (**b**) demonstrate a small polypoid lesion within the posterior ethmoid sinus (*arrows*) projecting into the sphenoid sinus. The lesion has hyperintense signal on TSE T2, and bright enhancement

In the head and neck, about 60% of lymphomas have an extranodal origin (QURAISHI et al. 2000). Sinonasal tract may be involved by primary lesions (nasal cavity T-NK lymphoma and marginal zone B-cell lymphoma) and secondary lesions. For primary neoplasms, it is possible an exclusive localization within the sinonasal tract; conversely, all secondary lesions should be considered as a systemic disease. Sinonasal lesions, either primary or secondary, are mostly non-Hodgkin lymphomas, while Hodgkin lymphoma is very rarely encountered.

A difference in terms of neoplastic cells subtype, epidemiology, and site of origin between Western World and Far East is well known. In the Western World, non-Hodgkin lymphomas are mainly B-cell subtype and sinonasal tract involvement varies between 0.2 and 2% of all non-Hodgkin lymphomas (QURAISHI et al. 2000). In Far East and South America instead, the most frequent cell subtype is T or NK (NAKAMURA et al. 1997). In the Western World, non-Hodgkin lymphomas tend to affect paranasal sinuses in the elderly, whereas in Far East and South America the nasal cavity in younger people is mainly involved (QURAISHI et al. 2000).

In relation to the etiopathogenesis, viruses such as Epstein-Barr and HTLV-1 are considered important agents, especially for specific lymphomas (i.e., Burkitt lymphoma and nasal NK-T lymphoma).

At presentation, non-Hodgkin lymphomas of the sinonasal tract are often bulky, with possible involve-ment of the surrounding structures. They may display a tendency to destroy bony walls of the sinonasal tract, just like other aggressive malignancies; however, it is noteworthy that the lesion may also infiltrate and expand the bone (NAKAMURA et al. 1997) with a permeative rather than a destructive pattern.

Involvement of regional lymph nodes is commonly observed; their distribution varies in relation of the location of the primary lesion within the sinonasal tract. Involvement of the skin, Waldeyer's ring, and extranodal organs has also been described, especially in the advanced stages of the disease.

Plasmacytoma, a lesion included among plasma-cell derived tumors, is more frequently observed in the sinonasal tract in the extramedullary form, while its solitary form is extremely rare. Extramedullary plasmacytoma develops in the head and neck area in up to 90% of cases, with an elective localization in the submucosa of the upper aerodigestive tract (SUSNERWALA et al. 1997; MAJUMDAR et al. 2002). Most patients are elderly, and half of them have the lesion located within the sinonasal tract. According to SUSNERWALA et al. (1997), diagnostic criteria for extramedullary plasmacytoma are considered: 1) a biopsy proven plasma cell tumor involving a single extramedullary site with or without lymph node involvement; 2) a bone marrow biopsy showing less than 5% plasma cells, 3) normal skeletal survey. Extramedullary plasmacytoma cells may show a wide range of cell differentiation which goes from mature cells clones (Grade 1) to intermediate (Grade 2) and completely immature (Grade 3) ones (KAPADIA et al. 1982).

9.7.2
Clinical and Endoscopic Findings

In about 30% of patients, systemic symptoms (i.e., weight loss, temperature, night sweat) should suggest the diagnosis of lymphoma; also hepatosplenomegaly is a frequent presenting sign. Apart from symptoms typical of an expansile lesion of the sinonasal tract, non-Hodgkin lymphomas may also present as midline destructive lesions, with possible palate perforation (FAJARDO-DOLCI et al. 1999).

At nasal endoscopy, the lesion shows no macroscopic peculiarity, since it may appear as a submucosal mass covered by healthy mucosa, as a polypoid mass, or as a frankly neoplastic mass, with superficial necrosis, hemorrhages, and ulcers.

From the clinical standpoint, lymphomas should be differentiated from benign conditions such as Wegener's granulomatosis, sarcoidosis, cocaine addiction, tuberculosis, and from other sinonasal malignancies.

Since non-Hodgkin lymphomas often present as systemic diseases, with possible involvement of other anatomic areas, like chest, abdomen, and/or bone marrow, different staging systems have been put forward. The Ann Arbor staging system (Table 9.6), orig-

inally used only for Hodgkin's lymphoma, and subsequently adopted even for non-Hodgkin lymphomas, is based upon the number of sites involved by the disease (nodal and extranodal [E]), their distribution in relation to the diaphragm, and the absence (A) or presence (B) of systemic symptoms (CARBONE et al. 1971; MEDINA 1985).

This staging system is not fully reliable as a prognostic predictor, since it does not take into account the local extension of the lesion. For this reason, some authors prefer the classification criteria of TNM staging system (ROBBINS et al. 1985).

Pre-treatment diagnostic work-up includes total body CT, blood count and chemistry, and bone marrow biopsy

Diagnosis of lymphomas is mainly established upon biopsy. Cyto-architectural features, immunohistochemical and molecular profile (chromosomal translocations, rearrangement of T-cell receptor or immunoglobulin light chains) are the parameters currently studied to establish a proper diagnosis (JAFFE et al. 2001). Aspiration cytology on a lymph node may only suggest the diagnosis which in most cases is definitively achieved by the histological analysis of a lymph node.

Endoscopic appearance is nonspecific even for extramedullary plasmacytoma, since it may present as a sessile, polypoid or pedunculated lesion, with a color varying from yellowish gray to dark red (SUSNERWALA et al. 1997). It is worth remembering that 10-20% of patients have lymph node involvement at diagnosis. With regard to growth pattern, a tendency of extramedullary plasmacytoma to bone destruction has been described (SUSNERWALA et al. 1997).

Diagnosis of extramedullary plasmacytoma is based on histology but also on serum and urine evaluation, since about 25% of patients show a gamma monoclonal band at electrophoresis and Bence-Jones protein in the urine. Bone marrow biopsy and scintigraphy should consequently be performed in order to rule out bone involvement. Up to 20-30% of cases of extramedullary plasmacytoma can turn to multiple myeloma (SUSNERWALA et al. 1997).

Differential diagnosis includes other pathologic entities in whom a rich plasma-cell infiltrate is detectable, such as reactive plasmacytic hyperplasia, plasma cell granuloma and rhinoscleroma, hemopoietic neoplasms, sinonasal malignancies (such as olfactory neuroblastoma, melanoma, pituitary adenoma, and metastatic tumors) (MAJUMDAR et al. 2002).

Table 9.6. Ann Arbor staging system

	Stage
Stage I	Involvement of a single lymph node or a single extra-lymphatic organ or site
Stage II	Involvement of two or more lymph node regions on the same site of the diaphragm, or localized involvement of a single extra-lymphatic organ or site and one or more lymph node regions on the same side of the diaphragm
Stage III	Involvement of lymph node regions on both sides of the diaphragm
Stage IV	Diffuse or disseminated involvement of one or more extralymphatic organs or tissues with or without lymph node enlargement

	Systemic symptoms
1.	Not otherwise explainable weight loss (> 10%) in the six months before
2.	Not otherwise explainable fever with temperature > 38° C
3.	Night sweat

9.7.3
Treatment Guidelines and Outcome

Extranodal non-Hodgkin lymphomas with primary sinonasal localization are characterized by an aggressive behavior and a dismal prognosis (LI et al. 1998). Radiotherapy and chemotherapy are the mainstay of lymphoproliferative neoplasms treatment, alone or as a part of a combined protocol. Nevertheless, sinonasal non-Hodgkin lymphoma appears less responsive to chemotherapy than lesions with different anatomic localization (LI et al. 1998).

In the early stages or in presence of small lesions (limited IE), radiotherapy is the only treatment modality required. In extensive IE lesions, chemotherapy may be added, even though a single modality treatment (radiotherapy or chemotherapy) is also possible (LI et al. 1998). In case of advanced lesions, combined protocols including concomitant chemotherapy and radiotherapy (IIE) or chemotherapy followed by adjuvant radiotherapy are advised (LI et al. 1998). Radiotherapy dose varies from 40 to 70 Gy (LI et al. 1998; QURAISHI et al. 2000). Palliation may be ensured by chemotherapy alone. Chemotherapeutic regimen, according to different protocols, is based upon agents such as vincristine, cyclophosphamide, bleomycin, adriamycin, etoposide (YU et al. 1997).

Sinonasal lymphomas are characterized by a poor prognosis, with a 5-year overall survival ranging from 24% (YU et al. 1997) to 65% (LI et al. 1998). Poor prognostic factors are advanced age (over 60 years), advanced Ann Arbor stage, and presence of B symptoms (YU et al. 1997). According to the results of a very recent report, complete remission after treatment was the only significant positive prognostic factor in a multivariate analysis (LI et al. 2004).

Patterns of failure for non-Hodgkin lymphomas of the sinonasal tract include local, regional and distant progression or recurrence (LI et al. 1998). Local and/or regional failures account for about 43%, whereas systemic recurrences, which mainly occur in the skin, lung and liver (LI et al. 1998), are detected in 30% of patients (LI et al. 2004). Early stage lesions have a higher propensity for local relapse (YU et al. 1997).

Extramedullary plasmacytoma is a highly radiosensitive tumor (MAJUMDAR et al. 2002), with a 94% local control rate for localized disease if more than 40 Gy in 4 weeks are delivered (MENDENHALL et al. 1980). For low-grade solitary extramedullary plasmacytoma, a dose of 35-40 Gy in 3 weeks is recommended (SUSNERWALA et al. 1997). Elective treatment on the neck is instead considered unnecessary (SUSNERWALA et al. 1997), since nodal metastases at

presentation or during the course of the disease appear not to affect the overall prognosis or the possibility of conversion to multiple myeloma (SUSNERWALA et al. 1997). Chemotherapy should be reserved for invasive (SOESAN et al. 1992) and/or poorly differentiated lesions (MAJUMDAR et al. 2002). Since late recurrences are possible, local failure may be effectively re-treated by irradiation. Surgery instead should be reserved for resectable recurrences after radiotherapy (SUSNERWALA et al. 1997).

The rarity of extramedullary plasmacytoma makes identification of prognostic factors and evaluation of treatment outcomes quite difficult (SUSNERWALA et al. 1997). However, the high grade of the lesion seems to be the most important negative prognostic factor (MAJUMDAR et al. 2002). The risk of recurrence or conversion to a multiple myeloma, even 15 years after treatment, supports the need for a prolonged, even life-long follow up (SUSNERWALA et al. 1997). Periodic examinations should include nasal endoscopy and MR for the primary site and ultrasonography for the neck. Also blood and urine analysis are recommended in order to detect monoclonal paraprotein and Bence Jones protein, respectively.

9.7.4
Key Information to Be Provided by Imaging

- Assessment of critical extents and volume of the primary lesion (see section 9.1.6)
- Presence of nodal involvement
- Presence of extranodal involvement

9.7.5
Imaging Findings

Sinonasal lymphomas are almost exclusively non-Hodgkin lymphomas (GUFLER et al. 1997), their imaging appearance is rather nonspecific. CT and MR findings consist of a diffusely infiltrating soft tissue mass with ill-defined borders (GUFLER et al. 1997) (Fig. 9.37). On MR, slightly non-homogeneous signal may be observed, hyperintense on T2 and intermediate on T1 sequences (HAN et al. 1993; GUFLER et al. 1997; OOI et al. 2000). Variable degrees of enhancement can be observed both on CT and MR after contrast administration (NAKAMURA et al. 1997) (Fig. 9.38). Calcifications are not present, whereas tumor necrosis has been reported in T-cell natural killer lymphoma (JAFFE et al. 1996), more commonly in lesions with volume greater than $15mm^3$ (KING et al. 2000).

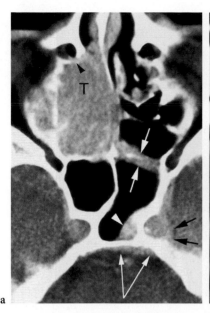 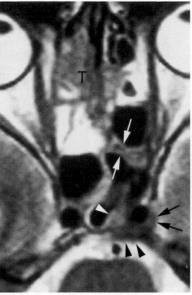

a   b

Fig. 9.37a,b. Sinonasal non-Hodgkin lymphoma. The patient complained of right side nasal obstruction associated with sixth left cranial nerve palsy. Axial enhanced CT (**a**) and T2 (**b**) images show a soft tissue mass occupying the right ethmoid sinus (*T*). Spread into both anterior sphenoid sinus walls is present, with a thicker plaque on left side (*short white arrows*). Via osseous spread, tumor invades the left posterior sphenoid sinus (*arrowhead*), and extends into posterior cranial fossa probably invading the foramen of Dorello (*long white arrows on* **a**, *black arrowheads on* **b**) where sixth nerve runs. Cavernous sinus invasion is also present with tumor surrounding left internal carotid artery (*black arrows*). Erosion of right nasolacrimal duct is demonstrated by CT (*black arrowhead on* **a**)

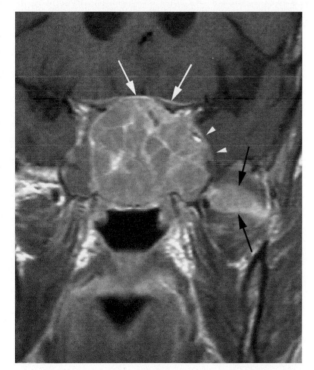

Fig. 9.38. Sinonasal non-Hodgkin lymphoma involving left sphenoid sinus and masticator space (*black arrows*). Roof and left wall (*arrowheads*) of the sphenoid are remodeled, the roof is also invaded with upwards displacement of the optic chiasm (*white arrows*)

T-cell NK lymphoma accounts for approximately 45% of all sinonasal lymphomas. This variant more commonly arises from midfacial structures (septum, nasal cavity, and hard palate) and provokes bone destruction in up to 78% of cases, mainly at the level of septum, the medial maxillary sinus wall and the lamina papyracea (Ooi et al. 2000). Due to its natural history, T-cell NK lymphoma, before the advent of immunophenotypic characterization, has been labeled with a variety of different names, such as *midline lethal granuloma, polymorphic reticulosis, progressive lethal granulomatous ulceration*. According to KING et al. (2000), posterior extension to the nasopharynx is common, whereas encroachment of the cribriform plate is not to be expected.

An additional pattern of bone destruction is reported consisting of permeative infiltration, i.e. the presence of tumor tissue on both sides of a bone boundary in the absence of detectable cortical erosion (Fig. 9.39). This phenomenon, described on both CT and MR examinations, may occur in up to 60% of cases. The lack of histological sub-typing in the majority of published reports does not allow ascertaining whether permeative bone infiltration is more frequent in any of the subtypes of non-Hodgkin lymphoma.

The list of differential diagnosis for sinonasal lymphoma potentially includes any other malignant histotype. Permeative bone infiltration is uncommon in most neoplasms, nonetheless it found also in adenoid cystic carcinoma (see section 9.2.5). In addition, whenever midfacial destruction is detected, the list

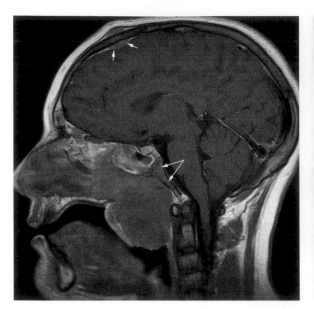

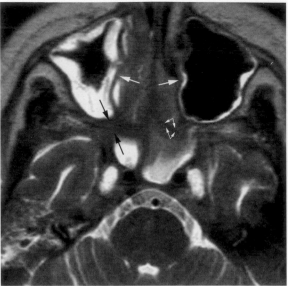

Fig. 9.39. Non-Hodgkin lymphoma extending from nasopharynx into the sinonasal tract. On the enhanced T1 in the sagittal plane, permeative invasion of the clivus is demonstrated (*long arrows*). A localization in the calvaria is also present. It is characterized by minimal changes in the diploic signal. Intracranial extent of this lesion appears as an epidural soft tissue mass, which - combined with thickening and enhancement of the adjacent dura mater – gives rise to the lenticular-like pattern of epidural lesions (*short arrows*). Extracranial extent with displacement of galea capitis is also seen

Fig. 9.40. Granulocytic sarcoma (chloroma) with invasion of both nasal fossae (*long white arrows*) and left sphenoid sinus, where the T2 axial image shows permeative invasion of the anterior wall (*short white arrows*). The mass extends into right pterygopalatine fossa (*black arrows*)

of differentials to be considered is even wider as such a pattern is shared also by infectious and non-infectious destructive diseases (such as fungal infections, Wegener's granulomatosis, sarcoidosis, and cocaine induced midline destructive lesions).

Granulocytic sarcoma (chloroma) is a rare complication of acute and chronic myeloid leukemia, which may easily be confused with lymphomas, particularly when extracranial sites are also involved. It is usually associated with a myeloproliferative disorder but may be seen preceding the onset of leukemia. Granulocytic sarcoma is formed of malignant myeloid precursor cells occurring at an extramedullary site. On CT, an enhancing soft tissue mass with slightly infiltrating appearance may be observed. On MR, variable signal intensity is shown on T2 and T1 sequences (FREEDY and MILLER 1991; PRADES et al. 2002) (Fig. 9.40).

Extramedullary plasmacytoma of the sinonasal tract does not have specific imaging features (Fig. 9.41). A soft tissue lesion with possible bone destruction has been reported (KONDO et al. 1986; CHING et al. 2002) (Fig. 9.42).

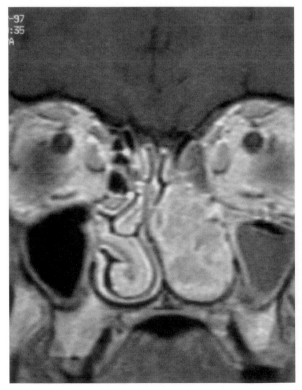

Fig. 9.41. Extramedullary plasmacytoma arising from left nasal cavity. The lesion presents as solid polypoid mass with heterogeneous enhancement on post-contrast T1 coronal image

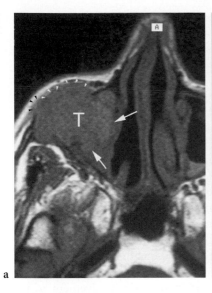
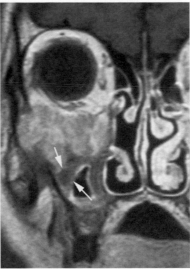

a   b

Fig. 9.42a,b. Extramedullary plasmacytoma arising from right maxillary sinus. **a** On unenhanced axial T1, the epicenter of the mass is located between anterior wall and zygomatic bone (*T*). Signal intensity of the lesion results slightly greater than retained mucus in the maxillary sinus. Extensive thinning with irregular remodeling of the anterior sinusal wall (*white arrowheads*) and also focal bone invasion (*black arrowheads*) are present. **b** Coronal enhanced T1 image demonstrates the submucosal location of the mass – as suggested by displacement of thickened mucosa by tumor (*white arrows*)

9.8
Secondary Tumors

9.8.1
Definition, Epidemiology, Pattern of Growth

Metastasis to nose and paranasal sinuses is an exceedingly rare occurrence, with approximately 100 cases reported in the literature (PIGNATARO et al. 2001). The highest incidence is in the sixth decade in men and the seventh decade in women (IZQUIERDO et al. 2000), which probably reflects the incidence of primary tumors.

Different pathogenetic mechanisms have been put forward to explain this exceptional event: hematogenous dissemination through the vertebral and epidural valveless venous plexus (BATSON 1995); neoplastic embolization (NAHUM and BAILEY 1963); spreading through hematic or lymphatic vessels (GOTTLIEB and ROLAND 1998; SIMO et al. 2000).

More than 50% of sinonasal metastases take origin from a renal carcinoma (SIMO et al. 2000; PIGNATARO et al. 2001). In up to 16% of patients with renal cell carcinoma, metastases are located above the clavicles (SIMO et al. 2000). However, an isolated head and neck metastasis is very rare, occurring in only 1% of all renal cell carcinomas (SIMO et al. 2000).

Less frequent malignant lesions metastasizing to the sinonasal area include thyroid gland (FREEMAN et al. 1996; ALTMAN et al. 1997), larynx (MORALES-ANGULO et al. 1994), breast (PIGNATARO et al. 2001; PITKARANTA et al. 2001), lung (CLARKSON et al. 2002), liver (IZQUIERDO et al. 2000), stomach (OWA et al. 1995), colon (CAMA et al. 2002), urinary blad-

der (KAWAI et al. 1989), ovary (CAMPISI and CHESKI 1998), and prostate carcinoma (SALEH 1996).

9.8.2
Clinical and Endoscopic Findings

Even though signs and symptoms of secondary tumors of the sinonasal tract do not differ from those of primary lesions, some peculiarities may be worth mentioning. The diagnosis of a sinonasal metastasis is often delayed, and in some cases it is recognized even years after the primary tumor (SIMO et al. 2000). Conversely, a metastasis may be the first presentation of a tumor otherwise clinically silent for a long period (ALTMAN et al. 1997; CAMA et al. 2002). Of course, the presence of a sinonasal mass in a patient already treated for a malignancy should always arouse the suspect of a secondary lesion. Since renal cell carcinoma is a highly vascularized tumor, epistaxis is the most frequent complaint. In these lesions, nasal bleeding may be catastrophic, thence surgeons should be aware of the risk of complications linked to simple procedures such as a biopsy under local anesthesia.

9.8.3
Treatment Guidelines

The presence of a metastasis into the sinonasal tract should be considered a poor prognostic factor, as the primary is usually advanced. Moreover, most metastases are extended beyond the limits of the sinonasal tract at diagnosis. According to these facts, in most cases treatment is palliative, only rarely curative, usually consisting of radio/chemotherapy. In selected cases, adjunctive treatments tailored to the biologic profile of the primary lesion, such as hormone therapy for breast cancer (PIGNATARO et al. 2001) or radioiodine therapy for thyroid carcinoma (FREEMAN et al. 1996) may be used. In some cases, treatment planning for metastases may differ from the primary, as in renal cell carcinoma. While the primary is considered radioresistant, metastatic disease appears to be responsive to external radiotherapy, at least for palliative purposes (SIMO et al. 2000). Transnasal endoscopic surgery may be an effective tool for obtaining a histological specimen and/or debulking the lesion for relieving patient's symptoms (SIMO et al. 2000). A more aggressive surgical treatment, including external approaches, such as lateral rhinotomy or craniofacial resection (SIMO et al. 2000), should be reserved to patients with a good performance status and with a single metastasis, especially if the lesion is scarcely invasive.

9.8.4
Imaging Findings

As most metastases primarily involve the bony walls of paranasal sinuses, the epicenter of lesions tends to be located about the margins of the sinus abutting the adjacent mucosa (MAFEE 1993). However, advanced lesions are usually indistinguishable from primary sinonasal tract tumors arising from the epithelial lining.

In a recent review of 123 cases reported, PRESCHER and BRORS (2001) noted that the incidence of metastases diminishes from maxillary sinus (33%) to sphenoid sinus (22%), ethmoid sinus (14%), and frontal sinus (9%). In approximately 22% of cases, two or more paranasal sinuses are affected.

Metastases from breast, gastrointestinal tract, and bronchogenic carcinomas are usually indistinguishable from a primary epithelial sinonasal carcinoma. In these lesions, cross sectional imaging shows a bone destroying soft tissue mass with slight enhancement (Fig. 9.43). Nevertheless, a peculiar pattern consisting of bilateral and symmetric involvement of the ethmoid sinuses mimicking inflammatory disease has been described in few patients with breast carcinoma (AUSTIN et al. 1995; MONSEREZ et al. 2001). Metastases from renal cell carcinoma and melanoma may show a relevant enhancement associated with bone remodeling or bone destruction (HAYES et al. 1985; SIMO et al. 2000).

In case of a highly vascularized renal cell carcinoma metastasis the differential diagnosis includes hypervascular masses of the sinonasal tract. Imaging features suggesting a hypervascularized lesion en-

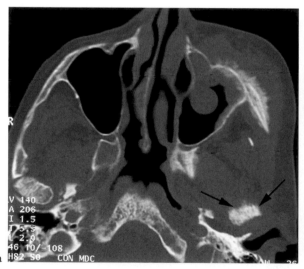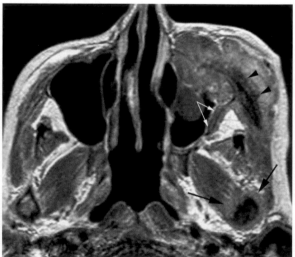

Fig. 9.43a,b. Metastasis from breast carcinoma. **a** Axial CT shows osteoblastic metastases in the left zygomatic-maxillary bone, mandibular condyle, and pterygoid process. Diffuse periosteal mineralization is present; lytic changes are observed in the mandibular condyle (*black arrows*). The zygomatic-maxillary bone metastasis is associated with a soft tissue mass invading the cheek and extending into the maxillary sinus. **b** On post-contrast T1 axial image, bone and periosteal changes are less evident, but recognizable (*arrowheads*). The soft tissue component destroying the left condyle and extending outside the bony boundaries is clearly shown (*black arrows*). Subperiosteal spread along postero-lateral maxillary sinus wall is detailed by MR with separation of the residual bone from the neoplastic tissue and from the sinusal mucosa (*white arrows*)

compass: enlargement of feeding vessels (compare the internal maxillary arteries in the masticator space or the pterygopalatine arteries within the pterygopalatine fossa), hypertrophy of peritumoral vessels, intratumoral flow voids, and early and intense enhancement on dynamic post-contrast T1-weighted images. Apart for juvenile angiofibroma, which has both peculiar imaging features (site of origin, pattern of growth) and patient's characteristics (adolescent male), neuroendocrine carcinoma, paraganglioma, ectopic meningioma, and olfactory neuroblastoma should be considered. In addition, Merkel cell carcinoma - a highly aggressive neoplasm of neuroendocrine origin, with a predilection for the head and neck skin in elderly patients - has been reported to arise also in the sinonasal tract. The origin of the Merkel cells in the sinonasal tract is controversial. There is evidence supporting their origin both from the neural crest and as from transitional cells in the basal layer of the epidermis (NGUYEN and McCULLOUGH 2002). On CT scan, Merkel cell carcinoma presents as a homogeneous soft-tissue mass without calcification; bone remodeling and/or bone destruction may also be noted. On MR, the tumor has been described to show homogeneous, intermediate signal on T1 and T2 sequences and to greatly enhance with a homogeneous pattern (AZIZI et al. 2001).

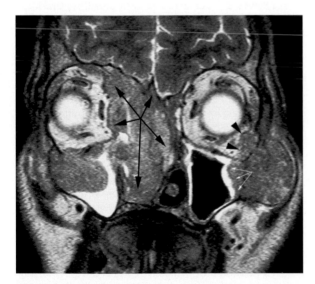

Fig. 9.44. Right naso-ethmoidal adenocarcinoma with synchronous metastasis in the facial bones. On T2 coronal image, a large tumor occupies the right naso-ethmoidal area with extent into ipsilateral frontal sinus (*black arrows*). Both remodeling and invasion of right medial orbital wall are present. Contralateral metastasis arising from zygomatic bone appears as a soft tissue mass with same signal features of the primary tumor. Intraorbital (*arrowheads*), and intrasinusal submucosal (*white arrows*) invasion is demonstrated

In case of metastasis from prostate carcinoma, CT appearance may range from a purely blastic pattern of bone involvement to a soft tissue mass with bone destruction with only minimal sclerotic changes (PRESCHER and BRORS 2001).

Nonetheless, as in most cases imaging findings of sinonasal tract metastases are nonspecific, the diagnosis is mainly suggested by other elements such as the presence of more than one soft tissue lesion eroding the bone with intervening normal bone. Patient's history is also important, although histologically confirmed metastatic renal cell carcinoma to sinonasal tract has been reported in the radiologic absence of a primary renal neoplasm (SGOURAS et al. 1995). Spontaneous regression of primary renal tumor is the more likely explanation (ABUBAKR et al. 1994; HAMID and POLLER 1998).

References

Abubakr YA, Chou TH, Redman BG (1994) Spontaneous remission of renal cell carcinoma: a case report and immunological correlates. J Urol 152:156–157

Aferzon M, Wood WE, Powell JR (2003) Ewing's sarcoma of the ethmoid sinus. Otolaryngol Head Neck Surg 128:897–901

Ahwal MA, Jha N, Nabholtz JM et al (1994) Olfactory neuroblastoma: report of a case associated with inappropriate antidiuretic hormone secretion. J Otolaryngol 23:437–439

Airoldi M, Pedani F, Succo G et al (2001) Phase II randomized trial comparing vinorelbine versus vinorelbine plus cisplatin in patients with recurrent salivary gland malignancies. Cancer 91:541–547

Altman KW, Mirza N, Philippe L (1997) Metastatic follicular thyroid carcinoma to the paranasal sinuses: a case report and review. J Laryngol Otol 111:647–651

August M, Magennis P, Dewitt D (1997) Osteogenic sarcoma of the jaws: factors influencing prognosis. Int J Oral Maxillofac Surg 26:198–204

Austin JR, Kershiznek MM, McGill D et al (1995) Breast carcinoma metastatic to paranasal sinuses. Head Neck 17:161–165

Azizi L, Marsot-Dupuch K, Bigel P et al (2001) Merkel cell carcinoma: a rare cause of hypervascular nasal tumor. AJNR Am J Neuroradiol 22:1389–1393

Barnes L (1986) Intestinal-type adenocarcinoma of the nasal cavity and paranasal sinuses. Am J Surg Pathol 10:192–202

Batra PS, Kern RC, Pelzer HJ et al (2001) Leiomyosarcoma of the sinonasal tract: report of a case. Otolaryngol Head Neck Surg 125:663–664

Batsakis JG (1979) Tumors of the head and neck: clinical and pathological considerations, 2nd edn. Williams and Wilkins, Baltimore

Batsakis JG, Mackay B, El-Naggar AK (1996) Ewing's sarcoma and peripheral primitive neuroectodermal tumor: an interim report. Ann Otol Rhinol Laryngol 105:838–843

Batsakis JG, Suarez P, El-Naggar AK (1998) Mucosal melanomas of the head and neck. Ann Otol Rhinol Laryngol 107:626–630

Beckhardt RN, Weber RS, Zane R et al (1995) Minor salivary gland tumors of the palate: clinical and pathologic correlates of outcome. Laryngoscope 105:1155–1160

Bennett JH, Thomas G, Evans AW et al (2000) Osteosarcoma of the jaws: a 30-year retrospective review. Oral Surg Oral Med Oral Pathol Oral Radiol Endod 90:323–332

Bhattacharyya N (2002) Factors predicting survival for cancer of the ethmoid sinus. Am J Rhinol 16:281–286

Bhattacharyya N (2003) Factors affecting survival in maxillary sinus cancer. J Oral Maxillofac Surg 61:1016–1021

Bhattacharyya N, Shapiro NL, Metson R (1997) Endoscopic resection of a recurrent sinonasal hemangiopericytoma. Am J Otolaryngol 18:341–344

Biller HF, Slotnick DB, Lawson W (1989) Superior rhinotomy for en bloc resection of bilateral ethmoid tumors. Arch Otolaryngol Head Neck Surg 115:1463–1466

Boor A, Jurkovic I, Friedman I et al (2001) Extraskeletal Ewing's sarcoma of the nose. J Laryngol Otol 115:74-76

Boyko OB, Cory DA, Cohen MD et al (1987) MR imaging of osteogenic and Ewing's sarcoma. AJR Am J Roentgenol 148:317–322

Bridger GP, Baldwin M (1989) Anterior craniofacial resection for ethmoid and nasal cancer with free flap reconstruction. Arch Otolaryngol Head Neck Surg 115:308–312

Bridger GP, Kwok B, Baldwin M et al (2000) Craniofacial resection for paranasal sinus cancer. Head Neck 22:772–780

Burdach S, Meyer-Bahlburg A, Laws HJ et al (2003) High-dose therapy for patients with primary multifocal and early relapsed Ewing's tumors: results of two consecutive regimens assessing the role of total-body irradiation. J Clin Oncol 21:3072–3078

Cakmak O, Ergin NT, Yilmazer C et al (2002) Endoscopic removal of esthesioneuroblastoma. Int J Pediatric Otorhinolaryngol 64:233–238

Caldemeyer KS, Mathews VP, Righi PD et al (1998) Imaging features and clinical significance of perineural spread or extension of head and neck tumors. Radiographics 18:97-110; quiz 147

Callender TA, Weber RS, Janjan N et al (1995) Rhabdomyosarcoma of the nose and paranasal sinuses in adults and children. Otolaryngol Head Neck Surg 112:252–257

Cama E, Agostino S, Ricci R et al (2002) A rare case of metastases to the maxillary sinus from sigmoid colon adenocarcinoma. ORL J Otorhinolaryngol Relat Spec 64:364–367

Campisi P, Cheski P (1998) Metastatic Sertoli-Leydig cell ovarian cancer manifested as a frontal sinus mass. J Otolaryngol 27:361–362

Cantù G, Solero CL, Salvatori P et al (1997) A new classification of malignant ethmoid tumors. 3rd European Skull Base Congress, London, 9-11 April 1997. Skull Base Surg 7 [Suppl 2]:33

Cantù G, Solero CL, Mariani L et al (1999a) Anterior craniofacial resection for malignant ethmoid tumors – a series of 91 patients. Head Neck 21:185–191

Cantù G, Solero CL, Mariani L et al (1999b) A new classification for malignant tumors involving the anterior skull base. Arch Otolaryngol Head Neck Surg 125:1252–1257

Cantù G, Bimbi F, Fabiani M et al (2002) Lymph node metastasis in paranasal sinus carcinomas: prognostic value and treatment. Acta Otorhinolaryngol Ital 22:273–279

Carbone PP, Kaplan HS, Mushoff K et al (1971) Report of the Committee on Hodgkin's disease staging classification. Cancer Res 31:1860–1861

Carney ME, O'Reilly RC, Sholevar B et al (1995) Expression of human Achaete-scute 1 gene in olfactory neuroblastoma (esthesioneuroblastoma). J Neurooncol 26:35–43

Carrau RL, Segas J, Nuss DW et al (1994) Role of skull base surgery for local control of sarcomas of the nasal cavity and paranasal sinuses. Eur Arch Otorhinolaryngol 251:350–356

Carrau RL, Segas J, Nuss DW et al (1999) Squamous cell carcinoma of the sinonasal tract invading the orbit. Laryngoscope 109:230–235

Casiano RR, Numa WA, Falquez AM (2001) Endoscopic resection of eshtesioneuroblastoma. Am J Rhinol 15:271–279

Castelnuovo P, Pagella F, Delù G et al (2003) Endoscopic resection of nasal haemangiopericytoma. Eur Arch Otorhinolaryngol 260:244–247

Catalano PJ, Brandwein M, Shah DK et al (1996) Sinonasal hemangiopericytomas: a clinicopathologic and immunohistochemical study of seven cases. Head Neck 18:42–53

Cheesman AD, Lund VJ, Howard DJ et al (1986) Craniofacial resection for tumors of the nasal cavity and paranasal sinuses. Head Neck 8:429–435

Chen CC, Hsu L, Hecht JL et al (2002) Bimaxillary chondrosarcoma: clinical, radiologic, and histologic correlation. AJNR Am J Neuroradiol 23:667–670

Chidambaram A, Sanville P (2000) Mesenchymal chondrosarcoma of the maxilla. J Laryngol Otol 114:536–539

Ching AS, Khoo JB, Chong VF (2002) CT and MR imaging of solitary extramedullary plasmacytoma of the nasal tract. AJNR Am J Neuroradiol 23:1632–1636

Clarkson JWH, Kirkland PM, Mady S (2002) Bronchogenic metastasis involving the frontal sinus and masquerading as a Pott's puffy tumour: a diagnostic pitfall. Br J Oral Maxillofac Surg 40:440–441

Coppit GL, Eustermann VD, Bartels J et al (2002) Endoscopic resection of chondrosarcomas of the nasal septum: a report of 2 cases. Otolaryngol Head Neck Surg 127:569–572

Cotran RS, Kumar V, Robbins SL (1989) Robbins pathologic basis of disease, 4th edn. Saunders, Philadelphia

Cottier JP, Destrieux C, Brunereau L et al (2000) Cavernous sinus invasion by pituitary adenoma: MR imaging. Radiology 215:463–469

Csokonai LV, Liktor B, Arato G et al (2001) Ewing's sarcoma in the nasal cavity. Otolaryngol Head Neck Surg 125:665–667

Curtin HD (1998) Detection of perineural spread: fat is a friend. AJNR Am J Neuroradiol 19:1385–1386

Curtin HD, Rabinov JD (1998) Extension to the orbit from paraorbital disease. The sinuses. Radiol Clin North Am 36:1201–1213, xi

Curtin HD, Williams R, Johnson J (1985) CT of perineural tumor extension: pterygopalatine fossa. AJR Am J Roentgenol 144:163–169

Derdeyn CP, Moran CJ, Wippold FJ 2nd et al (1994) MRI of esthesioneuroblastoma. J Comput Assist Tomogr 18:16–21

Douglas JG, Laramore GE, Austin-Seymour M et al (2000) Treatment of locally advanced adenoid cystic carcinoma of the head and neck with neutron radiotherapy. Int J Radiat Oncol Biol Phys 46:551–557

Downey TJ, Clark SK, Moore DW (2001) Chondrosarcoma of the nasal septum. Otolaryngol Head Neck Surg 125:98–100

Draf W, Schick B, Weber L et al (2000) Endonasal micro-endo-scopic surgery of nasal and paranasal sinuses tumors. In: Stamm AC, Draf W (eds) Micro-endoscopic surgery of the paranasal sinuses and the skull base. Springer, Berlin Heidelberg New York, pp 481–488

Dulguerov P, Calcaterra T (1992) Esthesioneuroblastoma: the UCLA experience 1970–1990. Laryngoscope 102:843–849

Dulguerov P, Allal AS, Calcaterra TC (2001) Esthesioneuroblastoma: a meta-analysis and review. Lancet Oncol 2:683–690

Dunst J, Sauer R, Burgers JM et al (1991) Radiation therapy as local treatment in Ewing's sarcoma. Cancer 67:2818–2825

Eich HT, Staar S, Micke O et al (2001) Radiotherapy of esthesioneuroblastoma. J Radiat Oncol Biol Physiol 49:155–160

Eisen MD, Yousem DM, Loevner LA et al (2000) Preoperative imaging to predict orbital invasion by tumor. Head Neck 22:456–462

El-Beltagi AH, Sobeih AA, Valvoda M et al (2002) Radiological appearances of sinonasal abnormalities. Clin Radiol 57:702–718

Ellingwood KE, Million RR (1979) Cancer of the nasal cavity and ethmoid/sphenoid sinus. Cancer 43:1517–1526

Enzinger FM, Smith BH (1976) Hemangiopericytoma: an analysis 106 cases. Hum Pathol 7:61–82

Evans RG, Nesbit ME, Gehan EA et al (1991) Multimodal therapy for the management of the localized Ewing's sarcoma of pelvic and sacral bones: a report from the second inter group study. J Clin Oncol 9:1173–1180

Fajardo-Dolci G, Magana RC, Bautista EL (1999) Sinonasal lymphoma. Otolaryngol Head Neck Surg 121:323–326

Ferlito A, Rinaldo A, Rhys-Evans PH (2003) Contemporary clinical commentary: Esthesioneuroblastoma: an update on management of the neck. Laryngoscope 113:1935–1938

Fischbein NJ, Kaplan MJ, Jackler RK et al (2001) MR imaging in two cases of subacute denervation change in the muscles of facial expression. AJNR Am J Neuroradiol 22:880–884

Fitzek MM, Thornton AF, Varvares M et al (2002) Neuroendocrine tumors of the sinonasal tract. Results of a prospective study incorporating chemotherapy, surgery, and combined proton-photon radiotherapy. Cancer 94:2623–2634

Fletcher BD (1991) Response of osteosarcoma and Ewing sarcoma to chemotherapy: Imaging evaluation. AJR Am J Roentgenol 157:825–833

Fordice J, Kershaw C, El-Naggar A et al (1999) Adenoid cystic carcinoma of the head and neck: predictors of morbidity and mortality. Arch Otolaryngol Head Neck Surg 125:149–152

Freedy RM, Miller KD Jr (1991) Granulocytic sarcoma (chloroma): sphenoidal sinus and paraspinal involvement as evaluated by CT and MR. AJNR Am J Neuroradiol 12:259–262

Freeman JL, Gershon A, Liavaag PG et al (1996) Papillary thyroid carcinoma metastasizing to the sphenoid-ethmoid sinuses and skull base. Thyroid 6:59–61

Freeman MP, Currie CM, Gray GF Jr et al (1988) Ewing sarcoma of the skull with an unusual pattern of reactive sclerosis: MR characteristics. J Comput Assist Tomogr 12:143–146

Frierson HF, Mills SE, Fechner RE et al (1986) Sinonasal undifferentiated carcinoma. An aggressive neoplasm derived from schneiderian epithelium and distinct from olfactory neuroblastoma. Am J Surg Pathol 10:771–779

Gadwal SR, Fanburg-Smith JC, Gannon FH et al (2000) Primary chondrosarcoma of the head and neck in pediatric population. Cancer 88:2181–2188

Gadwal SR, Gannon FH, Fanburg-Smith JC et al (2001) Primary osteosarcoma of the head and neck in pediatric patients. Cancer 91:598–605

Galera-Ruiz H, Sanchez-Calzado JA, Rios-Martin JJ et al (2001a) Sinonasal radition-associated osteosarcoma after combined therapy for rhabdomyosarcoma of the nose. Auris Nasus Larynx 28:261–264

Galera-Ruiz H, Villar-Rodriguez JL, Sanchez-Calzado JA et al (2001b) Sinonasal neuroendocrine carcinoma presenting as a nasopharyngeal mass. Otolaryngol Head Neck Surg 124:475–476

Garden AS, Weber RS, Morrison WH et al (1995) The influence of positive margins and nerve invasion in adenoid cystic carcinoma of the head and neck treated with surgery and radiation. Int J Radiat Oncol Biol Phys 37:51–58

Geirnaerdt MJ, Bloem JL, Eulderink F et al (1993) Cartilaginous tumors: correlation of gadolinium-enhanced MR imaging and histopathologic findings. Radiology 186:813–817

Giger R, Kurt AM, Lacroix JS (2002) Endoscopic removal of a nasal septum chondrosarcoma. Rhinology 40:96–99

Gilligan D, Slevin J (1991) Radical radiotherapy for 28 cases of mucosal melanoma in the nasal cavity and sinuses. Br J Radiol 64:1147–1150

Ginsberg LE (1992) Neoplastic diseases affecting the central skull base: CT and MR imaging. AJR Am J Roentgenol 159:581–589

Ginsberg LE (1999) Imaging of perineural tumor spread in head and neck cancer. Semin Ultrasound CT MR 20:175–186

Ginsberg LE (2002) MR imaging of perineural tumor spread. Magn Reson Imaging Clin North Am 10:511–525, vi

Ginsberg LE, De Monte F, Gillenwater AM (1996) Greater superficial petrosal nerve: anatomy and MR findings in perineural tumor spread. AJNR Am J Neuroradiol 17:389–393

Ginsberg LE, DeMonte F (1998) Imaging of perineural tumor spread from palatal carcinoma. AJNR Am J Neuroradiol 19:1417–1422

Goffart Y, Jorissen M, Daele J et al (2000) Minimally invasive endoscopic management of malignant sinonasal tumors. Acta Otorhinolaryngol Belg 54:221–232

Goldenberg D, Golz A, Fradis A et al (2001) Malignant tumors of the nose and paranasal sinuses: a retrospective review of 291 cases. Ear Nose Throat J 80:273–277

Gorelick J, Ross D, Martenette L et al (2000) Sinonasal undifferentiated carcinoma: case series and review of the literature. Neurosurgery 47:750–755

Gotte K, Hormann K, Schmoll J et al (1999) Congenital nasal hemangiopericytoma: intrauterine, intraoperative, and histologic findings. Ann Otol Rhinol Laryngol 108:589–593

Gottlieb MD, Roland JT (1998) Paradoxical spread of renal cell carcinoma to the head and neck. Laryngoscope 108:1301–1305

Greger V, Schirmacher P, Bohl J et al (1990) Possible involvement of the retinoblastoma gene in undifferentiated sinonasal carcinoma. Cancer 66:1954–1959

Griffin TW, Pajak TF, Laramopre GE et al (1988) Neutron vs photon irradiation of inoperable salivary gland tumor. Results of an RTOG-MRC cooperative randomized study. Int J Radiat Oncol Biol Phys 15:1085–1090

Gufler H, Laubenberger J, Gerling J et al (1997) MRI of lymphomas of the orbits and the paranasal sinuses. J Comput Assist Tomogr 21:887–891

Ha PK, Eisele DW, Frassica FJ et al (1999) Osteosarcoma of the head and neck: a review of the Johns Hopkins experience. Laryngoscope 109:964-969

Hagiwara A, Inoue Y, Nakayama T et al (2001) The "botryoid sign": a characteristic feature of rhabdomyosarcomas in the head and neck. Neuroradiology 43:331-335

Hamid Y, Poller DN (1998) Spontaneous regression of renal cell carcinoma: a pitfall in diagnosis of renal lesions. J Clin Pathol 51:334-336

Han MH, Chang KH, Kim IO et al (1993) Non-Hodgkin lymphoma of the central skull base: MR manifestations. J Comput Assist Tomogr 17:567-571

Hanna SL, Fletcher BD, Kaste SC et al (1994) Increased confidence of diagnosis of Ewing sarcoma using T2-weighted MR images. Magn Reson Imaging 12:559-568

Harman M, Kiroglu F, Kosem M et al (2003) Primary Ewing's sarcoma of the paranasal sinus with intracranial extension: imaging features. Dentomaxillofac Radiol 32:343-346

Hayashi T, Kuroshima Y, Yoshida K et al (2000) Primary osteosarcoma of the sphenoid bone with extensive periosteal extension – case report. Neurol Med Chir (Tokyo) 40:419-422

Hayes E, Weber AL, Davis KR et al (1985) Metastatic renal cell carcinoma manifesting as nasal mass: CT findings. J Comput Assist Tomogr 9:387-389

Hayes FA, Thompson E, Meyer WH et al (1989) Therapy for localized Ewing's sarcoma of bone. J Clin Oncol 7:208-213

Hekkenberg RJ, Davidson J, Kapusta L et al (1997) Hemangiopericytoma of the sinonasal tract. J Laryngol Otol 26:277-280

Hervé S, Abd Alsamad I, Beautru R et al (1999) Management of sinonasal hemangiopericytomas. Rhinology 37:153-158

Hicks J, Flaitz C (2002) Rhabdomyosarcoma of the head and neck in children. Oral Oncol 38:450-459

Horowitz ME, Kinsella TJ, Wexler LH et al (1993) Total-body irradiation and autologous bone marrow transplant in the treatment of high-risk Ewing's sarcoma and rhabdomyosarcoma. J Clin Oncol 11:1911-1918

Howard DJ, Daniels HA (1993) Ewing's sarcoma of the nose. Ear Nose Throat J 72:277-279

Howarth KL, Khodaei I, Karkanevatos A, et al (2004) A sinonasal primary Ewing's sarcoma. Int J Pediatr Otorhinolaryngol 68:221-224

Hyams VJ (1982) Olfactory neuroblastoma. In: Batsakis JG, Hyams VJ, Morales AR (eds) Special tumors of the head and neck. ASCP Press, Chicago, pp 24-29

Ichimura K, Sasaki T, Nakatsuka T et al (1998) Analysis of tumor recurrence following anterior skull base surgery. Eur Arch Otolaryngol 255:155-162

Imola MJ, Schramm VL Jr (2002) Orbital preservation in surgical management of sinonasal malignancy. Laryngoscope 112:1357-1365

Ishida H, Mohri M, Amatsu M (2002) Invasion of the skull base by carcinomas: histopathologically evidenced findings with CT and MRI. Eur Arch Otorhinolaryngol 259:535-539

Izquierdo J, Armengot M, Cors R et al (2000) Hepatocarcinoma: metastases to the nose and paranasal sinuses. Otolaryngol Head Neck Surg 122:932-933

Jaffe ES, Chan JK, Su IJ et al (1996) Report of the workshop on nasal and related extranodal angiocentric T/natural killer cell lymphomas. Definitions, differential diagnosis, and epidemiology. Am J Surg Pathol 20:103-111

Jaffe ES, Harris NL, Stein H et al (2001) World Health Organization classification of tumors. Pathology and genetics of tumors of hematopoietic and lymphoid tissues. IARC Press, Lyon (France)

Jeng YM, Sung MT, Fang CL et al (2002) Sinonasal undifferentiated carcinoma and nasopharyngeal-type undifferentiated carcinoma: two clinically, biologically, and histopathologically distinct entities. Am J Surg Pathol 26:371-376

Johnson RE, Pomeroy TC (1975) Evaluation of therapeutic results in Ewing's sarcoma. Am J Roentgenol 123:583

Jones HM (1973) Cartilaginous tumours of the head and neck. J Laryngol Otol 87:135-151

Junior AT, de Abreu Alves F, Pinto CA et al (2003) Clinicopathological and immunohistochemical analysis of twenty-five head and neck osteosarcomas. Oral Oncol 39:521-530

Kadish S, Goodman M, Wang CC (1976) Olfactory neuroblastoma. Cancer 37:1571-1576

Kairemo KJ, Jekunen AP, Kestila MS et al (1998) Imaging of olfactory neuroblastoma: an analysis of 17 cases. Auris Nasus Larynx 25:173-179

Kameya T, Shimosato Y, Adachi I et al (1980) Neuroendocrine carcinoma of the paranasal sinuses: a morphological and endoscrinological study. Cancer 45:330-339

Kanamalla US, Kesava PP, McGuff HS (2000) Imaging of nonlaryngeal neuroendocrine carcinoma. AJNR Am J Neuroradiol 21:775-778

Kapadia SB, Desai U, Cheng VS (1982) Extramedullary plasmacytoma of the head and neck. Medicine 61:317-329

Kassir RR, Rassekh CH, Kinsella JB et al (1997) Osteosarcoma of the head and neck: meta-analysis of nonrandomized studies. Laryngoscope 107:56-61

Kawai N, Asakura K, Sambe S et al (1989) Metastatic squamous cell carcinoma of the paranasal sinuses from a primary squamous cell carcinoma of the urinary bladder. J Laryngol Otol 103:602-604

Keck T, Mattfeldt T, Kuhnemann S (2001) Leiomyosarcoma of the ethmoidal cells. Rhinology 39:115-117

Khan AJ, Digiovanna MP, Ross DA et al (2001) Adenoid cystic carcinoma: a retrospective clinical review. Int J Cancer 96:149-158

Kim BS, Vongtama R, Juillard G (2004) Sinonasal undifferentiated carcinoma: case series and literature review. Am J Otolaryngol 25:162-166

Kim GE, Chung EJ, Lim JJ et al (1999a) Clinical significance of neck node metastasis in squamous cell carcinoma of the maxillary antrum. Am J Otolaryngol 20:383-390

Kim GE, Park HC, Keun KC et al (1999b) Adenoid cystic carcinoma of the maxillary antrum. Am J Otolaryngol 20:77-84

Kim KH, Sung MW, Chung PS et al (1994) Adenoid cystic carcinoma of the head and neck. Arch Otolaryngol Head Neck Surg 120:721-726

King AD, Lei KI, Ahuja AT et al (2000) MR imaging of nasal T-cell/natural killer cell lymphoma. AJR Am J Roentgenol 174:209-211

Kingdom TT, Kaplan MJ (1995) Mucosal melanoma of the nasal cavity and paranasal sinuses. Head Neck 17:184-189

Knegt PP, Ah-See KW, vd Velden LA et al (2001) Adenocarcinoma of the ethmoid sinus complex. Surgical debulking and topic fluorouracil may be the optimal treatment. Arch Otolaryngol Head Neck Surg 127:141-146

Knott PD, Gannon FH, Thompson LD (2003) Mesenchymal chondrosarcoma of the sinonasal tract: a clinico-pathologic study of 13 cases with a review of the literature. Laryngoscope 113:783-790

Koka VN, Julieron M, Bourhis J et al (1998) Aesthesioneuroblastoma. J Laryngol Otol 112:628–633

Komiyama M (1990) Magnetic resonance imaging of the cavernous sinus. Radiat Med 8:136–144

Kondo M, Hashimoto S, Inuyama Y et al (1986) Extramedullary plasmacytoma of the sinonasal cavities: CT evaluation. J Comput Assist Tomogr 10:841–844

Kraus DH, Roberts JK, Medendorf SV et al (1990) Nonsquamous cell malignancies of the paranasal sinuses. Ann Otol Rhinol Laryngol 90:5–11

Kuhel W, Goepfert H, Luna M et al (1992) Adenoid cystic carcinoma of the palate. Arch Otolaryngol Head Neck Surg 118:243–247

Kuhn UM, Mann WJ, Amedee RG (2001) Endonasal approach for nasal and paranasal sinus tumors removal. ORL J Otorhinolaryngol Relat Spec 63:366–371

Kuruvilla A, Wenig BM, Humphrey DM et al (1990) Leiomyosarcoma of the sinonasal tract. A clinicopathologic study of nine cases. Arch Otolaryngol Head Neck 116:1278–1286

Laine FJ, Braun IF, Jensen ME et al (1990) Perineural tumor extension through the foramen ovale: evaluation with MR imaging. Radiology 174:65–71

Lane S, Ironside JW (1990) Extra-skeletal Ewing's sarcoma of the nasal fossa. J Laryngol Otol 104:570–573

Latack JT, Hutchinson RJ, Heyn RM (1987) Imaging of rhabdomyosarcomas of the head and neck. AJNR Am J Neuroradiol 1987 8:353–359

Le QT, Fu KK, Kaplan M et al (1999) Treatment of maxillary sinus carcinoma: a comparison of the 1997 and 1977 American Joint Committee on cancer staging systems. Cancer 86:1700–1711

Lee JH, Lee MS, Lee BH et al (1996) Rhabdomyosarcoma of the head and neck in adults: MR and CT findings. AJNR Am J Neuroradiol 17:1923–1928

Lee YY, van Tassel P (1989) Craniofacial chondrosarcomas: imaging findings in 15 untreated cases. AJNR Am J Neuroradiol 10:165–170

Lee YY, Van Tassel P, Nauert C et al (1988) Craniofacial osteosarcomas: plain film, CT, and MR findings in 46 cases. AJR Am J Roentgenol 150:1397–1402

Levine PA, Gallagher R, Cantrell RW (1999) Esthesioneuroblastoma: reflections of a 21-year experience. Laryngoscope 109:1539–1543

Li C, Yousem DM, Hayden RE et al (1993) Olfactory neuroblastoma: MR evaluation. AJNR Am J Neuroradiol 14:1167–1171

Li CC, Tien HF, Tang JL et al (2004) Treatment outcome and pattern of failure in 77 patients with sinonasal natural killer/T cell or T-cell lymphoma. Cancer 100:366–375

Li YX, Coucke PA, Li JY et al (1998) Primary non-Hodgkin's lymphoma of the nasal cavity. Prognostic significance of paranasal extension and the role of radiotherapy and chemotherapy. Cancer 83:449–456

Lippert BM, Godbersen GS, Luttges J et al (1996) Leiomyosarcoma of the nasal cavity. Case report and literature review. ORL J Otorhinolaryngol Relat Spec 58:115–120

Lloyd G, Phelps PD, Michaels L (1992) The imaging characteristics of naso-sinus chondrosarcoma. Clin Radiol 46:189–192

Lloyd G, Lund VJ, Howard D et al (2000) Optimum imaging for sinonasal malignancy. J Laryngol Otol 114:557–562

Lund VJ (1993) Malignant melanoma of the nasal cavity and paranasal sinuses. Ear Nose Throat J 72:285–290

Lund VJ, Milroy C (1993) Olfactory neuroblastoma: clinical and pathological aspects. Rhinology 31:1–6

Lund VJ, Howard DJ, Wei WI et al (1998) Craniofacial resection for tumors of the nasal cavity and paranasal sinuses – a 17-year experience. Head Neck 20:97–105

Lund VJ, Howard DJ, Harding L et al (1999) Management options and survival in malignant melanoma of the sinonasal mucosa. Laryngoscope 109:208–211

Lund VJ, Howard D, Wei W et al (2003) Olfactory neuroblastoma: past, present, and future? Laryngoscope 113:502–507

Mafee MF (1993) Nonepithelial tumors of the paranasal sinuses and nasal cavity. Role of CT and MR imaging. Radiol Clin North Am 31:75–90

Majumdar S, Raghavan U, Jones NS (2002) Solitary plasmacytoma and extramedullary plasmacytoma of the paranasal sinuses and soft palate. J Laryngol Otol 116:962–965

Manolidis S, Donald PJ (1997) Malignant mucosal melanoma of the head and neck. Cancer 80:1373–1386

Manome Y, Yamaoka R, Yuhki K et al (1990) Intracranial invasion of neuroendocrine carcinoma: a case report. No Shinkei Geka 18:483–487

Mark RJ, Tran LM, Sercarz J et al (1993) Chondrosarcoma of the head and neck: the UCLA experience. Am J Clin Oncol 16:232–237

Maroldi R, Farina D, Battaglia G et al (1996) Risonanza Magnetica e Tomografia Computerizzata a confronto nello staging delle neoplasie rino-sinusali. Valutazione di costo-efficienza. Radiol Med (Torino) 91:211–218

Maroldi R, Farina D, Battaglia G et al (1997) MR of malignant nasosinusal neoplasms. Frequently asked questions. Eur J Radiol 24:181–190

Maroldi R, Battaglia G, Farina D et al (1999) Tumours of the oropharynx and oral cavity: perineural spread and bone invasion. JBR BTR 82:294–300

Marsot-Dupuch K, Matozza F, Firat MM et al (1990) Mandibular nerve: MR versus CT about 10 proved unusual tumors. Neuroradiology 32:492–496

Matias C, Corde J, Soares J (1988) Primary malignant melanoma of the nasal cavity: a clinicopathologic study on nine cases. J Surg Oncol 39:29–32

Matthews B, Whang C, Smith S (2002) Endoscopic resection of a nasal septal chondrosarcoma: first report of a case. Ear Nose Throat J 81:327–329

Matzko J, Becker DG, Phillips CD (1994) Obliteration of fat planes by perineural spread of squamous cell carcinoma along the inferior alveolar nerve. AJNR Am J Neuroradiol 15:1843–1845

McElroy EA Jr, Buckner JC, Lewis JE et al (1998) Chemotherapy for advanced esthesioneuroblastoma: the Mayo Clinic experience. Neurosurgery 42:1023–1028

Medina JE, Ferlito A, Pellittieri PK et al (2003) Current management of mucosal melanoma of the head and neck. J Surg Oncol 83:116–122

Medina R (1985) Linfoma non-Hodgkin. Medicine 8:474–483

Mendenhall WM, Thar TL, Million RR (1980) Solitary plasmacytoma of bone and soft tissue. Int J Radiat Oncol Biol Phys 6:1497–1501

Mendenhall WM, Morris CG, Amdur RJ et al (2004) Radiotherapy alone or combined with surgery for adenoid cystic carcinoma of the head and neck. Head Neck 26:154–162

Mills SE, Fechner RE (1989) „Undifferentiated" neoplasms of the sinonasal region: differential diagnosis based on clinical, light microscopic, immunohistochemical, and ultra-structural features. Semin Diagn Pathol 6:316-328

Miyaguchi M, Sakai S, Mori N et al (1990) Symptoms in patients with maxillary sinus carcinoma. J Laryngol Otol 104:557-559

Miyamoto RC, Gleich LL, Biddinger PW (2000) Esthesioneuroblastoma and sinonasal undifferentiated carcinoma: impact of histological grading and clinical staging on survival and prognosis. Laryngoscope 110:1262-1265

Monserez D, Vlaminck S, Kuhweide R et al (2001) Symmetrical ethmoidal metastases from ductal carcinoma of the breast, suggesting transcribrosal spread. Acta Otorhinolaryngol Belg 55:251-257

Morales-Angulo C, Gonzalez-Rodilla I, del Valle Zapico A et al (1994) Metástasis esfenoidal de un carcinoma de laringe. Acta Otorrinolaringol Esp 45:287-289

Morita A, Ebersold MJ, Olsen KD et al (1993) Esthesioneuroblastoma: prognosis and management. Neurosurgery 32:706-715

Musy PY, Reibel JF, Levine PA (2002) Sinonasal undifferentiated carcinoma: the search for a better outcome. Laryngoscope 112:1450-1455

Nahum AM, Bailey BJ (1963) Malignant tumors metastatic to the paranasal sinuses: case report and review of the literature. Laryngoscope 73:942-953

Nakamura K, Uehara S, Omagari J et al (1997) Primary non-Hodgkin lymphoma of the sinonasal cavities: correlation of CT evaluation with clinical outcome. Radiology 204:431-435

Nakhleh RE, Swanson PE, Dehner LP (1991) Juvenile (embryonal and alveolar) rhabdomyosarcoma of the head and neck in adults. A clinical, pathologic, and immunohistochemical study of 12 cases. Cancer 67:1019-1024

Nemzek WR, Hecht S, Gandour-Edwards R et al (1998) Perineural spread of head and neck tumors: how accurate is MR imaging? AJNR Am J Neuroradiol 19:701-706

Nguyen BD, McCullough AE (2002) Imaging of Merkel cell carcinoma. Radiographics 22:367-376

Nibu K, Sugasawa M, Asai M et al (2002) Results of multimodality therapy for squamous cell carcinoma of maxillary sinus. Cancer 94:1476-1482

Nishino H, Miyata M, Morita M et al (2000) Combined therapy with conservative surgery, radiotherapy, and regional chemotherapy for maxillary sinus carcinoma. Cancer 89:1925-1932

Oda D, Bavisotto LM, Schmidt RA et al (1997) Head and neck osteosarcoma at the University of Washington. Head Neck 19:513-523

Ooi GC, Chim CS, Liang R et al (2000) Nasal T-cell/natural killer cell lymphoma: CT and MR imaging features of a new clinicopathologic entity. AJR Am J Roentgenol 174:1141-1145

Oot RF, Parizel PM, Weber AL (1986) Computed tomography of osteogenic sarcoma of nasal cavity and paranasal sinuses. J Comput Assist Tomogr 10:409-414

Osguthorpe JD (1994) Sinus neoplasia. Arch Otolaryngol Head Neck Surg 120:19-25

Osterman J, Calhoun A, Dunham M et al (1986) Chronic syndrome of inappropriate antidiuretic hormone secretion and hypertension in a patient with olfactory neuroblastoma. Evidence of ectopic production of arginine vasopressin by the tumor. Arch Intern Med 146:1731-1735

Owa AO, Gallimore AP, Ajulo SO et al (1995) Metastatic adenocarcinoma of the ethmoids in a patient with previous gastric adenocarcinoma: a case report. J Laryngol Otol 109:759-761

Paling MR, Black WC, Levine PA et al (1987) Tumor invasion of the anterior skull base: a comparison of MR and CT studies. J Comput Assist Tomogr 11:824-830

Pandey M, Abraham EK, Mathew A et al (1999) Primary malignant melanoma of the upper aero-digestive tract. Int J Oral Maxillofac Surg 28:45-49

Park HR, Min SK, Cho HD et al (2004) Osteosarcoma of the ethmoid sinus. Skeletal Radiol 33:291-294

Park YK, Ryu KN, Park HR et al (2003) Low-grade osteosarcoma of the maxillary sinus. Skeletal Radiol 32:161-164

Parker GD, Harnsberger HR (1991) Clinical-radiologic issues in perineural tumor spread of malignant diseases of the extracranial head and neck. Radiographics 11:383-399

Patel SG, Meyers P, Huvos AG et al (2002a) Improved outcomes in patients with osteogenic sarcoma of the head and neck. Cancer 95:1495-1503

Patel SG, Prasad ML, Escrig M et al (2002b) Primary mucosal malignant melanoma of the head and neck. Head Neck 24:247-257

Patel SG, Singh B, Polluri A et al (2003) Craniofacial surgery for malignant shull base tumors. Cancer 98:1179-1187

Paulino AC, Marks JE, Bricker P et al (1998) Results of treatment of patients with maxillary sinus carcinoma. Cancer 83:457-465

Paulussen M, Frohlich B, Jurgens H (2001) Ewing tumour: incidence, prognosis and treatment options. Ped Drugs 3:899-913

Pellitteri PK, Ferlito A, Bradley PJ et al (2003) Management of sarcomas of the head and neck in adults. Oral Oncol 39:2-12

Perez-Ordonez B, Caruana SM, Huvos AG et al (1998) Small cell neuroendocrine carcinoma of the nasal cavity and paranasal sinuses. Hum Pathol 29:826-832

Phillips CD, Futterer SF, Lipper MH et al (1997) Sinonasal undifferentiated carcinoma: CT and MR imaging of an uncommon neoplasm of the nasal cavity. Radiology 202:477-480

Picci P, Rougraff BT, Bacci G et al (1993) Prognostic significance of histopathologic response to chemotherapy in non-metastatic Ewing's sarcoma of the extremities. J Clin Oncol 11:1763-1769

Pickuth D, Heywang-Kobrunner SH, Spielmann RP (1999) Computed tomography and magnetic resonance imaging features of olfactory neuroblastoma: an analysis of 22 cases. Clin Otolaryngol 24:457-461

Pignataro L, Peri A, Ottaviani F (2001) Breast carcinoma metastatic to the ethmoid sinus: a case report. Tumori 87:455-457

Pitkaranta A, Markkola A, Malmberg H (2001) Breast cancer metastasis presenting as ethmoiditis. Rhinology 39:107-108

Pontius KI, Sebek BA (1981) Extraskeletal Ewing's sarcoma arising in the nasal fossa. Light- and electron-microscopic observations. Am J Clin Pathol 75:410-415

Prades JM, Alaani A, Mosnier JF et al (2002) Granulocytic sarcoma of the nasal cavity. Rhinology 40:159-161

Prescher A, Brors D (2001) Die Metastasenabsiedlung in die Nasennebenhohlen: Fallmitteilung und Literaturubersicht. Laryngorhinootologie 80:583-594

Prokopakis EP, Snyderman CH, Hanna EY et al (1999) Risk factors for local recurrence of adenoid cystic carcinoma: the role of postoperative radiation therapy. Am J Otolaryngol 20:281-286

Quraishi MS, Bessell EM, Clark D et al (2000) Non-Hodgkin's lymphoma of the sinonasal tract. Laryngoscope 110:1489–1492

Ramos R, Som PM, Solodnik P (1990) Nasopharyngeal melanotic melanoma: MR characteristics. J Comput Assist Tomogr 14:997–999

Rassekh CH, Nuss DW, Kapadia SB et al (1996) Chondrosarcoma of the nasal septum: skull base imaging and clinicopathologic correlation. Otolaryngol Head Neck Surg 115:29–37

Regenbogen VS, Zinreich SJ, Kim KS et al (1988) Hyperostotic esthesioneuroblastoma: CT and MR findings. J Comput Assist Tomogr 12:52–56

Reiner SA, Siegel GJ, Clark KF et al (1990) Hemangiopericytoma of the nasal cavity. Rhinology 28:129–136

Rice DH (1999) Malignant salivary gland neoplasms. Otolaryngol Clin North Am 32:875–886

Rinaldo A, Shaha AR, Patel SG et al (2001) Primary mucosal melanoma of the nasal cavity and paranasal sinuses. Acta Otolaryngol 121:979–982

Rinaldo A, Ferlito A, Shaha AR et al (2002a) Esthesioneuroblastoma and cervical lymph node metastases: clinical and therapeutic implications. Acta Otolaryngol 122:215–221

Rinaldo A, Ferlito A, Shaha AR et al (2002b) Is elective neck treatment indicated in patients with squamous cell carcinoma of the maxillary sinus? Acta Otolaryngol (Stockh) 122:443–447

Rischin D, Porceddu S, Peters L et al (2004) Promising results with chemoradiation in patients with sinonasal undifferentiated carcinoma. Head Neck 26:435–441

Robbins KT, Fuller LM, Vlasak M et al (1985) Primary lymphoma of the nasal cavity and paranasal sinuses. Cancer 56:814–819

Roh HJ, Batra PS, Citardi MJ, et al (2004) Am J Rhinol 18:239–246

Rosenberg AE, Nielsen P, Keel SB et al (1999) Chondrosarcoma of the skull base. A clinicopathologic study of 200 cases with emphasis on its distinction from chordoma. Am J Surg Pathol 23:1370–1378

Roux FX, Brasnu D, Menard M et al (1991) Les abords combinès des tumeurs maligne de l'ethmoide et autres sinus paranasux. Principles et resultats. Ann Otol-Laryngol (Paris) 108:292–297

Roux FX, Pages JC, Nataf F et al (1997) Malignant ethmoid-sphenoidal tumors. 130 cases. Retrospective study. Neurochirurgie 43:100–110

Saleh HA (1996) A case of prostatic cancer metastatic to the orbit and ethmoid sinus. Ann Otol Rhinol Laryngol 105:584

Salvan D, Julieron M, Marandas P et al (1998) Combined transfacial and neurosurgical approach to malignant tumours of the ethmoid sinus. J Laryngol Otol 112:446–450

Sato Y, Morita M, Takhashi HO (1970) Combined surgery, radiotherapy, and regional chemotherapy in carcinoma of paranasal sinuses. Cancer 25:571–579

Schulz-Ertner D, Nikoghosyan A, Thilmann C et al (2004) Results of carbon ion radiotherapy in 152 patients. Int J Radiat Oncol Biol Phys 58:631–640

Schuster JJ, Phillips CD, Levine PA (1994) MR of esthesioneuroblastoma (olfactory neuroblastoma) and appearance after craniofacial resection. AJNR Am J Neuroradiol 15:1169–1177

Sercarz JA, Mark RJ, Traan L et al (1994) Sarcomas of the nasal cavity and paranasal sinuses. Ann Otol Rhinol Laryngol 103:699–704

Serrano E, Coste A, Percodani J et al (2002) Endoscopic sinus surgery for sinonasal haemangiopericytomas. J Laryngol Otol 116:951–954

Servenius B, Vernachio J, Price J (1994) Metastatizing neuroblastomas in mice transgenic for simian virus 40 large T (SV40T) under the olfactory marker protein gene promotor. Cancer Res 54:5198–5205

Sgouras ND, Gamatsi IE, Porfyris EA et al (1995) An unusual presentation of a metastatic hypernephroma to the frontonasal region. Ann Plast Surg 34:653–656

Shah JP, Kraus DH, Bilsky MH et al (1997) Craniofacial resection for malignant tumors involving the anterior skull base. Arch Otolaryngol Head Neck 123:1312–1317

Shapeero L, Vanel D, Couanet D et al (1993) Extraskeletal mesenchymal chondrosarcoma. Radiology 186:819–826

Sheehan JM, Sheehan JP, Jane JA Sr et al (2000) Chemotherapy for esthesioneuroblastomas. Neurosurg Clin North Am 11:693–670

Siegal GP, Oliver WR, Reinus WR et al (1987) Primary Ewing's sarcoma involving the bones of the head and neck. Cancer 60:2829–2840

Sigal R, Monnet O, de Baere T et al (1992) Adenoid cystic carcinoma of the head and neck: evaluation with MR imaging and clinical-pathologic correlation in 27 patients. Radiology 184:95–101

Silva EG, Butler JJ, Mackay B et al (1982) Neuroblastomas and neuroendocrine carcinomas of the nasal cavity: a proposed new classification. Cancer 50:2388–2405

Simo R, Sykes AJ, Hargreaves SP et al (2000) Metastatic renal cell carcinoma to the nose and paranasal sinuses. Head Neck 22:722–727

Simon JH, Zhen W, McCulloch TM et al (2001) Esthesioneuroblastoma: the University of Iowa experience 1978-1998. Laryngoscope 111:488–493

Singh P, Jain M, Singh DP et al (2002) MR findings of primary Ewing's sarcoma of greater wing of sphenoid. Austr Radiol 46:409–411

Smith SR, Som P, Fahmy A et al (2000) A clinicopathological study of sinonasal neuroendocrine carcinoma and sinonasal undifferentiated carcinoma. Laryngoscope 110:1617–1622

Sobin LH, Wittekind C, International Union against Cancer. eds. (2002), TNM classification of malignant tumours. (6th ed) Wiley-Liss, New York

Soesan M, Paccagnella A, Chiarion-Sileni V et al (1992) Extramedullary plasmacytoma: clinical behaviour and response to treatment. Ann Oncol 3:51–57

Sohaib SA, Moseley I, Wright JE (1998) Orbital rhabdomyosarcoma – the radiological characteristics. Clin Radiol 53:357–362

Som PM, Lawson W, Biller HF et al (1986) Ethmoid sinus disease: CT evaluation in 400 cases. Part III. Craniofacial resection. Radiology 159:605–609

Som PM, Shapiro MD, Biller HF et al (1988) Sinonasal tumors and inflammatory tissues: differentiation with MR imaging. Radiology 167:803–808

Som PM, Dillon WP, Sze G et al (1989) Benign and malignant sinonasal lesions with intracranial extension: differentiation with MR imaging. Radiology 172:763–766

Som PM, Lidov M (1994) The significance of sinonasal radiodensities: ossification, calcification, or residual bone? AJNR Am J Neuroradiol 15:917–922

Som PM, Lidov M, Brandwein M et al (1994) Sinonasal esthesioneuroblastoma with intracranial extension: marginal tumor cysts as a diagnostic MR finding. AJNR Am J Neuroradiol 15:1259–1262

Sorensen P, Liu X, Delattre O et al (1993 Reverse transcriptase PCR amplification of EWS/FL-1 fusion transcripts as a diagnostic test for peripheral primitive neuroectodermal tumors of childhood. Diagn Mol Pathol 2:147–157

Spaulding CA, Kranyak MS, Constable WC et al (1988) Esthesioneuroblastoma: a comparison of two treatment eras. Int J Radiat Oncol Biol Physiol 15:581–590

Spiro HR, Huvos AG (1992) Stage means more than grade in adenoid cystic carcinoma. Am J Surg 164:623–628

Stammberger H, Anderhuber W, Walch C et al (1999) Possibilities and limitations of endoscopic management of nasal and paranasal sinus malignancies. Acta Otorhinolaryngol Belg 53:199–205

Stern S, Guillamondegui OM (1991) Mucosal melanoma of the head and neck. Head Neck 13:22–27

Stout AP, Murray MR (1942) Hemangiopericytoma: vascular tumor featuring Zimmermann's pericytes. Ann Surg 116:26–33

Sumida T, Hamakawa H, Otsuka K et al (2001) Leiomyosarcoma of the maxillary sinus with cervical lymph node metastasis. J Oral Maxillofac Surg 59:568–571

Sur RK, Donde B, Levin V et al (1997) Adenoid cystic carcinoma of the salivary glands: a review of 10 years. Laryngoscope 107:1276–1280

Susnerwala SS, Shanks JH, Banerjee SS et al (1997) Extramedullary plasmacytoma of the head and neck region: clinicopathological correlation in 25 cases. Br J Cancer 75:921–927

Tanaka H, Westesson PL, Wilbur DC (1998) Leiomyosarcoma of the maxillary sinus: CT and MRI findings. Br J Radiol 71:221–224

Tiwari R, Hardillo JA, Mehta D et al (2000) Squamous cell carcinoma of maxillary sinus. Head Neck 22:164–169

Tomura N, Hirano H, Kato K et al (1999) Comparison of MR imaging with CT in depiction of tumour extension into the pterygopalatine fossa. Clin Radiol 54:361–366

Trapp KT, Fu YS, Calcaterra TC (1987) Melanoma of the nasal and paranasal sinus mucosa. Arch Otolaryngol Head Neck Surg 113:1086–1089

Tufano RP, Mokadam NA, Montone KT (1999) Malignant tumors of the nose and paranasal sinuses: Hospital of the University of Pennsylvania experience 1990-1997. Am J Rhinol 13:117–123

Vaccani JP, Forte V, de Jong AL et al (1999) Ewing's sarcoma of the head and neck in children. Int J Ped Otorhinolaryngol 48:209–216

Van der Wal JE, Snow GB, van der Waal I (1990) Intraoral adenoid cystic carcinoma. The presence of perineural spread in relation to site, size, local extension, and metastatic spread in 22 cases. Cancer 66:2031–2033

Van Es RJ, Keus RB, van der Waal I et al (1997) Osteosarcoma of the jaw bones. Long term follow up of 48 cases. Int J Oral Maxillofac Surg 26:191–197

Vasan NR, Medina JE, Canfield VA et al (2004) Sinonasal neuroendocrine carcinoma in association with SIADH. Head Neck 26:89–93

Vlasak R, Sim FH (1996) Ewing's sarcoma. Orthop Clin North Am 27:591–603

Vrielinck LJ, Ostyn F, van Damme B et al (1988) The significance of perineural spread in adenoid cystic carcinoma of the major and minor salivary glands. Int J Oral Maxillofac Surg 17:190–193

Walch C, Stammberger H, Anderhuber W et al (2000) The minimally invasive approach to olfactory neuroblastoma: combined endoscopic and stereotactic treatment. Laryngoscope 110:635–640

Wax KW, Yun KJ, Wetmore SJ et al (1995) Adenocarcinoma of the ethmoid sinus. Head Neck 17:303–311

Westerveld GJ, van Diest PJ, van Nieuwkerk EB (2001) Neuroendocrine carcinoma of the sphenoid sinus: a case report. Rhinology 39:52–54

Wexler LH, DeLaney TF, Tsokos M et al (1996) Ifosfamide and Etoposide plus Vincristine, Doxorubicin, and Cyclophosphamide for newly diagnosed Ewing's sarcoma family of tumors. Cancer 78:901–911

Williams LS (1999) Advanced concepts in the imaging of perineural spread of tumor to the trigeminal nerve. Top Magn Reson Imaging 10:376–383

Wiseman SM, Popat SR, Rigual NR et al (2002) Adenoid cystic carcinoma of the paranasal sinuses or nasal cavity: a 40-year review of 35 cases. Ear Nose Throat J

Wood RE, Nortje CJ, Hesseling P et al (1990) Ewing's tumor of the jaw. Oral Surg Oral Med Oral Pathol 69:120–127

Woodhead P, Lloyd GA (1988) Olfactory neuroblastoma: imaging by magnetic resonance, CT and conventional techniques. Clin Otolaryngol 13:387–394

Woodruff WW, Vrabec DP (1994) Inverted papilloma of the nasal vault and paranasal sinuses: spectrum of CT findings. AJR Am J Roentgenol 162:419–423

Woodruff WW Jr, Yeates AE, McLendon RE (1986) Perineural tumor extension to the cavernous sinus from superficial facial carcinoma: CT manifestations. Radiology 161:395–399

Yasumoto M, Taura S, Shibuya H et al (2000) Primary malignant lymphoma of the maxillary sinus: CT and MRI. Neuroradiology 42:285–289

Yoshida H, Nagao K, Ito H et al (1997) Chromosomal translocation in human soft tissue sarcomas by interphase fluorescence in situ hybridization. Pathol Int 47:222–229

Yousem DM, Lexa FJ, Bilaniuk LT et al (1990) Rhabdomyosarcomas in the head and neck: MR imaging evaluation. Radiology 177:683–686

Yousem DM, Li C, Montone KT et al (1996) Primary malignant melanoma of the sinonasal cavity: MR imaging evaluation. Radiographics 16:1101–1110

Yousem DM, Kraut MA, Chalian AA (2000) Major salivary gland imaging. Radiology 216:19–29

Yu KH, Yu SCH, Teo PML et al (1997) Nasal lymphoma: results of local radiotherapy with or without chemotherapy. Head Neck 19:251–259

Yu Q, Wang P, Shi H et al (2000) Central skull base invasion of maxillofacial tumors: computed tomography appearance. Oral Surg Oral Med Oral Pathol Oral Radiol Endod 89:643–650

Zimmermann KW (1923) Der feinere bau der blutcapillaren. Z Anat Entwicklungsgesch 68:26–109

10 Expansile Lesions Arising from Structures and Spaces Adjacent to the Paranasal Sinuses

Luca Oscar Redaelli de Zinis, Pietro Mortini, Davide Farina, and Francesca Mossi

CONTENTS

10.1   Introduction *221*
10.2   Skull Base Tumors Extending into the
         Sinonasal Tract *223*
10.2.1   Chordoma *223*
10.2.1.1 Definition, Epidemiology, Pattern of Growth *223*
10.2.1.2 Clinical Findings *223*
10.2.1.3 Treatment Guidelines and Prognosis *224*
10.2.1.4 Key Information to Be Provided by Imaging *224*
10.2.1.5 Imaging Findings *224*
10.2.2   Cartilaginous Tumors
         (Chondroma, Chondrosarcoma) *226*
10.2.2.1 Chondroma (or Osteochondroma) *226*
10.2.2.2 Chondrosarcoma *226*
10.2.3   Pituitary Tumors *228*
10.2.3.1 Definition, Epidemiology, Pattern of Growth *228*
10.2.3.2 Clinical Findings *229*
10.2.3.3 Treatment Guidelines and Prognosis *229*
10.2.3.4 Key Information to Be Provided by Imaging
         (see Section 10.2.1.4) *229*
10.2.3.5 Imaging Findings *229*
10.2.4   Craniopharyngioma *230*
10.2.4.1 Definition, Epidemiology, Pattern of Growth *230*
10.2.4.2 Clinical Findings *231*
10.2.4.3 Treatment Guidelines and Prognosis *231*
10.2.4.4 Key Information to Be Provided by Imaging
         (see Section 10.2.1.4) *232*
10.2.4.5 Imaging Findings *232*
10.2.5   Meningioma *233*
10.2.5.1 Definition, Epidemiology, Pattern of Growth *233*
10.2.5.2 Clinical Findings *234*
10.2.5.3 Treatment Guidelines and Prognosis *234*
10.2.5.4 Key Information to Be Provided by Imaging
         (see Section 10.2.1.4) *234*
10.2.5.5 Imaging Findings *234*
10.3   Masticator Space Tumors Extending into the
         Sinonasal Tract *235*
10.3.1   Definition, Epidemiology, Pattern of Growth *235*
10.3.2   Clinical Findings *236*
10.3.3   Treatment Guidelines and Prognosis *236*
10.3.4   Key Information to Be Provided by Imaging *237*
10.3.5   Imaging Findings *237*
10.4   Hard Palate Expansile Lesions *238*
10.4.1   Definition, Epidemiology, Pattern of Growth *238*
10.4.2   Clinical Findings *239*
10.4.3   Treatment Guidelines and Prognosis *239*
10.4.4   Key Information to Be Provided by Imaging *239*
10.4.5   Imaging Findings *240*
10.5   Odontogenic and Nonodontogenic
         Cysts and Tumors *240*
10.5.1   Introduction and Definition *240*
10.5.2   Epidemiology, Clinical Findings and
         Treatment Guidelines *242*
10.5.3   Key Information to be Provided by Imaging *245*
10.5.4   Imaging Findings *245*
         References *247*

L. O. Redaelli de Zinis, MD
Department of Otorhinolaryngology, University of Brescia, Piazzale Spedali Civili 1, Brescia, BS, 25123, Italy

P. Mortini, Professor, MD
Skull Base and Endocrinoneurosurgery Center, Department of Neurosurgery, University Vita e Salute, Via Olgettina 60, Milan, MI, 20132, Italy

D. Farina, MD; F. Mossi, MD
Department of Radiology, University of Brescia, Piazzale Spedali Civili 1, Brescia, BS, 25123, Italy

10.1 Introduction

Nose and paranasal sinuses can be involved by a variety of different neoplasms arising from adjacent spaces/structures and secondarily invading the bony framework composing the peripheral border of the sinonasal tract.

Upwards, the skull base separates the frontal sinus, the ethmoid and the sphenoid sinus from the anterior and middle cranial fossae. In exceedingly rare cases, meningioma or meningosarcoma can breach the cribriform plate, the fovea ethmoidalis and/or the planum sphenoidale (Rubinstein and Arbit 1985). Moving posteriorly, the list of lesions encompasses neoplasms arising from embryonic remnants (chordoma, craniopharyngioma), from bone and cartilage (chondroma, chondrosarcoma, osteosarcoma), and from the pituitary gland (adenoma) (Chakrabarty et al. 1998; DeMonte et al. 2000; Brown et al. 1994; Johnsen et al. 1991).

No real anatomic boundary separates nasal cavities from the nasopharynx. Thereby, nasopharyngeal tumors may have an unimpeded access to the nasal fossae through the choanae. Invasion of the paranasal sinuses is less common, probably because nasopharyngeal cancer typically takes origin from the vault or the lateral recess. As these areas are closer to the skull base, the preferential pathway of spread is towards the anterior foramen lacerum and the clivus (NG et al. 1997).

The posterolateral wall of the maxillary sinus is the boundary between the sinonasal tract and the masticator space. Neoplasms originating within this space are basically sarcomas or lymphomas, less frequently neurogenic tumors (YU et al. 1998).

The inferior boundary of the sinonasal tract (i.e., nasal cavity floor, alveolar recess of the maxillary sinus) may be involved by expansile lesions arising from the mucosa or submucosa lining the oral cavity. These lesions include epithelial neoplasms (basically squamous cell carcinoma) and tumors arising from minor salivary glands (GINSBERG and DEMONTE 1998). Several benign and malignant lesions arise from the alveolar process of maxillary bone and extend toward the sinonasal tract, mostly into the maxillary sinus and hard palate. Peculiar imaging findings may be observed in cysts and tumors arising from cells and tissues involved in odontogenesis. Finally, basal or squamous cell carcinoma of the face can invade adjacent sinonasal tract structures and further extend submucosally into bones or access the skull base via perineural spread (WILLIAMS et al. 2001) (Fig. 10.1–2).

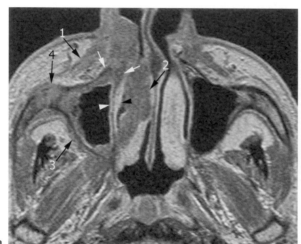

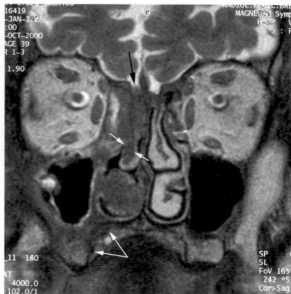

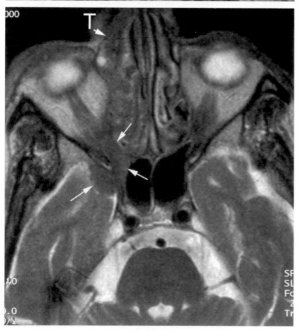

Fig. 10.1a–c. Basal cell carcinoma of the face. a Enhanced T1-weighted axial plane. Tumor spreads from the nasal skin into the muscles of the lip (*1*), and grows mainly along the bony framework of sinonasal structures into the inferior turbinate (*2*) (replacing the hyperintense signal of the vascularized tissue), anterior (*arrows*) and postero-lateral maxillary wall from which the hypointense tumor tissue penetrates the masticator space (*3*) and pterygopalatine fossa. Bone marrow invasion and cortical erosion of the zygomatic bone (*4*) is also present. At this level, the medial maxillary sinus wall is partially spared from the subperiosteal invasion (*arrowheads*). b The coronal plane (T2-weighted image) shows the hypointense tumor invading the hard palate (*long white arrows*), inferior and middle (*opposite white arrows*) turbinate. Spread through the cribriform plate appears with effacement of CSF signal on right side (*black arrow*). c A T2-weighted axial image demonstrates intracranial invasion through the superior orbital fissure (*white arrows*) with involvement of the foramen rotundum structures (*arrows*). Tumor (*T*)

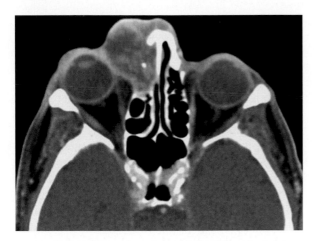

Fig. 10.2. Keratoacanthoma of the nasal skin with invasion of nasal bones, orbit, and anterior ethmoid

10.2
Skull Base Tumors Extending into the Sinonasal Tract

10.2.1
Chordoma

10.2.1.1
Definition, Epidemiology, Pattern of Growth

Chordoma, a tumor taking origin from embryonic remnants of the primitive notochord (BATSAKIS 1979) accounts for less than 1% of central nervous system tumors (WEBER et al. 1995). The most common locations are the sacrococcygeal region (45%–49%), the base of the skull (36%–39%), and the spinal axis (8%–15%) (HARRISON and LUND 1993). In the cranio-cervical region, seven points of origin have been identified: dorsum sellae, Blumenbach's clivus, retropharyngeal notochord vestiges, remnants in the apical ligament of the dens, nuclei pulposi of the cervical vertebrae, vestiges in the squama occipitalis, and ectopic localizations (BINKHORST et al. 1957). Primitive chordomas of the sinonasal tract, which have been rarely reported (LOUGHRAN et al. 2000), are interpreted not as real ectopic localizations but more properly as lesions arising from embryonic remnants of the notochord (SHUGAR et al. 1980).

Male-to-female ratio is generally reported to be 2:1 (PERZIN and PUSHPARAJ 1986; WEBER et al. 1995). The lesion can be observed at any age, with a predominance for the third and fourth decades in intracranial localizations, while spinal chordomas

are generally diagnosed at an older age because of a late occurrence of signs and symptoms (PERZIN and PUSHPARAJ 1986; WEBER et al. 1995). No association with irradiation or any other environmental factors has been observed. A small percentage of cases have a familial pattern of inheritance (DALPRÀ et al. 1999).

Chordomas develop from the bone, so they initially grow extradurally with bone destruction and secondary extension into the adjacent soft tissues (Fig. 10.3a) (OIKAWA et al. 2001). They present some of the typical features of a malignant tumor, such as local invasiveness, tendency to recur, and a potential for developing distant metastases, which have been reported in up to 43% of patients (HIGINBOTHAM et al. 1967). This event is typical for sacrococcygeal localizations. The low rate of systemic spread of skull base chordomas, ranging from 0 to 10%, is considered related to the fact that patients die for local progression before developing metastases (GAY et al. 1995; HUG et al. 1999).

Chordoma generally presents as a whitish, soft, multilobulated mass with a fibrous pseudocapsule, sometimes filled by a mucoid substance (secondary to previous hemorrhage), sometimes with hemorrhages, necrosis and/or calcifications and fragments of bone (BATSAKIS 1979). Microscopically, it is characterized by vacuolated physaliphorous cells, which are translucent cells of different sizes, rich in mucin and glycogen (BATSAKIS 1979).

At histology, the differential diagnosis includes primary bone tumors, cartilaginous neoplasms such as chondromas or chondrosarcomas, epithelial neoplasms such as mucinous-forming adenocarcinoma or salivary neoplasms, metastases, schwannoma, neurofibroma, meningioma, neuroblastoma, hemangioma and lymphoma. Cytokeratin antibodies and epithelial membrane antigen positivity differentiates chordoma from cartilaginous neoplasms, while S-100 positivity, not a constant feature, may help the differentiation from epithelial neoplasms (BOTTLES and BECKSTEAD 1984; WALKER et al. 1991). Some chordomas stain positive for vimentin, which reflects a mesenchymal differentiation (BOUROPOULOU et al. 1989).

10.2.1.2
Clinical Findings

Headache and diplopia, more frequently due to abducens nerve involvement, are the most common presenting symptoms (VOLPE et al. 1993). The fifth cranial nerve is also frequently involved, due to the progressive neoplastic lateral growth with invasion of adjacent structures such as the cavernous sinus. Signs and symptoms also include visual loss and limitation of the visual field, and extraocular complaints such as dysphagia, dyspnea, dysphonia, facial pain, facial paresis, hearing loss, tinnitus, dizziness and ataxia, due to brain stem compression. Anterior extension of the lesion into the nasopharynx can explain pharyngolaryngeal and otological symptoms, whereas extension toward the sinonasal tract can cause nasal obstruction, hypo-anosmia, hyponasal speech, mucopurulent discharge, and, rarely, epistaxis (PERZIN and PUSHPARAJ 1986; HARRISON and LUND 1993).

10.2.1.3
Treatment Guidelines and Prognosis

The treatment of choice for chordoma is surgery and a wide spectrum of approaches (transoral, anterior transfacial, subfrontal transcranial, frontotemporal transcavernous, lateral transpetrosal, subtemporal transpetrous-transcavernous, subtemporal infratemporal, and extreme lateral retrocondylar-transcondylar) (STRUGAR and SEKHAR 2000) have been described. Selection of surgical access mainly depends on tumor location, which is grouped in upper-, mid-, and lower-clival. Postoperative radiotherapy, both by linear accelerator, or proton beam, can provide a better control of the disease (ROSENBERG et al. 1999; HUG et al. 1999; CROCKARD et al. 2001).

Prognosis of chordoma is related to the extent of surgical removal: 5-year survival of 35% is reported after incomplete resection combined with conventional radiation therapy (ZORLU et al. 2000). Better results are obtained with aggressive surgical treatment and proton-beam postoperative radiotherapy, with 5-year and 10-year disease-free survival rates ranging from 50% (COLLI and AL-MEFTY 2001) to 77% (CROCKARD et al. 2001) and from 45% to 69%, respectively (ROSENBERG et al. 1999; CROCKARD et al. 2001). No effective chemotherapeutic agents are available for the treatment of this disease.

The prognosis of chordoma is affected by a variety of clinical and pathologic characteristics. Important features include tumor location, size and resectability, as well as the age and the gender of the patient. Larger tumors, female gender, and age greater than 40 years are associated with a poorer outcome (FORSITH et al. 1993; O'CONNELL et al. 1994; GAY et al. 1995; HUG et al. 1999).

10.2.1.4
Key Information to Be Provided by Imaging

- Involvement of the sella turcica, clivus, sphenoid sinus, pyramid apex.
- Displacement or encasement of internal carotid artery, involvement of the cavernous sinus, displacement of the basilar artery.
- Compression of central nervous system structures, involvement of cranial nerves.
- Involvement of the ventricular system, presence of hydrocephalus.
- Extent toward other skull base areas (foramen lacerum, pterygopalatine fossa) or into the nasopharynx, the atlanto-occipital joint and proximal cervical spine.
- Presence of imaging features highly suggestive for this specific lesion.

10.2.1.5
Imaging Findings

The site of origin of most skull base chordomas is the basiocciput-basisphenoid where the terminal portion of the notochord ends reaching the sphenoid bone just inferior to the sella turcica and dorsum sellae. Nasopharyngeal and intracranial locations are rarely observed, their origin being explained by the extra-osseous path of the notochord, which may have short segments running outside the bone, either

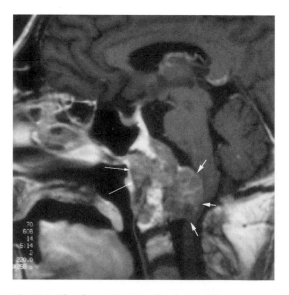

Fig. 10.3. Chordoma. On sagittal enhanced T1 sequence the lesion has a cervical location with invasion of the lower aspect of the atlanto-occipital joint; posteriorly the foramen magnum is invaded (*short arrows*). Anteriorly, the neoplasm extends into the nasopharynx (*long arrows*)

within nasopharyngeal soft tissues or within the posterior cranial fossa (Fig. 10.3).

On CT, chordoma appears as a midline clival soft tissue mass with bone destruction (OOT et al. 1988). Invasion of the body of the sphenoid usually occurs, accounting for the presence of coarse high densities within the mass, assumed to be remaining fragments of the eroded bone, rather than calcifications or new matrix formation (Fig. 10.4). No sclerotic changes are detected at the boundary with the invaded bone. Cystic components are frequently observed. Enhancement is present in at least some parts of the soft tissue component. When chordoma arises in nasopharynx or posterior fossa, the bone may or may not be eroded.

Intracranial extent frequently leads to posterior displacement of the basilar artery and mass effect on the brain stem. Lateral clival chordoma may present as a cerebello-pontine angle mass.

The MR appearance varies in relation to the composite histologic pattern of the tumor. In up to 80%

of lesions, MR shows heterogeneous hyperintensity on T2 - moderate to extreme (MEYERS et al. 1992) with possible dark areas, reflecting the presence of mucoid or old hemorrhagic areas, respectively. Soft tissue components show iso to hypointensity on T1, and variable degrees of contrast enhancement (SZE et al. 1988) (Fig. 10.5). Cystic areas may present bright signal on unenhanced T1.

Sagittal plain T1 sequences are particularly useful, as the hypointense chordoma replacing the hyperintensity of the clival bone marrow can be clearly seen (SZE et al. 1988). On all sequences, hypointense areas standing for large intratumoral calcifications can be identified. On T2, low intensity strands – composed of fibroconnective tissue – form hypointense septations enclosing lobulated hyperintense areas.

Though imaging findings of chordoma are rather nonspecific, the site of origin and patient's age may help in the differential diagnosis.

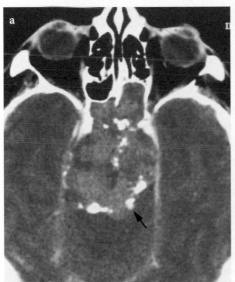

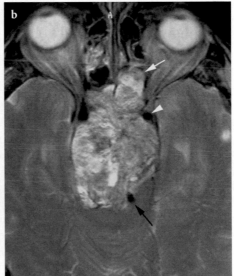

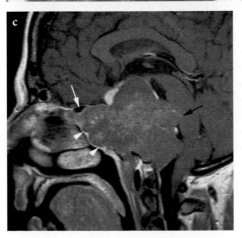

Fig. 10.4a-c. Chordoma. CT (a) and T2-weighted MR (b) show the tumor extending into the sphenoid sinuses (*white arrow*). Brain stem is compressed. Intratumoral coarse high densities are clearly shown by CT. Vessels displacement is demonstrated by both techniques. Basilar artery (*black arrow*), left internal carotid artery (*white arrowhead*). c The sagittal enhanced T1 image shows posterior cranial fossa invasion and brain stem compression (*black arrow*). Submucosal invasion of the nasopharynx/sphenoid (*arrowheads*) and extent into the posterior ethmoid (*white arrow*) is also detected

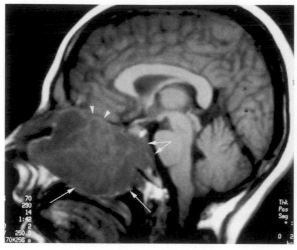

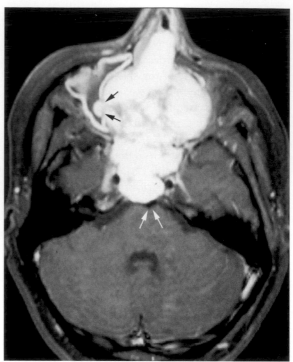

Fig.10.5 a,b. Chordoma. **a** Unenhanced T1-weighted sequence in the sagittal plane. A large extradural chordoma with invasion of the sphenoid sinus and ethmoid is shown. Replacement of bone marrow signal within the sphenoid bone (*double arrows*) with erosion of the posterior bony rim is detected. Intranasal extent reaches the planum sphenoidale from below (*arrowheads*). The mass projects into the nasopharynx (*white arrow*). **b** The chordoma shows relevant and heterogeneous enhancement. Extradural intracranial extent with basilar artery displacement (*white arrows*). Initial extent through the medial maxillary wall is present

10.2.2
Cartilaginous Tumors (Chondroma, Chondrosarcoma)

10.2.2.1
Chondroma (or Osteochondroma)

This benign neoplasm is composed of mature hyaline cartilage. It occurs as either solitary or multiple lesions. When the tumor arises within the medullary osseous cavity, it is termed enchondroma. As the tumor grows outward from the cortex, it develops on the external bone surface (osteochondroma) as a painless, slow-growing lesion producing symptoms and signs depending on the location. Surgical treatment has to be considered only for symptomatic tumors.

10.2.2.2
Chondrosarcoma

10.2.2.2.1
Definition, Epidemiology, Pattern of Growth

Chondrosarcoma of the skull base is a rare primary intraosseous neoplasm, which is frequently

included in the differential diagnosis of chordoma. It can be isolated or multiple, being part of one of the enchondromatosis syndromes (Ollier disease, Maffucci syndrome, metachondromatosis) (WEBER et al. 1995).

Prevalence of chondrosarcoma is less than 0.2% among intracranial tumors and 6% among skull base tumors (CIANFRIGLIA et al. 1978; KVETON et al. 1986). The peak incidence is in the second and third decades (HASSOUNAH et al. 1985), and the male-to-female ratio is 1:1 (GAY et al. 1995). Chondrosarcoma may arise from primitive mesenchymal cells or from embryonal rests of the cranium's cartilaginous matrix (GAY et al. 1995). Conventional chondrosarcomas are grouped in 3 grades, according to the degree of their cellularity, cytologic atypia, and mitotic activity. Grade 1 is the least aggressive neoplasm with features of a benign tumor, while grade 3 is the most aggressive type. Other histological types are clear cell, myxoid, mesenchymal, and dedifferentiated chondrosarcoma (DORFMAN and CZERNIAK 1998). Conventional chondrosarcoma is composed of hyaline, myxoid, or an mixture of hyaline and myxoid cartilage. Typically it grows with an infiltrative pattern, replacing the normal marrow elements, encasing preexisting cancellous bone, and permeating haversian channels. It is by this mechanism that the tumor frequently transgresses the cortex and forms a soft tissue mass.

The clivus, the sphenoid bone - particularly in the parasellar area and the petrous apex (KORTEN et al. 1998; ROSENBERG et al. 1999) - are the most frequent sites of localization of skull base chondrosarcomas, which are considered to arise from residual endochondral cartilage (NEFF et al. 2002). Chondrosarcomas have more commonly a paramedian location and they involve the sphenoethmoidal area in 33% of cases (SEKHAR and OLIVEIRA 1999).

10.2.2.2.2
Clinical Findings

Since chondrosarcoma is a slow growing tumor, signs and symptoms occur late and depend on the site of origin and pattern of growth. Usually, the clinical findings are undistinguishable from those of chordoma, the latter being more frequently asymptomatic, while chondrosarcoma is more commonly associated with visual loss, facial numbness, and multiple cranial nerves impairment (VOLPE et al. 1993).

10.2.2.2.3
Treatment Guidelines and Prognosis

Surgical treatment is the first line therapy, generally followed by proton-beam postoperative radiotherapy. In a group of 200 patients who received proton beam irradiation after biopsy or surgical treatment, the 5- and 10-year local control rates were 99% and 98%, respectively, and 5- and 10-year disease-specific survival rates were both 99% (ROSENBERG et al. 1999). As the outcome is significantly better than that of chordoma, this finding emphasizes the importance of an accurate distinction between the two neoplasms.

10.2.2.2.4
Key Information to Be Provided by Imaging (see Section 10.2.1.4)

10.2.2.2.5
Imaging Findings

Most frequent sites of origin of skull base chondrosarcoma include the spheno-occipital, spheno-petrosal and petro-occipital synchondroses, and a large part of the petrous bone where the tumor is hypothesized to develop from residual enchondral cartilage (LEE and VAN TASSEL 1989; WATTERS and BROOKES 1995; NEFF et al. 2002)

The quantity of chondroid matrix within the lesion influences the appearance on CT. The soft tissue component appears hypodense on CT and shows variable degrees of enhancement.

Calcifications largely vary, ranging from small and scattered, often arranged as a peripheral rim, to large, dense, and diffuse. They tend to have an interrupted ring-like shape (Fig. 10.6). Nonetheless, intratumoral calcifications may be absent (BROWN et al. 1994). Bone destruction is a rather constant finding (LEE and VAN TASSEL 1989).

MR shows moderately high to very high hyperintense T2 signal within the nonmineralized portion of the lesion (Fig. 10.7). The signal is non-homogeneous in about 60% of cases, due to intratumoral areas of hypointensity corresponding to coarse chondroid mineralization or fibrocartilaginous areas on CT. Otherwise to CT, small calcifications may be undetected on MR. Chondrosarcoma appears iso to hypointense on T1, and may show marked non-homogeneous contrast enhancement (immediately after contrast agent administration), partly related to the presence of calcifications and chondroid matrix (MEYERS et al. 1992) (Fig. 10.8).

Based on pathologic findings, it is often difficult to discriminate low-grade chondrosarcoma from its benign counterpart. Imaging may play a role providing information about cortical bone destruction.

The imaging based differential diagnosis in the skull base includes a variety of lesions, the most challenging of which is represented by chordoma. Some

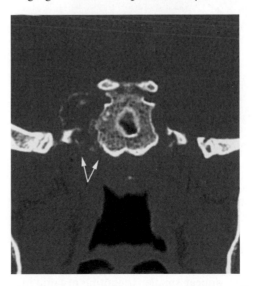

Fig. 10.6. Chondrosarcoma of the right petro-clival suture. Unenhanced CT in the coronal plane shows small, thin calcifications 1s lining the boundary of the mass that extends submucosal through the foramen lacerum into the nasopharynx (*arrows*)

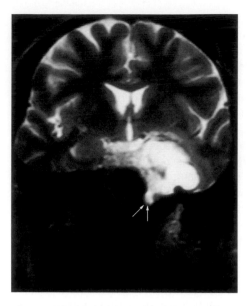

Fig. 10.7. Chondrosarcoma of the left petro-clival suture, highly hyperintense on the coronal T2-weighted image. Left cavernous sinus and internal carotid artery are involved. Downward extent toward the nasopharynx is shown (*arrows*)

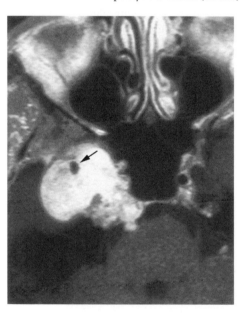

Fig. 10.8. Chondrosarcoma of the right petrous apex with internal carotid artery encasement (*black arrow*), cavernous sinus and Meckel cave involvement. Part of the lesion extends into left pre-pontine cistern

clues are offered by calcifications, which are larger (probably representing residual bone) in chordoma, whereas they appear smaller (denoting organic matrix production) in chondrosarcoma. Nonetheless, the site of origin (midline for chordoma, paramedian for chondrosarcoma) is probably the most reliable criterion (BOURGOUIN et al. 1992).

10.2.3
Pituitary Tumors

10.2.3.1
Definition, Epidemiology, Pattern of Growth

Pituitary tumors are frequent neoplasms representing about 8%-10% of all intracranial tumors (KAYE 1997). They are incidentally found in 10% of autopsies (NAMMOUR et al. 1997; FAJFR et al. 2002). Most pituitary tumors occur in young adults, with a predilection for females, and the highest incidence in the third and the sixth decades. The pathogenesis of pituitary tumors can be sometimes related to oncogenes anomalies (G-protein, ras gene, p53) and to the syndrome of multiple endocrine neoplasia (CORBETTA et al. 1997; SPADA et al. 1998; SUHARDJA et al. 1999). Most pituitary tumors are benign, but some of them may show a high growth rate and aggressiveness. Central nervous system and distant metastases are exceptionally described (PICHARD et al. 2002). Hardy's radiological classification distinguishes tumors on the basis of the size and gross features (bone changes, extent) (HARDY 1969). According to the size, tumors are divided in microadenomas (less than 10 mm) and macroadenomas (greater than 10 mm). On the basis of imaging features, 5 classes of tumors are identified. Microadenomas are designated as being either grade 0 or grade I, depending on whether the sella appears normal, or minor focal sellar changes are present. Macroadenomas causing diffuse sellar enlargement, focal sellar erosion or extensive sellar and skull base destruction are classified as grade II, grade III, and grade IV, respectively. Macroadenomas are further subclassified by the degree of suprasellar extension (HARDY 1969). Pituitary adenomas have also been classified by their staining in chromophobic and chromophilic, but this classification is disused because of the overwhelming importance of immunohistochemistry and electron microscopy, that sometimes show the hormone production and also multiple hormonal production in the same tumor.

Differential diagnosis includes many other intracranial neoplasms such as craniopharyngioma, meningioma, germinoma, and secondary tumors. Granulomatous and infectious disorders involving the intrasellar region should also be considered. In case of sphenoid invasion by a pituitary adenoma or ectopic sphenoid localization, the differential diagnosis includes mucocele and fungus ball.

10.2.3.2
Clinical Findings

Clinical findings depend on the local extent of the tumor and on the possible endocrine disorders due to hormonal overproduction and/or hypopituitarism. In about 70% of cases, the clinical picture is dominated by features of anterior pituitary hypersecretion resulting in a characteristic hypersecretory syndrome. (ZERVAS and MARTIN 1980). Acromegaly, Cushing's disease, amenorrhea-galactorrhea syndrome and, rarely, secondary hyperthyroidism represent the classical paradigms of GH, ACTH, PRL and TSH hypersecretion, respectively. It is important to recognize that hyperprolactinemia is not always a feature specific for PRL-producing adenomas. Moderate hyperprolactinemia (<120 ng/ml) can occur in a variety of lesions involving the sellar region. This phenomenon, frequently referred to as the "stalk section effect", is the result of compressive or destructive lesions involving the hypothalamus or the pituitary stalk. Pituitary tumors can also present with symptoms suggesting partial or total hypopituitarism (fatigue, weakness, hypogonadism, regression of sexual secondary characteristics, hypothyroidism). This often occurs insidiously in association with pituitary macroadenomas which compress and impair the secretory capability of the adjacent nontumorous pituitary gland. Pituitary insufficiency can also acutely occur in the context of pituitary apoplexy. A progressively enlarging pituitary mass can also generate a constellation of neurologic signs and symptoms, depending on its growth path.

Headache, due to stretching of the enveloping dura or of the diaphragma sellae, may be an early finding. However, the single most common neurologic sign is visual loss, which is related to suprasellar extension of the tumor, with compression of the optic nerves and chiasm. The classic and most common pattern of visual loss is that of a bitemporal hemianopic field deficit, often in association with decreased visual acuity. Large pituitary adenomas can encroach upon the hypothalamus, causing alteration of sleep, alertness, behavior, eating and emotion. These tumors can extend into the region of the third ventricle, where obstruction to effluent CSF flow can result in obstructive hydrocephalus. Quite commonly, the tumor extends laterally in the region of the cavernous sinus. With progressive cavernous sinus invasion, cranial nerves (oculomotor, trochlear, trigeminal, abducens) can occasionally be affected. Finally, some pituitary adenomas can reach a giant size, extending into the anterior, middle and posterior cranial fossae. Neuro-ophthalmologic examination together with hormones testing are indicated prior to imaging (LISSETT and SHALET 2000).

10.2.3.3
Treatment Guidelines and Prognosis

Therapy for pituitary tumors should be directed at the following goals: reversal of endocrinopathy and restoration of the normal pituitary function; removal of tumor mass and restoration of normal neurologic function. Nowadays, these goals can be more frequently achieved due to the evolution of microsurgical techniques, the development of receptors-mediate pharmacotherapy, and refinements in the delivery of radiation therapy. Each of these treatment modalities has specific advantages and limitations, therefore treatment selection should be thoughtfully individualized to each patient (WILSON 1984).

Medical management can sometimes control endocrine manifestations, particularly in case of prolactinomas and growth hormone secreting adenomas. Two classes of pharmacologic agents have emerged as primary or adjuvant therapies for pituitary tumors: dopamine agonists and somatostatin analogues. Surgical treatment is advised to control local expansion signs and symptoms and to release the patient from chronic drug treatment. Transsphenoidal access (microscopic or endoscopic) is the approach of choice (CAPPABIANCA et al. 2002; CHO and LIAU 2002; ZADA et al. 2003). A transcranial approach can be added in larger lesions (LANDOLT 2001). Transsphenoidal surgery is associated with low morbidity (CIRIC et al. 1983). Currently, more than 95% of pituitary tumors are approached transsphenoidally, with conventional transcranial approaches reserved for the remaining few cases in which anatomic features of the sella or unusual intracranial tumor extension (dumb-bell shape) limit the transsphenoidal accessibility (MAC CARTY et al. 1973; MORTINI and GIOVANELLI 2002). Prognosis of pituitary tumors is generally good (REES et al. 2002). Whenever residual neoplasm is left, medical treatment adequately controls the disease. Radiosurgery has also been proposed for small residual lesions or for the cavernous sinus invasion (SHEEHAN et al. 2002; LOSA et al. 2004).

10.2.3.4
Key Information to Be Provided by Imaging
(see Section 10.2.1.4)

10.2.3.5
Imaging Findings

Pituitary adenoma may have an extrasellar extension, laterally into the cavernous sinus, inferiorly into the sphenoid sinus. The latter may occasionally occur in the absence of a suprasellar growth. In this case, the floor may be the only bony boundary of the sella to be disrupted. Such a pattern of growth may hinder the discrimination between pituitary adenoma, chordoma, chondrosarcoma, and superior extension of a nasopharyngeal carcinoma.

More than CT and MR appearance, correlation of site of the lesion with laboratory tests and clinical history may help to properly address the diagnosis (COTTIER et al. 2000).

MR is the technique of choice in the diagnosis of pituitary adenomas, as its high contrast resolution allows to detect even small microadenomas, which are not identified on CT (THUOMAS 1999). In addition, in the preoperative work-up of macroadenomas, MR allows to demonstrate lateral extension toward the cavernous sinus, internal carotid artery, middle and anterior cerebral arteries as well as vertical extension towards the suprasellar cistern, optic chiasm and nerves (upwards) and sphenoid sinus (downwards) (Fig. 10.9) (DAVIS et al. 1987).

Pituitary adenomas share some common MR features regardless of their size (micro- or macroadenomas). T1 sequence is the most appropriate tool to identify these lesions – generally hypointense – and to discriminate them from the adjacent normal parenchyma – more hypointense – unless totally compressed. In this sequence, spontaneous hyperintensity is the hallmark of the presence of blood (OSTROV et al. 1989). On T2 sequence, hyperintensity is more commonly observed in macroadenomas; according to IUCHI et al. (1998) high T2 signal indicates a softer tumor and, therefore, better predicts resectability.

Cystic degeneration of pituitary adenomas is heralded by the presence of T1 hypo-and T2 hyperintense areas, which are infrequently associated with fluid on fluid levels.

Sphenoid sinus invasion can be demonstrated when the iso- to hypointense signal of the adenoma protrudes into the air-containing sinus. Expectedly, subtle abnormalities of cortical bone of the sella may be complex to identify on MR. As a result, the interpretation of MR findings may be sometimes difficult, particularly when the sphenoid sinus shows inflammatory changes (mucosal thickening, retained secretions with variable degrees of dehydration, fungal superinfection). Narrow display windows are recommended to identify subtle sinus septa, as these may represent valuable landmarks during transsphenoidal surgery. The intra-sphenoidal portion of the pituitary adenoma has been reported to result less intense on both T1 and T2 images and on contrast-enhanced images when compared with the sellar/suprasellar solid portion of the adenoma, which show marked contrast enhancement. Histological examination of adenoma specimens demonstrate some degree of fibrosis within the portion extending into the sphenoid sinus (ISHII et al. 1996). Rarely, isolated ectopic pituitary adenomas arising within sphenoid sinus have been reported, showing nonspecific MR findings such as soft tissue mass, isointense with gray matter on T1-weighted images with heterogeneous enhancement (SLONIM et al. 1993).

10.2.4
Craniopharyngioma

10.2.4.1
Definition, Epidemiology, Pattern of Growth

ERDHEIM in 1904 contributed the first adequate histological description of the lesion (ERDHEIM 1904). However, the term craniopharyngioma was introduced by CUSHING in 1932 (CUSHING 1932). Craniopharyngioma is thought to arise from small ectodermal cellular clusters, which are usually found in the transition area of the pituitary stalk with the pars distalis of the adenohypophysis, but may also be detected in the pars tuberalis along the upper part of the stalk. Two main hypotheses about the origin of

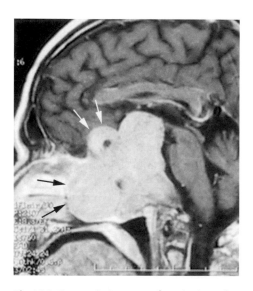

Fig. 10.9. Large pituitary non-functioning adenoma in a 48 years old male who experienced decreased visual acuity on both eyes with bitemporal hemianopsia. The tumor inferiorly extends through the sphenoid sinus into the nasopharynx and posterior nasal cavity (*black arrows*). Anteriorly, the pituitary adenoma extends into the anterior cranial fossa (*white arrows*)

the tumor exist in the literature. According to the first one, craniopharyngioma develops from the ectodermal clusters of primitive craniopharyngeal duct and adenohypophysis (embryologic theory). The second one hypothesizes an origin from metaplasia of the residual squamous epithelium found in the adenohypophysis and anterior infundibulum (metaplastic theory). Although the origin of craniopharyngioma is still controversial, some authors believe that it may have a dual origin (GIANGASPERO et al. 1984). They attribute the so-called childhood (adamantinous) craniopharyngioma to embryonic remnants, and the adulthood (squamous papillary) craniopharyngioma to metaplastic foci of adenohypophysis cells.

Craniopharyngioma accounts for 1%–4% of intracranial tumors (5–10% in children) and has a bimodal age distribution with a peak in childhood (5–10 years) and in the middle-aged patients (50–60 years). There is no difference in distribution between males and females or among races (EINHAUS and SANFORD 2000). Primitive or secondary sinonasal involvement has been exceptionally observed (AKIMURA et al. 1989; BRET and BEZIAT 1993; CHAKRABARTY et al. 1998; JIANG et al. 1998; FALAVIGNA and KRAEMER 2001).

Craniopharyngioma typically arises in the infundibulo-hypophyseal axis in the sella and suprasellar area, frequently occupying the suprasellar cisterns, but it may grow in any direction. A better topographic classification of craniopharyngioma was established by MR, recognizing four major types: intrasellar, infundibulum-tuberian, intraventricular, and dumbbell-shaped craniopharyngioma (RAYBAUD et al. 1991). Important surgical classifications have been proposed by SAMII and BIN, (1991) and YASARGIL et al. (1990). They are based on the vertical extension of the tumor and its relationship with the third ventricle.

Craniopharyngioma is an epithelial neoplasm with solid and cystic components with frequent calcifications, which has a tendency to infiltrate and to produce a glial reaction causing strong adherences (EINHAUS and SANFORD 2000). Child and adult types have a different growth pattern, with a higher tendency for brain infiltration in the adamantinous type. Differential diagnosis encompasses other tumors, infectious or inflammatory processes and other congenital anomalies (SHIN et al. 1999).

10.2.4.2
Clinical Findings

Since craniopharyngioma is a slow-growing tumor, it may reach even a large size before causing symptoms.

In the majority of cases, the time interval between the onset of symptoms and the diagnosis ranges from 1 to 2 years.

Most frequently, craniopharyngiomas have an intrasellar and suprasellar localization. Their growth usually is associated with involvement of surrounding structures in all directions, eventually resulting in intracranial hypertension, endocrine dysfunction and neurologic signs and symptoms (ROHRER et al. 2002). Increased intracranial pressure results from an enlarging intracranial mass or obstructive hydrocephalus. Visual deficits may be related to direct compression of the optic pathways or may be secondary to intracranial hypertension. Endocrine abnormalities, which appear in men as decreased sexual drive (88%) and in women as amenorrhea (82%) (CARMEL 1990), are caused by compression of the hypothalamic-hypophyseal axis. In case of large tumors of the adult, psychiatric, cognitive, and complex neurologic symptoms have been described (DONNET et al. 1999; FITZGERALD and MORGENSTERN 2000).

Children frequently present with symptoms of increased intracranial pressure (65–75%), such as headache and vomiting. About 20% of them have papilloedema. Obstructive hydrocephalus is present in about one third of the cases. Visual deficits are commonly well tolerated by children. PANG (1993) described the typical child with a craniopharyngioma as being short, obese, dull, half-blind, and with a poor school record.

10.2.4.3
Treatment Guidelines and Prognosis

There is general agreement that surgery plays a major role in the treatment of craniopharyngioma. A transsphenoidal approach is elected when the lesion is mostly intrasellar, while a pterional or a subfrontal approach is appropriate for suprasellar lesions, and a transcallosal approach is used for third ventricle floor lesions (infundibulum and tuber cinereum) (NORRIS et al. 1998; FAHLBUSCH et al. 1999; CHEN 2002; VAN EFFENTERRE and BOCH 2002; WANG et al. 2002). Radiotherapy is added when an incomplete tumor excision is obtained (KALAPURAKAL et al. 2003). Limited surgery with postoperative radiotherapy have been proposed with the aim of limiting the sequelae of a more extended surgery (ISAAC et al. 2001; MERCHANT et al. 2002). In addition, stereotactic radiosurgery has been used as exclusive treatment (SCHULZ-ERTNER et al. 2002; ULFARSSON et al. 2002).

Perioperative morbidity is mainly related to intracranial complications (KALAPURAKAL et al.
2003). Endocrine deficits are frequently expected
(HONEGGER et al. 1999).

Five-year survival rates ranging from 92% to
100% have been reported (FAHLBUSCH et al. 1999;
VAN EFFENTERRE and BOCH 2002; KALAPURAKAL et
al. 2003). Owing to the young age at diagnosis and
the potential clinical impact of treatment sequelae,
a longer survival estimation shows the 10-year and
15-year survival rates to decrease down to 68% and
59%, respectively (BULOW et al. 1998). Tumor recurrence, which accounts for about 28% (CHOUX et al.
1991), often occurs along the operative track. Factors
associated with an increased risk of recurrence are
preoperative visual symptoms, tumor adhesiveness
at surgery, and subtotal resection (DUFF et al. 2000).

10.2.4.4
Key Information to Be Provided by Imaging
(see Section 10.2.1.4)

10.2.4.5
Imaging Findings

Because it arises from the pituitary stalk axis, craniopharyngioma is usually located on the midline, most
frequently within an area extending from the third
ventricle to the sphenoid body. Moreover, due to its
origin from remnants of the craniopharyngeal duct,
it shares a common embryologic origin from oral
ectoderm. This feature accounts for the histological
and imaging similarity with ameloblastoma and with
keratinizing and calcifying odontogenic cyst, which
is characterized by proliferating ameloblastic epithelium, ghost keratin, calcification, and cyst formation.
The term itself *adamantinous* craniopharyngioma
derives from this histological similarity (BERNSTEIN
and BUCHINO 1983).

Adamantinous craniopharyngioma, which is the
most common form, typically presents as a mass
with both cystic and solid components. On CT, a cyst
with nodular or rim calcifications (90% of cases) and
some solid enhancing components is the most typical feature (GUPTA et al. 1999). Though variable, the
density of the cystic part is generally superior to cerebrospinal fluid. Site of the lesion is both suprasellar and sellar in 60% of cases, entirely intrasellar or
suprasellar in 10% and 20% of cases, respectively.

The most typical MR finding is a heterogeneous
suprasellar-sellar signal mass containing a cystic
component, well defined, with internal uniform
signal, hyperintense on both T1 and T2 sequences

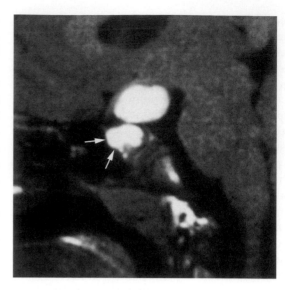

Fig. 10.10. Sellar and suprasellar craniopharyngioma showing
a double cystic component which has a bright signal on the
T1-weighted sagittal plane (*arrows*)

(Fig. 10.10). Nonetheless, a variety of different MR
patterns may be present, including solid, calcified,
CSF-like, hematin-like, and protein-like signals. A
solid component is also invariably present, often
partially calcified. In up to 92% of cases, more than
one pattern coexists in the same lesion, reflecting the histopathologic complexity of the lesion
(MOLLÀ et al. 2002; WARAKAULLE et al. 2003). It is
important to note that the adamantinous craniopharyngioma often elicits a relevant inflammatory
reaction from adjacent tissues. At the interface with
brain, this results in a dense gliosis that may be very
difficult to separate from the neoplasm. Infrasellar
extension is rare (HILLMAN et al. 1988; BRET and
BEZIAT 1993; CHAKRABARTY et al. 1998; FUJIMOTO
et al. 2002; CHEDDADI et al. 1996). The solid component of the infrasellar lesion may extend into the
sinonasal tract or into the nasopharynx. Cystic signals are present both within and at the boundaries
of the mass. Sclerotic changes within the sphenoid
bone are also observed (BRET and BEZIAT 1993).

Papillary craniopharyngioma, typically found in
adulthood, is more frequently located within the floor
of third ventricle, in up to 41% of cases. It appears
more solid, calcifications are usually absent, cystic
components are less relevant than in the adamantinous type, and do not show hyperintensity on T1.
Post contrast studies show a partially cystic mass that
enhances peripherally, mural nodules are detected in
about 70% of lesions (CROTTY et al. 1995). The mass

is usually encapsulated and readily separable from adjacent structures.

Imaging features useful for differentiating the two tumor types are the encasement of vessels, the lobulated shape, and the presence of hyperintense cysts in adamantinous type, and the more round shape, the presence of hypointense cysts, and the predominantly solid appearance in squamous-papillary tumors (SARTORETTI-SCHEFER et al. 1997).

Differential diagnosis includes the *Rathke's pouch or cleft cyst* which shares the same common embryologic origin of craniopharyngioma, but is lined by a single layer of epithelial cells (cuboidal or columnar), filled by mucoid or – less commonly serous – fluid, or cellular debris. Mucoid contents accounts for the hyperintensity on both T1 and T2 sequences, making the distinction with craniopharyngioma difficult. Serous content results in CSF-like findings on CT and MR. Those cysts containing cellular debris are more dense on CT and show heterogeneous signal on MR: focal components with low signal on T2 that become iso- to slightly hyperintense on T1 (KUCHARCZYK et al. 1987). Unlike craniopharyngioma, Rathke's cleft cyst does not enhance except for a thin, peripheral enhancement of its wall. Only large lesions are symptomatic. Most are intrasellar, though they can be confined to the sphenoid bone, making the differential diagnosis with mucocele very difficult.

10.2.5
Meningioma

10.2.5.1
Definition, Epidemiology, Pattern of Growth

Meningioma is thought to take origin from arachnoidal cap cells (GREENBERG 2001). It accounts for more than 20% of all intracranial neoplasms (LONGSTRETH et al. 1993; D'ALESSANDRO et al. 1995; SURAWICZ et al. 1999), with an annual incidence rate ranging from 2 to 13 new cases per 100,000 inhabitants (BONDY and LIGON 1996; HELSETH 1997; CORDERA et al. 2002). There is a female predominance of about 2:1 (HELSETH 1997; SURAWICZ et al. 1999; CORDERA et al. 2002), with a predominance in African people (BONDY and LIGON 1996). Every age can be involved, with a peak incidence in the seventh and eighth decades (BONDY and LIGON 1996).

There are many hypotheses for the etiology of meningioma. Previous radiation therapy – latency period inversely proportional to the dose of radiations

(SADETZKI et al. 2002) –, viruses (SV-40, adenovirus, and papovavirus) (BONDY and LIGON 1996), chromosomal abnormalities (long arm chromosome 22, but also other chromosomes have been considered) (BONDY and LIGON 1996; ARSLANTAS et al. 2003), hormonal alterations (estrogen, progesterone, androgens, epidermal growth factor, platelet derived growth factor, fibroblast growth factor) (DETTA et al. 1993; BLACK et al. 1994; FIGARELLA-BRANGER et al. 1994; LAMBE et al. 1997), and various occupational exposures (LONGSTRETH et al. 1993; HU et al. 1999) have been suggested to play a role in the pathogenesis of meningioma. Also head traumas have been considered (PHILLIPS et al. 2002), but many controversies exist about this hypothesis (LONGSTRETH et al. 1993; BONDY and LIGON 1996).

Meningioma can arise from many different intracranial sites. Among these, tuberculum sellae (12.8% of intracranial locations) (GREENBERG 2001), olfactory groove (9.8% of intracranial meningiomas) (GREENBERG 2001), and petroclival meningiomas (2% of intracranial meningiomas) (PIEPER and AL-MEFTY 1999) can potentially extend toward the sinonasal tract and the nasopharynx (MORRIS et al. 1990; MAIURI et al. 1998), an event observed in 3% of cases (FARR et al. 1973).

Primary sinonasal meningioma has also been observed (PERZIN and PUSHPARAJ 1984; THOMPSON and GYURE 2000; HATFIELD et al. 2001; SWAIN et al. 2001), accounting in a large series for 0.17% of sinonasal and nasopharyngeal neoplasms (THOMPSON and GYURE 2000).

The World Health Organization histological classification includes three types of meningiomas: benign, atypical and malignant (KLEIHUES et al. 1993). The vast majority of cases belong to the benign type. Histologic subtypes of meningiomas are the meningothelial (syncytial), fibroblastic and transitional (GREENBERG 2001). The latter type, which encompasses features of the other types, is frequently characterized by the typical psammoma bodies. Papillary growth pattern is one of the features of malignancy, which is associated with brain infiltration and distant metastases (lung, liver, lymph nodes, heart) (GREENBERG 2001). Hyperostosis can be due to bony reaction to the tumor or more frequently to direct invasion (PIEPER et al. 1999). However, one should keep in mind that even primary intraosseous meningioma may be associated with either hyperostotic or osteolytic changes (ARANA et al. 1996; DEVI et al. 2001). In the "en-plaque meningioma", which is more commonly found in the sphenoid wings, the amount of hyperostotic bone is disproportionate to the volume of the intradural tumor, thereby appearing as a thin layer of tissue investing the inner table of the skull (DEROME 1991).

10.2.5.2
Clinical Findings

Primary intracranial meningioma can silently, but relentlessly grow and eventually results in a variety of signs and symptoms. Apart from general complaints induced by cortical irritation (i.e. seizures) or hydrocephalus (i.e., headache), specific signs (cranial nerves paralysis, hormonal deficiency, specific brain stem compression syndromes, head and face deformity secondary to hyperostosis, exophthalmos) related to tumor location may be the clinical hallmarks.

Clinical findings of sinonasal tract meningioma, either primary or secondary, are similar to those of other benign and malignant neoplasms (PERZIN and PUSHPARAJ 1984; THOMPSON and GYURE 2000). Specific locations may be associated with a typical clinical presentation. Meningioma of the olfactory groove may present with anosmia and Foster-Kennedy syndrome (optic atrophy, scotoma in the ipsilateral eye, papilloedema in the contralateral); tuberculum sellae meningioma with early visual loss; cavernous sinus meningioma with proptosis and diplopia; foramen magnum meningioma with nuchal and suboccipital pain, stepwise appendicular sensory and motor deficits.

10.2.5.3
Treatment Guidelines and Prognosis

The mainstay of treatment for meningioma is still surgical resection. Critical parameters affecting resectability include tumor location, size, consistency, vascular and neural involvement, and, in recurrent lesions, prior surgery and/or radiotherapy. New and innovative approaches have been devised to reach and widely expose meningiomas in any location. Furthermore, a better knowledge of risk factors for tumor recurrence changed the philosophy of surgical management. In order to decrease the incidence of recurrences, resection of a meningioma should include not only the gross lesion, but also the involved dura, soft tissue, and bone. Postoperative radiotherapy is advisable for atypical and malignant meningiomas and in selected cases of incomplete resection. Instead of a standard fractionated radiation therapy, stereotactic radiosurgery is indicated for residual tumor (KONDZIOLKA et al. 1991), particularly when cavernous sinus invasion is present (NICOLATO et al. 2002). However, the size of the lesion should not exceed 35–40 mm. The morbidity of meningioma treatment is strongly related to its location and extension. Overall, 5-year survival for benign and malignant meningiomas is about 70%; and 55%, respectively (McCARTHY et al. 1998). A more favorable prognosis with a 5-year and 10-year disease-free survival of 82% and 79% has been reported for sinonasal meningiomas (THOMPSON and GYURE 2000).

10.2.5.4
Key Information to Be Provided by Imaging (see Section 10.2.1.4)

10.2.5.5
Imaging Findings

Approximately 33% of benign intracranial meningiomas arise from the skull base, mostly at the level of sphenoid wings. Extracranial spread more frequently occurs along skull base foramina or through direct destruction of middle cranial fossa floor.

CT findings consist of a plaque-like enhancing mass along with hyperostosis of the adjacent bone, particularly at the level of sphenoid wings, being due more frequently to neoplastic invasion rather than reactive sclerosis (GINSBERG 1992).

Relative to cerebral white matter, meningioma is generally hyperintense on T2 and hypointense on T1 images. In comparison with the cortex, it is isointense to hyperintense on T2, more often isointense than hypointense on T1 (SPAGNOLI et al. 1986). T2 signal is the least predictable, as 50% of lesions are described to be isointense to brain, 40% hyperintense and the remaining 10% hypointense. A certain degree of signal heterogeneity is reported, basically related to tumor vascularity, calcifications, or the presence of cystic areas. Since on unenhanced MR images meningioma may have a signal intensity similar to the brain, its detection is improved by indirect signs such as mass effect, white matter edema, dural thickening, bone hyperostosis (BRADAC et al. 1987; YEAKLEY et al. 1988; CASTILLO et al. 1989).

Relevant enhancement is invariably obtained after contrast agent administration, even when the lesion is densely calcified. The enhancement is related to the absence of blood barrier in meningioma capillaries. Frequently, thickening and enhancement of the adjacent dura may be observed (*dural tail sign*), a finding that can be due either to direct dural infiltration with accompanying dural congestion or to nonspecific inflammatory changes (TOKUMARU et al. 1990; KAWAHARA et al. 2001).

Meningioma may involve the paranasal sinuses either through skull base encroachment or as ectopic lesions. When the lesion arises from the planum sphenoidale or from the sphenoid sinus roof the bone may be sclerotic or show a characteristic *blistering* consisting of upward expansion; an associated pneumosinus dilatans has been described (Fig. 10.11) (MILLER et al. 1996). Primary intranasal meningioma has been reported to have slow growth and to exhibit high degree of enhancement (SPINDLER et al. 1989; WOLTERS and KLEINSASSER 1985).

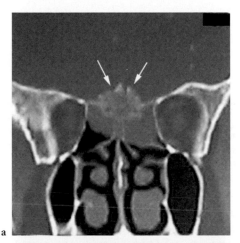

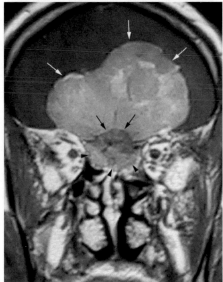

Fig. 10.11a,b. Meningioma of the planum sphenoidale in a 60 years old male who complained anosmia, visual acuity loss and mental changes. **a** Coronal CT shows a large olfactory groove meningioma with *blistering* of the bone toward the inner cranium (*white arrow* on **a**, *black arrow* on **b**) and invasion of the ethmoid. **b** On postcontrast coronal T1-weighted image, both the intracranial (*white arrows*) and extra-cranial (*black arrowheads*) components remarkably enhance. Bone blistering at the olfactory groove is hypointense than the surrounding soft component

10.3
Masticator Space Tumors Extending into the Sinonasal Tract

10.3.1
Definition, Epidemiology, Pattern of Growth

From an anatomical and surgical perspective, an ideal line drawn from the medial pterygoid plate to the glenoid fossa subdivides the extracranial surface of the middle cranial fossa into two compartments, infratemporal and petrotemporal (KUMAR et al. 1986). The infratemporal compartment is anterior-lateral located and corresponds to the roof of masticator space, whereas petrotemporal compartment is posterior-medial located and corresponds to the roof of parapharyngeal space.

The masticator space is an irregularly shaped pyramidal space including the temporal and the infratemporal fossae. Two leaflets originating from the superficial layer – which invests the mandible – of the deep cervical fascia and extending upwards to envelope masticatory muscles are considered to limit the masticator space. The roof of the masticator space is made up of the extracranial surface of sphenoid wing and a part of the temporal bone. The anterior-medial limit is the posterior wall of the maxillary sinus. The posterior-medial limit is the medial pterygoid fascia, which separates the masticator space from the prestyloid compartment of the parapharyngeal space. The superficial layer of the temporalis muscle, the zygomatic arch and the superficial layer of the masseter muscle can be considered the lateral limit of the masticator space.

Masticator space tumors have been classified by CONLEY (1964) according to their site of origin in primary, secondarily extending into the space from adjacent site, and metastases.

Primary tumors account for about 30%, lesions spreading from adjacent sites for about 70%, while metastases are exceedingly rare (JOHNSON and MARAN 1982; SHAHEEN 1982; KAPLAN and DUCKERT 1984; COHEN and ROSENHECK 1998; HSU et al. 2002).

Each anatomic structure contained within the masticator space may give origin to a tumor so that a great variety of different pathological entities have been observed in this area. Most of them are soft tissue tumors (LORIGAN et al. 1989; TORIUMI et al. 1989; ABDEL-FATTAH et al. 1990; KNOX et al. 1990; COLMENERO et al. 1991; DOHAR et al. 1991; GRUNDFAST et al. 1991; OGREN et al. 1991; PAPAGEORGE et al. 1992; RUBIN and SADOFF 1992; UMMAT and NASSER 1992; SHINOHARA et al. 1993; WOOLFORD et al. 1994;

KORNFEHL et al. 1996; SIMSIR et al. 1996; GOTO et al. 1998; KRISHNAMURTHY et al. 1998; LEE et al. 1998; HERMAN et al. 1999; LOPES et al. 1999; VAJRAMANI et al. 1999; SARAC et al. 2000; KANAZAWA et al. 2001; RANGHEARD et al. 2001; BIANCHI et al. 2002; HICKS and FLAITZ 2002); but bone, cartilaginous, epithelial, neuroendocrine, neurogenic, odontogenic, and lymphoreticular neoplasms have also been described (MENDELSOHN et al. 1983; CANTRELL et al. 1984; TASHIRO et al. 1988; AKIMURA et al. 1989; SCHREIBER et al. 1991; EAVEY et al. 1992; KOO et al. 1992; CURRIE et al. 1993; WEISSMAN et al. 1993; ZHAO et al. 1993; HOCHBERG et al. 1994; SALEH et al. 1994; SICHEL et al. 1994; GORMLEY et al. 1995; McCLUGGAGE et al. 1995; HIRABAYASHI et al. 1997; GALANT et al. 1998; KAWAI et al. 1998; JUNG et al. 1999; PIEPER and AL-MEFTY 1999; MINODA et al. 2001; VOGL et al. 2001). About 20% of primitive tumors are benign (SHAHEEN 1982). Differential diagnosis should also include non-neoplastic expansile lesions, which have been rarely observed in the masticator space (O'RYAN et al. 1987; WEISMAN and OSGUTHORPE 1988; PATEL et al. 1998; FLACKE et al. 1999; REITER et al. 2000; ACARTURK and STOFMAN 2001; UPPAL et al. 2002).

Maxillary sinus, orbit, oral cavity, pharynx and parapharyngeal space, parotid gland, middle ear and middle cranial fossa are the sites of origin of other tumors secondarily involving the masticator space (CONLEY 1964; SHAHEEN 1982), which are mostly epithelial in origin (BOUAZIZ et al. 1991).

10.3.2
Clinical Findings

During the early phase of growth, masticator space tumors are asymptomatic or they may be associated with subtle, nonspecific signs and symptoms such as headache, paresthesia or facial pain, unnoticeable paresis of masticator muscles or taste modifications (SHAPSHAY et al. 1976). Trigeminal sensory dysfunction can be determined by testing corneal sensation with blink reflex, but it is easily underestimated. Eustachian tube dysfunction due to compression can be present for a long time before the lesion is identified. Only when the neoplasm considerably increases in size, a cheek swelling can develop. Lateral deviation of the jaw upon opening may be due to paralysis or tumor invasion of the pterygoid muscles or to dysfunction of the temporomandibular joint. Similarly, trismus may be due to several causes: mechanical effect of the tumor, muscle adhesions due to scar-

ring, neoplastic ankylosis of the temporomandibular joint, or pain.

As a general rule, benign tumors tend to respect anatomic boundaries and they expand along soft-tissue planes, or preexisting pathways (i.e., foramen ovale, foramen spinosum, pterygomaxillary fissure, inferior orbital fissure) (SOM et al. 1997). Conversely, malignant tumors tend to infiltrate surrounding structures. Symptoms clearly reflect the dominant pattern of spread (SOM et al. 1997).

10.3.3
Treatment Guidelines and Prognosis

Due to the heterogeneity of tumors involving the masticator space, therapeutic planning greatly depends on the histology of the lesion. Instead of an open biopsy, which may be indicated only when there is skin involvement, fine needle aspiration cytology or needle biopsy have to be preferred.

Surgery is indicated for most masticator space tumors. Contraindications include patients with lymphoreticular tumors, which are best treated by radiation and/or chemotherapy, patients who are poor surgical candidates due to pulmonary, cardiac, renal, or other significant comorbidities, and patients with disseminated disease.

A major surgical procedure is usually required even for small tumors, in order to obtain a wide exposure, which is essential to perform an en bloc resection of the lesion and to preserve at the same time uninvolved vascular and neural structures, thus optimizing functional and aesthetic results. As a consequence of the location and complexity of the masticator space, several surgical approaches have been developed. They can be summarized as follows: anterior transfacial, lateral preauricular, lateral postauricular, and combined antero-lateral approach (FISCH 1978; CONLEY and PRICE 1979; FRIEDMAN et al. 1981; KRESPI and SISSON 1984; WETMORE et al. 1986; GATES 1988; KRESPI 1989; LAWSON et al. 1990; SMITH et al. 1990; HOWARD and LUND 1992; CATALANO and BILLER 1993; BIGELOW et al. 1999; SHAHINIAN et al. 1999). Each technique can be associated to a frontal or temporal craniotomy and to a transorbital approach (SEKHAR et al. 1987; SEIFERT and DIETZ 1992; LEONETTI et al. 1993) to have a better control of critical extensions of the tumor into the cranial fossa/e and into the orbit, respectively.

Anterior transfacial approaches are indicated for sinonasal tumors invading the masticator space, while indications for lateral preauricular approaches include tumors taking origin from the masticator space and involving the anterior aspect of the temporal bone or the greater wing of the sphenoid bone. Postauricular approaches are designed for lesions extended to the posterior aspect of the temporal bone.

The reconstructing part of the surgical procedure is meant to correct functional and cosmetic deficits and to minimize complications. A water-tight dural closure is required when resection of the dura has been performed. The surgical defect is usually filled by rotating the temporalis muscle or, less frequently, by using a free flap (SEKHAR et al. 1987; BIGELOW et al. 1999).

The most important sequelae of these procedures can be facial paralysis, face and corneal anesthesia, loss of motor and sensitive functions of the mandibular nerve with asymmetry of jaw opening; further impairment of mastication may derive from resection of the temporo-mandibular join or mandibular ramus (GUINTO et al. 1999; LEONETTI et al. 2001). Infections and wound necrosis of the reconstructive flap, neurovascular endocranial complications or CSF leak are uncommon events (SEKHAR et al. 1987; BIGELOW et al. 1999; GUINTO et al. 1999).

Only a few data regarding the prognosis of patients with tumors of the masticator space, mostly coming from single case reports or from very small series, are available in the literature (SEKHAR et al. 1987; BIGELOW et al. 1999; GUINTO et al. 1999; SHAHINIAN et al. 1999). Generally, benign tumors have an excellent prognosis with a low recurrence rate (LEONETTI et al. 2001). Conversely, prognosis of malignant tumors is poor and strongly influenced by histology and by the radicality of the resection (SEKHAR et al. 1987;

BIGELOW et al. 1999; GUINTO et al. 1999; SHAHINIAN et al. 1999). Nevertheless, even aggressive malignant neoplasms with a low chance of cure may be candidate to surgery with the intent to palliate symptoms such as pain or trismus (ROSENBLUM et al. 1990).

10.3.4
Key Information to Be Provided by Imaging

- Differentiation between primary masticator space masses/metastases and neoplasms from adjacent sites secondarily invading the space
- Identification of imaging features suggesting the nature (benign or malignant) or content (solid, cystic, adipose, vascular) of the lesion.
- Assessment of tumor extent and relationship with adjacent critical anatomical structures (pterygopalatine fossa, skull base foramina and fissures, orbit, middle cranial fossa, internal carotid artery)
- Guidance for a needle biopsy
- Identification of regional and distant metastases in aggressive malignant tumors.

10.3.5
Imaging Findings

Some important hallmarks on CT and MR studies help to indicate the masticator space as the site of origin of a lesion. The center of the mass is expected to be within masticator muscles or in the mandible,

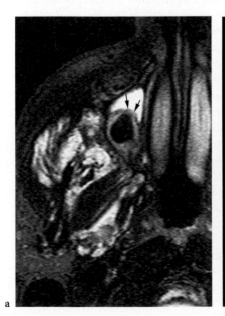
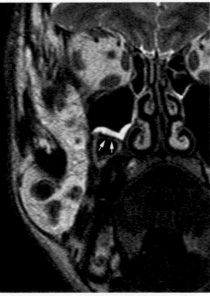

Fig. 10.12a,b. Masticator space hemangioma appears hyperintense on fat-saturated axial T2-weighted sequences, extending around masticator muscles. **a** A double posterior sinus wall with a sharp boundary (*arrows*) is apparently subdividing the maxillary sinus into an anterior hyperintense and posterior hypointense compartments. **b** The *double posterior sinusal wall* sign is related to upward displacement of the sinusal floor by a radicular cyst

a   b anterior to the prestyloid compartment of parapharyngeal space (Fig. 10.12) (ASPESTRAND and BOYSEN 1992). As a consequence, the latter is generally posteriorly displaced (CHONG and FAN 1996). Secondary invasion by lesions arising from adjacent structures is suggested by the identification of the most probable epicenter of the mass (Fig. 10.13).

As the medial pterygoid muscle fascia attaches to the skull base medial to foramen ovale, the mandibular nerve and its inferior alveolar branch run within the masticator space. This accounts for the need to thoroughly scrutinize this nerve, as it may represent the route for perineural spread into the middle cranial fossa, towards the cavernous sinus (LAINE et al. 1990). Perineural spread may also occur when the lesion extends medially into the pterygopalatine fossa, a crossroads between intra and extracranial course of multiple nerve structures.

Destruction of posterolateral maxillary sinus wall is the most common pathway of tumor invasion into the sinonasal tract.

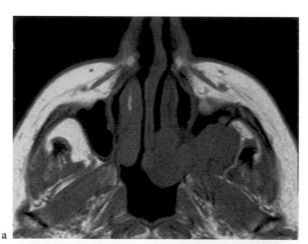

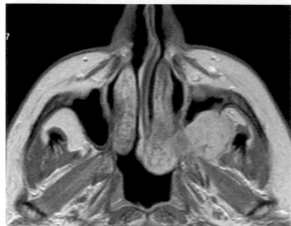

Fig.10.13a,b. Maxillary sinus squamous cell carcinoma invading the left masticator space and pterygopalatine fossa

10.4
Hard Palate Expansile Lesions

10.4.1
Definition, Epidemiology, Pattern of Growth

The palate is an anatomical region which is included into the oral cavity (hard palate) and the oropharynx (soft palate). The hard palate represents the inferior boundary of the nasal cavities and the maxillary sinuses. Malignant neoplasms of the hard palate have been included in this chapter because they can extend into the nose and paranasal sinuses. Malignant neoplasms of the hard palate are rare, accounting for about 2%–5% of oral cavity cancers, they represent about 50% of hard palate neoplasms (KROLLS and HOFFMAN 1976; POGREL 1994; INAGI et al. 2002). Most tumors have an epithelial origin with squamous cell carcinoma accounting for about half to two thirds of cases (CHUNG et al. 1980; PETRUZZELLI and MYERS 1994; TRUITT et al. 1999; YOROZU et al. 2001). Salivary gland tumors are also frequently observed, being the hard palate the most common localization of minor salivary gland neoplasms (CHUNG et al. 1980; TRAN et al. 1987; LOPES et al. 1998; TRUITT et al. 1999; HYAM et al. 2004). Among minor salivary gland tumors of the hard palate, adenoid cystic carcinoma and mucoepidermoid carcinoma are the most common histotypes (TRAN et al. 1987; LOPES et al. 1998; TRUITT et al. 1999; YOROZU et al. 2001; JANSISYANONT et al. 2002; HYAM et al. 2004). Non-epithelial or secondary neoplasms have been rarely reported in the hard palate (CHUNG et al. 1980; FLORIO and HURD 1995; HEFER et al. 1998; LAHOZ ZAMARRO et al. 2001; MORIYA et al. 2001; PRITCHYK et al. 2002; CHANG et al. 2003). The peak incidence is in the second half of the sixth decade for squamous cell carcinoma and in the first half of the same decade for salivary tumors. There is a male predominance in squamous cell carcinoma of about 2:1, whereas salivary tumors are equally distributed in males and females or there is a slight female predominance (LOPES et al. 1998; TRUITT et al. 1999; INAGI et al. 2002).

Extension beyond the hard palate is a frequent finding, in particular for squamous cell carcinoma, which is more rapidly growing than salivary tumors, which have a more subtle long-standing clinical history (KORNBLUT 1987; POGREL 1994; BECKHARDT et al. 1995). Posterior mucosal extension to the soft palate and the nasopharynx is more typical for squamous cell carcinoma, whereas posterosuperior submucosal perineural spread to the sphenopalatine foramen, then to the pterygopalatine fossa, the infratemporal fossa and through the foramen rotundum, foramen ovale, or inferior orbital fissure to the skull base is a feature of adenoid cystic carcinoma (BECKHARDT et al. 1995). Invasion of the floor of the nasal cavity or of the maxillary sinus by direct bone infiltration or through dental sockets is another frequent route of spread for squamous cell cancer (KORNBLUT 1987). Lymph node metastases are infrequent (TRUITT et al. 1999; YOROZU et al. 2001) and the first echelon of nodal drainage are the submandibular and upper deep jugular nodes (I and II levels) (ROUVIERE 1932).

10.4.2
Clinical Findings

Squamous cell carcinoma usually presents as an infiltrative ulcerated lesion, while salivary tumors are mostly submucosal with a smooth, normal mucosal swelling, sometimes with a bluish appearance (POGREL 1994; MANGANARO et al. 1997). In both cases, the patient can be asymptomatic in the early stage. Squamous cell carcinoma is typically associated with poor oral hygiene in heavy smokers and drinkers. Bleeding, foul odor, dental numbness, ill-fitting dentures, malocclusion, or loose teeth are other manifestation of neoplastic growth. Signs and symptoms of local advanced growth are velopharyngeal insufficiency and hypernasal speech, palatal hypoesthesia, middle ear effusion, hypoesthesia along the mandible or wasting of the temporalis or masseter muscles, trismus, and absence of corneal reflex.

10.4.3
Treatment Guidelines and Prognosis

Surgery is the mainstay for treatment of hard palate neoplasms. Even though radiotherapy can be considered effective for squamous cell carcinoma, the high risk of osteoradionecrosis justifies why it is rarely recommended as a primary treatment. Its use as a complementary post-operative treatment is indicated in advanced diseases.

The extent of the resection is dictated by the local spread of tumor, particularly by perineural extent, which can be suggested by imaging findings but has to be looked for and checked especially in adenoid cystic carcinoma. To this purpose, multiple frozen sections are strongly recommended. Tumors of limited extent not invading the bone may be removed

by a simple transoral excision; on the other site, major procedures with a skull base and/or a cervical access and temporary tracheotomy may be required to manage advanced tumors (FUTRAN and HALLER 1999; TRUITT et al. 1999). When a maxillectomy (inferior, subtotal or total) is required, the oroantral defect can be occluded by a prosthetic obturator, or it can be definitively closed by a temporalis flap or by more sophisticated reconstructive techniques using free flaps (see Chapter 5) (BERNHART et al. 2003). Owing to the low rate of neck metastases, a neck dissection is performed only when there is clinical evidence of lymph node involvement (SHAH and LYDIATT 1999).

Conventional postoperative radiation therapy is performed for involved or uncertain surgical margins, perineural invasion, for multiple lymph node metastases or extracapsular spread of at least one metastatic lymph node (BECKHARDT et al. 1995; TRUITT et al. 1999). A controversy still exists about the efficacy of radiotherapy for adenoid cystic carcinoma: promising results have been obtained with fast neutrons radiotherapy, which is expected to be more effective in this specific tumor than the conventional treatment (DOUGLAS et al. 1996; PROTT et al. 2000; HUBER et al. 2001).

Survival of patients with malignant tumors of the hard palate is strictly dependent on the local extent and the presence of nodal metastases (CHUNG et al. 1980; TRAN et al. 1987; TRUITT et al. 1999; YOROZU et al. 2001). Usually, 5-year survival is higher for adenoid cystic carcinoma and minor salivary gland malignancies. However, when a longer follow-up is considered, a progressive decrease of disease-specific survival for adenoid cystic carcinoma is observed: 5-year survival generally ranges from 87% to 93% and 10-year survival from 75% to 80% (TRAN et al. 1987; BECKHARDT et al. 1995; TRUITT et al. 1999). In squamous cell carcinoma, a better survival is reported when surgery is used as a primary modality treatment, with a 5-year survival up to 76% (TRUITT et al. 1999) compared to 48% for radiotherapy (YOROZU et al. 2001).

10.4.4
Key Information to Be Provided by Imaging

- Identification and assessment of bony invasion as well as of submucosal, subperiosteal and perineural spread in malignant tumors
- Identification of regional and distant metastases in aggressive malignant tumors.

10.4.5
Imaging Findings

Salivary gland carcinomas and squamous cell carcinoma which arise from the palate can spread along the greater and lesser palatine nerves to reach the skull base and eventually extend intracranially. MR imaging is superior to CT either in primary tumor detection and in the assessment of perineural extent (GINSBERG and DeMONTE 1998; CALDEMEYER et al. 1998; MAROLDI et al. 1999; TOMURA et al. 1999; BLANDINO et al. 2000). Proper selection of the imaging technique and of the MR parameters is essential for detecting both small hard or soft palate tumors and, particularly, for the identification of the subtle changes associated with perineural spread (GINSBERG 1999). Unenhanced T1 coronal images increase the detectability of even small palatal lesions because the hypointense tumor stands upon the high signal intensity of the hard palate, its fat tissue component acting as a natural contrast (Fig. 10.14). Similarly, on contrast-enhanced MR sequences fat saturation improves the identification of both the primary tumor and of the involved nerves. Thin slices are necessary in all cases. Sagittal MR planes are useful in case of soft palate carcinoma.

Particular attention has to be paid to the inferior opening of the greater and lesser palatine canals, where tumor can gain access to the palatine nerves. Axial and coronal unenhanced T1 and fat-saturated post-contrast images should be carefully scrutinized to detect the effacement of fat surrounding the opening of the canal by the hypointense tumor, or the enhancing nerve or the neoplastic tissue replacing the fat within the pterygopalatine fossa (Fig. 10.15). Sub-millimetric VIBE sequences are well suited at identifying subtle nerve abnormalities at this level.

While MR findings are based on direct signs of nerve involvement, CT has to rely on indirect findings, such as effacement of fat tissue within fissures, canals and foramina or the occurrence of bone erosion, which is usually late (CURTIN 1998). Once the palatine nerves have been involved, perineural spread can progress toward the sphenopalatine ganglion, and from this step can further extend either toward the skull base foramina or canals (*centripetal* direction), or perineural tumor can grow along the opposite direction (*centrifugal*). Detailed description of the patterns of growth, intracranial extent and imaging findings is reported in Chapter 9, section 9.2.5.1.

10.5
Odontogenic and Nonodontogenic Cysts and Tumors

10.5.1
Introduction and Definition

A wide range of cystic lesions and tumors of odontogenic origin involving the mandible and the maxilla have been described in the literature.

This chapter will not provide a detailed description of any of them, but instead an overview of the common clinical aspects together with some peculiarities of those lesions which more often involve the adjacent structures of the sinonasal tract.

According to pathogenesis, epithelial cysts of the jaws are classified in developmental and inflammatory. Developmental cysts are subdivided in odontogenic and non odontogenic (KRAMER et al. 1992). Since their epithelial lining is composed by squamous cells, the developmental odontogenic cysts are further divided by their topographic relation to specific structures, rather than by histologic features.

Fig. 10.14a–f. Adenoid cystic carcinoma with perineural spread in a 32 years old female who complained hypoesthesia of right cheek for 8 months. Unenhanced coronal T1-weighted images show a small hypointense neoplasm of the hard palate (**a**) (*double arrows*) associated with fat signal effacement at the opening of the greater palatine canal (*arrow*) and hypointense signal in the adjacent alveolar process (*arrowheads*). **b** At the level of the upper pterygopalatine fossa, a soft tissue mass (*arrowheads*) replaces the fat content, effacing the pterygopalatine artery, clearly demonstrated on the contralateral side (*black arrow*). **c** Thickening of right maxillary and vidian nerves is present (*arrows*). **d** Postcontrast images show enhancement of tumor tissue, which becomes less detectable in the hard palate (when compared to unenhanced image), stands out at the greater palatine canal opening (*arrow*) and give rise to *mild* bone marrow enhancement in the adjacent alveolar process. Enhancement of pterygopalatine neoplastic component (*arrowheads* in **e**) and both maxillary and vidian nerve (*arrows* in **f**) is clearly demonstrated. Contralateral vidian nerve (*arrowhead*). Note that the pterygopalatine mass is larger than the primitive tumor in the hard palate

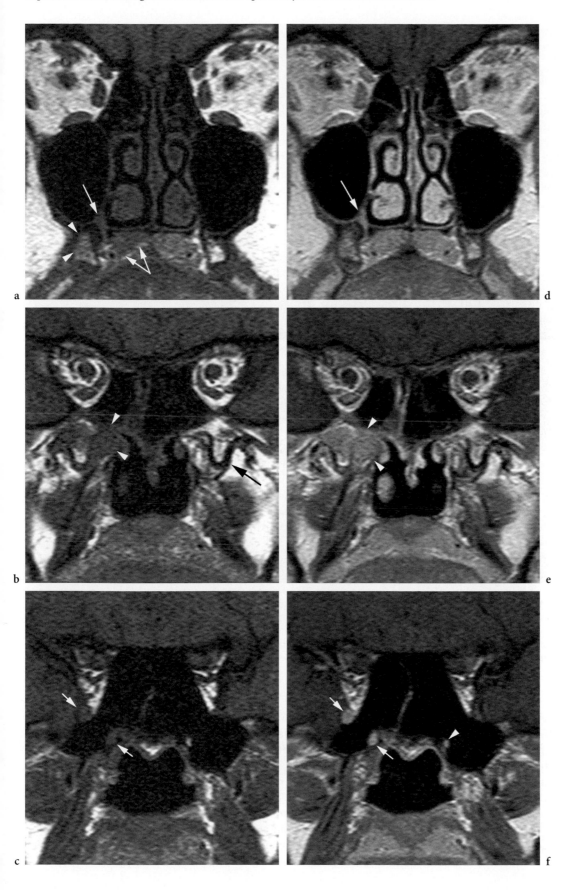

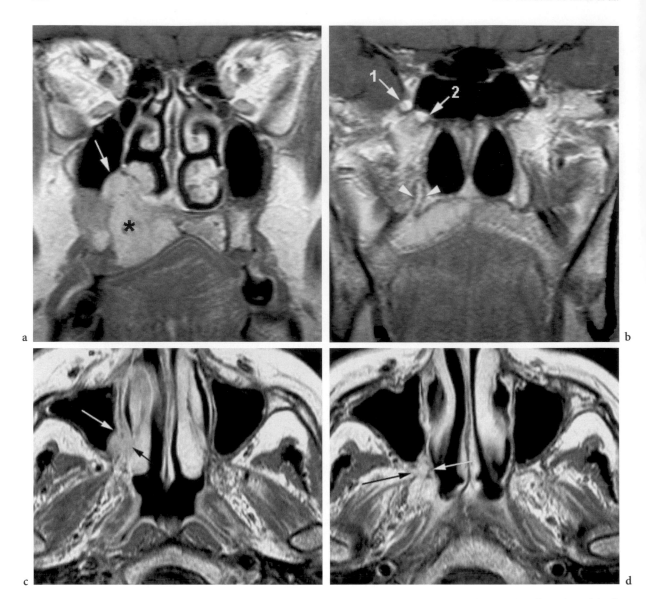

Fig. 10.15a–d. Adenoid cystic carcinoma with perineural spread Contrast enhanced T1-weighted coronal (**a–b**) and axial (**c–d**) planes. **a** The neoplasm (*asterisk*) arise from the right hard palate, abutting the alveolar recess of maxillary sinus (*arrow*). **b** Perineural spread is detected along palatine nerves (*arrowheads*) and more centrifugally along both the maxillary nerve (*1*) and vidian nerve (*2*). **c** Submucosal tumor growth is shown along both surfaces of medial antral wall (*arrows*) reaching posteriorly the pterygopalatine fossa. **d** Solid and enhancing tissue fills the widened pterygopalatine fossa (*arrows*)

Odontogenic tumors are very rare lesions arising from the tissues of developing teeth. They are believed to result from an interruption of odontogenesis or from the reactivation of special tissues participating into odontogenesis. Many histologic variants with different presentation and behavior have been recognized. Their classification is based on histogenetic, organogenetic, and embryologic aspects of tooth development.

10.5.2
Epidemiology, Clinical Findings and Treatment Guidelines

The most frequent jaw cyst is the apical radicular cyst, followed by dentigerous cyst and odontogenic keratocyst (MOSQUEDA-TAYLOR et al. 1997).

Radicular cyst results from pulp necrosis due to inflammation. The Malassez epithelial rests in the periodontal ligament are stimulated to produce a periapical granuloma, which subsequently evolves in a cyst (apical radicular cyst). Rarely, are these cysts found laterally to the root (lateral radicular cyst). Radicular cysts are most frequently seen between 10 and 40 years, with a 60% male preponderance. Most of them develop in the anterior maxillary region (37%–82% are found in the maxilla) (McDANIEL 1999). They are often asymptomatic, while pain and swelling are present if the cyst becomes inflamed. Radicular cysts are lined by stratified nonkeratinizing squamous epithelium, with a dense infiltrate of chronic inflammatory cells. Most lesions are treated by endodontic therapy of the involved tooth. Surgical removal can be added in cases of failure.

Dentigerous (follicular) cyst is the most common developmental odontogenic cyst (MOSQUEDA-TAYLOR et al. 1997). Its location surrounding the crown of an impacted or partially unerupted tooth is quite typical. The cyst is commonly observed in the second, third and fourth decades with a male predominance. The most frequent sites are the region of impacted teeth (mandibular and maxillary third molars, maxillary canines, and mandibular premolars, in decreasing order of frequency). Most of them are small and asymptomatic although they can grow to reach even remarkable size. Owing to their origin from the follicular epithelium, which has a great potential for degeneration, dentigerous cysts are sometimes associated with benign or malignant neoplasms. In view of this peculiarity, removal of impacted teeth with a large pericoronal radiolucency is recommended.

Odontogenic keratocyst is an aggressive lesion characterized by the production of keratin, without a specific topographic location. It is the second most common developmental odontogenic cyst (MOSQUEDA-TAYLOR et al. 1997; REGEZI 2002). Multiple odontogenic keratocysts can be part of the basal cell nevus syndrome, also known as Gorlin syndrome (5% of cases of parakeratinized type) (ODA et al. 2000; REGEZI 2002). There is an age predominance from the second to the fourth decade, and males are most frequently affected than women (McDANIEL 1999). The posterior region of the mandible is the preferred site of origin, followed by the posterior region of the maxilla (McDANIEL 1999). Swelling and drainage are the most frequent findings (50% of patients are symptomatic) followed by pain, paresthesia and trismus (BRANNON 1976). Cysts producing orthokeratin have a lower tendency to recur compared to those producing parakeratin (2.2% versus 42.6%) (CROWLEY et al. 1992). Surgical excision with free margins is the treatment of choice (BATAINEH and AL QUDAH 1998; ZHAO et al. 2002).

Nasopalatine duct cyst (incisive canal cyst) taking origin from embryonic epithelial remnants of the nasopalatine duct or incisive canal, is the most frequent developmental non-odontogenic cyst (DALEY et al. 1994). It is generally observed in the middle age (fourth to sixth decade) with a slight predilection for males (VASCONCELOS et al. 1999a). Palatal swelling is the most common complaint, rarely associated with root resorption of incisor teeth; most cases are asymptomatic (VASCONCELOS et al. 1999a). The cyst is lined by stratified squamous epithelium and/or respiratory epithelium. Differential diagnosis includes odontogenic keratocyst and periapical cyst, when located in the midline (NEVILLE et al. 1997). Enucleation is generally sufficient to avoid recurrences, which are reported in less than 10% of cases (SPINELLI et al. 1994).

Nasolabial (nasoalveolar) cyst is a developmental non-odontogenic cyst originating from the epithelial remnants of the nasolacrimal duct and developing in soft tissues (VASCONCELOS et al. 1999b). Most cases are observed in the middle-aged females (VASCONCELOS et al. 1999b). The most common clinical finding is an asymptomatic soft tissue swelling involving the canine fossa/nasal alar base region. Microscopically, this cystic structure is composed of a fibrous capsule with an unremarkable layer of pseudostratified columnar epithelium (VASCONCELOS et al. 1999b). The treatment of choice is surgical excision by sublabial approach rarely followed by recurrence (VASCONCELOS et al. 1999b; CHOI et al. 2002). Also transnasal endoscopic marsupialization has been described (SU et al. 1999).

Benign odontogenic tumors are rare. The most frequent is *odontoma*, which accounts for about 50% of all odontogenic tumors. It is considered quite similar to a malformative lesion, since all dental tissues can be observed within it. Odontomas are subdivided in compound and complex in relation to the distribution of dental tissues (more or less ordered). The second most common benign odontogenic tumor is *ameloblastoma*, which is the most aggressive. Adenomatoid odontogenic tumor, which preferably arises in the maxilla, is the third most frequent lesion.

Most benign odontogenic tumors are observed in the middle age, and there is a various distribution among males and females. Compound odontoma is more frequently observed in the anterior part of the maxilla. A painless swelling is the only complaint in almost all type of tumors with the exception of odontoma and cementoblastoma. If tumors reach a relevant size, pain, loss of teeth, malocclusion, ulceration, rhinorrhea and nasal obstruction (in upper jaw locations), can be observed.

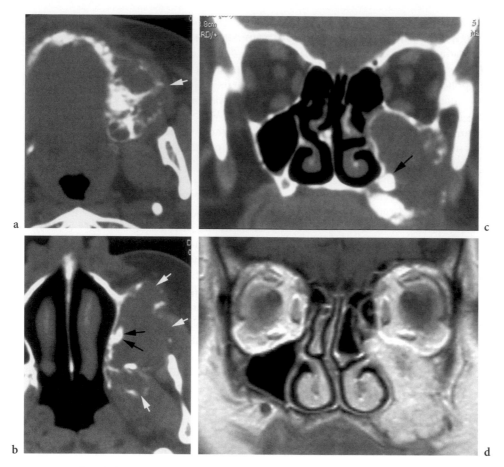

Fig. 10.16a-d. Calcifying odontogenic cyst (Pindborg tumor). **a** Axial CT scans show the irregular destruction of the alveolar process with spread into the buccal fat pad (*arrow*). **b** The lesion extends into the masticator space (*arrows*), irregular intratumoral densities are shown (*black arrows* in **b** and **c**). Mottled enhancing appearance of the lesion on post-contrast T1 coronal plane (**d**).

Enucleation or limited surgical excision is a proper treatment for most benign odontogenic tumors. On the other site, ameloblastoma, ameloblastic fibroma, odontoameloblastoma, calcifying epithelial odontogenic tumor (FIG. 10.16) and myxoma require wide free margins to avoid recurrences.

Malignant odontogenic tumors are divided in carcinomas and sarcomas (KRAMER et al. 1992). The most frequent odontogenic malignant neoplasm is the *primary intraosseous carcinoma* (MCDANIEL 1999). The diagnosis requires that metastatic disease had been excluded (EVERSOLE 1999). It is observed in elderly patients, with a predilection for the mandibular body (SUEI et al. 1994). Pain and paresthesia can derive from compression of the alveolar nerve. Regional and distant metastases are frequent and a 30% to 40% 5-year survival is reported (To et al. 1991).

Malignant ameloblastic tumors include *malignant ameloblastoma*, which shows the same histologic fea-

tures of benign ameloblastoma, but it is usually associated with late distant metastases to the lung (less frequently to the brain, viscera, skin, and bone), and ameloblastic carcinoma, in which clear histologic signs of malignancy are evident (EVERSOLE 1999). The latter has no gender predilection, is more common in the mandible, and generally displays a local aggressiveness rather than a tendency to metastasize (EVERSOLE 1999).

Odontogenic sarcoma is the malignant counterpart of the ameloblastic fibroma (ameloblastic fibrosarcoma), being characterized by benign epithelium with a malignant fibrous stroma. When it exhibits dysplastic dentin, it is called ameloblastic fibrodentinosarcoma, and when focal deposits of dysplastic enamel proteins are present, it is called ameloblastic fibro-odontosarcoma (BREGNI et al. 2001). Finally, when a jaw tumor with an ameloblastic fibroma-like pattern displays both a carcinomatous and a malignant spindle cell component it is defined as odontogenic carcinosarcoma (SLATER 1999; SLAMA et al. 2002).

10.5.3
Key Information to be Provided by Imaging

- Differentiation between cystic and solid lesions
- Presence of imaging features highly suggestive for a specific lesion
- Relationship with adjacent anatomical structures (hard palate, masticator space structures, pterygopalatine fossa)
- Assessment of distant metastases for malignant tumors

10.5.4
Imaging Findings

Maxillary sinus and hard palate can be encroached by a variety of lesions of odontogenic origin; the most commonly observed are radicular cyst, dentigerous cyst, odontogenic keratocyst, ameloblastoma, and non-odontogenic (developmental cysts), such as nasopalatine and nasolabial cyst .

All the odontogenic lesions share some common imaging features, such as radiolucency on plain films and hypodensity on CT. Ameloblastoma and, less frequently, odontogenic keratocyst may have a multilocular appearance being crossed by coarse and curved

internal septa. Dystrophic calcifications may be detected, especially in radicular cysts. At their periphery, all these lesions are usually bordered by a thin corticated rim. Nonetheless, this outer boundary may be effaced or may appear sclerotic (particularly after secondary infections in cystic lesions), thus making identification of the site of origin of the lesion – inside or outside the maxillary sinus – extremely difficult. On coronal native or reconstructed MPR coronal images, the identification of such a thin bony plate between the lesion and maxillary sinus cavity is the hallmark to distinguishing extra-antral odontogenic lesions from antral lesions (HAN et al. 1995).

Evaluation of the site of origin of the lesion and assessment of its relationship with adjacent teeth is useful in distinguishing among some of the more frequent odontogenic lesions involving the adjacent sinonasal tract structures.

Radicular cyst arises from epithelial cells rests after inflammatory stimulation. It is located close to the apex of a non-vital tooth. In the maxilla, it is more frequently located around incisors and canines roots. CT findings and signal intensities on MR are nonspecific, they mainly consist of a unilocular, purely cystic pattern, with homogeneous fluid (Fig. 10.17) (MINAMI et al. 1996).

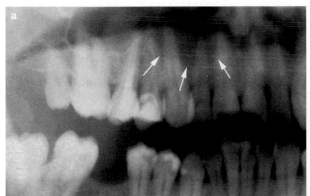

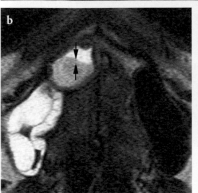
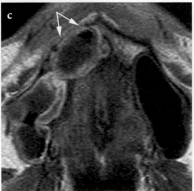
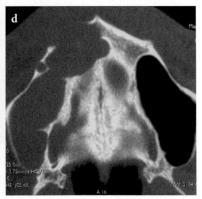

Fig. 10.17a-d. Large radicular cyst. **a** The orthopanoramic film shows a periapical radiolucency with thin and regular lobulated rim occupying the right maxilla (*arrows*). **b** Fluid-fluid (*black arrow*) level is demonstrated in the axial T2 weighted image. Displacement and thinning of the cortical rim of the maxillary bone is shown either by the post-contrast T1 (*double arrow* in **c**) and by the bone-window axial CT (**d**).

Otherwise than radicular cyst, *dentigerous cyst* develops around – eventually "containing" – the crown of an unerupted tooth, which is more frequently a canine in the maxilla, or supernumerary tooth (Som et al. 1992). It has to be distinguished from a normal dental follicle. If more than 20 mm in size, a dental follicle is probably developing a dentigerous cyst. When the dentigerous cyst grows upwards, the maxillary sinus floor is remodeled; its bone content can be reabsorbed. Typically, the floor is posteriorly and superiorly displaced, accounting for a *double posterior sinus wall* on axial CT images, where the posterior one is the true sinusal wall and the anterior one is actually the displaced floor. Sagittal or coronal sections improve this distinction. The displaced tooth is clearly demonstrated within the cyst (Okita et al. 1991). Except for the tooth, which appears hypointense, or totally signal void, on MR sequences, the cyst has a homogeneous signal content, hyperintense on T2 and hypo to intermediate on T1 (Hisatomi et al. 2003).

Odontogenic keratocyst is far most common in the posterior body or ramus of the mandible than in the maxilla. This lesion, which arises from dental lamina, may have a pericoronal position, thus being difficult to distinguish from dentigerous cyst on radiographic films. On CT a unilocular or multilocular cystic lesion is seen, invading the adjacent "scalloped" bone and presenting thin, reactive and smooth bony walls (Fig. 10.18). MR images of odontogenic keratocyst show a unilocular or multilocular lesion, the

appearance of cyst walls can greatly vary: they can be absent or thin or even thick. The cystic contents usually is heterogeneous, the signal can be predominantly intermediate to low on T2, and intermediate to high on T1 (Hisatomi et al. 2003; Minami et al. 1996). Contrast enhanced MR is superior to CT in detecting features that enable to distinguish the odontogenic keratocyst from other cysts, such as focal rim enhancement and iso-intense intraluminal soft-tissue components which correlate with the histological findings of focal inflammatory ulceration of the cyst lining, orthokeratosis and cell debris (Janse van Rensburg et al. 1997). MR findings are particularly useful in the diagnosis of nevoid basal cell carcinoma syndrome, characterized by multiple odontogenic keratocysts, by the early development of multiple basal cell carcinomas and skeletal development abnormalities (Palacios et al. 2004).

Nasopalatine and nasolabial are the most frequent non-odontogenic developmental cysts of the maxilla (Holtmann et al. 1985). The nasopalatine cyst develops from the nasopalatine-incisive canal area to present as a well-defined radiolucency above or between the root apices of the central incisors, exceeding 0.6 mm in size (Verbin and Barnes 2001). On CT the cyst has a midline location, shows smooth expansion with sclerotic margins and displacement of teeth apices. Radicular cysts differ in that the teeth apices are within the cyst rather than being displaced (Pevsner et al. 2000). On MR, its keratin and viscous fluid contents account for high signal intensity on T1 (Hisatomi et al. 2001).

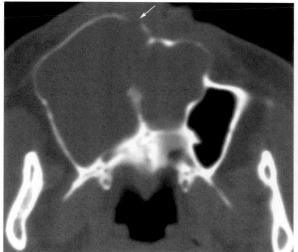 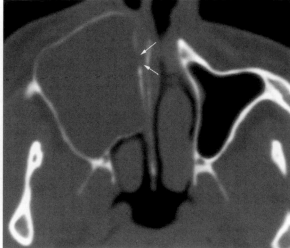

a   b

Fig. 10.18a,b. a A large odontogenic keratocyst arises from right maxilla and grows towards the contralateral side. b The cyst fills the right maxillary sinus. Extensive remodeling and thinning of bone is observed. Focal bony dehiscences are demonstrated (*arrows* in a and b)

Nasolabial cyst, thought to origin fro the nasolacrimal duct apparatus, is generally located in the nasal vestibule or ala or in the upper lip (SOM and NORTON 1991). It is an extra-osseous soft tissue mass that may remodel the adjacent bone (CURE et al. 1996).

Ameloblastoma is a locally invasive but almost invariably slow growing benign tumor arising from remnants of odontogenic epithelium (dental lamina, dental organ). In the maxilla, ameloblastoma more frequently develops in the third molar region, it behaves more aggressively than in its mandibular counterpart (JACKSON et al. 1996). Radiographically, the most typical finding includes a multiloculated lytic lesion, in which the number and arrangement of internal "septa" may give the lesion a honeycomb-like appearance. On CT, maxillary ameloblastoma appears as a multilocular solid and cystic lesion, non-enhancing, with well-defined thin cystic borders (HERTZANU et al. 1984) MR findings encompass: mixed solid and cystic pattern, irregularly thick walls, papillary projections, and strong enhancement of solid components including papillary projections, walls, and septa (MINAMI et al. 1996). Unilocular lesions are more frequent in the mandible (PHILIPSEN and REICHART 1998).

References

Abdel-Fattah HM, Adams GL, Wick MR. Hemangiopericytoma of the maxillary sinus and skull base. Head Neck 1990;12:77-83.

Acarturk TO, Stofman GM (2001) Posttraumatic epidermal inclusion cyst of the deep infratemporal fossa. Ann Plast Surg 46:68-71

Akimura T, Kameda H, Abiko S et al (1989) Infrasellar craniopharyngioma. Neuroradiology 31:180-183

Arana E, Diaz C, Latorre FF et al (1996) Primary intraosseous meningiomas. Acta Radiol 37:937-942

Arslantas A, Artan S, Oner U et al (2003) Detection of chromosomal imbalances in spinal meningiomas by comparative genomic hybridization. Neurol Med Chir (Tokyo) 43:12-18; discussion 19

Aspestrand F, Boysen M (1992) CT and MR imaging of primary tumors of the masticator space. Acta Radiol 33:518-522

Bataineh AB, al Qudah M (1998) Treatment of mandibular odontogenic keratocysts. Oral Surg Oral Med Oral Pathol Oral Radiol Endod 86:42-47

Batsakis JG (1979) Tumors of the head and neck : clinical and pathological considerations. 2d edition Baltimore: Williams & Wilkins

Beckhardt RN, Weber RS, Zane R et al (1995) Minor salivary gland tumors of the palate: clinical and pathologic correlates of outcome. Laryngoscope 105:1155-1160

Bernhart BJ, Huryn JM, Disa J et al (2003) Hard palate resection, microvascular reconstruction, and prosthetic restoration: a 14-year retrospective analysis. Head Neck 25:671-680

Bernstein ML, Buchino JJ (1983) The histologic similarity between craniopharyngioma and odontogenic lesions: a reappraisal. Oral Surg Oral Med Oral Pathol 56:502-511

Bianchi B, Poli T, Bertolini F et al (2002) Malignant hemangiopericytoma of the infratemporal fossa: report of a case. J Oral Maxillofac Surg 60:309-312

Bigelow DC, Smith PG, Leonetti JP et al (1999) Treatment of malignant neoplasms of the lateral cranial base with the combined frontotemporal-anterolateral approach: five-year follow-up. Otolaryngol Head Neck Surg 120:17-24

Binkhorst CD, Schierbeek P, Petten GJW (1957) Neoplasms of the notochord. Acta Otolaryngol 47:10-20

Black PM, Carroll R, Glowacka D et al (1994) Platelet-derived growth factor expression and stimulation in human meningiomas. J Neurosurg 81:388-393

Blandino A, Gaeta M, Minutoli F et al (2000) CT and MR findings in neoplastic perineural spread along the vidian nerve. Eur Radiol 10:521-526

Bondy M, Ligon BL (1996) Epidemiology and etiology of intracranial meningiomas: a review. J Neurooncol 29:197-205

Bottles K, Beckstead JH (1984) Enzyme histochemical characterization of chordomas. Am J Surg Pathol 8:443-447

Bouaziz A, Chabardes E, Laccourreye O et al (1991) Extension to the infratemporal fossa of malignant tumors of the face. Ann Otolaryngol Chir Cervicofac 108:113-118

Bourgouin PM, Tampieri D, Robitaille Y et al (1992) Low-grade myxoid chondrosarcoma of the base of the skull: CT, MR, and histopathology. J Comput Assist Tomogr 16:268-273

Bouropoulou V, Bosse A, Roessner A et al (1989) Immunoistochemical investigation of chordomas: Histogenetic and differential diagnostic aspects. Current Topics in Pathology 80:183-203

Bradac GB, Riva A, Schorner W et al (1987) Cavernous sinus meningiomas: an MRI study. Neuroradiology 29:578-581

Brannon RB (1976) The odontogenic keratocyst. A clinicopathologic study of 312 cases. Part I. Clinical features. Oral Surg Oral Med Oral Pathol 42:54-72

Bregni RC, Taylor AM, Garcia AM (2001) Ameloblastic fibrosarcoma of the mandible: report of two cases and review of the literature. J Oral Pathol Med 30:316-320

Bret P, Beziat JL (1993) Craniopharyngiome sphenoido-nasopharynge. Un cas avec exerese radicale par maxillotomie de Le Fort I. Neurochirurgie 39:235-240

Brown E, Hug EB, Weber AL (1994) Chondrosarcoma of the skull base. Neuroimaging Clin N Am 4:529-541

Bulow B, Attewell R, Hagmar L et al (1998) Postoperative prognosis in craniopharyngioma with respect to cardiovascular mortality, survival, and tumor recurrence. J Clin Endocrinol Metab 83:3897-3904

Caldemeyer KS, Mathews VP, Righi PD et al (1998) Imaging features and clinical significance of perineural spread or extension of head and neck tumors. Radiographics 18:97-110; quiz 147

Cantrell RW, Kaplan MJ, Atuk NO et al (1984) Catecholamine-secreting infratemporal fossa paraganglioma. Ann Otol Rhinol Laryngol 93:583-588

Cappabianca P, Cavallo LM, Colao A et al (2002) Endoscopic endonasal transsphenoidal approach: outcome analysis of 100 consecutive procedures. Minim Invasive Neurosurg 45 193-200

Carmel PW (1990) Brain tumors of disordered embryogenesis.

In: Youmans JR (ed) Neurological surgery : a comprehensive reference guide to the diagnosis and management of neurosurgical problems. Saunders, Philadelphia, pp 3223-3249

Castillo M, Davis PC, Ross WK et al (1989) Meningioma of the chiasm and optic nerves: CT and MR findings. J Comput Assist Tomogr 13:679-681

Catalano PJ, Biller HF (1993) Extended osteoplastic maxillotomy. A versatile new procedure for wide access to the central skull base and infratemporal fossa. Arch Otolaryngol Head Neck Surg 119:394-400

Chakrabarty A, Mitchell P, Bridges LR (1998) Craniopharyngioma invading the nasal and paranasal spaces, and presenting as nasal obstruction. Br J Neurosurg 12:361-363

Chang CC, Rowe JJ, Hawkins P et al (2003) Mantle cell lymphoma of the hard palate: a case report and review of the differential diagnosis based on the histomorphology and immunophenotyping pattern. Oral Surg Oral Med Oral Pathol Oral Radiol Endod 96:316-320

Cheddadi D, Triki S, Gallet S et al (1996) Obstruction rhinopharyngee neonatale par craniopharyngiome. Arch Pediatr 3:348-351

Chen HJ (2002) The neurological abnormalities and operative findings in the transcallosal approach for large juxtasellar-ventricular craniopharyngiomas. J Clin Neurosci 9:159-163

Cho DY, Liau WR (2002) Comparison of endonasal endoscopic surgery and sublabial microsurgery for prolactinomas. Surg Neurol 58:371-6

Choi JH, Cho JH, Kang HJ et al (2002) Nasolabial cyst: a retrospective analysis of 18 cases. Ear Nose Throat J 81:94-96

Chong VF, Fan YF (1996) Pictorial review: radiology of the masticator space. Clin Radiol 51:457-465

Choux M, Lena G, Genitori L. Le craniopharyngiome de l'enfant. Neurochirurgie (Paris) 1991;37(suppl1):12-165.

Chung CK, Johns ME, Cantrell RW et al (1980) Radiotherapy in the management of primary malignancies of the hard palate. Laryngoscope 90:576-584

Cianfriglia F, Pompili A, Occhipinti E (1978) Intracranial malignant cartilaginous tumours. Report of two cases and review of literature. Acta Neurochir (Wien) 45:163-175

Ciric I, Mikhael M, Stafford T et al (1983) Transsphenoidal microsurgery of pituitary macroadenomas with long-term follow-up results. J Neurosurg 59:395-401

Cohen HV, Rosenheck AH (1998) Metastatic cancer presenting as TMD. A case report. J N J Dent Assoc 69:17-19

Colli B, Al-Mefty O (2001) Chordomas of the craniocervical junction: follow-up review and prognostic factors. J Neurosurg 95:933-943

Colmenero C, Rivers T, Patron M et al (1991) Maxillofacial malignant peripheral nerve sheath tumours. J Craniomaxillofac Surg 19:40-46

Conley J, Price JC (1979) Sublabial approach to the nasal and nasopharyngeal cavities. Am J Surg 138:615-618

Conley JJ (1964) Tumors of the Infratemporal Fossa. Arch Otolaryngol 79:498-504

Corbetta S, Pizzocaro A, Peracchi M et al (1997) Multiple endocrine neoplasia type 1 in patients with recognized pituitary tumours of different types. Clin Endocrinol (Oxf) 47:507-512

Cordera S, Bottacchi E, D'Alessandro G et al (2002) Epidemiology of primary intracranial tumours in NW Italy, a population based study: stable incidence in the last two decades. J Neurol 249:281-284

Cottier JP, Destrieux C, Brunereau L et al (2000) Cavernous sinus invasion by pituitary adenoma: MR imaging. Radiology 215:463-469

Crockard HA, Steel T, Plowman N et al (2001) A multidisciplinary team approach to skull base chordomas. J Neurosurg 95:175-183

Crotty TB, Scheithauer BW, Young WF, Jr. et al (1995) Papillary craniopharyngioma: a clinicopathological study of 48 cases. J Neurosurg 83:206-214

Crowley TE, Kaugars GE, Gunsolley JC (1992) Odontogenic keratocysts: a clinical and histologic comparison of the parakeratin and orthokeratin variants. J Oral Maxillofac Surg 50:22-26.

Cure JK, Osguthorpe JD, Van Tassel P (1996) MR of nasolabial cysts. AJNR Am J Neuroradiol 17:585-588

Currie WJ, Thompson WD, Stassen LF (1993) Adenocarcinoma: the use of computed tomography and magnetic resonance imaging for investigation of a tumour in the infratemporal fossa. Dentomaxillofac Radiol 22:155-158

Curtin HD (1998) Detection of perineural spread: fat is a friend. AJNR Am J Neuroradiol 19:1385-1386

Cushing H (1932) The craniopharyngiomas. In: Cushing H (ed) Intracranial tumours; notes upon a series of two thousand verified cases with surgical-mortality percentages pertaining thereto. C. C. Thomas, Springfield, 93-98

D'Alessandro G, Di Giovanni M, Iannizzi L et al (1995) Epidemiology of primary intracranial tumors in the Valle d'Aosta (Italy) during the 6-year period 1986-1991. Neuroepidemiology 14:139-146

Daley TD, Wysocki GP, Pringle GA (1994) Relative incidence of odontogenic tumors and oral and jaw cysts in a Canadian population. Oral Surg Oral Med Oral Pathol 77:276-280

Dalprà L, Malgara R, Miozzo M et al (1999) First cytogenetic study of a recurrent familial chordoma of the clivus. Int J Cancer 81:24-30

Davis PC, Hoffman JC, Jr., Spencer T et al (1987) MR imaging of pituitary adenoma: CT, clinical, and surgical correlation. AJR Am J Roentgenol 148:797-802

DeMonte F, Ginsberg LE, Clayman GL (2000) Primary malignant tumors of the sphenoidal sinus. Neurosurgery 46:1084-1091

Derome PJ (1991) Bony reaction and invasion in meningiomas. In: Al-Mefty O (ed) Meningiomas. Raven Press, New York, pp 169-174

Detta A, Kenny BG, Smith C et al (1993) Correlation of proto-oncogene expression and proliferation and meningiomas. Neurosurgery 33:1065-1074

Devi B, Bhat D, Madhusudhan H et al (2001) Primary intraosseous meningioma of orbit and anterior cranial fossa: a case report and literature review. Australas Radiol 45:211-214

Dohar JE, Marentette LJ, Adams GL (1991) Rhabdomyosarcoma of the infratemporal fossa: diagnostic dilemmas and surgical management. Am J Otolaryngol 12:146-149

Donnet A, Schmitt A, Dufour H et al (1999) Neuropsychological follow-up of twenty two adult patients after surgery for craniopharyngioma. Acta Neurochir (Wien) 141:1049-1054

Dorfman HD, Czerniak B (1998) Bone tumors. Mosby , St. Louis:

Douglas JG, Laramore GE, Austin-Seymour M et al (1996) Neutron radiotherapy for adenoid cystic carcinoma of minor salivary glands. Int J Radiat Oncol Biol Phys 36:87-93

Duff JM, Meyer FB, Ilstrup DM. (2000) Long-term outcomes for surgically resected craniopharyngiomas. Neurosurgery; 46:291-305.

Eavey RD, Janfaza P, Chapman PH et al (1992) Skull base dumbbell tumor: surgical experience with two adolescents. Ann Otol Rhinol Laryngol 101:939-945

Einhaus SL, Sanford RA (2000) Craniopharyngiomas. In: Robertson JT, Coakham HB, Robertson JH (eds) Cranial base surgery. Churchill Livingstone, London, pp 417-429

Erdheim J (1904) Uber Hypophysenganggeschwülste und Hirncholesteatome. Sitzungsbericht der Kaiserlichen Akademie der Wissenshaften. Mathematisch-naturwissenschaftliche Classe (Wien) 113:537-726

Eversole LR (1999) Malignant epithelial odontogenic tumors. Semin Diagn Pathol 16:317-324

Fahlbusch R, Honegger J, Paulus W et al (1999) Surgical treatment of craniopharyngiomas: experience with 168 patients. J Neurosurg 90:237-250

Fajfr R, Muller B, Diem P (2002) Hypophysares Inzidentalom bei Patientin mit autosomal dominanter polyzystischer Nierenerkrankung. Schweiz Rundsch Med Prax 91:1123-1126

Falavigna A, Kraemer JL (2001) Infrasellar craniopharyngioma: case report. Arq Neuropsiquiatr 59:424-430

Farr HW, Gray GF, Jr., Vrana M et al (1973) Extracranial meningioma. J Surg Oncol 5:411-420

Figarella-Branger D, Vagner-Capodano AM, Bouillot P et al (1994) Platelet-derived growth factor (PDGF) and receptor (PDGFR) expression in human meningiomas: correlations with clinicopathological features and cytogenetic analysis. Neuropathol Appl Neurobiol 20:439-447

Fisch U (1978) Infratemporal fossa approach to tumours of the temporal bone and base of the skull. J Laryngol Otol 92:949-967

Fitzgerald SG, Morgenstern E (2000) Global improvement in intellectual and neuropsychological functioning after removal of a suprasellar cystic craniopharyngioma. Mil Med 165:496-499

Flacke S, Pauleit D, Keller E et al (1999) Infantile fibromatosis of the neck with intracranial involvement: MR and CT findings. AJNR Am J Neuroradiol 20:923-925

Florio SJ, Hurd TC (1995) Gastric carcinoma metastatic to the mucosa of the hard palate. J Oral Maxillofac Surg 53:1097-1098

Forsith PA, Cascino TL, Shaw EG et al (1993) Intracranial chordomas: a clinicopathological and prognostic study of 51 cases. J Neurosurg 78:741-747

Friedman WH, Katsantonis GP, Cooper MH et al (1981) Stylohamular dissection: a new method for en bloc reaction of malignancies of the infratemporal fossa. Laryngoscope 91:1869-1879

Fujimoto Y, Matsushita H, Velasco O et al (2002) Craniopharyngioma involving the infrasellar region: a case report and review of the literature. Pediatr Neurosurg 37:210-216

Futran ND, Haller JR (1999) Considerations for free-flap reconstruction of the hard palate. Arch Otolaryngol Head Neck Surg 125:665-669

Galant C, Rombaux P, Hamoir M et al (1998) Meningioma of the infratemporal fossa: report of a case. Acta Clin Belg 53:282-284

Gates GA (1988) The lateral facial approach to the nasopharynx and infratemporal fossa. Otolaryngol Head Neck Surg 99:321-325

Gates GA. The lateral facial approach to the nasopharynx and infratemporal fossa. Otolaryngol Head Neck Surg 1988;99:321-5.

Gay E, Sekhar LN, Rubinstein E et al (1995) Chordomas and chondrosarcomas of the cranial base: results and follow-up of 60 patients. Neurosurgery 36:887-897

Giangaspero F, Burger PC, Osborne DR et al (1984) Suprasellar papillary squamous epithelioma („papillary craniopharyngioma"). Am J Surg Pathol 8:57-64

Ginsberg LE (1992) Neoplastic diseases affecting the central skull base: CT and MR imaging. AJR Am J Roentgenol 159:581-589

Ginsberg LE (1999) Imaging of perineural tumor spread in head and neck cancer. Semin Ultrasound CT MR 20:175-186

Ginsberg LE, DeMonte F (1998) Imaging of perineural tumor spread from palatal carcinoma. AJNR Am J Neuroradiol 19:1417-1422

Gormley WB, Beckman ME, Ho KL et al (1995) Primary craniofacial chordoma: case report. Neurosurgery 36:1196-1199

Goto TK, Yoshiura K, Tanaka T et al (1998) A follow-up of rhabdomyosarcoma of the infratemporal fossa region in adults based on the magnetic resonance imaging findings: case reports. Oral Surg Oral Med Oral Pathol Oral Radiol Endod 86:616-625

Greenberg MS (2001) Handbook of Neurosurgery. 5th Edition, Thieme, New York:.

Grundfast K, Healy G, Richardson M (1991) Fibrosarcoma of the infratemporal fossa in an 8-year-old girl. Head Neck 13:156-159

Guinto G, Abello J, Molina A et al (1999) Zygomatic-transmandibular approach for giant tumors of the infratemporal fossa and parapharyngeal space. Neurosurgery 45:1385-1398

Gupta K, Kuhn MJ, Shevlin DW et al (1999) Metastatic craniopharyngioma. AJNR Am J Neuroradiol 20:1059-1060

Han MH, Chang KH, Lee CH et al (1995) Cystic expansile masses of the maxilla: differential diagnosis with CT and MR. AJNR Am J Neuroradiol 16:333-338

Hardy J (1969) Transsphenoidal microsurgery of the normal and pathological pituitary. Clinical Neurosurgery 16:185-217

Harrison DFN, Lund VJ (1993) Tumours of the upper jaw Edinburgh; New York: Churchill Livingstone

Hassounah M, Al-Mefty O, Athar M et al (1985) Primary cranial and intracranial chondrosarcoma, a survey. Acta Neurochir 78:123-132

Hatfield DL, White M, Araoz C (2001) Nasal meningioma: report of one case and review. J Ark Med Soc 97:416-417

Hefer T, Manor R, Zvi Joachims H et al (1998) Metastatic follicular thyroid carcinoma to the maxilla. J Laryngol Otol 112:69-72

Helseth A (1997) Incidence and survival of intracranial meningioma patients in Norway 1963-1992. Neuroepidemiology 16:53-59

Herman P, Lot G, Chapot R et al (1999) Long-term follow-up of juvenile nasopharyngeal angiofibromas: analysis of recurrences. Laryngoscope 109:140-147

Hertzanu Y, Mendelsohn DB, Cohen M (1984) Computed tomography of mandibular ameloblastoma. J Comput Assist Tomogr 8:220-223

Hicks J, Flaitz C (2002) Rhabdomyosarcoma of the head and neck in children. Oral Oncol 38:450-459

Higinbotham NL, Phillips RF, Farr HW et al (1967) Chordoma: thirty-five year study at the Memorial Hospital. Cancer 20:1841-1850

Hillman TH, Peyster RG, Hoover ED et al (1988) Infrasellar craniopharyngioma: CT and MR studies. J Comput Assist Tomogr 12:702-704

Hirabayashi S, Yanai A, Muraishi Y (1997) Huge pleomorphic adenoma of the upper retromolar area. Ann Plast Surg 38:184-186

Hisatomi M, Asaumi J, Konouchi H et al (2001) MR imaging of nasopalatine duct cysts. Eur J Radiol 39:73-76

Hisatomi M, Asaumi J, Konouchi H et al (2003) MR imaging of epithelial cysts of the oral and maxillofacial region. Eur J Radiol 48:178-182

Hochberg MG, Currie WR, Rafetto LK (1994) Osteotomy technique for accessing a meningioma in the infratemporal fossa: report of a case. J Oral Maxillofac Surg 52:499-502

Holtmann S, Martin F, Permanetter W (1985) Die dysontogenetischen, medianen Oberkieferzysten. Laryngol Rhinol Otol (Stuttg) 64:331-334

Honegger J, Buchfelder M, Fahlbusch R (1999) Surgical treatment of craniopharyngiomas: endocrinological results. J Neurosurg 90:251-257

Howard DJ, Lund VJ (1992) The midfacial degloving approach to sinonasal disease. J Laryngol Otol 106:1059-1062

Hsu HC, Huang EY, Eng HL (2002) Cheek mass as a presentation of metastatic rectal cancer. Chang Gung Med J 25:345-348

Hu J, Little J, Xu T et al (1999) Risk factors for meningioma in adults: a case-control study in northeast China. Int J Cancer 83:299-304

Huber PE, Debus J, Latz D et al (2001) Radiotherapy for advanced adenoid cystic carcinoma: neutrons, photons or mixed beam? Radiother Oncol 59:161-167

Hug EB, Loredo LN, Slater JD et al (1999) Proton radiation therapy for chordomas and chondrosarcomas of the skull base. J Neurosurg 91:432-439

Hyam DM, Veness MJ, Morgan GJ (2004) Minor salivary gland carcinoma involving the oral cavity or oropharynx. Aust Dent J 49:16-19

Inagi K, Takahashi H, Okamoto M et al (2002) Treatment effects in patients with squamous cell carcinoma of the oral cavity. Acta Otolaryngol Suppl (547):25-29

Isaac MA, Hahn SS, Kim JA et al (2001) Management of craniopharyngioma. Cancer J 7:516-520

Ishii K, Ikeda H, Takahashi S et al (1996) MR imaging of pituitary adenomas with sphenoid sinus invasion: characteristic MR findings indicating fibrosis. Radiat Med 14:173-178

Iuchi T, Saeki N, Tanaka M et al (1998) MRI prediction of fibrous pituitary adenomas. Acta Neurochir (Wien) 140:779-786

Jackson IT, Callan PP, Forte RA (1996) An anatomical classification of maxillary ameloblastoma as an aid to surgical treatment. J Craniomaxillofac Surg 24:230-236

Janse van Rensburg L, Nortje CJ, Thompson I (1997) Correlating imaging and histopathology of an odontogenic keratocyst in the nevoid basal cell carcinoma syndrome. Dentomaxillofac Radiol 26:195-199

Jansisyanont P, Blanchaert RH, Jr., Ord RA (2002) Intraoral minor salivary gland neoplasm: a single institution experience of 80 cases. Int J Oral Maxillofac Surg 31:257-261

Jiang RS, Wu CY, Jan YJ et al (1998) Primary ethmoid sinus craniopharyngioma: a case report. J Laryngol Otol 112:403-405

Johnsen DE, Woodruff WW, Allen IS et al (1991) MR imaging of the sellar and juxtasellar regions. Radiographics 11:727-758

Johnson AT, Maran AG (1982) Extra-cranial tumours of the infratemporal fossa. J Laryngol Otol 96:1017-1026

Jung SL, Choi KH, Park YH et al (1999) Cemento-ossifying fibroma presenting as a mass of the parapharyngeal and masticator space. AJNR Am J Neuroradiol 20:1744-1746

Kalapurakal JA, Goldman S, Hsieh YC et al (2003) Clinical outcome in children with craniopharyngioma treated with primary surgery and radiotherapy deferred until relapse. Med Pediatr Oncol 40:214-218

Kanazawa T, Nishino H, Miyata M et al (2001) Haemangiopericytoma of infratemporal fossa. J Laryngol Otol 115:77-79

Kaplan JN, Duckert LG (1984) Lesions metastatic to the infratemporal fossa: report of a case and review of the literature. Otolaryngol Head Neck Surg 92:241-246

Kawahara Y, Niiro M, Yokoyama S et al (2001) Dural congestion accompanying meningioma invasion into vessels: the dural tail sign. Neuroradiology 43:462-465

Kawai T, Murakami S, Kishino M et al (1998) Diagnostic imaging in two cases of recurrent maxillary ameloblastoma: comparative evaluation of plain radiographs, CT and MR images. Br J Oral Maxillofac Surg 36:304-310

Kaye AH (1997) Essential neurosurgery. 2nd edition. Churchill Livingstone, New York

Kleihues P, Burger PC, Scheithauer BW et al (1993) Histological typing of tumours of the central nervous system. 2nd edition. Springer-Verlag, Berlin

Knox RD, Pratt MF, Garen PD et al (1990) Intramuscular hemangioma of the infratemporal fossa. Otolaryngol Head Neck Surg 103:637-641

Kondziolka D, Lunsford LD, Coffey RJ et al (1991) Stereotactic radiosurgery of meningiomas. J Neurosurg 74:552-559

Koo JY, Kadonaga JN, Wintroub BV et al (1992) The development of B-cell lymphoma in a patient with psoriasis treated with cyclosporine. J Am Acad Dermatol 26:836-840

Kornblut AD (1987) Clinical evaluation of tumors of the oral cavity In: Thawley SE, Panjie WR, Batsakis JG, Lindberg RD (eds) Comprehensive Management of Head and Neck Tumors. Saunders, Philadelphia, pp 460-479.

Kornfehl J, Gstottner W, Kontrus M et al (1996) Transpalatine excision of a cavernous hemangioma of the infratemporal fossa. Eur Arch Otorhinolaryngol 253:172-175

Korten AG, Berg HJ, Spincemaille GH et al (1998) Intracranial chondrosarcoma: review of the literature and report of 15 cases. J Neurol Neurosurg Psychiatry 65:88-92

Kramer IRH, Pindborg JJ, Shear M (1992) Histological typing of odontogenic tumours. 2nd edition. Springer-Verlag, Berlin

Krespi YP (1989) Lateral skull base surgery for cancer. Laryngoscope 99:514-524

Krespi YP, Sisson GA (1984) Transmandibular exposure of the skull base. Am J Surg 148:534-538

Krishnamurthy S, Holmes B, Powers SK (1998) Schwannomas limited to the infratemporal fossa: report of two cases. J Neurooncol 36:269-277

Krolls SO, Hoffman S (1976) Squamous cell carcinoma of the oral soft tissues: a statistical analysis of 14,253 cases by age, sex, and race of patients. J Am Dent Assoc 92:571-574

Krolls SO, Hoffman S. Squamous cell carcinoma of the oral soft tissues: a statistical analysis of 14,253 cases by age, sex, and race of patients. J AM Dent Assoc 1976;92:571-4.

Kucharczyk W, Peck WW, Kelly WM et al (1987) Rathke cleft cysts: CT, MR imaging, and pathologic features. Radiology 165:491-495

Kumar A, Valvassori G, Jafar J et al (1986) Skull base lesions: a classification and surgical approaches. Laryngoscope 96:252-263

Kveton JF, Brackmann DE, Glasscock ME 3rd et al (1986) Chondrosarcoma of the skull base. Otolaryngol Head Neck Surg 94:23-32

Lahoz Zamarro MT, Martinez Subias J, Muniesa Soriano JA et al (2001) Melanoma de paladar duro. Acta Otorrinolaringol Esp 52:422-425

Laine FJ, Braun IF, Jensen ME et al (1990) Perineural tumor extension through the foramen ovale: evaluation with MR imaging. Radiology 174:65-71

Lambe M, Coogan P, Baron J (1997) Reproductive factors and the risk of brain tumors: a population-based study in Sweden. Int J Cancer 72:389-393

Landolt AM (2001) History of pituitary surgery from the technical aspect. Neurosurg Clin North Am 12:37-44

Lawson W, Naidu RK, Le Benger J et al (1990) Combined median mandibulotomy and Weber-Fergusson maxillectomy. Arch Otolaryngol Head Neck Surg 116:596-599

Lee RJ, Smith SH, Hicks WL, Jr. et al (1998) Management of extraosseous ewing sarcoma of the infratemporal fossa. Med Pediatr Oncol 31:31-35

Lee YY, Van Tassel P (1989) Craniofacial chondrosarcomas: imaging findings in 15 untreated cases. AJNR Am J Neuroradiol 10:165-170

Leonetti JP, al-Mefty O, Eisenbeis JF et al (1993) Orbitocranial exposure in the management of infratemporal fossa tumors. Otolaryngol Head Neck Surg 109:769-772

Leonetti JP, Wachter B, Marzo SJ, Petruzzelli G (2001) Extracranial lower cranial nerve sheath tumors. Otolaryngol Head Neck Surg 125:640-644.

Lissett CA, Shalet SM (2000) Management of pituitary tumours: strategy for investigation and follow-up. Horm Res 53 Suppl 3:65-70

Longstreth WT, Jr., Dennis LK, McGuire VM et al (1993) Epidemiology of intracranial meningioma. Cancer 72:639-648

Lopes M, Duffau H, Fleuridas G (1999) Primary spheno-orbital angiosarcoma: case report and review of the literature. Neurosurgery 44:405-407; discussion 407-408

Lopes MA, Santos GC, Kowalski LP (1998) Multivariate survival analysis of 128 cases of oral cavity minor salivary gland carcinomas. Head Neck 20:699-706

Lorigan JG, O'Keeffe FN, Evans HL et al (1989) The radiologic manifestations of alveolar soft-part sarcoma. AJR Am J Roentgenol 153:335-339

Losa M, Valle M, Mortini P et al. (2004) Gamma Knife surgery for treatment of residual nonfunctioning pituitary adenomas after surgical debulking. J Neurosurg 100:438-444

Loughran S, Badia L, Lund V (2000) Primary chordoma of the ethmoid sinus. J Laryngol Otol 114:627-629

Mac Carty CS, Hanson EJ Jr, Randall RV et al (1973) Indications for and results of surgical treatment of pituitary tumors by the transfrontal approach. International Congress Series 303. Diagnosis and teratment of pituitary tumors. Excerpta Medica, Amsterdam

Maiuri F, Salzano FA, Motta S et al (1998) Olfactory groove meningioma with paranasal sinus and nasal cavity extension: removal by combined subfrontal and nasal approach. J Craniomaxillofac Surg 26:314-317

Manganaro AM, Will MJ, Ragno JR, Jr. et al (1997) Red-blue lesion of the hard palate. J Oral Maxillofac Surg 55:159-165

Maroldi R, Battaglia G, Farina D et al (1999) Tumours of the oropharynx and oral cavity: perineural spread and bone invasion. Jbr-Btr 82:294-300

McCarthy BJ, Davis FG, Freels S et al (1998) Factors associated with survival in patients with meningioma. J Neurosurg 88:831-839

McCluggage WG, McBride GB, Primrose WJ et al (1995) Giant cell tumour of the temporal bone presenting as vertigo. J Laryngol Otol 109:538-541

McDaniel RK (1999) Odontogenic cyst and tumors: clinical evaluation and pathology,. In: Thawley SE, Panje WR, Batsakis JG, Lindberg RD (eds) Comprehensive Management of Head and Neck Tumors. 2nd edn. Saunders, Philadelphia, pp 1566-1610.

Mendelsohn DB, Hertzanu Y, Glass RB (1983) Computed tomographic findings in primary mandibular osteosarcoma. Clin Radiol 34:153-155

Merchant TE, Kiehna EN, Sanford RA et al (2002) Craniopharyngioma: the St. Jude Children's Research Hospital experience 1984-2001. Int J Radiat Oncol Biol Phys 53:533-542.

Meyers SP, Hirsch WL, Jr., Curtin HD et al (1992) Chordomas of the skull base: MR features. AJNR Am J Neuroradiol 13:1627-1636

Miller NR, Golnik KC, Zeidman SM et al (1996) Pneumosinus dilatans: a sign of intracranial meningioma. Surg Neurol 46:471-474

Minami M, Kaneda T, Ozawa K et al (1996) Cystic lesions of the maxillomandibular region: MR imaging distinction of odontogenic keratocysts and ameloblastomas from other cysts. AJR Am J Roentgenol 166:943-949

Minoda R, Masako M, Masuyama K et al (2001) Malignant myoepithelioma arising within the masticator space ectopically. Otolaryngol Head Neck Surg 124:342-343

Molla E, Marti-Bonmati L, Revert A et al (2002) Craniopharyngiomas: identification of different semiological patterns with MRI. Eur Radiol 12:1829-1836

Moriya S, Tei K, Notani K et al (2001) Malignant hemangiopericytoma of the head and neck: a report of 3 cases. J Oral Maxillofac Surg 59:340-345

Morris KM, Campbell D, Stell PM et al (1990) Meningiomas presenting with paranasal sinus involvement. Br J Neurosurg 4:511-515

Mortini P, Giovanelli M (2002) Transcranial Approaches to Pituitary Tumors. Operative Techniques in Neurosurgery 3:1-14

Mosqueda-Taylor A, Ledesma-Montes C, Caballero-Sandoval S et al (1997) Odontogenic tumors in Mexico: a collaborative retrospective study of 349 cases. Oral Surg Oral Med Oral Pathol Oral Radiol Endod 84:672-675

Nammour GM, Ybarra J, Naheedy MH et al (1997) Incidental pituitary macroadenoma: a population-based study. Am J Med Sci 314:287-291

Neff B, Thayer Sataloff R, Storey L et al (2002) Chondrosarcoma of the skull base. Laryngoscope 112: 134-139

Neville BW, Damm DD, Brock T (1997) Odontogenic keratocysts of the midline maxillary region. J Oral Maxillofac Surg 55:340-344

Ng SH, Chang TC, Ko SF et al (1997) Nasopharyngeal carcinoma: MRI and CT assessment. Neuroradiology 39:741-746

Nicolato A, Foroni R, Alessandrini F et al (2002) Radiosurgical treatment of cavernous sinus meningiomas: experience with 122 treated patients. Neurosurgery 51:1153-1159; discussion 1159-1161

Norris JS, Pavaresh M, Afshar F (1998) Primary transsphenoidal microsurgery in the treatment of craniopharyngiomas. Br J Neurosurg 12:305-312

O'Connell JX, Renard LG, Liebsch NJ (1994) Base of skull chordoma: a correlative study of hystologic and clinical features of 62 cases. Cancer 74:2261-2267

Oda D, Rivera V, Ghanee N et al (2000) Odontogenic keratocyst: the northwestern USA experience. J Contemp Dent Pract 1:60-74

Ogren FP, Wisecarver JL, Lydiatt DD et al (1991) Ancient neurilemmoma of the infratemporal fossa: a case report. Head Neck 13:243-246

Oikawa S, Kyoshima K, Goto T et al (2001) Histological study on local invasiveness of clival chordoma. Case report of autopsy. Acta Neurochir (Wien) 143:1065-1069

Okita W, Ichimura K, Iinuma T (1991) Dentigerous cyst of the maxilla and its image diagnosis. Rhinology 29:307-314

Oot RF, Melville GE, New PF et al (1988) The role of MR and CT in evaluating clival chordomas and chondrosarcomas. AJR Am J Roentgenol 151:567-575

O'Ryan F, Eversole LR, Alikpala A (1987) Juvenile fibromatosis of the infratemporal fossa. Oral Surg Oral Med Oral Pathol 64:603-608

Ostrov SG, Quencer RM, Hoffman JC et al (1989) Hemorrhage within pituitary adenomas: how often associated with pituitary apoplexy syndrome? AJR Am J Roentgenol 153:153-160

Palacios E, Serou M, Restrepo S et al (2004) Odontogenic keratocysts in nevoid basal cell carcinoma (Gorlin's) syndrome: CT and MRI evaluation. Ear Nose Throat J 83:40-42

Pang D. Surgical management of craniopharyngioma. (1993) In: Sekhar LN, Janecka IP (eds) Surgery of cranial base tumors. Raven Press, New York, pp 787-807

Papageorge MB, Doku HC, Lis R (1992) Solitary neurofibroma of the mandible and infratemporal fossa in a young child. Report of a case. Oral Surg Oral Med Oral Pathol 73:407-411

Patel PC, Pellitteri PK, Vrabec DP et al (1998) Tumefactive fibroinflammatory lesion of the head and neck originating in the infratemporal fossa. Am J Otolaryngol 19:216-219

Perzin KH, Pushparaj N (1984) Nonepithelial tumors of the nasal cavity, paranasal sinuses, and nasopharynx. A clinicopathologic study. XIII: Meningiomas. Cancer 54:1860-1869

Perzin KH, Pushparaj N (1986) Nonepithelial tumors of the nasal cavity, paranasal sinuses, and nasopharynx. A clinicopathologic study. XIV: Chordomas. Cancer 57:784-796

Petruzzelli GJ, Myers EN (1994) Malignant neoplasms of the hard palate and upper alveolar ridge. Oncology (Huntingt) 8:43-48; discussion 50, 53

Pevsner PH, Bast WG, Lumerman H et al (2000) CT analysis of a complicated nasopalatine duct cyst. N Y State Dent J 66:18-20

Phillips LE, Koepsell TD, van Belle G et al (2002) History of head trauma and risk of intracranial meningioma: population-based case-control study. Neurology 58:1849-1852

Pichard C, Gerber S, Laloi M et al (2002) Pituitary carcinoma: report of an exceptional case and review of the literature. J Endocrinol Invest 25:65-72

Pieper DR, Al-Mefty O (1999) Management of intracranial meningiomas secondarily involving the infratemporal fossa: radiographic characteristics, pattern of tumor invasion, and surgical implications. Neurosurgery 45:231-237; discussion 237-238

Pieper DR, Al-Mefty O, Hanada Y et al (1999) Hyperostosis associated with meningioma of the cranial base: secondary changes or tumor invasion. Neurosurgery 44:742-746; discussion 746-747

Pogrel MA (1994) The management of salivary gland tumors of the palate. J Oral Maxillofac Surg 52:454-459

Pritchyk KM, Schiff BA, Newkirk KA et al (2002) Metastatic renal cell carcinoma to the head and neck. Laryngoscope 112:1598-1602

Prott FJ, Micke O, Haverkamp U et al (2000) Results of fast neutron therapy of adenoid cystic carcinoma of the salivary glands. Anticancer Res 20:3743-3749

Rangheard AS, Vanel D, Viala J et al (2001) Synovial sarcomas of the head and neck: CT and MR imaging findings of eight patients. AJNR Am J Neuroradiol 22:851-857

Raybaud C, Rabehanta P, Girard N (1991) Aspects radiologiques des craniopharyngiomes. In: Choux M, Lena G, Genitori L (eds) Le craniopharyngiome de l'enfant. Neurochirurgie (Paris) 37(suppl1):12-165.

Rees DA, Hanna FW, Davies JS et al (2002) Long-term follow-up results of transsphenoidal surgery for Cushing's disease in a single centre using strict criteria for remission. Clin Endocrinol (Oxf) 56:541-551

Regezi JA (2002) Odontogenic cysts, odontogenic tumors, fibroosseous, and giant cell lesions of the jaws. Mod Pathol 15:331-341

Reiter ER, Varvares MA, August M et al (2000) Mucocele of the infratemporal fossa as an unusual complication of midfacial fracture. Ann Otol Rhinol Laryngol 109:522-525

Rohrer T, Gassmann K, Buchfelder M et al (2002) Klinische Symptome und Befunde zum Zeitpunkt der Diagnosestellung bei Kindern und Jugendlichen mit Kraniopharyngeom. Klin Padiatr 214:285-290

Rosenberg AE, Nielsen GP, Keel SB et al (1999) Chondrosarcoma of the base of the skull: a clinicopathologic study of 200 cases with emphasis on its distinction from chordoma. Am J Surg Pathol 23:1370-1378

Rosenblum BN, Katsantonis GP, Cooper MH et al (1990) Infratemporal fossa and lateral skull base dissection: long-term results. Otolaryngol Head Neck Surg 102:106-110

Rouviáere H (1932) Anatomie des lymphatiques de l'homme. Masson, Paris

Rubin MM, Sadoff RS (1992) Rhabdomyosarcoma of the infratemporal fossa. N Y State Dent J 58:32-35

Rubinstein AB, Arbit E (1985) Intracranial meningiomas presenting with epistaxis--case report and literature review. J Otolaryngol 14:248-250

Sadetzki S, Flint-Richter P, Ben-Tal T et al (2002) Radiation-induced meningioma: a descriptive study of 253 cases. J Neurosurg 97:1078-1082

Saleh EA, Taibah AK, Naguib M et al (1994) Giant cell tumor of the lateral skull base: a case report. Otolaryngol Head Neck Surg 111:314-318.

Samii M, Bini W (1991) Surgical treatment of craniopharyngiomas. Zentralbl Neurochir 52:17-23

Sarac S, Koybasi S, Kaya S (2000) Transmaxillary excision of a rare cavernous hemangioma of the infratemporal fossa. Ear Nose Throat J 79:448-449, 452

Sartoretti-Schefer S, Wichmann W, Aguzzi A et al (1997) MR

differentiation of adamantinous and squamous-papillary craniopharyngiomas. AJNR Am J Neuroradiol 18:77-87

Schreiber A, Kinney LA, Salman R (1991) Large-cell lymphoma of the infratemporal fossa presenting as myofacial pain. J Craniomandib Disord 5:286-289

Schulz-Ertner D, Frank C, Herfarth KK et al (2002) Fractionated stereotactic radiotherapy for craniopharyngiomas. Int J Radiat Oncol Biol Phys 54:1114-1120

Seifert V, Dietz H (1992) Combined orbito-frontal, sub- and infratemporal fossa approach to skull base neoplasms. Surgical technique and clinical application. Acta Neurochir (Wien) 114:139-144

Sekhar LN, Oliveira ED (1999) Cranial microsurgery: approaches and techniques. Thieme, New York

Sekhar LN, Schramm VL, Jr., Jones NF (1987) Subtemporal-preauricular infratemporal fossa approach to large lateral and posterior cranial base neoplasms. J Neurosurg 67:488-499

Shah JP, Lydiatt WM Buccal mucosa, alveolus, retromolar trigone, floor of mouth, hard palate, and tongue tumors (1999) In: Thawley SE, Panjie WR, Batsakis JG, Lindberg RD (eds) Comprehensive Management of Head and Neck Tumors. 2nd edn. Saunders, Philadelphia, pp 686-694

Shaheen OH (1982) Swellings of the infratemporal fossa. J Laryngol Otol 96:817-836

Shahinian HK, Suh RH, Jarrahy R (1999) Combined infratemporal fossa and transfacial approach to excising massive tumors. Ear Nose Throat J 78:350, 353-356.

Shapshay SM, Elber E, Strong MS (1976) Occult tumors of the infratemporal fossa: report of seven cases appearing as preauricular facial pain. Arch Otolaryngol 102:535-538

Sheehan JP, Kondziolka D, Flickinger J et al. (2002) Radiosurgery for residual or recurrent nonfunctioning pituitary adenoma. J Neurosurg 97 (Suppl 5):408-414

Shin JL, Asa SL, Woodhouse LJ et al (1999) Cystic lesions of the pituitary: clinicopathological features distinguishing craniopharyngioma, Rathke's cleft cyst, and arachnoid cyst. J Clin Endocrinol Metab 84:3972-3982

Shinohara Y, Uchida A, Hiromatsu T et al (1993) A case of neurilemmoma in the infratemporal fossa showing the antral bowing sign. Dentomaxillofac Radiol 22:214-215

Shugar JM, Som PM, Krespi YP, Arnold LM, Som ML (1980) Primary chordoma of the maxillary sinus. Laryngoscope 90:1825-1830

Sichel JY, Monteil JP, Elidan J (1994) Skull base chondroma of extracranial origin. Head Neck 16:578-581

Simsir A, Osborne BM, Greenebaum E (1996) Malignant granular cell tumor: a case report and review of the recent literature. Hum Pathol 27:853-858

Slama A, Yacoubi T, Khochtali H et al (2002) Carcinosarcome odontogene mandibulaire. Rev Stomatol Chir Maxillofac 103:124-127

Slater LJ (1999) Odontogenic sarcoma and carcinosarcoma. Semin Diagn Pathol 16:325-332

Slonim SM, Haykal HA, Cushing GW et al (1993) MRI appearances of an ectopic pituitary adenoma: case report and review of the literature. Neuroradiology 35:546-548

Smith PG, Grubb RL, Kletzker GR et al (1990) Combined pterional-anterolateral approaches to cranial base tumors. Otolaryngol Head Neck Surg 103:357-363

Som PM, Curtin HD, Silvers AR (1997) A re-evaluation of imaging criteria to assess aggressive masticator space tumors. Head Neck 19:335-341

Som PM, Norton KI (1991) Lesions that manifest as medial cheek and nasolabial fold masses. Radiology 178:831-835

Som PM, Shangold LM, Biller HF (1992) A palatal dentigerous cyst arising from a mesiodente. AJNR Am J Neuroradiol 13:212-214

Spada A, Lania A, Ballare E (1998) G protein abnormalities in pituitary adenomas. Mol Cell Endocrinol 142:1-14

Spagnoli MV, Goldberg HI, Grossman RI et al (1986) Intracranial meningiomas: high-field MR imaging. Radiology 161:369-375

Spindler MB, Philipp A, Laszig R (1989) Das extrakranielle Meningeom: eine seltene Differentialdiagnose eines intranasalen Tumors. Hno 37:162-164

Spinelli HM, Isenberg JS, O'Brien M (1994) Nasopalatine duct cysts and the role of magnetic resonance imaging. J Craniofac Surg 5:57-60

Strugar J, Sekhar LN (2000) Chordomas and chondrosarcomas. In: Robertson JT, Coakham HB, Robertson JH (eds) Cranial base surgery. Churchill Livingstone, London, pp 397-415

Su CY, Chien CY, Hwang CF (1999) A new transnasal approach to endoscopic marsupialization of the nasolabial cyst. Laryngoscope 109:1116-1118

Suei Y, Tanimoto K, Taguchi A et al (1994) Primary intraosseous carcinoma: review of the literature and diagnostic criteria. J Oral Maxillofac Surg 52:580-583

Suhardja AS, Kovacs KT, Rutka JT (1999) Molecular pathogenesis of pituitary adenomas: a review. Acta Neurochir (Wien) 141:729-736

Surawicz TS, McCarthy BJ, Kupelian V et al (1999) Descriptive epidemiology of primary brain and CNS tumors: results from the Central Brain Tumor Registry of the United States 1990-1994. Neuro-oncol 1:14-25

Swain RE, Jr., Kingdom TT, DelGaudio JM et al (2001) Meningiomas of the paranasal sinuses. Am J Rhinol 15:27-30

Sze G, Uichanco LS 3rd, Brant-Zawadzki MN et al (1988) Chordomas: MR imaging. Radiology 166:187-191

Tashiro M, Nagase M, Nakajima T et al (1988) Malignant paraganglioma. Report of a case and review of the Japanese literature. J Craniomaxillofac Surg 16:324-329

Thompson LD, Gyure KA (2000) Extracranial sinonasal tract meningiomas: a clinicopathologic study of 30 cases with a review of the literature. Am J Surg Pathol 24:640-650

Thuomas KA (1999) Pituitary microadenoma. MR appearance and correlation with CT. Acta Radiol 40:663

To EH, Brown JS, Avery BS et al (1991) Primary intraosseous carcinoma of the jaws. Three new cases and a review of the literature. Br J Oral Maxillofac Surg 29:19-25

Tokumaru A, O'Uchi T, Eguchi T et al (1990) Prominent meningeal enhancement adjacent to meningioma on Gd-DTPA-enhanced MR images: histopathologic correlation. Radiology 175:431-433

Tomura N, Hirano H, Kato K et al (1999) Comparison of MR imaging with CT in depiction of tumour extension into the pterygopalatine fossa. Clin Radiol 54:361-366

Toriumi DM, Shermetaro CB, Pecaro BC (1989) Cavernous hemangioma of the infratemporal fossa. Ear Nose Throat J 68:252 258-259

Tran L, Sadeghi A, Hanson D et al (1987). Salivary gland tumors of the palate: the UCLA experience. Laryngoscope 97:1343-1345

Truitt TO, Gleich LL, Huntress GP et al (1999) Surgical management of hard palate malignancies. Otolaryngol Head Neck Surg 121:548-552

Ulfarsson E, Lindquist C, Roberts M et al (2002) Gamma knife radiosurgery for craniopharyngiomas: long-term results in the first Swedish patients. J Neurosurg 97:613-622

Ummat S, Nasser JG (1992) Fibrosarcoma of the infratemporal fossa in childhood: a challenging problem. J Otolaryngol 21:441-446

Uppal HS, D'Souza AR, De R et al (2002) Dermoid cyst of the infratemporal fossa. J Laryngol Otol 116:150-152

Vajramani G, Devi I, Santosh V et al (1999) Benign triton tumor of the trigeminal nerve. Childs Nerv Syst 15:140-144

Van Effenterre R, Boch AL (2002) Craniopharyngioma in adults and children: a study of 122 surgical cases. J Neurosurg 97:3-11

Vasconcelos R, de Aguiar MF, Castro W et al (1999a) Retrospective analysis of 31 cases of nasopalatine duct cyst. Oral Dis 5:325-328

Vasconcelos RF, Souza PE, Mesquita RA (1999b) Retrospective analysis of 15 cases of nasolabial cyst. Quintessence Int 30:629-632

Verbin R., Barnes L. (2001) Cyst and cystic like lesions of the oral cavity, jaws, and neck. In: Barnes L (ed) Surgical pathology of the head and neck. M. Dekker, New York, pp 1437-1555

Vogl TJ, Mack MG, Straub R et al (2001) MR-guided laser-induced thermotherapy of the infratemporal fossa and orbit in malignant chondrosarcoma via a modified technique. Cardiovasc Intervent Radiol 24:432-435

Volpe NJ, Liebsch NJ, Munzenrider JE et al (1993) Neuro-ophthalmologic findings in chordoma and chondrosarcoma of the skull base. Am J Ophthalmol 115:97-104

Walker WP, Landas SK, Bromley CM et al (1991) Immunohistochemical distinction of classic and chondroid chordomas. Mod Pathol 4:661-666

Wang KC, Kim SK, Choe G et al (2002) Growth patterns of craniopharyngioma in children: role of the diaphragm sellae and its surgical implication. Surg Neurol 57:25-33

Warakaulle DR, Anslow P (2003) Differential diagnosis of intracranial lesions with high signal on T1 or low signal on T2-weighted MRI. Clin Radiol 58:922-933

Watters GW, Brookes GB (1995) Chondrosarcoma of the temporal bone. Clin Otolaryngol 20:53-58

Weber AL, Brown EW, Hug EB et al (1995) Cartilaginous tumors and chordomas of the cranial base. Otolaryngol Clin North Am 28:453-471

Weisman RA, Osguthorpe JD (1988) Pseudotumor of the head and neck masquerading as neoplasia. Laryngoscope 98:610-614

Weissman JL, Snyderman CH, Yousem SA et al (1993) Ameloblastoma of the maxilla: CT and MR appearance. AJNR Am J Neuroradiol 14:223-226

Wetmore SJ, Suen JY, Snyderman NL (1986) Preauricular approach to infratemporal fossa. Head Neck Surg 9:93-103

Wetmore SJ, Suen JY, Snyderman NL. Preauricular approach to infratemporal fossa. Head Neck Surg 1986;9:93-103.

Williams LS, Mancuso AA, Mendenhall WM (2001) Perineural spread of cutaneous squamous and basal cell carcinoma: CT and MR detection and its impact on patient management and prognosis. Int J Radiat Oncol Biol Phys 49:1061-1069

Wilson CB (1984) A decade of pituitary microsurgery. The Herbert Olivecrona Lecture. J Neurosurg 61:814-833

Wolters B, Kleinsasser O (1985) Intranasale extradurale meningeome. Fallbericht und Literaturzusammenstellung. Laryngol Rhinol Otol (Stuttg) 64:198-201

Woolford TJ, Birzgalis AR, Ramsden RT (1994) An extensive vestibular schwannoma with both intracranial spread and lateral extension to the external auditory canal. J Laryngol Otol 108:149-151

Yasargil MG, Curcic M, Kis M et al (1990) Total removal of craniopharyngiomas. Approaches and long-term results in 144 patients. J Neurosurg 73:3-11

Yeakley JW, Kulkarni MV, McArdle CB et al (1988) High-resolution MR imaging of juxtasellar meningiomas with CT and angiographic correlation. AJNR Am J Neuroradiol 9:279-285

Yorozu A, Sykes AJ, Slevin NJ (2001) Carcinoma of the hard palate treated with radiotherapy: a retrospective review of 31 cases. Oral Oncol 37:493-497

Yu Q, Wang P, Shi H et al (1998) The lesions of the pterygopalatine and infratemporal spaces: computed tomography evaluation. Oral Surg Oral Med Oral Pathol Oral Radiol Endod 85:742-751

Zada G, Kelly DF, Cohan P et al (2003) Endonasal transsphenoidal approach for pituitary adenomas and other sellar lesions: an assessment of efficacy, safety, and patient impressions. J Neurosurg 98:350-358

Zervas NT, Martin JB (1980) Current concepts in cancer: management of hormone-secreting pituitary adenomas. N Engl J Med 302:210-214

Zhao K, Liu N, Qi DY et al (1993) Primary meningioma of the infratemporal fossa: a clinicopathologic and immunohistochemical study. J Oral Maxillofac Surg 51:597-601

Zhao YF, Wei JX, Wang SP (2002) Treatment of odontogenic keratocysts: a follow-up of 255 Chinese patients. Oral Surg Oral Med Oral Pathol Oral Radiol Endod 94:151-156

Zorlu F, Gurkaynak M, Yildiz F et al (2000) Conventional external radiotherapy in the management of clivus chordomas with overt residual disease. Neurol Sci 21:203-207

11 Normal and Abnormal Appearance of Nose and Paranasal Sinuses After Microendoscopic Surgery, Open Surgery, and Radiation Therapy

Roberto Maroldi, Piero Nicolai, Laura Palvarini, Vanessa Portugalli, and Andrea Borghesi

CONTENTS

11.1 Introduction 255
11.2 Imaging of Perioperative Complications 256
11.3 Imaging After Microendoscopic Surgery 258
11.3.1 Inflammatory Diseases 259
11.3.1.1 Imaging After Endonasal Surgery for Rhinosinusitis Without Nasal Polyposis 259
11.3.1.2 Imaging After Endonasal Surgery for Rhinosinusitis With Nasal Polyposis 261
11.3.2 Expansile and Benign Lesions 268
11.4 Imaging After Treatment of Malignant Neoplasms 270
11.4.1 Clinical Issues in the Immediate Postoperative and Intermediate Phases 270
11.4.2 Clinical Issues in the Late Phase 270
11.4.3 Imaging Strategies in the Follow-up 271
11.4.4 CT and MR Imaging Findings 271
11.4.4.1 Normal Postoperative Imaging Changes 271
11.4.4.2 Normal Post-radiation Therapy Imaging Changes 277
11.4.4.3 Imaging the Complications of Post-radiation Therapy 278
11.4.4.4 Imaging of Local Recurrences 280
References 291

11.1 Introduction

CT and MR are imaging techniques routinely used before treatment to assess the extent of inflammatory and neoplastic lesions, to detail the anatomy of sinonasal tract structures, and to suggest a possible diagnosis.

Indications to post-treatment imaging by means of CT or MR include the evaluation of acute and late complications of surgery and radiation therapy, assessment of response to radiation therapy and/ or chemotherapy, and early detection or detailed mapping of known recurrences (SCHUSTER et al. 1994; JANKOWSKI et al. 1997; MAROLDI et al. 1997;

R. MAROLDI, MD, Professor; L. PALVARINI, MD; V. PORTUGALLI, MD; A. BORGHESI, MD
Department of Radiology, University of Brescia, Piazzale Spedali Civili 1, Brescia, BS, 25123, Italy
P. NICOLAI, MD, Professor
Department of Otorhinolaryngology, University of Brescia, Piazzale Spedali Civili 1, Brescia, BS, 25123, Italy

CHAGNAUD et al. 1998; SAIDI et al. 1998). Possibilities and limitations of PET in this area are far to be established (LIU et al. 2004; NINOMIYA et al. 2004).

It is important to note that follow up of inflammatory and neoplastic lesions shares some common problems that post-treatment cross sectional imaging has to solve. Among these, the knowledge of the nature of the previously treated lesion, and of the type of treatment(s) is essential and should be provided by the referring physician or by the patient. Moreover, most patients treated for neoplasms undergoing MR or CT follow up studies tend to be uncooperative, particularly because of nasal discharge or dripping, or because of frequent swallowing. In this setting, MR technique – rather than CT, which is generally less time-consuming - should be adjusted in order to reduce the overall examination time (see chapter 1, section 1.3.2.1).

In the follow up of patients treated for malignancies, knowledge of the intraoperative findings and of pathological data is a key point in identifying areas at higher risk for relapse. In addition, the most frequent known patterns of local recurrence for any specific histotype have to be carefully taken into account. Among these are perineural and perivascular spread, and permeative bone invasion (WILLIAMS et al. 2001; GINSBERG 2002). Whenever a reconstruction with local or revascularized free flaps tissue has been done, meticulous analysis of the areas at the interface between native tissues and flap is necessary, as most relapses arise at that level (HUDGINS 2002).

While few data is available about the pattern of response of sinonasal tract neoplasms to radiation therapy or chemotherapy, more knowledge has been accumulated regarding normal changes of tissues adjacent to neoplasms after radiation treatment (GONG et al. 1991).

In inflammatory and neoplastic lesions the typical pattern of post-surgical changes of mucosa and underlying tissues has to be known. Both endonasal and open approaches usually result in a large nasal cavity, facilitating the endoscopic detection of lesions involving the mucosa.

Finally, the availability of previous studies and the careful matching with current imaging and clinical findings is certainly a key point in minimizing the chance of missing early relapsing lesions.

The choice of the most appropriate imaging technique and the timing of follow up studies are dictated by the nature of the treated lesion.

11.2
Imaging of Perioperative Complications

Because of the strategic location of the sinonasal tract, the risk of damaging critical structures is high with both a microendoscopic or an open surgical approach. As a result, early cross sectional imaging after microendoscopic or open surgery is required only when an acute complication is suspected. The onset of severe headache, orbital signs as proptosis, alteration in pupil diameter, ophthalmoplegia, vision loss, severe nasal hemorrhage, and confusion or changes in behavior should prompt the surgeon to obtain an immediate CT study and consultation with an ophthalmologist and/or a neurologist (VASSALLO et al. 2001; YOUNIS et al. 2002; GRAHAM and NERAD 2003).

According to their severity, complications are classified as *major*, bearing relevant morbidity and the potential for mortality, and *minor*, which have modest morbidity and no possibility of mortality. In addition, complications are further classified - according to their onset - as immediate and delayed (STAMM 2000).

The most frequent immediate major complications after microendoscopic sinus surgery requiring imaging encompass: diplopia, impairment or vision loss, perioperative bleeding, rhinorrhea, severe neurologic symptoms and signs.

Diplopia is more often related to damage to the medial rectus or superior oblique muscles, which are those closest to the lamina papyracea (HUDGINS 1993). Anatomic conditions that predispose to medial orbital wall injury include dehiscence of the lamina papyracea and abnormal configuration of the middle meatus. The latter can result from a reduced size of either the maxillary or the ethmoid sinus, from an exceeding lateral bending of the uncinate process, from a large concha bullosa or from a paradoxical middle turbinate (SALIB et al. 2001). In these cases, the medial orbital wall and the maxillary sinus ostium are not aligned on a vertical plane, as it occurs normally (BOLGER et al. 1990; MAY et al.

1990; MEYERS and VALVASSORI 1998). This anatomic arrangement is reported to bring an increased risk of orbital damage.

The risk of orbital penetration and muscle injury is higher when an ethmoidectomy is performed, particularly in patients previously treated and/or with extensive nasal polyposis. In that case, disruption of the periosteum may facilitate the penetration of the orbit with possible damage to the muscles (ROUVIERE and PEYNEGRE 2000). Immediate CT may show the hematoma associated with the damaged muscle, where retraction of the stumps is less frequently imaged. Delayed MR study is indicated to precise the extent of the damage, which influences the type of reparative surgery (Fig. 11.1).

In the event that impairment/loss of vision is manifested on awakening, the association with proptosis indicates intraorbital hematoma, which requires emergency decompression of the orbit, high-dose steroid therapy and monitoring of visual acuity. Conversely, if proptosis is not present, impairment/loss of vision prompts an emergency CT, which can reveal damage to the lamina papyracea with displacement of bony fragments impinging the optic nerve or section of the optic nerve.

Both the anterior and posterior ethmoidal arteries run in thin osseous canals, which enter the lamina papyracea. Iatrogenic damage to the artery can lead to its retraction into the orbit, causing intraorbital hematoma. Because of its location and course, the anterior ethmoidal artery is more frequently injured than the posterior one. It may be that the posterior ethmoidal artery is closer to the optic nerve and that at its level, the orbital diameter is smaller, but damage to this artery is associated with an increased risk of optic nerve injury, possibly due to an earlier rise of intraorbital pressure, even in case of a little hematoma (HUDGINS 1993).

Post-operative evaluation of bone and soft tissue orbital damage requires axial and coronal or reformatted high quality images (i.e., those obtained with multislice CT). CT signs suggesting orbital penetration include: proptosis, effacement of fat tissue planes, orbital emphysema, retrobulbar hematoma, and distortion of the extraocular muscles or of the optic nerve (HUDGINS 1993; DUBRULLE et al. 2003). When evaluating the CT study, the radiologist should carefully trace the optic nerve from the posterior globe to the chiasm and accurately search for the presence of bony fragments.

If an infectious complication is suspected, contrast agent should be administered.

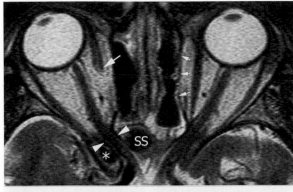
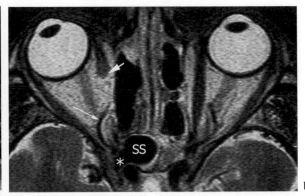
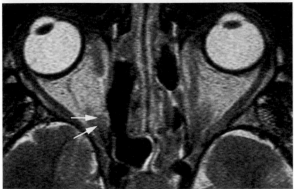

Fig. 11.1a-c. Iatrogenic laceration of right medial rectus occurred during ethmoidotomy. Postoperative axial TSE T2 axial sequences show the interruption of the muscle with the distal stump easily detectable (*short arrow on* **a** *and* **b**), while the proximal one is smaller and shorter (*white arrows on* **c**). The whole course of the right optic nerve is shown. *Arrowheads* (**a**) indicate the walls of the orbital canal. Pneumatization of right clinoid is present (*asterisk on* **a** *and* **b**). On the opposite side the lamina papyracea is clearly demonstrated (*short arrows on* **a**) as the air on the ethmoid side is partly replaced by mucosal thickening. Right sphenoid sinus (*SS*). Ophthalmic artery (*long arrow on* **b**)

Pre-operative CT is also relevant in preventing possible orbital damage. The radiologist should clearly warn about the presence of particular anatomic variants (Onodi Cell, anterior clinoid pneumatization, dehiscence of optic canal bony walls) which favor the occurrence of a direct optic nerve damage.

Damage to the anterior cranial fossa floor can result in *intracranial lesions,* which range from the acute onset of CSF leakage to the occurrence of a brain hematoma, tension pneumocephalus, encephalitis or meningo-encephalitis, abscess, cephalocele, damage to the anterior communicating or anterior cerebral artery, and death (ROUVIERE and PEYNEGRE 2000).

Most iatrogenic CSF leaks occur for a lesion at the level of the vertical portion of the cribriform plate, they should be immediately repaired during the same session (Fig. 11.2). Failure to control the leak or delayed onset (24-48 hours) eventually require cross sectional imaging (see chapter 7), which in very rare instances may also show the presence of a pneumocephalus (OPHIR et al. 1994; BENDET et al. 1995). Tension pneumocephalus can be detected by conventional x-ray imaging, though it is more accurately assessed by CT (or MR) (Fig. 11.3) (HUDGINS et al. 1992).

Injuries caused by penetration of instruments into the brain can range from local edema to sub-arach-noid hemorrhage, and may be associated with transitory or permanent neurological deficits or death. CT is the technique of choice to evaluate the patient in case of possible intracranial major complications, and to monitor the response to treatment of iatrogenic lesions.

Severe nasal bleeding, requiring transfusion, is infrequent and can occur during or just after the operation. It should be distinguished from a diffuse oozing, which is typical of patients with extensive polyposis or under treatment with aspirin.

Most common sources of bleeding are injuries to the internal maxillary artery branches (the spheno-palatine arteries feed turbinates and nasal septum) and the anterior and posterior ethmoidal arteries (STANKIEWICZ 1987).

Direct injury to the internal carotid artery rarely occurs, particularly in case of sphenoid sinus surgery (DUBRULLE et al. 2003). Angiography and endovascular procedures can be indicated in case surgery fails to control bleeding or a pseudoaneurysm develops.

Among minor orbital complications requiring imaging is the development of epiphora. This is caused by a lesion of the nasolacrimal duct (with subsequent development of stenosis or occlusion), which usually occurs while enlarging anteriorly the natural maxillary sinus ostium. Once epiphora devel-

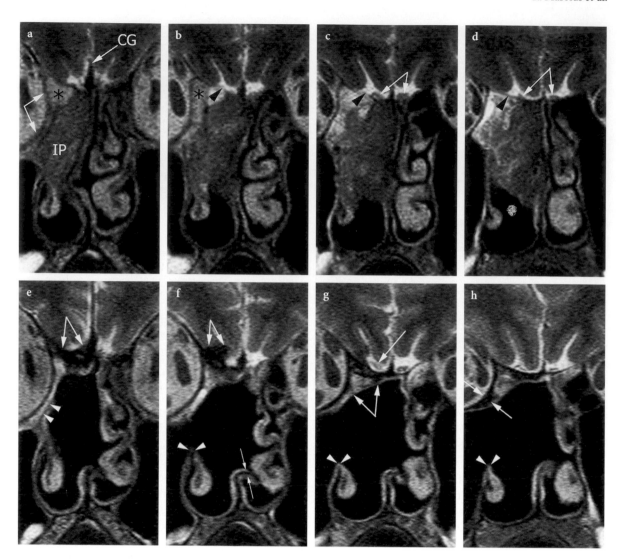

Fig. 11.2 a-h Iatrogenic damage to the dura with CSF leak treated in the same session. **a-d** Preoperative TSE T2 coronal images show an inverted papilloma (*IP*) occupying the right ethmoid and part of the nasal fossa. The tumor abuts the horizontal and part of the vertical laminae of the cribriform plate. Retention of mucus with intermediate intensity within an anterior ethmoid cell facing both the lamina papyracea (*white arrow* on **a**) and ethmoid roof (*asterisk* on **a** and **b**). The hypointense interface is identified on all planes (*arrowheads* on b-d). The olfactory bulbs (*white arrows* on **c**) and tracts (*white arrows* on **d**) are detailed. **e-h** Postoperative TSE T2 coronal images. Underlay technique was used by placing graft material (bone from the nasal septum) between the dura and the skull base (*double arrows* on **e** and **f**). Extensive resection of the nasal septum is demonstrated (*opposite arrows* on **f**). A right ethmoidotomy with middle antrostomy and total resection of the horizontal uncinate process was also performed (*arrowheads* on **f** to **h**). Normal thickening of the mucosa investing the right lamina papyracea (*arrowheads* on **e**) and ethmoid roof (*arrows* on **g**). No signal consistent with residual/relapsing inverted papilloma beneath the healed mucosa. Right olfactory bulb (*long arrow* on **g**) has a brighter signal. No abnormality of the gray and white matter is seen. **h** Mild bone thickening of the medial orbital wall is demonstrated (*opposite arrows*).

ops, exploration of the duct may be attempted by an ophthalmologist. If unsuccessful, dacryocystography is generally indicated to differentiate stenosis from total occlusion, and to identify the level of the occlusion. Recanalization and dilatation of the duct with balloon dacryocystoplasty may be attempted before going to an endoscopic dacryocystorhinostomy (Metson et al. 1994; Janssen et al. 1997).

11.3
Imaging After Microendoscopic Surgery

Although microendoscopic sinus surgery is mainly performed in the treatment of inflammatory diseases, in the last two decades the indications have been expanded to include most benign lesions of the sinonasal tract (Schick et al. 2001; Tomenzoli et al.

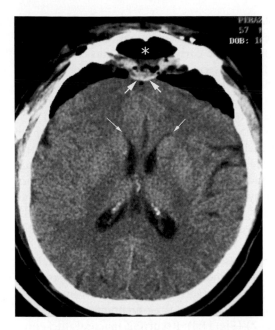

Fig. 11.3. Tension pneumocephalus secondary to anterior craniofacial resection. Increased intracranial pressure is suspected because of the amount of intradural gas and the presence of signs indicating compression of the anterior part of brain: bilateral reduced size of the frontal ventricles (*long arrows*). Part of the meningo-galeal complex is seen (*short arrows*). A residual frontal sinus cavity is filled by air (*asterisk*)

2004), nasopharynx (ROGER et al. 2002; NICOLAI et al. 2003), and even selected cases of early malignant tumors (STAMMBERGER et al. 1999; GOFFART et al. 2000).

As a consequence, both the indications to follow patients with cross sectional imaging and the choice between CT and MR greatly differ, depending on the nature of the treated lesion, and on the patient's characteristics. Since only a few malignant neoplasms are treated by endonasal surgery, the normal appearance and patterns of local recurrence after microendoscopic sinus surgery will be included in the section dealing with post treatment imaging of malignant lesions. The present section will specifically focus on the follow up of inflammatory lesions and expansile lesions (including benign neoplasms).

11.3.1
Inflammatory Diseases

Which are the indications for CT after microendoscopic sinus surgery for rhinosinusitis?

Since CT implies patient's irradiation – though minimal, but very often to a young subject - it should

be only used when the data provided is expected to influence medical decision.

Unfortunately, discordances have been reported between patient's referred symptoms and CT findings. In a series of patients examined by CT before and 3 months after microendoscopic surgery, MANTONI et al. (1996) reported that regardless the very modest objective improvement observed at CT, up to 91% of patients found clinical relief of symptoms. That means that both negative and positive CT studies can result unrelated to patient status (LEVINE 1990).

Given these limitations, relapsing sinogenic headache, which is a possible, frequent indication, should be carefully evaluated by the clinician to confirm that it is likely to origin from recurrent inflammatory sinus disease, before asking for a follow up CT examination. A key feature for the diagnosis of sinogenic headache is the demonstration of purulent discharge coming from on or more sinuses. Clearer indications to follow up CT are represented by persisting symptoms, recurrent acute or chronic rhinosinusitis, recurrent polyposis with nasal obstruction or infection requiring surgical revision (LEVINE 1990).

It is important to note that in patients treated for nasal polyposis, symptoms tend to recur more frequently - up to 40% (KENNEDY 1992) of cases - than in those operated on for rhinosinusitis without nasal polyposis. Therefore, two groups of patients will be considered in the analysis of post treatment imaging for inflammatory disease.

Finally, whilst follow up CT can result unrelated to patient's clinical status, data obtained by pre-operative CT is predictive of the probability of relapse (FRIEDMAN et al. 1995; STEWART et al. 2000).

11.3.1.1
Imaging After Endonasal Surgery for Rhinosinusitis Without Nasal Polyposis

Despite restoration of sinus ventilation, diffuse thickening of the mucosa may persist for some months at CT in patients treated for rhinosinusitis without nasal polyposis, even in case of improvement of symptoms (MANTONI et al. 1996).

In this group of patients, recurrent symptoms occur in about 4% to 8% of cases. Synechiae and scar formation - particularly between the lateral nasal wall and the middle turbinate or the nasal septum - are the most frequent causes (RAYNAL et al. 1999). Inadequate drainage of frontal or maxillary sinus may develop.

Patients are usually clinically evaluated with endoscopy, first. If a surgical revision is considered, or a retention mucocele, or an infectious complication are suspected, CT is required.

The CT protocol does not differ from the pre-operative study; contrast agent administration can be required on suspect of an infectious complication. Information regarding the symptoms or signs for which CT is required should be accurately matched with imaging findings.

Imaging interpretation should begin with a detailed description of the anatomic structures partially or completely resected, one side after the other.

Knowledge of the basic aspects (which structure/s was/were resected, in which sequence, for which purpose) related to the five main microendoscopic surgical procedures (uncinectomy; middle antrostomy; ethmoidotomy; sphenoidotomy; clearance of the frontal recess) is essential for a proper interpretation (see chapter 5, section 5.2).

Of course, the extent of bony framework resection performed during the different microendoscopic procedures may vary, according to the specific needs of each patient. Moreover, healing of soft tissues is quite unpredictable.

Soft tissue thickening should be thoroughly evaluated and reported. Unfortunately, CT does not permit to distinguish (KATSANTONIS et al. 1990) between scar, fibrosis, and inflamed mucosa. Since sinus ventilation is related to the patency of natural or surgically-created openings, a practical suggestion is to consider abnormal any soft tissue thickening which reduces or blocks sinus openings. Consequently, any thickening in the corresponding sinus cavity should be considered secondary to stenosis or obstruction. Specific attention should be given to the status of frontal and sphenoid sinuses, which are less readily accessible to endoscopy (DUBRULLE et al. 2003).

As for the pre-operative CT, careful assessment of the integrity of the lamina papyracea, the cribriform plate, the ethmoid roof and sphenoid walls should be provided. Anatomic variants of structures uninvolved by previous surgery and predisposing to an increased risk of intraoperative complications to the optic nerve and carotid artery should be reported as well.

In patients with recurrent symptoms, the most common CT findings include focal or diffuse thickening of mucosa (CHU et al. 1997) either in presence or absence of predisposing anatomic variants (see chapter 2) (Fig. 11.4). Recurrent mucosal thickening is reported to decrease in frequency from anterior ethmoid to maxillary sinus, posterior ethmoid, and to frontal sinus (VLEMING et al. 1993; CHU et al. 1997). Particular attention should be paid to the appearance of the middle turbinate, which is a key structure in the ethmoid. Management of the middle turbinate during ethmoid surgery is one of the major sources of debates among rhinosurgeons. An unstable residual middle turbinate may result from resection

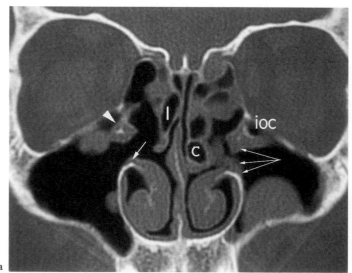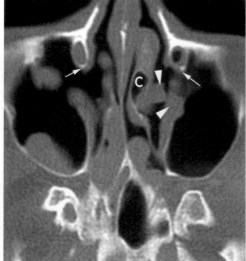

a   b

Fig. 11.4a,b. Bilateral relapsing rhinosinusitis without polyposis since one year. Coronal (**a**) and axial (**b**) CT. The patient was treated with bilateral uncinectomy, right ethmoidotomy. (**a**) Absence of the uncinate process on right side (*short arrow*). Clinically recurrent disease is associated with mild mucosal thickening around the walls of bilateral residual infraorbital cells (*arrowhead on right side; ioc on the left*) and at the surgically created opening of left maxillary sinus (*long arrows*). Concha bullosa is detected on left side (*c*), lamellar concha (*l*) on the right one. **b** The axial plane shows resection of both uncinate processes (*arrows*) and mild recurrent mucosal thickening more pronounced in the left middle meatus (*arrowheads*)

of the inferior part of the ground lamella, eventually entailing a high risk of lateralization and secondary closure of frontal recess and maxillary ostium (CHU et al. 1997; SAIDI et al. 1998) (Fig. 11.5).

After uncinectomy, a variable part of the medial wall of the ethmoid infundibulum is lacking in relation to the extent of uncinate process resection. Synechiae and scars are frequently seen at the level of the natural maxillary sinus ostium, especially in case of subtotal resection of the uncinate process (CHAMBERS et al. 1997). After middle antrostomy, CT commonly shows that the ostium has been enlarged posteriorly at the expense of the posterior fontanelle, to preserve the anterior lining which is close to the naso-lacrimal duct.

After ethmoidotomy, the variable resection of ethmoid cells can result in a large common cavity, in which the presence of any residual cell should be reported, as these cells account for most microendoscopic sinus surgery failures (KATSANTONIS et al. 1990).

Sagittal reformatted images are important to evaluate if recurrent mucosal disease in the ethmoid sinus involves the frontal recess and causes stenosis or blockage, or to detect recurrent frontal sinus disease (Fig. 11.6). Causes of frontal sinus obstruction after endonasal surgery include residual agger nasi, supraorbital, or frontal cells, obstruction of the infundibulum ethmoidalis, or of the frontal recess itself.

In case of previous frontal recess clearance, normal ventilation is expected, particularly after extensive endonasal surgery as for Draf's type III median drainage (DRAF et al. 1995). On coronal CT, imaging findings of Draf's III procedure include resection of the antero-superior portion of the nasal septum together with the intersinus septum and of the floor of both frontal sinuses, resulting in a wide common drainage for both frontal sinuses (Fig. 11.7).

As sphenoidotomy can be performed via transnasal or transethmoid approach, post surgical changes may be quite different (Fig. 11.8). Microendoscopic surgery may be indicated in case of complications secondary to transsphenoidal resection of hypophyseal neoplasms. Rarely, relevant sclerotic changes of the bony walls develop after transsphenoidal approach, similar to those observed in the maxillary sinus after intraoral antrostomy (Caldwell Luc's procedure) (Fig. 11.9).

Mucoceles can develop from chronic obstruction of sinuses, more frequently they arise from frontal recess or anterior ethmoid sinus (Fig. 11.10).

11.3.1.2
Imaging After Endonasal Surgery for Rhinosinusitis With Nasal Polyposis

Recurrent polyposis is characterized by the presence of polyps in the nasal cavity after previous surgical removal of polyps. If medical treatment fails to control the progression of the relapsing disease and related symptoms, surgical revision may be necessary. In this setting, it is important to note that the useful anatomical landmarks such as the middle turbinate and the uncinate process may be absent. Moreover, critical bony structures which line the sinonasal tract – particularly the lamina papyracea and the ethmoid roof – are often abnormal secondary to compression and distortion by polyps or to previous surgery, and may present significant bony dehiscences (ROUVIERE and PEYNEGRE 2000).

In that case, the surgical approach entails a high risk of orbital or intracranial complications or of significant nasal bleeding. Apart from a thorough documentation of previous treatment, particularly of the complications occurred, CT examination is mandatory. However, since CT does not distinguish between polyps, scar and inflammatory thickening of mucosa, it cannot replace clinical examination for the identification of early recurrent disease (BATTEUR et al. 1994). Nevertheless, data provided by CT is useful to assess the extent of disease, and it is particularly relevant to detail the status of sinonasal tract bony framework (i.e., the presence of thickened or dehiscent areas).

According to the clinical findings and to the extent of the relapsing disease demonstrated by endoscopic examination and CT, recurrent nasal polyposis may be grouped into three patterns, all requiring different treatments (ROUVIERE and PEYNEGRE 2000).

Limited recurrence usually develops after few months or within two years from primary surgery. When asymptomatic, it is detected during clinical follow up. Onset of anosmia, even transitory, may arouse the suspect of recurrent disease. Limited recurrence may be associated with two different endoscopic patterns: *localized polyposis* and *polypoid edema*. The former, which is less frequent; prevalently involves the anterior ethmoid (Fig. 11.11); the latter, which is usually addressed at endoscopy as "cobblestone appearance", is more often observed. In this case, the entire sagittal extent of the ethmoid mucosa is involved. Limited recurrent polyposis can be treated either by medical therapy or by endonasal surgery.

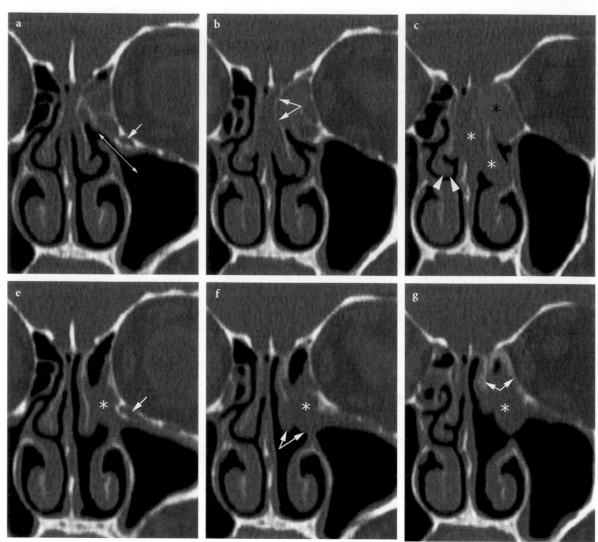

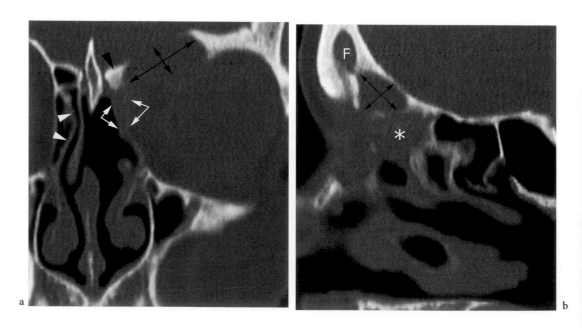

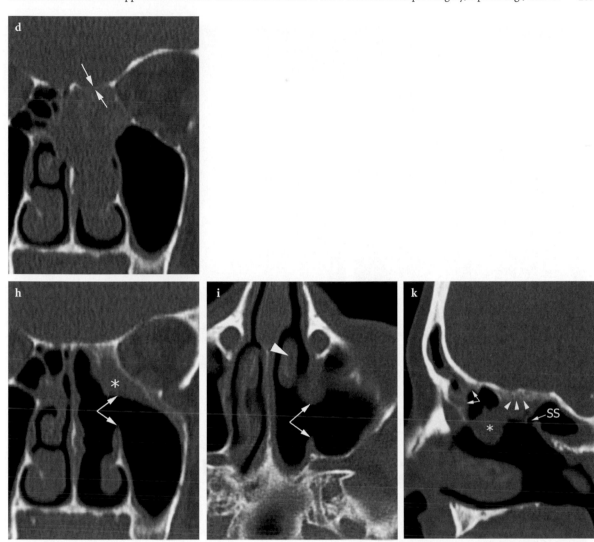

Fig. 11.5a-k. The 57 years old female patient complained of left nasal obstruction for one year. **a-d** Coronal preoperative refor-matted images (multislice CT)show a left ethmoid polypoid lesion filling ethmoid cells (*short arrow in* **a** *indicates a small infraorbital cell*) but sparing (**a**) the ethmoid infundibulum (*double arrowheads arrow*). **b** Medial displacement of middle turbinate is present (*arrows*). **c** High densities within the ethmoid part of the lesion (*black asterisk*) suggest association with mycotic disease. The pol-ypoid thickening of the mucosa extends into the nasal fossa, between middle turbinate and septum (*white asterisks*) parodoxically curved middle turbinate (*arrowheads*). **d** Focal dehiscence of left ethmoid roof is demonstrated (*opposite arrows*). **e-h** Postoperative reformatted images (multislice CT) obtained for recurrent sinogenic headache. Microendoscopic procedure included left uncinectomy, ethmoidotomy, middle antrostomy and subtotal resection of the middle turbinate. Medially to the residual middle turbinate relevant mucosal thickening (*asterisk*) occupies the ex-middle meatus/anterior ethmoid area. Thickening is located laterally to the infraorbital cell (*arrow in* **e**), extends posteriorly between lateral nasal wall and residual middle turbinate (*arrows in* **f** *and* **g**) with a minimal re-duction in size of the middle antrostomy (*arrows in* **h**). Focal bone thickening of the residual vertical lamella of the middle turbinate and of the lamina papyracea is seen in **g**. Site and extent of middle antrostomy are shown (*arrows in* **i**). Part of the residual middle turbinate is seen (*arrowhead*). **k** Apart from projecting into middle meatus, mucosal thickening (*asterisk*) is associated with partial involvement of the frontal recess (*arrows*). Bone thickening of the residual portion of middle turbinate (*arrowheads*). Sphenoid sinus (*SS*) and sphenoethmoid recess (*arrow*)

◁ ◁ **Fig. 11.6a,b.** Recurrent fronto-ethmoid mucocele after microendoscopic surgery: left uncinectomy, ethmoidotomy and subtotal resection of middle turbinate. **a** CT in coronal plane shows the frontal component of the mucocele (*black arrows*), which reab-sorbs the surrounding bone. Reactive sclerosis of the ethmoid roof is present (*black arrowheads*). A synechia is seen between residual middle turbinate and lateral nasal wall (*white arrows*). Nasal septum was partially resected. By comparison, on the opposite side the vertical portion of the uncinate process is intact (*white arrowhead*). **b** Mucosal thickening obstructing the frontal recess (*asterisk*) explains the development of the mucocele, whose ethmoidal component (*black arrows*) is clearly seen in the sagittal reformatted CT. Blocked frontal sinus (*F*)

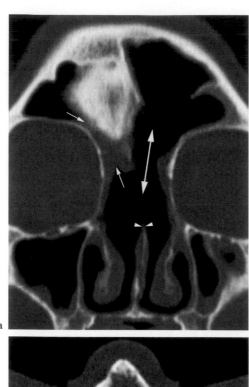

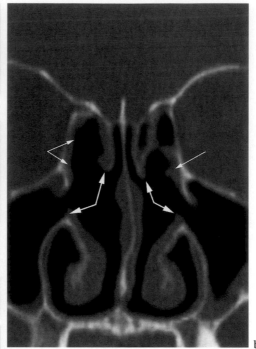

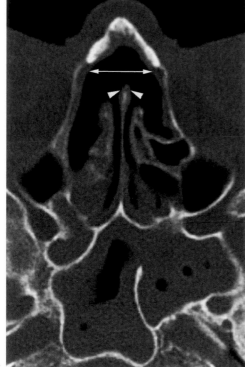

Fig. 11.7a-c. Postoperative CT. After Draf III median's drainage a large surgical opening of the floor of frontal sinuses was obtained (*double arrowheads arrow*). On left side minimal mucosa thickening is seen. Though a mild mucosal thickening is present on right side (*arrows*), the sinus is normally ventilated. Residual portion of the nasal septum (*arrowheads*). **b** Bilateral uncinectomy and subtotal middle turbinectomy (*thick arrows*) is demonstrated. No significant mucosal thickening post bilateral ethmoidotomy (*thin arrows*). **c** The axial CT plane show the anterior partial resection of nasal septum performed in the Draf III procedure (*arrowheads*) to obtain a large common anterior chamber (*double arrowheads arrow*). Mucosal thickening in the sphenoid sinuses is present

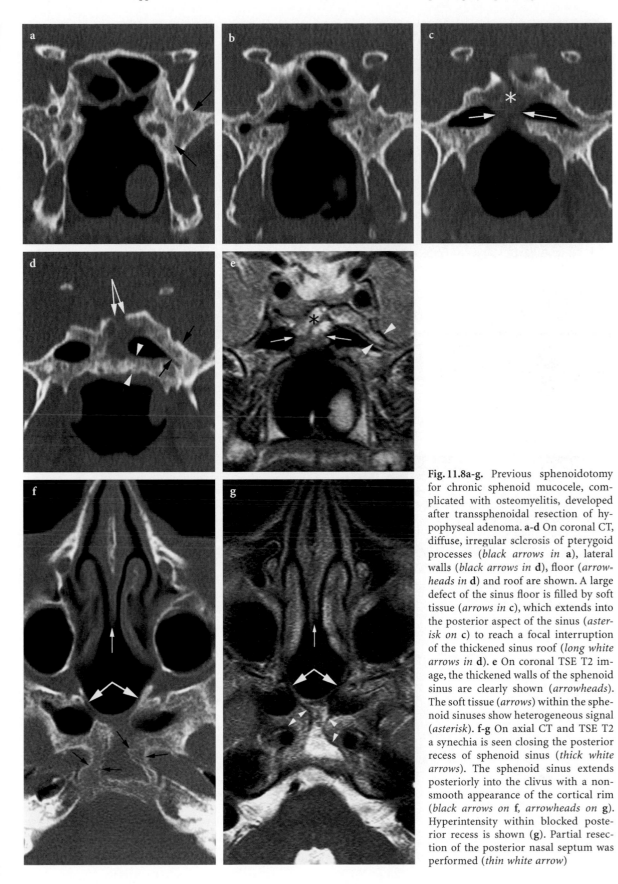

Fig. 11.8a-g. Previous sphenoidotomy for chronic sphenoid mucocele, complicated with osteomyelitis, developed after transsphenoidal resection of hypophyseal adenoma. **a-d** On coronal CT, diffuse, irregular sclerosis of pterygoid processes (*black arrows in* **a**), lateral walls (*black arrows in* **d**), floor (*arrowheads in* **d**) and roof are shown. A large defect of the sinus floor is filled by soft tissue (*arrows in* **c**), which extends into the posterior aspect of the sinus (*asterisk on* **c**) to reach a focal interruption of the thickened sinus roof (*long white arrows in* **d**). **e** On coronal TSE T2 image, the thickened walls of the sphenoid sinus are clearly shown (*arrowheads*). The soft tissue (*arrows*) within the sphenoid sinuses show heterogeneous signal (*asterisk*). **f-g** On axial CT and TSE T2 a synechia is seen closing the posterior recess of sphenoid sinus (*thick white arrows*). The sphenoid sinus extends posteriorly into the clivus with a nonsmooth appearance of the cortical rim (*black arrows on* **f**, *arrowheads on* **g**). Hyperintensity within blocked posterior recess is shown (**g**). Partial resection of the posterior nasal septum was performed (*thin white arrow*)

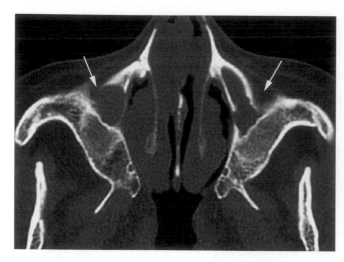

Fig. 11.9. Previous bilateral intraoral antrostomy (Caldwell Luc's procedure) for nasal polyposis. Marked reactive enlargement of posterolateral maxillary sinus walls with thick spongiotic bone. Sinus cavity is quite small and fills by soft tissue. Retraction of the anterior walls is appreciated (*arrows*)

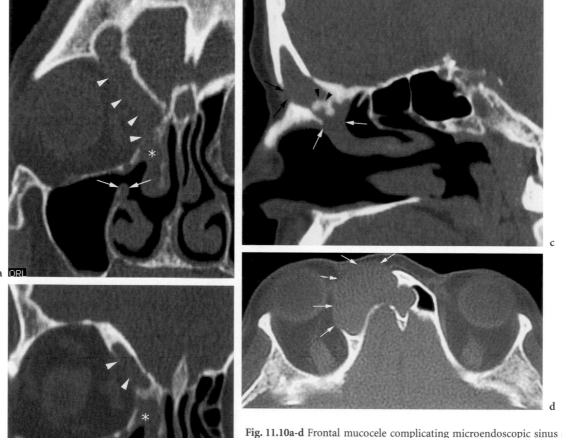

Fig. 11.10a-d Frontal mucocele complicating microendoscopic sinus surgery (right uncinectomy and ethmoidotomy). **a-b** On coronal CT, a mucosal thickening (*asterisk*) occupies the space between middle turbinate and lateral nasal wall to continue on adjacent maxillary sinus roof (synechia). The medial orbital wall and the roof are reabsorbed (*arrowheads*). Soft tissue density occupies the frontal sinus. Uncinectomy (*white arrows*). **c** On sagittal plane the frontal recess is occupied by soft tissue (synechia, *white arrows*). Bone thickening of the walls of a residual cell close to frontal ostium is present (*arrowheads*). Focal erosion of the anterior wall of the frontal sinus is indicated (*black arrows*). **d** The large frontal mucocele causes remodelling and reabsorption of the sinus wall (*arrows*) and lateral displacement of the globe.

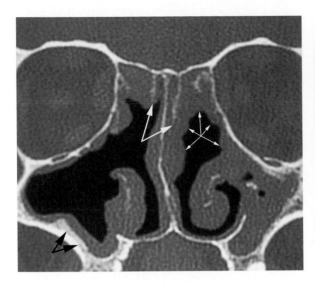

Fig. 11.11. Limited recurrent polyposis. Polypoid-lining soft tissue thickening in the large nasal cavities, more evident on the left side (*thin white arrows*). On both sides the residual vertical lamella of the middle turbinate is detected (*thick white arrows*). A synechia between the left one and septum is probably present. Chronic inflammatory bone reaction in the right maxillary sinus floor is shown (*black arrows*)

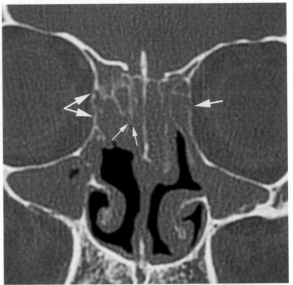

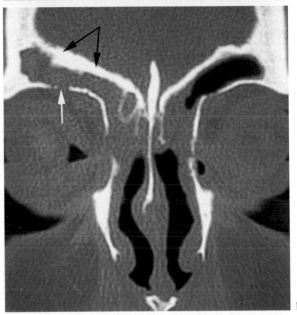

Fig. 11.12a,b. Widespread recurrent polyposis in both ethmoids with partial resorption of right middle turbinate, which (**a**) appears "truncated" (*short arrows*). Mild lateral bowing of both medial orbital walls is a typical finding secondary to chronic pressure of the growing polyps (*thick arrows*). **b** CT cannot distinguish polyps from thickened mucosa. Bilateral soft tissue thickening without polypoid appearance occupies the frontal sinus ostia; on right side it is associated with both thickening of bone (roof of the sinus, *black arrows*) and focal erosions (floor of the sinus *white arrow*)

In case of *widespread recurrence*, the entire ethmoid is occupied by polyps which, extending into the nasal cavity, compress and distort the middle turbinate or other residual bony landmarks. Truncation of the middle turbinate may be observed on CT examination (LIANG et al. 1996) (Fig. 11.12, 11.13). This form of recurrent polyposis usually requires aggressive surgery, such as total ethmoidectomy, which consists in the removal of all bony lamellae and mucosa of the ethmoid, resulting in nasalization of the sinuses (JANKOWSKI et al. 1997).

The third pattern refers to the recurrence of polyposis combined with iatrogenic lesions, as the development of synechiae causing stenosis. The most serious and common complication is the stenosis of the frontal recess, which may eventually result in a frontal or fronto-ethmoidal mucocele. More rarely, stenosis of the sphenoid sinus occurs.

Apart from recurrent severe mucosal and polypoid thickening and possible middle turbinate truncation, dense sclerotic new bone formation appears as a typical feature of patients who have undergone repeated microendoscopic sinus surgery for nasal polyposis. Bony changes may be widespread or focal. On CT, a proper bone window is necessary to correctly assess abnormalities (Fig. 11.10, 11.12). Since several findings suggesting chronic osteomyelitis have been demonstrated by histopathologic studies in patients with recurrent nasal polyposis, the hypothesis of recurrent sinusitis sustained by bone infection has been advanced, but not confirmed (KENNEDY et al. 1998).

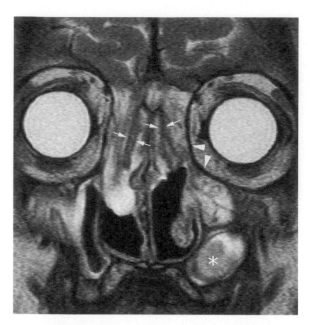

Fig. 11.13. Widespread recurrent polyposis associated with left maxillary sinus mucocele (*asterisk*) arising within a concameration. On TSE T2 coronal image, the polyps show various signal intensity, probably reflecting different degrees of edema. The hypointensity of the bony laminae of the middle turbinate permits their identification (*white arrows*). Thickening of the hypointense medial orbital wall suggests reactive bone (*arrowheads*)

11.3.2
Expansile and Benign Lesions

The most common expansile non-inflammatory lesions and non-malignant neoplasms treated by microendoscopic sinus surgery include inverted papilloma and juvenile angiofibroma. In both lesions, a large cavity usually results after surgical resection, facilitating the survey of the mucosal surface. On the other hand, the two lesions differ in the patterns of relapsing or persistent disease. Since inverted papilloma develops from mucosa, recurrences tend to be recognized early by endoscopic examination. Therefore, imaging is indicated only to detail the extent towards not assessable areas, either because extramucosal (anterior cranial fossa, orbit), blocked (by the tumor or by post surgical synechiae) (PETIT et al. 2000), or located in less easily accessible areas as the frontal sinus. Conversely, juvenile angiofibroma is a submucosal lesion, which relapse (i.e., the growth of residual disease) is often subclinical, and, as a consequence, detected earlier by follow up imaging than by clinical examination. Less frequently, relapse is suspected because of the onset of new symptoms or the presence of indirect signs, such as submucosal

bulging. Not only is imaging required to identify the submucosal growth of a residual lesion into diploic bone, or intracranially, or into the masticator space, but it is also essential either to detail the extent of disease or to monitor its progression (NICOLAI et al. 2003).

Furthermore, MR is the imaging technique recommended in the follow up of both inverted papilloma and juvenile angiofibroma, although with different roles: to integrate a diagnosis already obtained by endoscopy in the inverted papilloma; to be the mainstay follow up tool, in case of juvenile angiofibroma. In addition, MR is preferable because it avoids patient's irradiation, particularly in case of juvenile angiofibroma. Nevertheless, in those patients who undergo CT, post treatment changes are quite similar to those observed in the group of patients treated for rhinosinusitis without nasal polyposis. Major differences are given more extended resections, which is frequently required by expansile and benign lesions.

Detailed analysis of imaging findings suggestive of recurrent inverted papilloma or persisting juvenile angiofibroma are reported in chapter 8, in section 8.3.6 and 8.4.6, respectively.

Apart from the peculiar features of these two lesions, the interpretation of follow up MR studies requires the knowledge of the normal appearance of sinonasal structures after endonasal surgery so that post-operative changes can be distinguished from recurrences.

As after microendoscopic sinus surgery for inflammatory lesions, a variable number of bony structures appears partially or totally resected. Differently from CT, only high resolution MR images may identify the hypointense signal indicating the bony wall, which is more easily detected on condition that mucosa, mucus, or fat separate the wall from air (see chapter 4) (MAROLDI et al. 1999).

Unlike CT, the reactive changes of mucosa are more easily distinguished from fibrosis on MR. A key point is the presence of signals consistent with fluid within the thickened, inflamed mucosa. As a general rule, the abnormal mucosa appears hyperintense on T2 sequences, hypointense on plain T1, and shows a thin and regular rim enhancement on post contrast T1 images (Fig. 11.14). The signal pattern of retained secretions within the sinusal cavity is also important. It is related to the composition of the entrapped fluid. On MR, an inverse correlation is observed between protein concentration and T2 signal, resulting in signal hypointensity in case of "old" dehydrated mucus, which has a high protein concentration. On plain T1 sequence, signal rises to a maximal hyperintensity

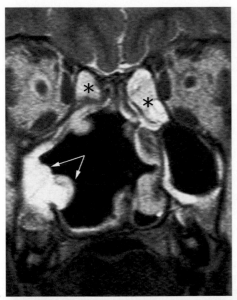

a

Fig. 11.14a-c. Follow up of juvenile angiofibroma 4 months after resection of a large lesion via microendoscopic surgery. **a** Coronal TSE T2. A wide naso-ethmoid cavity results after surgery. Persistent post treatment changes are characterized by relevant and asymmetric thickening of mucosa, especially in the right maxillary sinus cavity (*arrows*). Bright edematous mucosa fills the spared posterior ethmoid cells (*asterisks*). The edematous mucosa *in* the sphenoid floor (*single asterisk*), and in the residual right maxillary sinus cavity (*double asterisks*) has bright signal on TSE T2 (**b**), internal non-enhancing core and peripheral enhancing rim of variable thickness on post contrast T1 (**c**). The thick lining of right choana (*1*) is flatter, hypointense on TSE T2, and slightly enhances on T1, indicating non-mature scar. Conversely, the residual turbinate abutting the left nasal wall (*2*) shows the typical bright enhancement. On TSE T2 a clear separation of scar from masticator space is traced by a hypointense linear signal (*long arrows* on **b** and **c**). While the residual posterolateral maxillary sinus wall is clearly detected on TSE T2, both the sinusal wall and the hypointense linear signal enhance on T1, indicating, respectively, inflammation and persistent vascularization. This immature scar tissue replaces fat within the masticator space (*3*) and surrounds (*S*) a distorted medial pterygoid muscle (*white arrowheads on* **b**, *black arrowheads on* **c**). Focal enhancement within residual posterolateral maxillary sinus wall can suggest granuloma (*black arrow*)

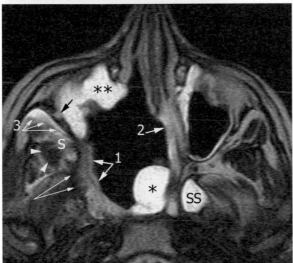

b

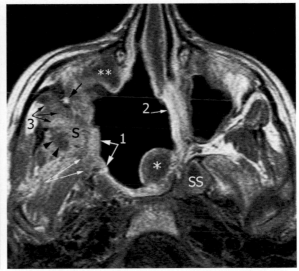

c

at about 40% protein concentration, and then progressively decreases to hypointensity (Som et al. 1989).

If the lesion previously extended beyond the bony boundaries of the sinonasal tract, the scar tissue replacing tumor at the involved site or developed at the edge with adjacent structures - orbit, pterygopalatine fossa, masticator space – over the time usually undergoes changes in thickness and signal pattern,. Progressive reduction in tissue thickness is observed, often combined with the tendency to assume a less convex and flatter shape (retraction). After months, and mostly within one year, scar tissue appears more or less hypointense on both T1 and T2 and should not enhance on MR after contrast agent administration (Fig. 11.15) (Gong et al. 1991).

Likewise open surgery, radical excision of the benign lesion has to be achieved by the microendoscopic approach to fulfil the principles of oncologic surgery. This requires a careful dissection of lesions along the subperiosteal plane, on condition that no sign of bony resorption is present. Resection of the underlying bone is needed whenever cross sectional imaging suggests bony thinning or resorption. Subtotal drilling of thick bones, especially the pterygoid process, is frequently associated with development of sclerosis, which appears as a diffuse, heterogeneous hypointensity on both T2 and plain T1 sequences. Similarly to the signal behavior of fibrotic tissue, absence of enhancement should rule out intraosseous recurrences. Fat saturation sequences improve MR sensitivity.

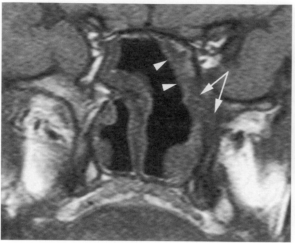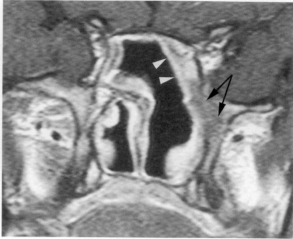

a

b

Fig. 11.15a,b, Follow up of juvenile angiofibroma one year after microendoscopic surgery. Resection of left middle turbinate, sphenoid sinus floor is noted. **a** On pre-contrast T1 image, thickening of the mucosa along the lateral wall of the sphenoid sinus and the choana (*arrowheads*) is seen. The resected left pterygoid process has been replaced by hypointense signal (*white arrows*), which on post-contrast T1 image (**b**) does not show any significant enhancement (*black arrows*), appearing clearly hypointense when compared with the adjacent enhancing mucosa (*arrowheads*)

11.4
Imaging After Treatment of Malignant Neoplasms

In the follow up of malignant neoplasms of the sinonasal tract, the main purpose of imaging consists in detecting early and late complications due to treatment, and persisting or relapsing lesions. If time is taken as the keynote, clinical problems are ordered into three different periods: an immediate post-operative phase (hours to day/s); an intermediate phase (weeks to few months); a late phase (months to years).

11.4.1
Clinical Issues in the Immediate Postoperative and Intermediate Phases

Clinical problems arising in the immediate post-operative and in the intermediate phase are usually largely dependent on the type of surgery performed. In general, limited resections are less prone to cause relevant complications. Conversely, extended procedures with wide tissue resection and complex reconstruction, as anterior craniofacial resection, give more frequently rise to severe complications. Similarly to what occurs after microendoscopic surgery, only a minority of early complications requires imaging studies. Among the most frequent ones are those which involve the brain or the orbit: brain edema or hemorrhage, de-

hiscences of the duraplasty of the restored anterior cranial fossa floor, tension pneumocephalus, thrombophlebitis, meningitis, exophthalmos (RICHTSMEIER et al. 1992; CATALANO et al. 1994).

CT is the technique of choice, as the examination time is reduced, permitting to study even poorly cooperative patients. Only in case a brain stem lesion is suspected, or the detailed extent of an intracranial venous thrombosis is required, is MR indicated.

11.4.2
Clinical Issues in the Late Phase

The most common clinical problems arising months to years from surgery, radiation therapy, or chemotherapy include late inflammatory complications, more often mucoceles caused by synechiae limiting or blocking sinus drainage, and persistent or recurrent malignant neoplasm.

In the late phase, the onset or the worsening of symptoms or signs is particularly relevant. More specifically, it is important to know how symptoms developed and which progression curve over the time they had. In fact, for a similar symptom or sign, different lesions can be inferred according to these issues. A trismus, which develops during radiation treatment, and gets progressively worse for months after the end of RT, is probably caused by radiation damage to masticator space structures, and needs an imaging study to rule out osteonecrosis of the mandible. Conversely, the onset of progressive trismus some months after treatment suggests recurrent disease.

Furthermore, the presence of a subcutaneous or submucosal (endoscopic finding) mass, the onset of pain (headache, neuralgia), or neurologic/ophthalmologic signs are clear indications for an anticipated follow up imaging study.

When designing a strategy for following up patients treated for malignant sinonasal tract neoplasms, two critical issues should be thoroughly considered.

- Apart from rare histotypes, the rate of nodal metastases is very low. On the other hand, the probability of systemic metastases is not negligible, with lung, liver and bone accounting for the most frequently involved sites. The biological aggressiveness of the different tumors is usually expressed by the course of the disease: undifferentiated carcinoma and squamous cell carcinoma are very aggressive, with early metastasization, whereas adenoid cystic carcinoma has a much slower progression, but it eventually spreads locally along nerves, and very often gives metastases to the lung.
- Submucosal recurrence is frequently undetected at clinical examination or endoscopy. When symptoms develop or a submucosal mass is suspected, the recurrent tumor is usually rather advanced.

Therefore, the critical goal of cross sectional imaging consists in detecting sub-clinical recurrences, and differentiate relapsing disease from late complications. Clinical assessment and cross sectional imaging play complementary roles (LELL et al. 2000; LOEVNER et al. 2002).

11.4.3
Imaging Strategies in the Follow-up

In general, the interpretation of post treatment CT or MR studies of the sinonasal tract can result quite challenging due to the changes induced by treatment (surgery, RT, chemotherapy). These consist of:

- changes in the anatomy due to surgical resection and reconstruction;
- presence of reactive mucosal changes, more pronounced than in rhinosinusitis because subperiosteal dissection is extensively required and irradiation effect is added;
- changes in density and signal intensity of tissues caused by the different treatments;

Overall, the compound of these elements greatly reduces the differences both in morphology and signal features (CT density or MR intensity) between the recurrent tumor and adjacent tissues. Clearly, MR is preferred to CT because contrast resolution is definitely superior, and – in this critical setting – any strategy capable of maximizing signal differences between recurrent lesion and surrounding tissue should be pursued. Given the fact that the differences in shape or signal are less relevant than in the preoperative MR, a second strategy is to record the new anatomy resulting from treatment to be used as baseline. Careful matching of baseline data with current imaging and clinical findings is certainly a key point in minimizing the chance of missing early relapsing lesions.

An interval of 3 to 4 months from surgery or radiotherapy is recommended in order to minimize the influence of post treatment inflammatory changes on the baseline study.

Timing of further follow up studies depends on post treatment outcome and tumor type. As a general rule, MR are scheduled every 4 months for the first two years, than twice a year until the fifth year after treatment. Adenoid cystic carcinoma and olfactory neuroblastoma usually requires a more prolonged follow up (BELY et al. 1997; LELL et al. 2000).

11.4.4
CT and MR Imaging Findings

One of the most critical factors affecting the effects of imaging studies on clinical decision during the follow up is the cooperation between the radiologist and the otorhinolaryngologist, the maxillo-facial surgeon, or the radiotherapist, which permits to access critical information. We consider indispensable conditions for interpreting CT or MR the following information:

- tumor type and extent prior to treatment;
- type of treatment. If surgery: type of approach, extent of resection, materials used for reconstruction. If radiation treatment: irradiation portals, boost areas, overall dose;
- areas at higher risk for persistent/recurrent disease, as intraoperatively assessed;
- post treatment course, complications;
- present symptoms and signs.

11.4.4.1
Normal Postoperative Imaging Changes

Surgical resection, reconstruction, and inflammatory tissue reaction account for three main categories of post-operative imaging changes.

Changes secondary to resection can be predicted based on the surgical report. However, the extent of each resection may vary, according to the actual spread of tumor. Acknowledge of variations from standard procedures helps to make a proper interpretation. For example, knowing that an ethmoido-maxillectomy required removal of the lamina papyracea because remodeled or invaded by tumor is important, as this variation accounts for a partial "collapse" into the nasal cavity of the orbital content (SOM et al. 1986a,b).

After orbital sparing surgical procedures entailing removal of a variable extent of orbital wall(s), enophthalmos or hypophthalmos can occur. Imaging may precise the status of the orbital walls (IMOLA and SCHRAMM 2002) (Fig. 11.16).

In extended resections and reconstructions, as in anterior craniofacial resection, one of the most important elements to be evaluated is the modality of restoring the separation of the inner cranium from the naso-ethmoidal cavity. In analyzing CT or MR follow up examinations, the assessment of these reconstructed interfaces is usually quite complex. The radiologist should know which materials have been used (dura mater, pericranium flap, in some cases bone or bone pâté), because duraplasty presents as a multiple-layer "sandwich" of signals (SCHUSTER et al. 1994; MAROLDI et al. 1997).

This meningo-galeal complex results from the need to remove a possibly invaded dura, along with the bony part of the anterior cranial fossa floor, and to restore the separation of cranium from nasal cavity. During anterior craniofacial resection, a small rectangle of dura (including the invaded area) is usually resected and replaced by autologous fascia lata or lyophilized dura. To obtain a better sealing and a more robust structure, a pedicled pericranium flap is used to reinforce the duraplasty and to offer a nicely vascularized barrier, which eventually divides the sinonasal tract from the cranium (OSGUTHORPE and PATEL 1995).

During the immediate post-operative phase, it is normal to observe a mild extradural air-fluid collection and a smaller intradural air collection on CT. Infrequently, a tension pneumocephalus may develop (Fig. 11.3) (WANAMAKER et al. 1995). Particular attention has to be given to even minimal frontal lobe lesions, though small contusions or mild edema may be considered expected findings (SOM et al. 1986b), but more extensive lesion may occur, yet sometimes asymptomatic since anosmia is a rule (Fig. 11.17). Months after surgery, the appearance of the meningo-galeal complex is characterized by a quite regular "plaque", 3-5 mm in thickness, which shows significant enhancement both on CT and on MR. Enhancement has been reported to be related to chronic inflammatory reaction and to increased vascularization of the dura.

A detailed evaluation of the overall extent of the meningo-galeal complex is obtained with sagittal MR

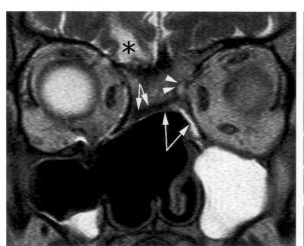
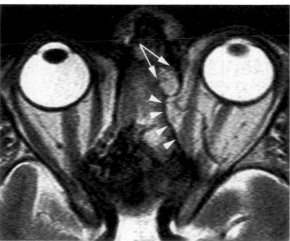

a   b

Fig. 11.16a,b. Follow up of ethmoid adenocarcinoma after anterior craniofacial resection. **a** On coronal TSE T2, bilateral medialization of medial orbital wall is seen. Dehiscence of left medial orbital wall with fat content (*arrowheads*) is present. A quite thick duraplasty has a linear hypointense inner signal in its lower aspect (possible autologous bone, *short arrows*). The duraplasty is invested on nasal surface by a thickened mucosa (*long arrows*). Post-surgical focal encephalomalacia is seen on right side (*asterisk*). **b** On axial TSE T2, the medial prolapse of left medial orbital wall results more evident (*arrowheads*). A small fluid collection faceting the anterior portion of left lamina papyracea is also present. The lesion has the potential to mucocele development (*arrows*)

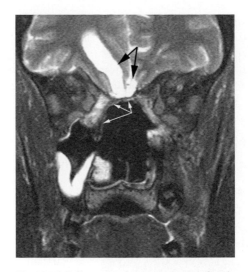

Fig. 11.17. Follow up of anterior craniofacial resection nine years after removal of an ethmoid recurrent inverted papilloma with foci of squamous cell carcinoma. The coronal Fat sat T2 image show two large cavities within the frontal lobes with fluid content (*black arrows*). Both reach the anterior cranial fossa floor. Quite regular lining of the nasal surface of the meningo-galeal complex is seen (*white arrows*)

sequences. By combining sagittal with coronal T2 and enhanced T1 images, a clear demonstration of the integration of the meningo-galeal complex with the adjacent dura is obtained (Fig. 11.18. 11.19). Moreover, its relationship with frontal bone, planum sphenoidale, and nasal cavity are detailed. On T2 sequences, the meningo-galeal complex has a continuous, thick, and quite regular hypointense signal. On high resolution post contrast T1, multiple layers with slightly different signals are usually detected. The whole complex of duraplasty can be disassembled into its singular components, which show different signal intensity. Moreover, the identification of the single components by their specific signal on MR sagittal and coronal planes help to differentiate the meningo-galeal complex from recurrent disease.

After extensive resection of the maxilla or of the orbit, the resulting large defect is reconstructed by means of a local or revascularized flap (muscular, myo-cutaneous, or fascio-cutaneous) (Fig. 11.20–11.23). Frequently, the temporalis muscle is used. The muscle can be easily recognized by identifying two

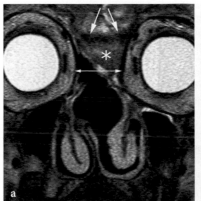
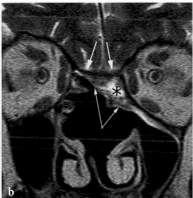
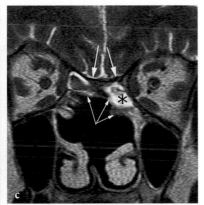

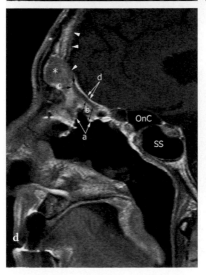

Fig. 11.18a-d. Follow up of anterior craniofacial resection one year after removal of a left ethmoid olfactory neuroblastoma. On coronal TSE T2 (**a-c**), the meningo-galeal complex is not cut perpendicularly on all images, therefore appearing with apparent different thickness and a more hypointense signal in the most anterior plane (**a**), because of the oblique course of the complex at this level (*asterisk*). For the same reason the superior limit of the complex has an unsharp appearance (*arrows*). Removal of the ethmoid associates with mild medial prolapse of the orbits (*double arrowheads arrow*). **b-c** The meningo-galeal complex has an asymmetric mild thickness, three main layers, which are all demonstrated only on the most perpendicular plane (**b,c**). The nasal mucosal lining (*thin arrows*) is quite hypointense and borders an intermediate layer with heterogeneous hyperintense signal (*asterisk*), which is limited superiorly by the inner layer (*thick arrows*), which faces the CSF. **d** On the contrast sagittal T1 plane, the meningo-galeal complex separable in its different components: nasal mucosa (*a*); intermediate layers (*b and c*), dura (*d*). At the integration with the posterior wall of the marsupialized frontal sinus (*asterisk*) the dura is thicker (*arrowheads*). Sphenoid sinus (*SS*), Onodi cell (*OnC*)

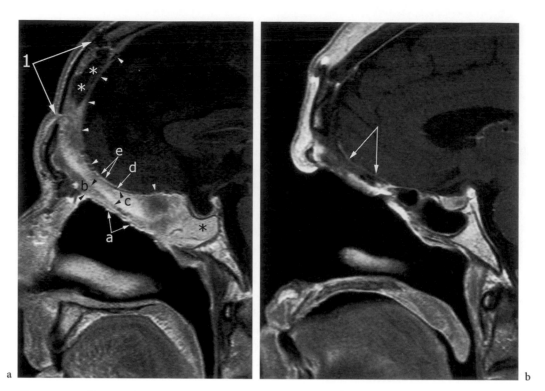

Fig. 11.19. a Follow up of anterior craniofacial resection and left rhinotomy nine months after removal of an ethmoid adeno-carcinoma invading the skull base, olfactory fila, and nasal septum. The sagittal post-contrast T1 image permits to separate the thicker than usual meningo-galeal complex into separate layers: nasal mucosa (*a*); more (*b*) and less mature (*c*) fibrotic scar; residual bone ad the periphery of the resection (*d*); restored dura mater (*e*). The thickened dura lines the restored anterior cranial fossa and the posterior aspect of frontal bone (*arrowheads*). Clear cur resection of the frontal bone cortical rim is seen (*1*). Small fluid collection between dura and facial bone (*double asterisks*). Mucus retention within the blocked sphenoid sinus has high signal intensity (*asterisk*). **b** Follow up of anterior craniofacial resection and total rhinectomy for squamous cell car-cinoma 10 years before, sagittal post-contrast T1 image. The thickness of the meningo-galeal complex is mild; the dural lining (*arrows*) is similar for enhancement and thickness to non-involved areas

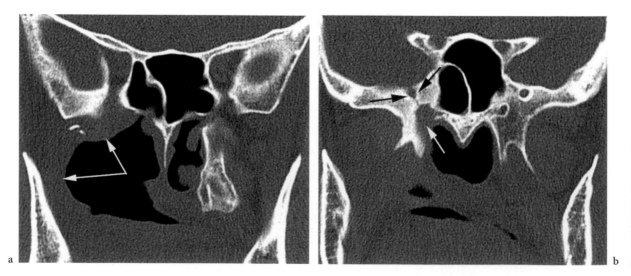

Fig. 11.20a,b. Follow up CT after radical maxillectomy for adenoid cystic carcinoma of right hard palate three years before. In the absence of the prosthetic obturator, a large defect results in a single oro-nasal cavity. Smooth surface is seen (*white arrows on* **a**). Resection of the right maxillary and vidian nerve with exploration of the respective canals was performed at surgery. Dense sclerosis of right pterygoid process is demonstrated by CT around the foramen rotundum (*black arrows on* **b**). Soft tissue fills the area previously occupied by the vidian canal (*white arrow*)

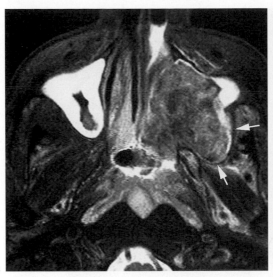
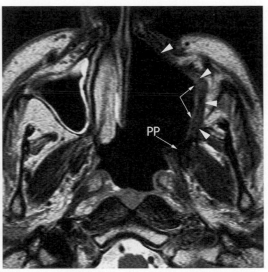

a   b

Fig. 11.21. a Squamous cell carcinoma of left maxillary sinus. Remodeling of posterolateral wall is clearly shown on fat saturated T2 axial image (*arrows*). **b** Three years after treatment with radical maxillectomy, the TSE T2 axial image shows a regular double layer lining of the cavity: the internal one corresponding to the mucosa (*arrows*); the external one to the mature scar (*arrowheads*). Hypointensity is shown at the level of pterygoid process (*PP*) possibly consistent with sclerotic changes

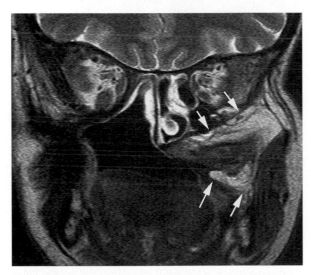

Fig. 11.22. Temporalis muscle flap. The patient had been treated with right radical maxillectomy and left subtotal maxillectomy for an adenoid cystic carcinoma of right hard palate two years before. Adjuvant radiation therapy was delivered (56Gy). A free flap had to be removed for necrosis after irradiation. On TSE T2 coronal image the muscle is partially replaced by fat (*white arrows*).

elements: the aponeurosis and the striated pattern (HUDGINS 2002). The aponeurosis, besides appearing denser on CT and more hypointense on MR in respect to the surrounding muscular bundles, indicates also the direction of the bulk of the muscle. The second element consists in the fan-shaped inner structure of the muscle, which is clearly detectable on condition that more than a single MR plane is evaluated. Progressive atrophy of flap leads to replacement of muscular bundles by fat tissue signal.

During immediate to intermediate phase, edema and enhancement surrounding the flap are usually present. A variable reduction of both abnormalities is observed during the late phase. Characteristic features of myo-cutaneous flaps are the presence of skin and subcutaneous fat, which show typical findings on MR and CT.

A third category of post-operative changes encompasses the modifications of the mucosal surface resulting from either subperiosteal dissection or from bone resection. Mucosal reactive changes and scar formation can be relevant, accounting for diffuse changes of the sinonasal tract mucosa, which can assume a polypoid configuration due to increased thickening, and usually shows abnormal density and signal (Fig. 11.24). The resulting general pattern includes a polypoid aspect of the mucosa lining the sinonasal cavities, with rim enhancement and low inner signal (density, intensity). Deviations from that pattern may be very difficult to separate from recurrent disease. Particularly, scar tissue may show imaging features at CT similar to mucosal thickening. Early scar and granulation tissue usually have hyperintense signal on T2 and enhance after contrast agent administration (LOEVNER and SONNERS 2002). Fibrosis is a hallmark of mature scar, it accounts for

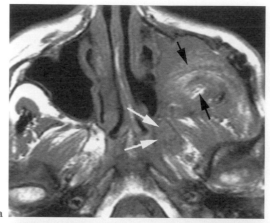

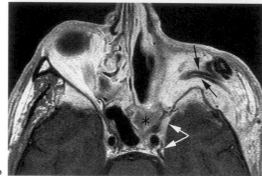

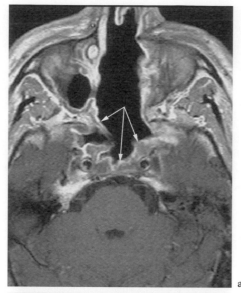

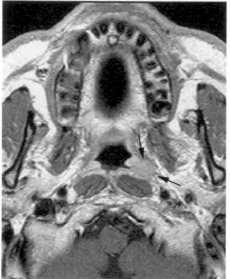

Fig. 11.23a,b. Temporalis muscle flap. **a** The patient had been treated with left radical maxillectomy extended to infratemporal fossa for an adenoid cystic carcinoma of the hard palate. Three years after surgery, on the plain T1 axial image the muscle is clearly detected, its architecture well preserved (*black arrows*). Sclerotic changes of left pterygoid process are present (*white arrows*) **b** The patient was operated on with left radical maxillectomy, ethmoidectomy, orbital exenteration, the defect reconstructed with temporalis muscle, for a squamous cell carcinoma arising from maxillary sinus. Adjuvant radiation therapy was given (60Gy). Trismus developed about one month after irradiation. Follow up MR one year after surgery. On the post-contrast T1 axial image, the enhancing fatty muscle enters the cavity left by orbital exenteration running behind the sclerotic frontal orbital process of frontal bone. The hypointense aponeurosis is well appreciated (*black arrows*). Asymmetric enlargement of cavernous sinus is seen after orbital exenteration (*white arrows*). The straight external outline does not suggest perineural spread (confirmed on subsequent MR studies). Blockage of left sphenoid sinus is present (*asterisk*)

Fig. 11.24a,b. Follow of a patient treated for ethmoid inverted papilloma with foci of squamous cell carcinoma nine years after surgery (same patient of figure 11.7). Post-contrast T1 in the axial plane. **a** Marked thickening of the mucosa lining the sinonasal cavities (*arrows*). **b** Incidental detection of a T1 undifferentiated carcinoma within left Rosenmüller fossa (*arrows*)

a more hypointense signal on T2 and a less tendency to enhance.

Synechiae can lead to stenosis of sinus drainage pathways or blockage. Stenosis or occlusion of the lacrimal pathways account for the onset of epiphora. Dilation of the lacrimal sac should be noted and reported.

Post-operative bone changes are frequent, being related both to resection and to subperiosteal mu-

cosa dissection. On CT, sclerotic changes can be compounded to focal areas of bone dehiscence, or erosion. On MR, thickening of the cortical hypointense rim is observed, sometimes associated with focal more intense areas, and periosteal thickening. This can be detected on the masticator space surface of the posterolateral wall as a thin solid stripe lining the hypointense bone.

11.4.4.2
Normal Post-radiation Therapy Imaging Changes

Since radiation therapy is seldom used as the exclusive treatment in malignant sinonasal tract neoplasms, changes due to irradiation damage are in most patients added to those occurring after surgery. The pattern of the most frequent effects of radiotherapy on paranasal sinuses has been reported in patients treated for nasopharyngeal carcinoma, as part of the sinuses are routinely included within the irradiation portals (CHANG et al. 2000). In these patients, nasal symptoms - in the form of persistent nasal obstruction, purulent discharge, posterior nasal dripping, and stuffy nose - are common.

Mucociliary damage by irradiation accounts for deterioration of the clearance function, which very often causes fluid retention and mucosal thickening. Pathologic findings show squamous metaplasia of the sinusal mucosa and thickening of the basement membrane, with disappearance of cilia. Fibrosis and thickening of the vessel walls within the stroma are also detected (CHANG et al. 2000) (Fig. 11.25). In pre-irradiation disease-free sinuses, mucosal abnormalities are detected in up to 60% of patients on post treatment CT (CHANG et al. 2000). Mucosal changes are similar to those observed after surgery, they develop early, are reversible, lasting for at least 4 years in about 50% of patients (PORTER et al. 1996).

In our experience, patients operated on for malignant neoplasm undergoing subsequent completion radiotherapy develop less pronounced mucosal changes in the first year from treatment. It may be that extensive subperiosteal dissection does not leave any mucosa, so that irradiation usually leads to development of a fibrotic lining of the treated sinonasal cavities. Only when mucosa regrows is reactive thickening usually observed.

Apart from changes in the sinonasal tract, irradiation effects modify the imaging findings of adjacent tissues, particularly those located in the masticator space or in the nasopharynx.

Likewise mucosal abnormalities, the two most prominent masticator space tissues (fat, muscles) show dynamic changes which reflect the acute and late effects of irradiation on tissues.

A few weeks after the completion of radiation treatment, inflammatory changes and edema are prevalent, giving rise to diffuse heterogeneity of the MR signal of fat (which becomes denser at CT) and to thickening and diffuse enhancement of masticator muscles. Bone marrow changes are also present

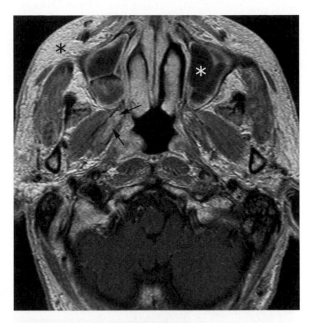

Fig. 11.25. Follow up after exclusive radiation therapy for a sphenoid sinus adenoid cystic carcinoma. The axial post-contrast T1 image is obtained four months after adjuvant of therapy. Subcutaneous and deep fat tissue (buccal fat pad, *black asterisk*) show a diffuse increase of *reticulations* indicating thickening. Reactive mucosal changes are seen in the maxillary sinuses (*white asterisk in the left*), asymmetric enhancement is observed in the right medial pterygoid muscle (*arrows*)

(hyperintensity on T2, hypointensity on plain T1, enhancement).

Approximately 6 to 8 months after treatment, subacute inflammatory modifications are replaced by the development of mature fibrosis, which is less vascularized. Masticator muscles progressively reduce in volume to normal size, while fatty changes may develop. The typical striation of muscular bundles provides reassurance that the muscle is "normal" (Fig. 11.26). While increased CT density of fat tissue persists, the hyperintensity observed on T2 reduces. Major salivary gland abnormalities include volume reduction and relevant enhancement on both CT and MR images (BECKER et al. 1997; NOMAYR et al. 2001).

Changes in the nasopharynx are characterized by reduction in size of the lymphoid tissue at the adenoid tonsil and along lateral recesses, variable thickening of the mucosa, and thickening of submucosal layers and fat planes surrounding the walls. A stiffer nasopharynx results, with hypointense (T2, plain T1) and non enhancing stripe of fat tissue surrounding its walls.

Within one year from radiation treatment, most imaging changes of masticator space, salivary glands

and nasopharynx are stable, except for mucosal abnormalities, which can still regress. Fatty replacement
of bone marrow within the sphenoid bone, especially
at the pterygoid process level, the clivus, and the vertebral bodies is a well known side effect of radiation
treatment, which is related to the transformation of
red into yellow bone marrow. Variable hyperintensity
of bone marrow on plain T1 sequences may be seen.

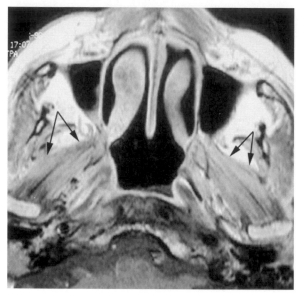

Fig. 11.26. Post-radiation changes in both lateral pterygoid
muscles (*arrows*) are characterized by non homogeneous enhancement; the typical muscular striation is preserved

11.4.4.3
Imaging the Complications of Post-radiation Therapy

Apart from mucosal scars, which may sometimes lead
to the formation of a mucocele (REJAB et al. 1991)
(Fig. 11.27), the most common complications of radiation therapy include cranial neuropathies –optic
neuritis being the most critical target, CNS radiation
abnormalities, osteoradionecrosis – the mandible being most frequently involved -, and development of
radiation-associated tumors.

Optic neuritis secondary to irradiation and radiation retinopathy may present with progressive visual
loss. This complication developed in up to 30% of
a group of 78 patients treated by radiation therapy
alone with curative intent (KATZ et al. 2002). Although
in most patients unilateral blindness was anticipated
because of disease extent, in 5% of cases it developed
unexpected due to optic neuropathy. On MR, thickening and enhancement of the involved nerve, optic
tract or chiasm are observed (Fig. 11.28).

In case of ethmoid or sphenoid sinus neoplasms,
radiation treatment portals do necessarily include
a portion of CNS. *Central nervous system involvement* has been reported in less than 3% of patients
treated for ethmoidal neoplasms (GAUCHER et al.
2002). Nevertheless, its incidence is probably higher,
as some patients may be asymptomatic and their lesions go undetected. The time interval for the onset of
symptoms ranges from a few weeks to several years.

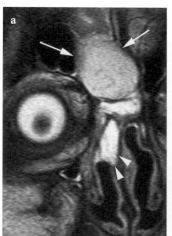
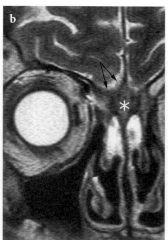
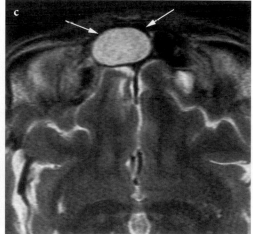

Fig. 11.27a-c. Frontal mucocele arising after radiation therapy for undifferentiated carcinoma of the right ethmoid. On TSE T2
coronal images, mucosal thickening involves both anterior naso-ethmoid cavities, thicker on the right side (*arrowhead in* **a**).
a A frontal right frontal mucocele is demonstrated (*arrows*). **b** Diffuse changes of the cribriform plates, perpendicular lamina
(*asterisk*) and crista galli are seen. They are characterized by bone thickening and unsharp outlines, especially at the bone/CSF
interface (*arrows*). Findings are related to previous invasion of the ethmoid by tumor. **c** On the axial plane remodeling of sinusal
wall by the mucocele is shown (*arrows*)

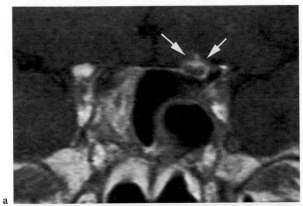

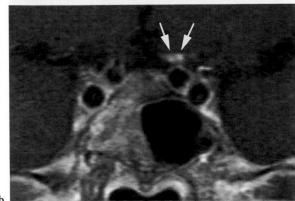

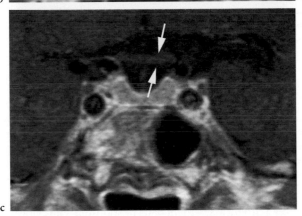

Fig. 11.28a-c. Optic neuritis after radiation therapy, same patient of Figure 11.27. Severe, progressive vision impairment on left side. Post-contrast coronal T1 images show peripheral irregular enhancement of the intracranial portion of the left optic nerve (*arrows in* **a** and **b**). **c** No abnormality is seen at the level of the chiasm (*arrows*)

Total dose, duration and fractionation influence the risk of developing such a complication. Depending on the interval from treatment, brain lesions due to irradiation are classified into early, early-delayed and late-delayed. The deep white matter is typically involved with relative sparing of the cortex (BECKER et al. 1997). Early lesions may develop during the pe-

riod of radiation treatment itself, probably caused by damage to brain capillaries with rupture of the blood brain barrier and subsequent development of edema. Early-delayed changes occurs weeks to months after treatment, while late-delayed abnormalities appears months to years after therapy.

Early and early-delayed necrosis are characterized by hyperintense T2 signal indicating edema and demyelination, which is often reversible. If the damage to the white matter progresses, radiation induced necrosis occurs. Late-delayed necrosis of the brain is generally irreversible, and sometimes fatal. Besides the presence of hyperintense T2 signals, which indicates demyelination foci in the white matter, imaging findings include punctate, gyriform or serpiginous enhancement on post-contrast T1, consistent with frank necrosis in the white matter (GAUCHER et al. 2002). Mass effect, usually with variable enhancement at the periphery, is also noted (RABIN et al. 1996; CHONG et al. 2000b, 2002). Sometimes, it may be difficult to differentiate radiation necrosis from recurrent intracranial ethmoidal or sphenoidal tumors with intracerebral invasion or from hematogenous metastases (CHONG et al. 1997). Careful analysis should permit to identify the pattern of a recurrent tumor, which is characterized by a mainly extradural location or epicenter and a minor intradural intracerebral component, from the exclusive intradural location of radiation necrosis (CHONG et al. 2000b).

Radiation therapy can also induce in the brain *mineralizing microangiopathy and telangiectasia* (VALK and DILLON 1991). Microangiopathy appears as multiple punctate calcifications in the cerebral cortex, brainstem, and basal ganglia. If deep perforating arteries are involved, ischemia of the basal ganglia, thalamus, and deep white matter may occur. Telangiectasia, probably secondary to the development of collateral circulation, may lead to brain hemorrhage (GAENSLER et al. 1994).

Osteoradionecrosis of the mandible, though more often observed after treatment of oral carcinoma, may occur also after irradiation of sinonasal tract neoplasms, especially for maxillary sinus carcinoma. The imaging findings are similar to bone necrosis in other areas. CT reveals the typical osseous findings of cortical disruption, trabecular disorganization, and fragmentation. Abnormal T1 hypointensity, T2 hyperintensity, and intense enhancement of the bone marrow in the involved mandible is usually shown on MR. Post-contrast fat saturated sequences can show the enhancing inflamed reaction surrounding the necrotic medullary bone (Fig. 11.29).

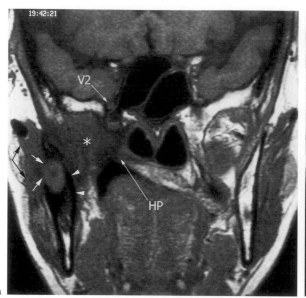 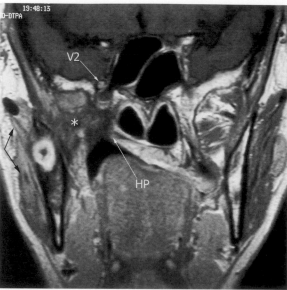

Fig. 11.29a,b. Follow up after right radical maxillectomy and adjuvant radiation therapy for a squamous cell carcinoma three years after treatment. The patient complained of progressive trismus for 3 months. Coronal plain (**a**) and post-contrast (**b**) T1 images show increased thickness of right mandibular ramus. **a** A lesion arises from cancellous bone, destroys the cortical (*white arrows*), surrounded by remarkably sclerotic spongiosa and thickened cortical rim (*arrowheads*). Abnormal hypointense signal of the adjacent masseter muscle is seen (*black arrows*). Masticator space structures and fat signal are replaced by homogeneous hypointense signal (*asterisk*), which is associated with retraction of adjacent common nasal-oral cavity structure. Hard Palate (*HP*). **b** The osteonecrotic bone shows marked, heterogeneous enhancement. Inflammatory changes of the adjacent masseter muscle give rise to mild enhancement (*black arrow*). The detectability of the muscular striation reassures about the non-neoplastic nature. Non homogenous enhancement of the scar replacing masticator space structures is demonstrated (*asterisk*). Asymmetric enhancement of the right maxillary nerve (*V2*) compared to the opposite side, requires further studies to rule out perineural spread

In addition, abnormal diffuse enhancement in surrounding tissues and in the adjacent masseter and pterygoid muscles may be noted. Those muscles can be irregularly enlarged, appearing as space-occupying lesions adjacent to the abnormal bone, mimicking recurrent disease. Abnormal T2 hyperintensity and relevant diffuse enhancement is usually present (CHONG et al. 2000a).

Radiation-associated neoplasms of the head and neck occur in the radiation portal area, with a frequency ranging from 0.4 to 0.7% (STEEVES and BATAINI 1981; VAN DER LAAN et al. 1995) (Fig. 11.30). Other criteria for the diagnosis of a post-irradiation tumor include a histology different from that of the primary tumor and a latency period of at least 5 years (KING et al. 2000).

A wide range of radiation-associated tumors has been reported, including sarcoma, meningioma, schwannoma, glioma, and squamous cell carcinoma (RUBINSTEIN et al. 1989; HARRISON et al. 1991; MARK et al. 1993). Osteosarcoma and malignant fibrous histiocytoma are the most frequent (RABIN et al. 1996).

11.4.4.4
Imaging of Local Recurrences

In the follow up, the radiologist may be faced with an asymptomatic recurrence or an already known relapse. In the first case, which is the most challenging situation, knowledge of the most probable site of recurrence and of the imaging features of early recurrences is essential. A known local relapse raises different issues, specifically a careful assessment of its relationship with critical structures such as the orbit, the skull base, the brain, the cavernous sinus, and the internal carotid artery (LACCOURREYE et al. 1994; LELL et al. 2000).

In general, asymptomatic extra-mucosal recurrences are more frequently expected close to the resection area or at its boundary with flaps.

Unlike primary tumors, abnormalities in symmetry (in comparison with the opposite side) due to treatment are so frequent to be commonly of limited usefulness. The resulting distorted anatomy is compounded of post treatment changes in residual structures, presence of a flap, and fibrous scar (Fig. 11.31-34). Therefore, the first step in the interpretation of CT or MR consists in a careful identification of the expected changes due

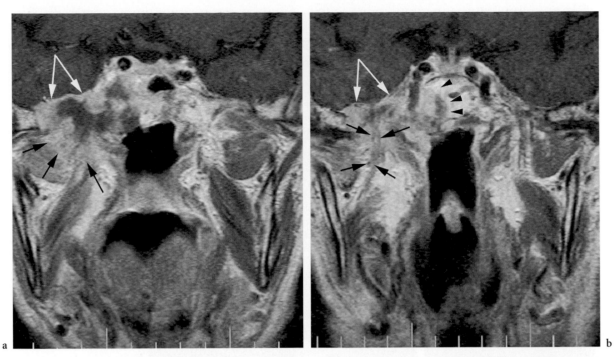

Fig. 11.30a,b. Radiation-associated leiomyosarcoma eleven years after irradiation for nasopharyngeal undifferentiated carcinoma. On contrast enhanced coronal T1 image, the neoplasm arises from the masticator space muscles and invades the right sphenoid (*white arrows on* **a** *and* **b**). **a** Both the medial and lateral pterygoid muscles are invaded (*black arrows*). **b** The epicenter of tumor is located at the level of the foramen ovale. Although the mandibular nerve is thickened and shows slight enhancement (*black arrows*) only minor changes in the ipsilateral masticator muscles are noted. Invasion of the clivus is present (*arrowheads*)

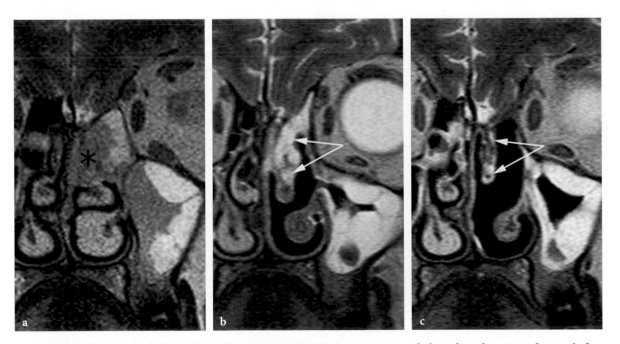

Fig. 11.31a,c. Follow up of left ethmoid rhabdomyosarcoma. TSE T2 images on coronal plane show the extent of tumor before (**a**) two months (**b**) and four months after treatment (**c**). Progressive shrinkage of tumor (*asterisk*) leads to total disappearance of the lesion, leaving an abnormally remodeled middle turbinate (*arrows in* **b** *and* **c**)

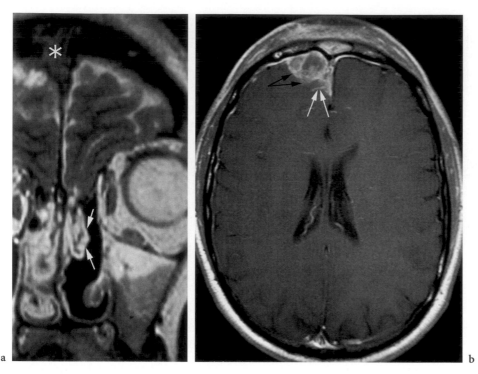

a   b

Fig. 11.32a,b. Same patient of Figure 11.31. Nine months after the follow up study of Figure 11.31c, the onset of persisting head-ache, leads the patient to an new study, which shows an extra-axial mass in the right frontal lobe (*asterisk on* **a**) corresponding to an epidural metastasis. Any recurrent lesion is seen in left ethmoid (*arrows*). **b** The post-contrast axial image shows the enhancing epidural nodule (*black arrows*), associated with adjacent linear enhancement which may suggest leptomeningeal metastasis (*white arrows*)

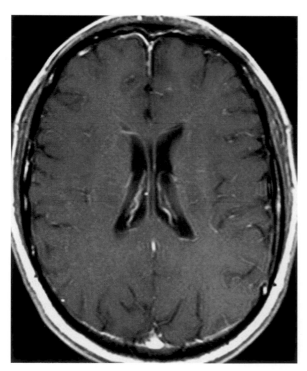

Fig. 11.33. Same patient of Figure 11.31-32, subsequently treated with chemotherapy. The study obtained eight months after the one of Figure 11.32b does not show any recurrent

to previous therapy. Once expected changes and the corresponding structures (mucosa lining the sinuses, bony framework, fat, muscles, dura) are detected, any other abnormal signal should be carefully evaluated, especially focal masses. In case of previous surgery with/without adjuvant radiotherapy, the resulting fibrous scar should be distinguished from recurrent tumor; whereas in case of exclusive radiotherapy, is the tumor shrinkage with its transformation into immature/mature scar to be differentiated from a relapse.

A combination of diagnostic strategies is generally recommended. Since MR has a superior contrast resolution, it is commonly preferred to CT. If the abnormal signal cannot be differentiated from fibrosis, a subsequent MR study may result definitive, otherwise a biopsy should be obtained.

However, MR imaging has been reported to be superior to CT only in differentiating recurrent tumor from mature fibrous scar, which has low signal intensity on all sequences and does not enhance (GONG et al. 1991; LELL et al. 2000). Immature fibrosis, viable tumor, tumor necrosis may all show homogenous to heterogeneous hyperintense signal on T2 (CHONG and FAN 1997; LELL et al. 2000). Nor can result decisive the pattern on post-contrast T1 sequences, as

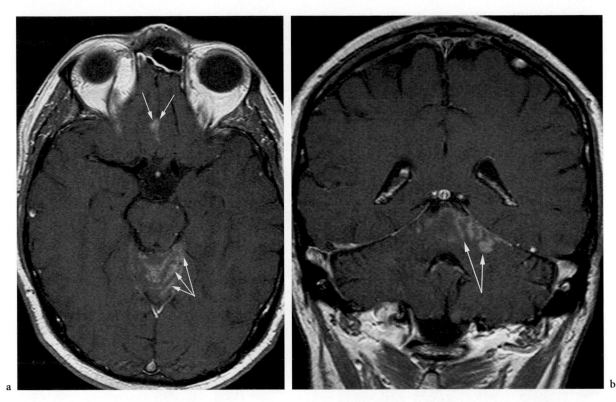

a   b

Fig. 11.34a,b. Same patient of Figure 11.31-33, only one month after the MR examination of Figure 11.33. Diffuse leptomeningeal metastasis is present (*arrows*)

the recurrent tumor can exhibit various degrees of contrast enhancement (NG et al. 1999).

Dynamic contrast-enhanced MR imaging can potentially improve the diagnostic yield (Fig. 11.35). Data provided reflects capillary blood flow, permeability, and the relative volume of extravascular extracellular space, resulting in quantitative parameters related to tumor angiogenesis (TAYLOR et al. 1999). Two quantitative parameters have been demonstrated to improve relapse detection in several areas of the body: the slope of enhancement over 60 seconds, which is related to tissue vascularization – i.e., the number of vessels, the degree of perfusion, and capillary permeability; and the maximum average enhancement which is dependent on the volume of the extracellular space (MOEHLER et al. 2001; FISCHBEIN et al. 2003; RAHMOUNI et al. 2003). In the follow-up after surgery and/or radiotherapy of 27 head and neck and skull base tumors, we recently observed that the slope of enhancement and maximum intensity averages of recurrences were significantly steeper and higher, respectively, than in negative lesions (PIAZZALUNGA et al. 2004).

The baseline MR examination remains a cornerstone reference for comparing areas with abnormal signal to previous findings (Fig. 11.36). MR

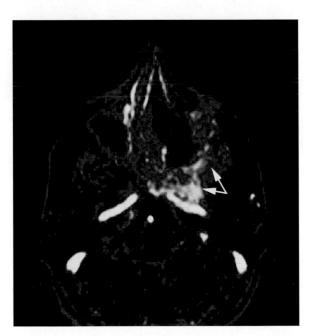

Fig. 11.35. Recurrent squamous cell carcinoma of left ethmoid after surgery (left radical maxillectomy with orbital exenteration), radiotherapy and chemotherapy. Color-coded image based on a pixel-by-pixel analysis of the slope of the enhancement curve. Yellow areas in the previous area of the pterygoid process (*white arrows*) indicate the relapse

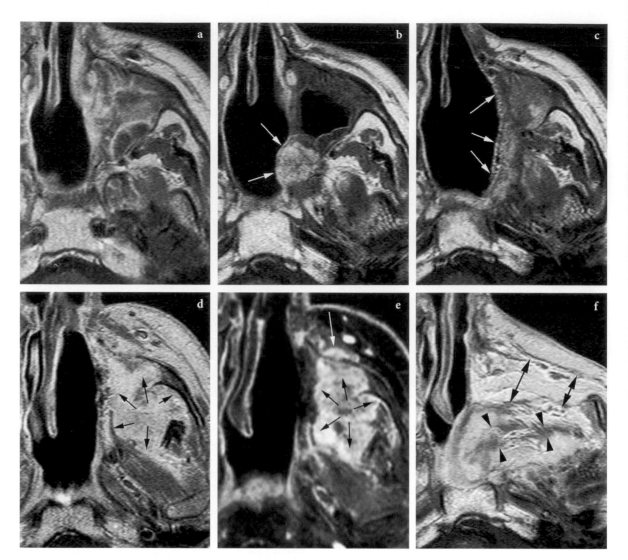

Fig. 11.36 a-f Multiple recurrences in a patient initially treated with craniofacial resection and adjuvant radiotherapy for an ethmoid adenocarcinoma. Post-contrast T1 (a-d, f) and VIBE (e) images in the axial plane, obtained four months after the end of radiation treatment (a), seven months after previous image (b), four months after left medial maxillectomy (c), eight months after the previous study (d and e), four months after radical maxillectomy with myo-cutaneous and fascio-cutaneous flaps (f). a The first follow up study shows only marked inflammatory reaction of the mucosa within the left maxillary sinus. b Submucosal recurrence is arising from left pterygopalatine fossa (*arrows*), with mucosal bulging. c The follow up after maxillectomy shows findings consistent with post surgical changes, a smooth lining of the cavity is seen (*arrows*). d-e A second recurrent lesion develops from the interface between the maxillary sinus and the masticator space with extensive involvement of adjacent structures (*arrows*). Both recurrent tumor and invasion of anterior maxillary sinus wall are more evident on VIBE image (e). f The temporalis myo-cutaneous flap (*arrowheads*) is clearly distinguished from the fascio-cutaneous (*double arrowheads arrows*) by means of its partially degenerated muscular architecture

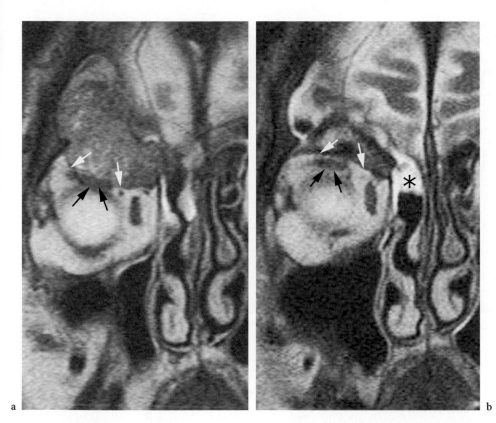

a

b

Fig. 11.37a-b. Follow up of right frontal sinus undifferentiated carcinoma four months after radiation therapy and chemotherapy. TSE T2 on coronal plane show the extent of tumor before (**a**) and after treatment (**b**). **a** Marked deformation of the orbital roof is caused by tumor, which is still separated from the orbital fat by the residual bone/periorbital lining (*white arrows*). The superior rectus muscle (*black arrows*) is compressed and displaced inferiorly. **b** The shrinkage of tumor after treatment is associated with partial restoration of the normal position of the orbital roof (*white arrows*). At surgery, the orbit was spared, being intraoperative frozen sections negative. The superior rectus muscle (*black arrows*) has a more normal position. Thickened mucosa in the anterior ethmoid is seen (*asterisk*)

imaging might be quite reassuring if the areas under questions undergo stabilization or continuous shrinkage or show a diminishing degree of enhancement (LOEVNER and SONNERS 2002; NG et al. 2002) (Fig. 11.37). These findings are particularly useful in case tumor was treated by exclusive radiotherapy and the location does not allow an easy assessment by endoscopy or it was totally extramucosal.

An additional key issue to improve early detection of recurrences encompasses the careful analysis of anatomically related cranial nerve branches to rule out perineural spread, which – though more frequent in malignant glandular carcinomas and in lymphomas – is also likely in squamous cell carcinoma. Perivascular spread is also possible, although rarer than perineural spread (Fig. 11.38).

It is important to note that in case of treatment of repeated local recurrences, mostly by combined therapies, the chance of developing relapses in unusual sites increases. Whereas the occurrence within neck fat tissue may be theoretically explained by intraoperative seeding (Fig. 11.39-43), the development of lesions in contralateral facial bony framework or in the epidural location does probably account for metastasis through the vascular system (Fig. 11.44).

Although single photon emission computed tomography and positron emission computed tomography with 18F-2-fluoro-deoxyglucose - without and with CT - appear promising for detecting recurrent or residual disease, their role in the follow up of malignant neoplasms of the sinonasal tract is not yet established (NINOMIYA et al. 2004).

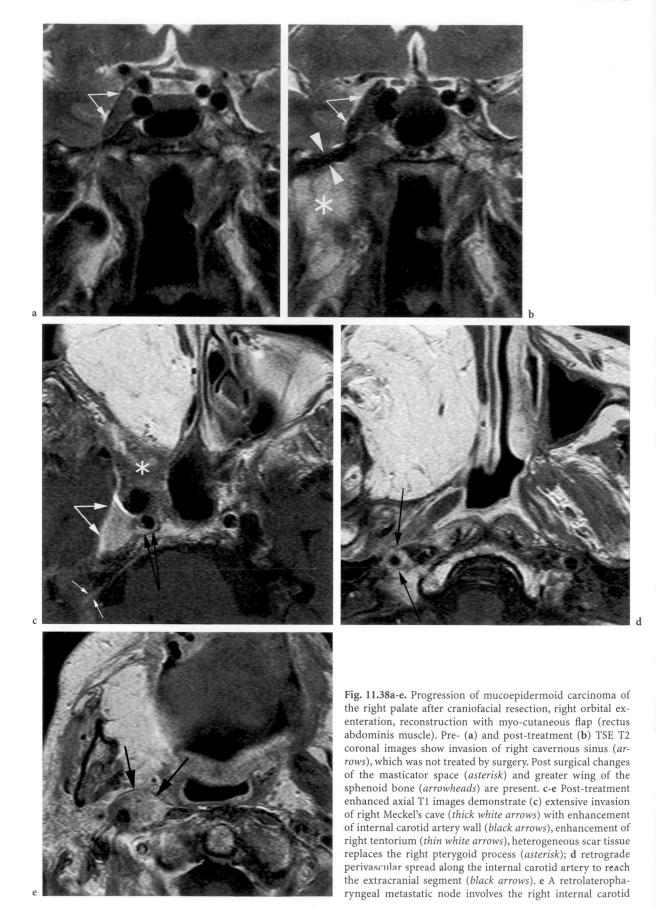

Fig. 11.38a-e. Progression of mucoepidermoid carcinoma of the right palate after craniofacial resection, right orbital exenteration, reconstruction with myo-cutaneous flap (rectus abdominis muscle). Pre- (**a**) and post-treatment (**b**) TSE T2 coronal images show invasion of right cavernous sinus (*arrows*), which was not treated by surgery. Post surgical changes of the masticator space (*asterisk*) and greater wing of the sphenoid bone (*arrowheads*) are present. **c-e** Post-treatment enhanced axial T1 images demonstrate (**c**) extensive invasion of right Meckel's cave (*thick white arrows*) with enhancement of internal carotid artery wall (*black arrows*), enhancement of right tentorium (*thin white arrows*), heterogeneous scar tissue replaces the right pterygoid process (*asterisk*); **d** retrograde perivascular spread along the internal carotid artery to reach the extracranial segment (*black arrows*). **e** A retrolateropharyngeal metastatic node involves the right internal carotid

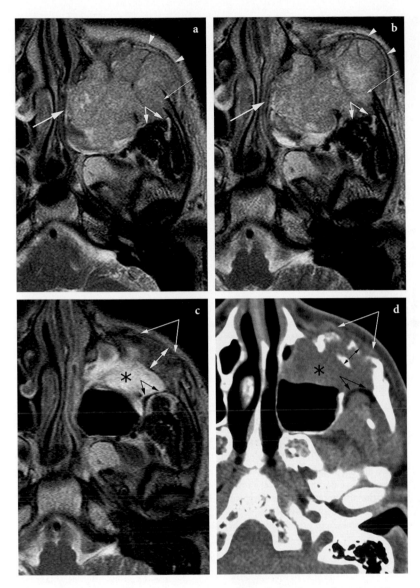

Fig. 11.39a-d. Left maxillary sinus squamous cell carcinoma in a male patient 31 years old. TSE T2 (**a-c**) and CT (**d**) in the axial plane, obtained before treatment (**a**), after the first cycle of chemotherapy (**b**), after radiation and chemotherapy, four (**c**), and six (**d**) months from treatment beginning. **a** Baseline study shows that the tumor has four major pathways of spread: marked displacement of the anterior sinus wall (*arrowheads*); invasion of the cortical and cancellous zygomatic bone (*long thin white arrow*); disruption of the most anterior part of the posterolateral sinus wall (*coupled white arrows*); remodeling and displacement of the medial sinus wall towards the nasal cavity (*thick white arrow*). **b** After the first cycle of chemotherapy, a very limited decrease of volume is observed, and the tumor signal is unchanged. **c** After adjuvant of radiation and chemotherapy, shrinkage of tumor is observed, resulting in residual questionable hyperintense tissue located in the anterior portion of maxillary sinus (*asterisk*). Relevant thickening of the previously invaded anterior sinus wall (*coupled thin white arrows*) is associated with diffuse signal hypointensity and clearly detectable outlines (*double white arrowheads arrow*). **d** On CT, the residual thickened bone cannot be clearly separated from the intrasinusal questionable tissue (*asterisk*). While any progression of zygomatic bone erosion is observed, shrinkage of tumor enables the eroded posterolateral wall to retract. MR is more precise than CT in demonstrating that a residual wall separates intrasinusal tissue from masticator space fat. In fact a continuous hypointense signal corresponding to the demineralized bone and periosteum is demonstrated (*black arrows*)

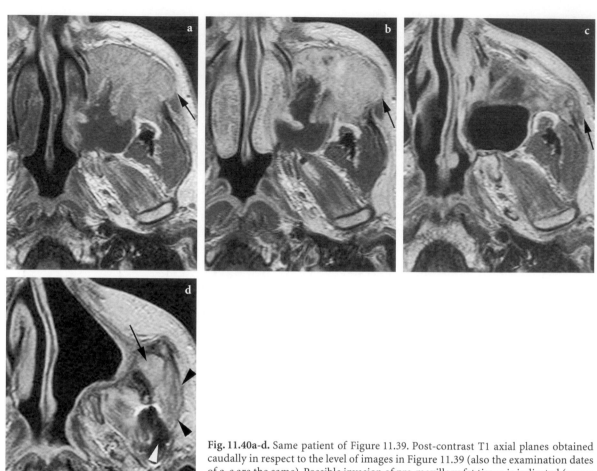

Fig. 11.40a-d. Same patient of Figure 11.39. Post-contrast T1 axial planes obtained caudally in respect to the level of images in Figure 11.39 (also the examination dates of a-c are the same). Possible invasion of pre-maxillary fat tissue is indicated (*arrow in* **a-c**) Image **d,** obtained after radical left maxillectomy (seven months after **c**) besides the normal post surgical appearance shows fatty degeneration of the masticator muscles (*black arrowheads*), reduced hyperintensity of fat within the masticator space (*arrow*), and artifacts due to mandible resection (*white arrowheads*)

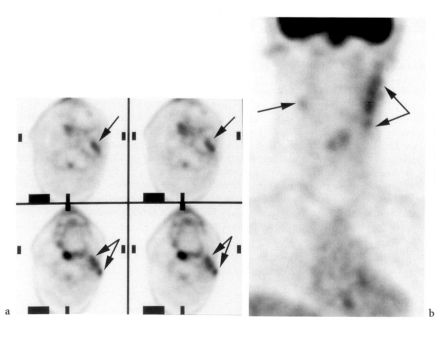

Fig. 11.41a,b. Same patient of Figures 11.39-40. Before maxillectomy, the patient had left superficial parotidectomy and selective neck dissection for metastasis. A PET study five months after maxillectomy shows hypermetabolic foci in the parotid area where a lamina of Silastic was placed. Multiple foci are seen on both the axial and coronal images (*arrows*). A contralateral lesion was suspected, not confirmed by fine needle aspiration cytology

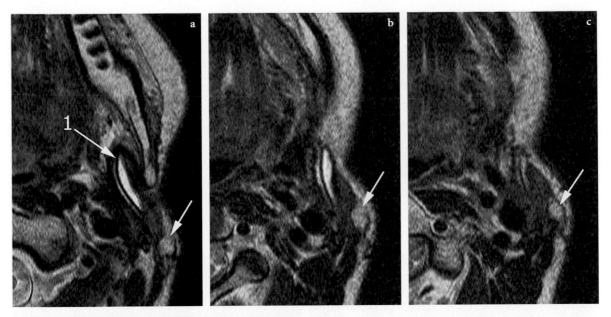

Fig. 11.42a-c. Same patient of Figures 11.39-41. The hypermetabolic foci detected by PET reveal to be multiple nodules disseminated along the sternocleidomastoid muscle (*white arrows*). Silastic lamina (*1*)

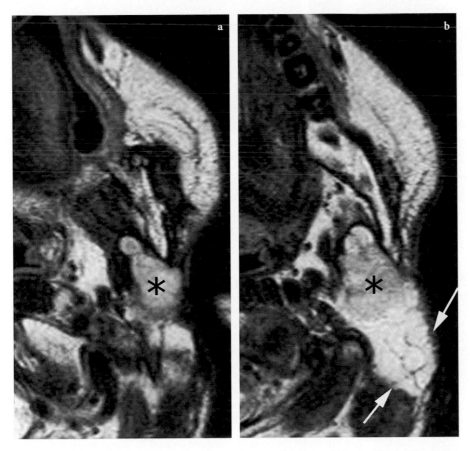

Fig. 11.43a,b. Same patient of Figures 11.39-42. Nine months after revision surgery with reconstruction by mean of a vascularized flap (*arrows*) local recurrence develops at the interface between flap and native tissues (*asterisk*)

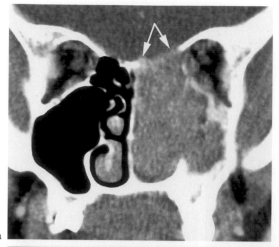

a

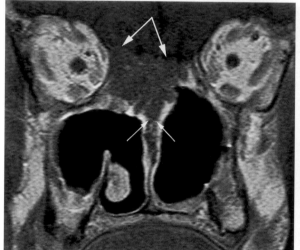

b

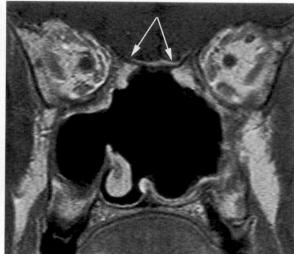

c

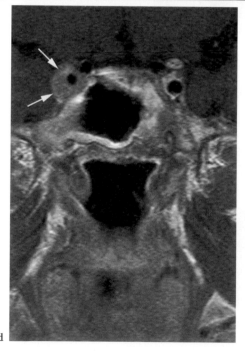

d

Fig. 11.44a-d. Follow up of left ethmoid squamous cell carcinoma developed two years after removal of an inverted papilloma at the same site. **a** Post-contrast coronal CT shows the mass occupying the whole left ethmoid and nasal fossa. Bone invasion of the ethmoid roof (*arrows*) and extent into maxillary sinus are noted. The patient was treated with left ethmoido-maxillectomy and radiation therapy. **b** The TSE T2 coronal image obtained two years after identifies a subclinical-submucosal recurrence (*thick arrows*) with intracranial extradural extent and invasion into the nasal septum (*thin arrows*) At surgery, the right lamina papyracea was normal. **c** The follow up TSE T2 study five months after anterior craniofacial resection shows only the normal pattern of the meningo-galeal complex (*arrows*). **d** Two months after, the onset of right side progressive impairment of vision prompted a new MR study. On contrast enhanced coronal T1 image, encasement of the internal carotid artery within the right cavernous sinus by a metastasis is demonstrated (*arrows*)

References

Batteur B, Strunski V, Caprio D et al (1994) Recurrence of nasosinusal polyposis after ethmoidectomy by endonasal approach. Functional, endoscopic, x-ray tomographic aspects and surgical implications. Ann Otolaryngol Chir Cervicofac 111:121–128

Becker M, Schroth G, Zbaren P et al (1997) Long-term changes induced by high-dose irradiation of the head and neck region: imaging findings. Radiographics 17:5–26

Bely N, Zanoun M, Laccourreye O et al (1997) Radiological surveillance of operated ethmoidal cancers. Practical points. Neurochirurgie 43:76–84

Bendet E, Eyal A, Kronenberg J (1995) Pneumocephalus as a complication of intranasal ethmoidectomy and polypectomy. Ann Otol Rhinol Laryngol 104:326–328

Bolger WE, Woodruff WW Jr, Morehead J et al (1990) Maxillary sinus hypoplasia: classification and description of associated uncinate process hypoplasia. Otolaryngol Head Neck Surg 103:759–765

Catalano PJ, Hecht CS, Biller HF et al (1994) Craniofacial resection. An analysis of 73 cases. Arch Otolaryngol Head Neck Surg 120:1203–1208

Chagnaud C, Petit P, Bartoli J et al (1998) Postoperative follow-up of juvenile nasopharyngeal angiofibromas: assessment by CT scan and MR imaging. Eur Radiol 8:756–764

Chambers DW, Davis WE, Cook PR et al (1997) Long-term outcome analysis of functional endoscopic sinus surgery: correlation of symptoms with endoscopic examination findings and potential prognostic variables. Laryngoscope 107:504–510

Chang CC, Chen MK, Wen YS et al (2000) Effects of radiotherapy for nasopharyngeal carcinoma on the paranasal sinuses: study based on computed tomography scanning. J Otolaryngol 29:23–27

Chong J, Hinckley LK, Ginsberg LE (2000a) Masticator space abnormalities associated with mandibular osteoradionecrosis: MR and CT findings in five patients. AJNR Am J Neuroradiol 21:175–178

Chong VF, Fan YF (1997) Detection of recurrent nasopharyngeal carcinoma: MR imaging versus CT. Radiology 202:463–470

Chong VF, Fan YF, Chan LL (1997) Temporal lobe necrosis in nasopharyngeal carcinoma: pictorial essay. Australas Radiol 41:392–397

Chong VF, Fan YF, Mukherji SK (2000b) Radiation-induced temporal lobe changes: CT and MR imaging characteristics. AJR Am J Roentgenol 175:431–436

Chong VF, Khoo JB, Chan LL et al (2002) Neurological changes following radiation therapy for head and neck tumours. Eur J Radiol 44:120–129

Chu CT, Lebowitz RA, Jacobs JB (1997) An analysis of sites of disease in revision endoscopic sinus surgery. Am J Rhinol 11:287–291

Draf W, Weber R, Keerl R et al (1995) Current aspects of frontal sinus surgery. I. Endonasal frontal sinus drainage in inflammatory diseases of the paranasal sinuses. HNO 43:352–357

Dubrulle F, Darras J, Khalil C (2003) Imagerie des sinus operes. J Radiol 84:945–959

Fischbein NJ, Noworolski SM, Henry RG et al (2003) Assessment of metastatic cervical adenopathy using dynamic contrast-enhanced MR imaging. AJNR Am J Neuroradiol 24:301–311

Friedman WH, Katsantonis GP, Bumpous JM (1995) Staging of chronic hyperplastic rhinosinusitis: treatment strategies. Otolaryngol Head Neck Surg 112:210–214

Gaensler EH, Dillon WP, Edwards MS et al (1994) Radiation-induced telangiectasia in the brain simulates cryptic vascular malformations at MR imaging. Radiology 193:629–636

Gaucher S, Viala J, Lusinchi A et al (2002) CT and MRI aspects of 28 patients with cerebral radiation necrosis irradiated for ORL tumors: correlation with the radiation technique. J Radiol 83:1749–1757

Ginsberg LE (2002) MR imaging of perineural tumor spread. Magn Reson Imaging Clin North Am 10:511–525, vi

Goffart Y, Jorissen M, Daele J et al (2000) Minimally invasive endoscopic management of malignant sinonasal tumors. Acta Otorhinolaryngol Belg 54:221–232

Gong QY, Zheng GL, Zhu HY (1991) MRI differentiation of recurrent nasopharyngeal carcinoma from postradiation fibrosis. Comput Med Imaging Graph 15:423–429

Graham SM, Nerad JA (2003) Orbital complications in endoscopic sinus surgery using powered instrumentation. Laryngoscope 113:874–878

Harrison MJ, Wolfe DE, Lau TS et al (1991) Radiation-induced meningiomas: experience at the Mount Sinai Hospital and review of the literature. J Neurosurg 75:564–574

Hudgins PA (1993) Complications of endoscopic sinus surgery. The role of the radiologist in prevention. Radiol Clin North Am 31:21–32

Hudgins PA (2002) Flap reconstruction in the head and neck: expected appearance, complications, and recurrent disease. Semin Ultrasound CT MR 23:492–500

Hudgins PA, Browning DG, Gallups J et al (1992) Endoscopic paranasal sinus surgery: radiographic evaluation of severe complications. AJNR Am J Neuroradiol 13:1161–1167

Imola MJ, Schramm VL Jr (2002) Orbital preservation in surgical management of sinonasal malignancy. Laryngoscope 112:1357–1365

Jankowski R, Pigret D, Decroocq F (1997) Comparison of functional results after ethmoidectomy and nasalization for diffuse and severe nasal polyposis. Acta Otolaryngol 117:601–608

Janssen AG, Mansour K, Bos JJ (1997) Obstructed nasolacrimal duct system in epiphora: long-term results of dacryocystoplasty by means of balloon dilation. Radiology 205:791–796

Katsantonis GP, Friedman WH, Sivore MC (1990) The role of computed tomography in revision sinus surgery. Laryngoscope 100:811–816

Katz TS, Hinerman RW, Amdur RJ et al (2002) Malignant tumors of the nasal cavity and paranasal sinuses. Head Neck 24:821–829

Kennedy DW (1992) Prognostic factors, outcomes and staging in ethmoid sinus surgery. Laryngoscope 102:1–18

Kennedy DW, Senior BA, Gannon FH et al (1998) Histology and histomorphometry of ethmoid bone in chronic rhinosinusitis. Laryngoscope 108:502–507

King AD, Ahuja AT, Teo P et al (2000) Radiation induced sarcomas of the head and neck following radiotherapy for nasopharyngeal carcinoma. Clin Radiol 55:684–689

Laccourreye O, Bely N, Halimi P et al (1994) Cavernous sinus involvement from recurrent adenoid cystic carcinoma. Ann Otol Rhinol Laryngol 103:822–825

Lell M, Baum U, Greess H et al (2000) Head and neck tumors: imaging recurrent tumor and post-therapeutic changes with CT and MRI. Eur J Radiol 33:239–247

Levine HL (1990) Functional endoscopic sinus surgery: evaluation, surgery, and follow-up of 250 patients. Laryngoscope 100:79–84

Liang EY, Lam WW, Woo JK et al (1996) Another CT sign of sinonasal polyposis: truncation of the bony middle turbinate. Eur Radiol 6:553–556

Liu SH, Chang JT, Ng SH et al (2004) False positive fluorine-18 fluorodeoxy-D-glucose positron emission tomography finding caused by osteoradionecrosis in a nasopharyngeal carcinoma patient. Br J Radiol 77:257–260

Loevner LA, Sonners AI (2002) Imaging of neoplasms of the paranasal sinuses. Magn Reson Imaging Clin North Am 10:467–493

Loevner LA, Tobey JD, Yousem DM et al (2002) MR imaging characteristics of cranial bone marrow in adult patients with underlying systemic disorders compared with healthy control subjects. AJNR Am J Neuroradiol 23:248–254

Mantoni M, Larsen P, Hansen H et al (1996) Coronal CT of the paranasal sinuses before and after functional endoscopic sinus surgery. Eur Radiol 6:920–924

Mark RJ, Bailet JW, Poen J et al (1993) Postirradiation sarcoma of the head and neck. Cancer 72:887–893

Maroldi R, Farina D, Battaglia G et al (1997) MR of malignant nasosinusal neoplasms. Frequently asked questions. Eur J Radiol 24:181–190

Maroldi R, Battaglia G, Farina D et al (1999) Tumours of the oropharynx and oral cavity: perineural spread and bone invasion. Jbr Btr 82:294–300

May M, Sobol SM, Korzec K (1990) The location of the maxillary os and its importance to the endoscopic sinus surgeon. Laryngoscope 100:1037–1042

Metson R, Woog JJ, Puliafito CA (1994) Endoscopic laser dacryocystorhinostomy. Laryngoscope 104:269–274

Meyers RM, Valvassori G (1998) Interpretation of anatomic variations of computed tomography scans of the sinuses: a surgeon's perspective. Laryngoscope 108:422–425

Moehler TM, Hawighorst H, Neben K et al (2001) Bone marrow microcirculation analysis in multiple myeloma by contrast-enhanced dynamic magnetic resonance imaging. Int J Cancer 93:862–868

Ng SH, Chang JT, Ko SF et al (1999) MRI in recurrent nasopharyngeal carcinoma. Neuroradiology 41:855–862

Ng SH, Liu HM, Ko SF et al (2002) Posttreatment imaging of the nasopharynx. Eur J Radiol 44:82–95

Nicolai P, Berlucchi M, Tomenzoli D et al (2003) Endoscopic surgery for juvenile angiofibroma: when and how. Laryngoscope 113:775–782

Ninomiya H, Oriuchi N, Kahn N et al (2004) Diagnosis of tumor in the nasal cavity and paranasal sinuses with [11C]choline PET: comparative study with 2-[18F]fluoro-2-deoxy-D-glucose (FDG) PET. Ann Nucl Med 18:29–34

Nomayr A, Lell M, Sweeney R et al (2001) MRI appearance of radiation-induced changes of normal cervical tissues. Eur Radiol 11:1807–1817

Ophir D, Shapiro M, Ruchvarger E et al (1994) Pneumocephalus following nasal polypectomy. Ann Otol Rhinol Laryngol 103:576–577

Osguthorpe JD, Patel S (1995) Craniofacial approaches to sinus malignancy. Otolaryngol Clin North Am 28:1239–1257

Petit P, Vivarrat-Perrin L, Champsaur P et al (2000) Radiological follow-up of inverted papilloma. Eur Radiol 10:1184–1189

Piazzalunga B, Moraschi Y, Ghirardi C et al (2004) Enhancement pattern of recurrent head and neck neoplasms: dynamic MR measurement. Eur Radiol 14:191

Porter MJ, Leung SF, Ambrose R et al (1996) The paranasal sinuses before and after radiotherapy for nasopharyngeal carcinoma: a computed tomographic study. J Laryngol Otol 110:19–22

Rabin BM, Meyer JR, Berlin JW et al (1996) Radiation-induced changes in the central nervous system and head and neck. Radiographics 16:1055–1072

Rahmouni A, Montazel JL, Divine M et al (2003) Bone marrow with diffuse tumor infiltration in patients with lymphoproliferative diseases: dynamic gadolinium-enhanced MR imaging. Radiology 229:710–717

Raynal M, Peynegre R, Beautru R et al (1999) Mucoceles sinusiennes et iatrogenie chirurgicale. Ann Otolaryngol Chir Cervicofac 116:85–91

Rejab E, Said H, Saim L et al (1991) Sphenoid sinus mucocoele: a possible late complication of radiotherapy to the head and neck. J Laryngol Otol 105:959–960

Richtsmeier WJ, Briggs RJ, Koch WM et al (1992) Complications and early outcome of anterior craniofacial resection. Arch Otolaryngol Head Neck Surg 118:913–917

Roger G, Tran Ba Huy P, Froehlich P et al (2002) Exclusively endoscopic removal of juvenile nasopharyngeal angiofibroma: trends and limits. Arch Otolaryngol Head Neck Surg 128:928–935

Rouviere P, Peynegre R (2000) Recurrence of polyposis: risk factors, prevention, treatment and follow-up. In: Stamm AC, Draf W (eds) Micro-endoscopic surgery of the paranasal sinuses and the skull base. Springer, Berlin Heidelberg New York, pp 286–307

Rubinstein AB, Reichenthal E, Borohov H (1989) Radiation-induced schwannomas. Neurosurgery 24:929–932

Saidi IS, Biedlingmaier JF, Rothman MI (1998) Pre- and postoperative imaging analysis for frontal sinus disease following conservative partial middle turbinate resection. Ear Nose Throat J 77:326–328, 330, 332 passim

Salib RJ, Chaudri SA, Rockley TJ (2001) Sinusitis in the hypoplastic maxillary antrum: the crucial role of radiology in diagnosis and management. J Laryngol Otol 115:676–678

Schick B, Steigerwald C, el Rahman el Tahan A, Draf W (2001) The role of endonasal surgery in the management of fronto-ethmoidal osteomas. Rhinology 39:667–670

Schuster JJ, Phillips CD, Levine PA (1994) MR of esthesioneuroblastoma (olfactory neuroblastoma) and appearance after craniofacial resection. AJNR Am J Neuroradiol 15:1169–1177

Som PM, Lawson W, Biller HF et al (1986a) Ethmoid sinus disease: CT evaluation in 400 cases, part II. Postoperative findings. Radiology 159:599–604

Som PM, Lawson W, Biller HF et al (1986b) Ethmoid sinus disease: CT evaluation in 400 cases, part III. Craniofacial resection. Radiology 159:605–609

Som PM, Dillon WP, Sze G et al (1989) Benign and malignant sinonasal lesions with intracranial extension: differentiation with MR imaging. Radiology 172:763–766

Stamm AC (2000) Complications of micro-endoscopic sinus surgery. In: Stamm AC, Draf W (eds) Micro-endoscopic surgery of the paranasal sinuses and the skull base. Springer, Berlin Heidelberg New York, pp 581–593

Stammberger H, Anderhuber W, Walch C et al (1999) Possibilities and limitations of endoscopic management of nasal and paranasal sinus malignancies. Acta Otorhinolaryngol Belg 53:199–205

Stankiewicz JA (1987) Complications of endoscopic intranasal ethmoidectomy. Laryngoscope 97:1270–1273

Steeves RA, Bataini JP (1981) Neoplasms induced by megavoltage radiation in the head and neck region. Cancer 47:1770–1774

Stewart MG, Donovan DT, Parke RB Jr et al (2000) Does the severity of sinus computed tomography findings predict outcome in chronic sinusitis? Otolaryngol Head Neck Surg 123:81–84

Taylor JS, Tofts PS, Port R et al (1999) MR imaging of tumor microcirculation: promise for the new millennium. J Magn Reson Imaging 10:903–907

Tomenzoli D, Castelnuovo P, Pagella F et al (2004) Different endoscopic surgical strategies in the management of inverted papilloma of the sinonasal tract: experience on 47 cases. Laryngoscope (in press)

Valk PE, Dillon WP (1991) Radiation injury of the brain. AJNR Am J Neuroradiol 12:45–62

Van der Laan BF, Baris G, Gregor RT et al (1995) Radiation-induced tumours of the head and neck. J Laryngol Otol 109:346–349

Vassallo P, Tranfa F, Forte R et al (2001) Ophthalmic complications after surgery for nasal and sinus polyposis. Eur J Ophthalmol 11:218–222

Vleming M, Middelweerd MJ, de Vries N (1993) Goede resultaten van endoscopische neusbijholtenchirurgie wegens chronische of recidiverende sinusitis en wegens polyposis nasi. Ned Tijdschr Geneeskd 137:1453–1456

Wanamaker JR, Mehle ME, Wood BG et al (1995) Tension pneumocephalus following craniofacial resection. Head Neck 17:152–156

Williams LS, Mancuso AA, Mendenhall WM (2001) Perineural spread of cutaneous squamous and basal cell carcinoma: CT and MR detection and its impact on patient management and prognosis. Int J Radiat Oncol Biol Phys 49:1061–1069

Younis RT, Lazar RH, Anand VK (2002) Intracranial complications of sinusitis: a 15-year review of 39 cases. Ear Nose Throat J 81:636–638, 640–632, 644

Legends of Anatomic Structures

A	agger nasi	MM	middle meatus
AC	anterior clinoid	MPP	medial pterygoid plate
aEC	anterior canal of the ethmoid	MS	maxillary sinus
ao	accessory ostium of maxillary sinus	MT	middle turbinate
arMS	alveolar recess of maxillary sinus	NLD	nasolacrimal duct
B	ethmoid bulla	NS	nasal septum
CB	concha bullosa	O	maxillary ostium
CC	carotid canal	oFS	ostium frontal sinus
CG	crista galli	OC	optic canal
EI	ethmoid infundibulum	OG	olfactory groove
ET	eustachian tube opening	ON	optic nerve
FE	fovea ethmoidalis	OnC	Onodi cell
FO	foramen ovale	oSS	ostium of sphenoid sinus
FS	frontal sinus	PEC	posterior ethmoid cells
FSp	foramen spinosum	PF	pterygoid (scaphoid) fossa
GL	ground lamella	PMF	pterygomaxillary fissure
GPC	greater palatine canal	PP	perpendicular plate of the ethmoid
GPF	greater palatine foramen	PPF	pterygopalatine fossa
H	hiatus semilunaris	PPr	pterygoid process
h	hamulus of the medial pterygoid plate	ppSS	sphenoid recess pneumatizing the pterygoid process
hlCP	horizontal lamella of the cribriform plate		
hUP	horizontal plate of the uncinate process	rs	rostrum of the sphenoid bone
HY	hypophisis	SL	sinus lateralis
IC	incisive canal	SOF	superior orbital fissure
ICA	internal carotid artery	SPF	sphenopalatine foramen
IEC	infraorbital ethmoid cell (Haller cell)	SS	sphenoid sinus
IF	incise foramen	ST	superior turbinate
IM	inferior meatus	suOC	supraorbital ethmoid cell
IOF	inferior orbital fissure	suR	suprabullar recess
ION	infraorbital nerve	SuT	supreme turbinate
IT	inferior turbinate	TR	terminal recess
L	common lamina of turbinates	UP	uncinate process
LB	lacrimal bone posterior crest	V2	maxillary nerve
LP	lamina papyracea	V3	mandibular nerve
LPC	lesser palatine canal	VC	vidian (pterygoid) canal
LPF	lesser palatine foramen	VN	vidian (pterygoid) nerve
LPP	lateral pterygoid plate	vlCP	vertical lamella of the cribriform plate
LS	lacrimal sac	vlMT	vertical lamella of the middle turbinate
MC	Meckel cave	vUP	vertical portion of the uncinate process

Subject Index

A

abscess   62
- brain   63–64, 95, 108, 257
- - epidural   63–64
- - intracerebral   60, 63
- - subdural   63
- orbital   60–63
- - intraconal extension   62–63
- - subperiosteal   60–62
acromegaly   229
adenocarcinoma   37, 40–43, 45, 119, 160, 165, 173–176, 195, 272, 274, 284
- intestinal type   176
adenoid cystic carcinoma   160, 170, 177–184, 238–239
- bone changes   37–39, 45
- distant metastasis   177
- follow-up   271
- perineural spread   178–184
- permeative bone invasion   178
- regional metastasis   177
- submucosal spread   178
agger nasi cells   19, 21, 52
ameloblastoma   232, 243–244, 247
anaplastic carcinoma   160
anastomosis, arterovenous   31
anatomic variants   62, 65, 68, 70, 257, 260
aneurysmal bone cyst   114–116
- classic   115
- differential diagnosis   116
- pathogenesis   114
- solid   115
anterior craniofacial resection   57, 164, 175, 186
- imaging findings   271, 272
arachnoid   93
- pits   93
- villi   93

B

basal cell carcinoma   222
benign fibrous histiocytoma   147
beta-1-transferrin   95
beta-2-transferrin   95
- assay   95, 98
beta-trace-protein   96
- assay   96, 98, 100, 102
bone
- cortical
- - breach   116
- - destruction   37, 133, 168, 179, 227, 279
- intra-medullary growth   37, 112, 133, 137, 268

- permeative invasion   37–38, 41, 168, 178–179, 192, 209
- remodeling   36–37, 69, 112, 116, 117, 121, 126, 129, 133, 137, 146, 150
- sclerosis   38–39, 76, 83, 99, 112, 114, 167–168, 179, 192, 213, 232, 234–235, 245, 261, 267, 269
brain
- abscess   95
- dysplastic   94, 99
- hematoma   257
- hernia   93, 94, 99
- lesions due to irradiation   278–279
- malformations   99
- mineralizing microangiopathy   279
- non-functioning   94
- pulsation   93, 99
- teleangiectasia   279
breathing, physiologic   29
calcification, intratumoral   205, 225
- ring-like   227

C

Caldwell's Luc procedure   261
cavernous sinus   75, 77
- invasion   132, 141, 161, 170, 180, 209, 286
- thrombophlebitis   61
- thrombosis   60, 63
cellulitis
- orbital   60, 62
- preseptal   60, 62
cephalocele   93, 257
- atretic   93
- fronto-ethmoidal   94–96
- meningocele   93, 99
- meningoencephalocele   93–94, 99
- nasopharyngeal   94–96
- spheno-maxillary   94, 96
- spheno-orbital   94–96
- spontaneous   94
- temporal   94
chemotherapy   163–164
chloroma see granulocytic sarcoma
chondroma   226
chondrosarcoma   162 196–197, 226–228, 230
- calcifications   201
- CT   227
- grade   196
- histogenesis   196
- lobular enhancement   202
- MR   228
- recurrence   197

chordoma   223–225, 227–228, 230
– CT   225
– MR   225
cisternography   102
– CT   104
– MR   98, 101, 104–105
– radionuclide   102, 104
cocaine abuse   80, 81, 86, 87
– differential diagnosis   80, 87
– MR findings   86, 87
concha bullosa see middle turbinate, pneumatized
conventional x-ray   1
– Caldwell projection   56
craniopharyngioma   230–232
– adamantinous   231–232
– MR classification   231
– papillary   232
CSF leak   22, 93, 95, 98, 100, 257
– endoscopy   95
– gyrus rectus sign   94
– intermittent   94
– persistent   95
– spontaneous   93–95, 102
– traumatic   93–94, 96, 100, 102
CT
– cisternography   102, 104
– contrast agent   3, 100, 104
– examination area   2, 3
– high resolution   98–100, 102
– radiation dose   1
– – low-dose protocols   1
– MPR (multiplanar reconstruction)   2
– patient positioning   2
– technique   1–3
Cushing's disease   229
cyst
– calcifying odontogenic   232
– dentigerous   243, 246
– follicular see dentigerous
– incisive canal see nasopalatine duct
– keratinizing   232
– nasopalatine duct   243
– radicular   242, 245
– Rathke's pouch   233
cystic fibrosis   66, 67
– ASA syndrome   66, 67
– asthma   66, 67
– Young's syndrome   66

D
dacryocystitis   79
dacryocystography   257
dacryocystoplasty   257
dacryocystorhinostomy   257
Dandy-Walker malformation   99
duct
– craniopharyngeal   231–232
– nasolacrimal   49, 257
dura mater   93
– MR imaging   35
– neoplastic invasion   42–43, 57
duraplasty   57, 96, 272–273
– overlay   96, 97

– tobacco pouch   96, 97
– underlay   96

E
emphysema, orbital   256
empty sella   94, 98, 102
empyema, subdural   60
encephalitis   257
epiphora   257
epithelium   30
– ciliated   30
– squamous   30
– olfactory   33
esthesioneuroblastoma see olfactory neuroblastoma
ethmoid   10–12
– atelectatic infundibulum   20
– bulla   10, 19, 21, 50
– concha bullosa   20
– cribriform plate   10, 15, 19, 22, 26
– crista galli   10
– embryologic development   9
– fovea   12, 57
– ground lamella   12, 50
– infraorbital cells   20
– infundibulum   12, 15, 18, 19, 20
– labyrinth   10–11
– lamellar concha   20
– lamina papyracea   11, 14, 18, 19, 23
– middle turbinate   12, 15, 19, 20
– perpendicular lamina   10
– roof   22
– superior turbinate   11
– supreme turbinate   11
ethmoiditis   68, 69
Ewing sarcoma   190–193
– permeative bone destruction   192

F
facial fracture   93
fibers, neural   31
– sensory   31
– parasympathetic   31
– autonomic   31
– vasomotor   31
fibrous dysplasia   110–114
flap
– composite   56
– free (soft tissues)   55, 239
– free (osseous)   55
– imaging findings   273
– pericranium   57
– temporalis muscle   55, 239
fluorescein
– leakage   101
– test   95, 96, 98, 102
follow-up, imaging
– baseline imaging study   271, 283
fontanelle, posterior   49
foramen cecum   99
frontal recess   12–16, 19
– surgical procedures   51
frontal sinus   12–16, 32–33
– bulla frontalis   15–16

– surgical approaches   52, 56, 57
fungal rhinosinusitis
– acute fulminant   72–73, 76
– allergic see eosinophilic fungal rhinosinusitis
– chronic invasive 72–73, 76
– cortical bone destruction 37
– eosinophilic 73–76
– fungus ball 72–76
– granulomatous invasive 72, 73
– mycetoma see fungus ball

G
gelfoam   97
glands   30, 31
– Bowman   32
– seromucous   30, 31
– serous   30
glioma, nasal   99
glucose, chemical methods   95
graft, in CSF leak   96
– fascia lata   97
– fat   97
– mucoperichondral   96, 97
granulocytic sarcoma   210
ground lamella see ethmoid

H
Haller cells see ethmoid, infraorbital cells
hemangioma, cavernous   147
hemangiopericytoma   205
hematoma
– brain   257
– intraorbital   256
hydrocephalus   94, 97, 102
hyperpneumatization   93
– paranasal sinuses   93, 102, 121–122
– – hypersinus   121–122
– temporal bone   93, 102
hypertelorism   95

I
inferior meatus   10
inferior turbinate   29
infratemporal approach   55
intracranial   93
– hypertension   94, 97, 102
– pressure   93
inverted papilloma   36, 37, 68, 122–131
– association with squamous cell carcinoma   123
– human papilloma virus   122
– lobulated surface contour   126
– staging systems   123–124
– striated inner pattern   126–129
– surgical resection, type   I–III 125

J
juvenile angiofibroma   131–144
– bone involvement   37, 137
– cystic changes   133
– embolization   139–141
– intracranial extent   132, 139, 141
– persistence   38, 141
– site of origin   133

L
lacrimal pathways
– stenosis   275
lamina papyracea
– collapse, post–surgical   272
– dehiscence   256
– erosion   40
– surgical dissection   50
lateral rhinotomy   54, 57
leiomyoma   147, 150–151
leiomyosarcoma   197, 198, 281
– cystic   203
– necrosis   203
– recurrence   198
lobular capillary hemangioma see pyogenic granuloma
Lothrop, modified procedure see microendoscopic surgery,
    Draf procedures
lumbar drainage   97, 102
Lund-Mackay staging system   72
lymphoma   162, 170, 180, 185, 205–210
- midline destructive lesions   207
– necrosis   208
– permeative bone invasion   37, 41, 209
– recurrence   208
– staging systems   207

M
mandibular nerve   170
masticator space   170, 235
mastoiditis   102
matrix, chondroid   227
maxillary sinus   17–18, 32–33
– fontanelle   17, 49
– hiatus semilunaris   17, 19
– infraorbital canal   17, 24
– infraorbital nerve   17, 23
– ostium   17, 18
– surgery for sinusitis   49
maxillectomy   239, 273
– inferior   53
– medial   54
– partial   54, 163
– radical   163
– – standard   55
– – extended   55–56
melanoma   180, 185, 193–195
– amelanotic   195
– melanotic   195
meningioma   233–235
– bone blistering   235
– CT   234
– dural tail sign   234
– MR   234
meningitis   60, 63, 94
– postoperative   97
– recurrent   94–95, 98, 102
meningo-encephalitis   257
meningo-galeal complex   272–273
Merkel cell carcinoma   213
metastasis
– to lymph nodes   160–161, 185, 189, 194, 197
– to sinonasal tract   211–213

microendoscopic surgery
- clearance of frontal recess   51, 260–261
- complications   256
- Draf procedures   52, 108, 118, 261
- ethmoidotomy   50, 260–261
- in CSF leak   93, 97–98, 102
- in malignant neoplasms   164
- middle antrostomy   49, 260–261
- sphenoidotomy   51, 260–261
- - transnasal approach   51
- - transethmoidal approach   51
- uncinectomy   49, 260–261
middle meatus
- anatomy   9–10, 12 , 17, 19, 30
- antrochoanal polyp   70
- inverted papilloma   124–126
- neoplastic invasion   201
- obstruction   66–68, 118
- polyposis   69
- surgery, complications   256
middle turbinate
- paradoxical   256
- pneumatized (concha bullosa)   50, 68, 256
- truncation   267
- unstable   50, 260
midfacial degloving   54, 57
mixed tumor see pleomorphic adenoma
mixosarcoma   38
MR technique
- CISS sequence   102
- dynamic GE T1sequence   6, 283
- fat-sat sequences   5, 101
- MR cisternography   98, 101, 104
- VIBE sequence   5
MSCT (Multislice CT)   3–4
- multiplanar reconstruction   100, 102
mucocele   83, 117–121
- calcification   119
- dehydration   119
- differential diagnosis   119
- frontal sinus, surgery   57
- infection   117
- post-radiation therapy   278
- post-surgery   260–261, 268, 270
- sinusitis   71
mucociliary clearance   48
mucoepidermoid carcinoma   160, 238, 286
mucosa   29–31
- inflammatory thickening   68, 71, 80, 100, 102
- nasal   30,31
- olfactory   29, 32–33
- reactive changes, post-treatment   267, 275, 277
- respiratory   30
- ulceration   80
myxoma   147

N
nasal
- airflow   29
- - laminar   29,31
- - turbulent   29, 30,31
- cavity   9–10, 29, 33
- pyramid collapse   80

- septum   9, 19, 26
- - deviation   68
- - perforation   59–60, 79, 80
- vessels   31
- - capacitance   31
- - exchange   31
- - resistance   31
nasalization   267
nasopharynx   94, 104
neuroendocrine carcinoma   185, 188–190
- chemotherapy   189
- imaging features   190
- local recurrence   189
- radiotherapy   189
notochord   223

O
odontogenic sarcoma   244
olfactory neuroblastoma   160, 185–188
- calcifications   187
- chemotherapy   186
- follow-up   271
- hyperostosis   187
- local recurrence   186
- marginal tumor cyst   187
- microendoscopic approach   186
- radiotherapy   186
Ollier disease   226
OMU see ostiomeatal unit
Onodi cell   21, 51, 257
optic nerve   60, 62, 63, 102
- neuritis, radiation induced   278
orbit
- exenteration   56, 163, 172
- reconstruction   56
ossifying fibroma   110–114
- cementiform   111
- classic   111
- differential diagnosis   114
- juvenile   111
osteitis   63
osteogenesis imperfecta   94
osteoma   57, 107–110
- intracranial   108
- intraorbital   108
- ivory   108
- mixed   108
- spongiosum   108
osteomyelitis   57, 63
osteoradionecrosis   279
osteosarcoma   197–198
- recurrence   198
- subtypes   197
- sunburst appearance   202
ostiomeatal unit   18–19, 20, 21, 48
otitis media   78

P
palate
- cleft   95
- hard, tumors   238–240
- perforation   80–81, 87
palatine canals   26

paraganglioma 147, 151
periorbita 40, 163, 172
periosteum, MR imaging 35
PET imaging 285
pituitary adenoma
– CT 230
– ectopic adenoma 230
– Hardy's classification 228
– macroadenoma 228
– microadenoma 228
– MR 230
– transsphenoidal access 229
plasmacytoma 185, 206 210
pleomorphic adenoma 147–149
– nasal septum 149
pneumatocele 121
pneumocele 121–122
pneumocephalus
– tension 257, 272
pneumosinus dilatans 121–122, 235
polyp 65, 66, 69, 79, 82
– angiomatous 129
– antrochoanal 66–70
polyposis 48, 66–70, 73–74, 76
– associated diseases 66
– CT 69
– MR 69, 70
– predisposing factors 66
– recurrent 257, 259, 261
pterygoid
– canal (Vidian)
– – anatomy 23–25
– – juvenile angiofibroma 132–133, 137
– – neoplastic invasion 166, 168
– hamulus 26
– process 22, 96
– – invasion 168
– – sclerosis 168
– scaphoid fossa 26
pterygopalatine fossa 23–26
– invasion 77, 168
pyogenic granuloma 145–147
– pathogenesis 145
– differential diagnosis 146

R
radiation-associated neoplasms 280
radiotherapy 163, 164
receptors, olfactory 32
retention cyst 70, 71
– CT 71
– MR 71
retrobullar recess 15
rhabdomyosarcoma 185, 196, 197, 281–283
– alveolar 196
– botryoid sign 199
– embryonal 196
– pleomorphic 196
– recurrence 198
rhinorrhea 93
– bilateral 94
– intermittent 95, 98, 104

– persistent 95, 98
– unilateral 94
– watery 94, 95
rhinosinusitis
– acute 57, 59–62, 66–67, 71, 74
– – CT 62–63
– chronic 59, 65–69, 71, 73, 76
– – CT 68–69, 72
– complications
– – intracranial 60, 61, 63
– – intraorbital 60, 61, 62, 63
– endoscopic appearance 61, 66
– fungi 65, 73
– predisposing factors 65, 68
– principles of endoscopic treatment 48
– recurrent 259
– staging systems 72

S
saddle nose 79
sarcoidosis 81–82, 84, 87
– CT 87
– differential diagnosis 82
– etiology 81
– MR 87, 88
– perineural spread 83
– stages 82, 83
scar tissue
– CSF leak 100
– CT 275
– MR 269, 275, 282–283
schwannoma 147, 149–150
secondary tumors to sinonasal tract 211–213
sinus lateralis 15
sinusoids, cavernous 31
sinusotomy
– Draf type III 108, 118, 261
– osteoplastic flap 56
skull base 33, 93–94
– dehiscences 100
– fracture 93
– invasion, imaging findings 42
– surgery 57, 93, 96
SPECT 285
sphenoid bone, dehiscence 100
sphenoid sinus 18, 22
– CSF leak 94–97
– sphenoethmoid recess 18, 19
spindle–cell carcinoma 41
spread
– perineural 240, 285
– perivascular 285
– sub-periosteal 38, 167
squamous cell carcinoma 160, 163–165, 175, 180, 271
– bone invasion 37, 40, 42
– inverted papilloma 123, 125, 129–130
– hard palate 239, 240
– perineural spread 285
– radiation induced 280
– recurrent 271
– skin 222
– signal intensity 167

subarachnoid   98
– cisterns   101
– space   98, 99,102
superior meatus   10
superior turbinate   11, 30, 51
suprabullar recess cell   15
supreme turbinate   11
surgical approach
– anterior transfacial   236
– canine fossa   50
– combined antero-lateral   236
– lateral preauricular   236
– lateral postauricular   237
– pterional   231
– subfrontal   231
– transorbital   236
– transsphenoidal   231, 261
syndrome
– ASA   66–67
– Foster-Kennedy   234
– Gardner   108
– Kartagener's   66
– Maffucci   226
– Marfan's   94
– Young's   66
synechia   276
– mucocele development   119, 270
– post-surgical   259
system, mucociliar   31

T
terminal recess   19
trauma, head   93
tumor
– inflammatory myofibroblastic   147
– Pindborg see cyst, calcifying odontogenic   246
turbinate, nasal see inferior, middle, superior, supreme turbinate

U
uncinate process
– anatomy   9, 10, 12, 15, 17–19
– post-surgical imaging findings   258, 260, 261
– surgical complications   256
– surgical resection   49, 52
– variants   20–21
undifferentiated carcinoma   44, 161, 185, 188–190
– recurrent   271, 285

V
valve, nasal   29,30
vein
– diploic veins thrombophlebitis   60, 63
– ophthalmic vein thrombosis   63
– superior sagittal sinus thrombosis   60
ventricles, cerebral   99
– elongated   99
– stretched   99
vidian canal see pterygoid canal

W
Wegener granulomatosis   77–81, 83, 85–86
– bone changes   83
– cranial nerve involvement   85
– CT   83, 84, 86
– endoscopic appearance   79
– laryngeal   78
– MR   83–87
– neurologic   85, 86
– ocular   79
– pseudotumor   79–80, 83–85
– sinonasal   78, 79
Wood lamp   102

List of Contributors

ANTONINO ROBERTO ANTONELLI, MD
Professor and Chairman,
Department of Otorhinolaryngology
University of Brescia
Piazzale Spedali Civili 1
25123 Brescia, BS
Italy

GIUSEPPE BATTAGLIA, MD
Department of Radiology
University of Brescia
Piazzale Spedali Civili 1
25123 Brescia, BS
Italy

MARCO BERLUCCHI, MD
Department of Otorhinolaryngology
University of Brescia
Piazzale Spedali Civili 1
25123 Brescia, BS
Italy

ANDREA BOLZONI, MD
Department of Otorhinolaryngology
University of Brescia
Piazzale Spedali Civili 1
25123 Brescia, BS
Italy

ANDREA BORGHESI, MD
Department of Radiology
University of Brescia
Piazzale Spedali Civili 1
25123 Brescia, BS
Italy

DAVIDE FARINA, MD
Department of Radiology
University of Brescia
Piazzale Spedali Civili 1
25123 Brescia, BS
Italy

DAVIDE LOMBARDI, MD
Department of Otorhinolaryngology
University of Brescia
Piazzale Spedali Civili 1
25123 Brescia, BS
Italy

PATRIZIA MACULOTTI, MD
Department of Radiology
University of Brescia
Piazzale Spedali Civili 1
25123 Brescia, BS
Italy

ROBERTO MAROLDI, MD
Professor, Department of Radiology
University of Brescia
Piazzale Spedali Civili 1
25123 Brescia, BS
Italy

ILENIA MORASCHI, MD
Department of Radiology
University of Brescia
Piazzale Spedali Civili 1
25123 Brescia, BS
Italy

PIETRO MORTINI, MD
Professor, Department of Neurosurgery
Skull Base and Endocrinoneurosurgery Center
University Vita e Salute
Via Olgettina 60
20132 Milano
Italy

FRANCESCA MOSSI, MD
Department of Radiology
University of Brescia
Piazzale Spedali Civili 1
25123 Brescia, BS
Italy

PIERO NICOLAI, MD
Professor, Department of Otorhinolaryngology
University of Brescia
Piazzale Spedali Civili 1
25123 Brescia, BS
Italy

LAURA PALVARINI, MD
Department of Radiology
University of Brescia
Piazzale Spedali Civili 1
25123 Brescia, BS
Italy

Luca Pianta, MD
Department of Otorhinolaryngology
University of Brescia
Piazzale Spedali Civili 1
25123 Brescia, BS
Italy

Cesare Piazza, MD
Department of Otorhinolaryngology
University of Brescia
Piazzale Spedali Civili 1
25123 Brescia, BS
Italy

Lorenzo Pinelli, MD
Department of Radiology, Neuroradiology Section
University of Brescia
Piazzale Spedali Civili 1
25123 Brescia, BS
Italy

Vanessa Portugalli, MD
Department of Radiology
University of Brescia
Piazzale Spedali Civili 1
25123 Brescia, BS
Italy

Luca Oscar Redaelli de Zinis, MD
Department of Otorhinolaryngology
University of Brescia
Piazzale Spedali Civili 1
25123 Brescia, BS
Italy

Davide Tomenzoli, MD
Department of Otorhinolaryngology
University of Brescia
Piazzale Spedali Civili 1
25123 Brescia, BS
Italy

MEDICAL RADIOLOGY Diagnostic Imaging and Radiation Oncology

Titles in the series already published

DIAGNOSTIC IMAGING

Innovations in Diagnostic Imaging
Edited by J. H. Anderson

Radiology of the Upper Urinary Tract
Edited by E. K. Lang

The Thymus - Diagnostic Imaging, Functions, and Pathologic Anatomy
Edited by E. Walter, E. Willich, and W. R. Webb

Interventional Neuroradiology
Edited by A. Valavanis

Radiology of the Pancreas
Edited by A. L. Baert, co-edited by G. Delorme

Radiology of the Lower Urinary Tract
Edited by E. K. Lang

Magnetic Resonance Angiography
Edited by I. P. Arlart, G. M. Bongartz, and G. Marchal

Contrast-Enhanced MRI of the Breast
S. Heywang-Köbrunner and R. Beck

Spiral CT of the Chest
Edited by M. Rémy-Jardin and J. Rémy

Radiological Diagnosis of Breast Diseases
Edited by M. Friedrich and E.A. Sickles

Radiology of the Trauma
Edited by M. Heller and A. Fink

Biliary Tract Radiology
Edited by P. Rossi, co-edited by M. Brezi

Radiological Imaging of Sports Injuries
Edited by C. Masciocchi

Modern Imaging of the Alimentary Tube
Edited by A. R. Margulis

Diagnosis and Therapy of Spinal Tumors
Edited by P. R. Algra, J. Valk, and J. J. Heimans

Interventional Magnetic Resonance Imaging
Edited by J.F. Debatin and G. Adam

Abdominal and Pelvic MRI
Edited by A. Heuck and M. Reiser

Orthopedic Imaging Techniques and Applications
Edited by A. M. Davies and H. Pettersson

Radiology of the Female Pelvic Organs
Edited by E. K.Lang

Magnetic Resonance of the Heart and Great Vessels Clinical Applications
Edited by J. Bogaert, A.J. Duerinckx, and F. E. Rademakers

Modern Head and Neck Imaging
Edited by S. K. Mukherji and J. A. Castelijns

Radiological Imaging of Endocrine Diseases
Edited by J. N. Bruneton in collaboration with B. Padovani and M.-Y. Mourou

Trends in Contrast Media
Edited by H. S. Thomsen, R. N. Muller, and R. F. Mattrey

Functional MRI
Edited by C. T. W. Moonen and P. A. Bandettini

Radiology of the Pancreas
2nd Revised Edition
Edited by A. L. Baert
Co-edited by G. Delorme and L. Van Hoe

Emergency Pediatric Radiology
Edited by H. Carty

Spiral CT of the Abdomen
Edited by F. Terrier, M. Grossholz, and C. D. Becker

Liver Malignancies Diagnostic and Interventional Radiology
Edited by C. Bartolozzi and R. Lencioni

Medical Imaging of the Spleen
Edited by A. M. De Schepper and F. Vanhoenacker

Radiology of Peripheral Vascular Diseases
Edited by E. Zeitler

Diagnostic Nuclear Medicine
Edited by C. Schiepers

Radiology of Blunt Trauma of the Chest
P. Schnyder and M. Wintermark

Portal Hypertension Diagnostic Imaging-Guided Therapy
Edited by P. Rossi
Co-edited by P. Ricci and L. Broglia

Recent Advances in Diagnostic Neuroradiology
Edited by Ph. Demaerel

Virtual Endoscopy and Related 3D Techniques
Edited by P. Rogalla, J. Terwissscha Van Scheltinga, and B. Hamm

Multislice CT
Edited by M. F. Reiser, M. Takahashi, M. Modic, and R. Bruening

Pediatric Uroradiology
Edited by R. Fotter

Transfontanellar Doppler Imaging in Neonates
A. Couture and C. Veyrac

Radiology of AIDS A Practical Approach
Edited by J.W.A.J. Reeders and P.C. Goodman

CT of the Peritoneum
Armando Rossi and Giorgio Rossi

Magnetic Resonance Angiography
2nd Revised Edition
Edited by I. P. Arlart, G. M. Bongratz, and G. Marchal

MEDICAL RADIOLOGY Diagnostic Imaging and Radiation Oncology

Titles in the series already published

Pediatric Chest Imaging
Edited by Javier Lucaya
and Janet L. Strife

**Applications of Sonography
in Head and Neck Pathology**
Edited by J. N. Bruneton
in collaboration with C. Raffaelli
and O. Dassonville

Imaging of the Larynx
Edited by R. Hermans

3D Image Processing
Techniques and Clinical Applications
Edited by D. Caramella
and C. Bartolozzi

**Imaging of Orbital and
Visual Pathway Pathology**
Edited by W. S. Müller-Forell

Pediatric ENT Radiology
Edited by S. J. King
and A. E. Boothroyd

**Radiological Imaging
of the Small Intestine**
Edited by N. C. Gourtsoyiannis

Imaging of the Knee
Techniques and Applications
Edited by A. M. Davies
and V. N. Cassar-Pullicino

Perinatal Imaging
From Ultrasound to MR Imaging
Edited by Fred E. Avni

**Radiological Imaging
of the Neonatal Chest**
Edited by V. Donoghue

**Diagnostic and Interventional
Radiology in Liver Transplantation**
Edited by E. Bücheler, V. Nicolas,
C. E. Broelsch, X. Rogiers,
and G. Krupski

Radiology of Osteoporosis
Edited by S. Grampp

Imaging Pelvic Floor Disorders
Edited by C. I. Bartram
and J. O. L. DeLancey
Associate Editors: S. Halligan,
F. M. Kelvin, and J. Stoker

Imaging of the Pancreas
Cystic and Rare Tumors
Edited by C. Procacci
and A. J. Megibow

**High Resolution Sonography
of the Peripheral Nervous System**
Edited by S. Peer and G. Bodner

Imaging of the Foot and Ankle
Techniques and Applications
Edited by A. M. Davies,
R. W. Whitehouse,
and J. P. R. Jenkins

Radiology Imaging of the Ureter
Edited by F. Joffre, Ph. Otal,
and M. Soulie

Imaging of the Shoulder
Techniques and Applications
Edited by A. M. Davies and J. Hodler

Radiology of the Petrous Bone
Edited by M. Lemmerling
and S. S. Kollias

Interventional Radiology in Cancer
Edited by A. Adam, R. F. Dondelinger,
and P. R. Mueller

**Duplex and Color Doppler Imaging
of the Venous System**
Edited by G. H. Mostbeck

Multidetector-Row CT of the Thorax
Edited by U. J. Schoepf

Functional Imaging of the Chest
Edited by H.-U. Kauczor

**Radiology of the Pharynx
and the Esophagus**
Edited by O. Ekberg

**Radiological Imaging
in Hematological Malignancies**
Edited by A. Guermazi

**Imaging and Intervention in
Abdominal Trauma**
Edited by R. F. Dondelinger

Multislice CT
2nd Revised Edition
Edited by M. F. Reiser, M. Takahashi,
M. Modic, and C. R. Becker

**Intracranial Vascular Malformations
and Aneurysms**
From Diagnostic Work-Up
to Endovascular Therapy
Edited by M. Forsting

Radiology and Imaing of the Colon
Edited by A. H. Chapman

Coronary Radiology
Edited by M. Oudkerk

**Dynamic Contrast-Enhanced Magnetic
Resonance Imaging in Oncology**
Edited by A. Jackson, D. L. Buckley,
and G. J. M. Parker

**Imaging in Treatment Planning
for Sinonasal Diseases**
Edited by R. Maroldi and P. Nicolai

Clinical Cardiac MRI
With Interactive CD-ROM
Edited by J. Bogaert,
S. Dymarkowski, and A. M. Taylor

Focal Liver Lesions
Detection, Characterization,
Ablation
Edited by R. Lencioni, D. Cioni,
and C. Bartolozzi

Multidetector-Row CT Angiography
Edited by C. Catalano
and R. Passariello

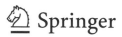

MEDICAL RADIOLOGY · Diagnostic Imaging and Radiation Oncology

Titles in the series already published

RADIATION ONCOLOGY

Lung Cancer
Edited by C.W. Scarantino

Innovations in Radiation Oncology
Edited by H. R. Withers
and L. J. Peters

**Radiation Therapy
of Head and Neck Cancer**
Edited by G. E. Laramore

**Gastrointestinal Cancer –
Radiation Therapy**
Edited by R.R. Dobelbower, Jr.

**Radiation Exposure
and Occupational Risks**
Edited by E. Scherer, C. Streffer,
and K.-R. Trott

**Radiation Therapy of Benign Diseases
A Clinical Guide**
S. E. Order and S. S. Donaldson

**Interventional Radiation
Therapy Techniques – Brachytherapy**
Edited by R. Sauer

Radiopathology of Organs and Tissues
Edited by E. Scherer, C. Streffer,
and K. R. Trott

**Concomitant Continuous Infusion
Chemotherapy and Radiation**
Edited by M. Rotman
and C. J. Rosenthal

**Intraoperative Radiotherapy –
Clinical Experiences and Results**
Edited by F. A. Calvo, M. Santos,
and L.W. Brady

**Radiotherapy of Intraocular
and Orbital Tumors**
Edited by W. E. Alberti and
R. H. Sagerman

**Interstitial and Intracavitary
Thermoradiotherapy**
Edited by M. H. Seegenschmiedt
and R. Sauer

**Non-Disseminated Breast Cancer
Controversial Issues in Management**
Edited by G. H. Fletcher and
S.H. Levitt

**Current Topics in
Clinical Radiobiology of Tumors**
Edited by H.-P. Beck-Bornholdt

**Practical Approaches to
Cancer Invasion and Metastases
A Compendium of Radiation
Oncologists' Responses to 40 Histories**
Edited by A. R. Kagan with the
Assistance of R. J. Steckel

Radiation Therapy in Pediatric Oncology
Edited by J. R. Cassady

Radiation Therapy Physics
Edited by A. R. Smith

Late Sequelae in Oncology
Edited by J. Dunst and R. Sauer

Mediastinal Tumors. Update 1995
Edited by D. E. Wood
and C. R. Thomas, Jr.

**Thermoradiotherapy
and Thermochemotherapy**

Volume 1:
Biology, Physiology, and Physics

Volume 2:
Clinical Applications

Edited by M.H. Seegenschmiedt,
P. Fessenden, and C.C. Vernon

**Carcinoma of the Prostate
Innovations in Management**
Edited by Z. Petrovich, L. Baert,
and L.W. Brady

**Radiation Oncology
of Gynecological Cancers**
Edited by H.W. Vahrson

**Carcinoma of the Bladder
Innovations in Management**
Edited by Z. Petrovich, L. Baert,
and L.W. Brady

**Blood Perfusion and
Microenvironment of Human Tumors
Implications for
Clinical Radiooncology**
Edited by M. Molls and P. Vaupel

**Radiation Therapy of Benign Diseases
A Clinical Guide
2nd Revised Edition**
S. E. Order and S. S. Donaldson

**Carcinoma of the Kidney and Testis, and
Rare Urologic Malignancies
Innovations in Management**
Edited by Z. Petrovich, L. Baert,
and L.W. Brady

**Progress and Perspectives in the
Treatment of Lung Cancer**
Edited by P. Van Houtte,
J. Klastersky, and P. Rocmans

**Combined Modality Therapy of
Central Nervous System Tumors**
Edited by Z. Petrovich, L. W. Brady,
M. L. Apuzzo, and M. Bamberg

**Age-Related Macular Degeneration
Current Treatment Concepts**
Edited by W. A. Alberti, G. Richard,
and R. H. Sagerman

**Radiotherapy of Intraocular
and Orbital Tumors
2nd Revised Edition**
Edited by R. H. Sagerman,
and W. E. Alberti

**Modification of Radiation Response
Cytokines, Growth Factors,
and Other Biolgical Targets**
Edited by C. Nieder, L. Milas,
and K. K. Ang

Radiation Oncology for Cure and Palliation
R. G. Parker, N. A. Janjan,
and M. T. Selch

**Clinical Target Volumes in
Conformal and Intensity Modulated
Radiation Therapy
A Clinical Guide to Cancer
Treatment**
Edited by V. Grégoire, P. Scalliet,
and K. K. Ang

**Advances in Radiation Oncology
in Lung Cancer**
Edited by Branislav Jeremić

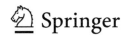 Springer

Printing and Binding: Stürtz GmbH, Würzburg